Worker and Public Health and Safety

Worker and Public Health and Safety: Current Views

Editors

Sara Lal

Thomas Penzel

Ann M Simpson

MDPI • Basel • Beijing • Wuhan • Barcelona • Belgrade • Manchester • Tokyo • Cluj • Tianjin

Editors
Sara Lal
University of Technology
Sydney
Australia

Thomas Penzel
Charité - Universitätsmedizin Berlin
Berlin
Germany

Ann M Simpson
University of Technology
Sydney
Australia

Editorial Office
MDPI
St. Alban-Anlage 66
4052 Basel, Switzerland

This is a reprint of articles from the Special Issue published online in the open access journal *International Journal of Environmental Research and Public Health* (ISSN 1660-4601) (available at: https://www.mdpi.com/journal/ijerph/special_issues/worker).

For citation purposes, cite each article independently as indicated on the article page online and as indicated below:

LastName, A.A.; LastName, B.B.; LastName, C.C. Article Title. *Journal Name* **Year**, *Volume Number*, Page Range.

ISBN 978-3-0365-0094-2 (Hbk)
ISBN 978-3-0365-0095-9 (PDF)

Contents

About the Editors

Sara Lal holds a BSc from Sydney University and M App Sc, PhD and Graduate Certificate in Higher Education (GCHE) from the University of Technology Sydney (UTS) and DipLaw from Legal Profession Admission Board, NSW, Australia. She held a National Medical and Health Research Council (NHMRC) Clinical Research Training Fellowship from 2001, and was appointed as an academic at UTS in 2004. Presently, she leads the Neuroscience Research Unit and is Deputy Leader of the Medical Science Discipline in the School of Life Sciences. Her main areas of research are in neurosciences, cognitive sciences, medical physiology, cardiovascular and diabetes research, psychophysiology, fatigue/sleepiness, worker safety and performance, including areas of digital and wearable medical/health technologies. She has attracted national and international competitive research grants and research consultation. She has published/presented over 200 varied types of scientific works including journal papers, refereed conference papers, books, chapters, reports, and abstracts.

Thomas Penzel graduated from physics (1986), human biology (1991), and physiology (1995) at the University Marburg, Germany. In 2006, he moved to Berlin where he is the Director of research of the Interdisciplinary Sleep Medicine Center at the Charité – Universitätsmedizin Berlin (Germany). In 2001, he received the Bial award for Clinical Medicine in Portugal, in 2008, the Bill Gruen Award for Innovations in Sleep Research by the American Sleep Research Society, and in 2014, the distinguished research award by the Chinese Sleep Research Society. He is secretary of the German Sleep Society and Adcom member of IEEE EMBS. He was IEEE EMBC 2019 conference chair, and co-chair of earlier conferences of EMBC, and World Sleep Society in 2005 in Berlin, and national conferences on sleep and biotelemetry. He is Editor-in-Chief of the journal Sleep and Breathing. He has published more than 300 journal papers (Pubmed), about 80 book chapters, and edited several books. His interests are sleep medicine, biomedical signals, and the cardiovascular and neural system related to sleep–wake regulation.

Ann M Simpson has a BSc (Hons) and a PhD (Veterinary Science) from the University of Sydney. Professor Simpson joined the staff at the University of Technology Sydney (UTS) in 1994 and since 2002 has held the position of Professor of Biochemistry. She is Director of the UTS Research Centre for Health Technologies. Her areas of expertise are biochemistry, molecular biology, and cell biology. Her main research interest is the gene therapy of diabetes mellitus. She was the first to show a liver cell can store insulin in granules and she has engineered two liver cell lines to store and secrete insulin to a glucose stimulus. One of these cell lines has reversed diabetes in an animal model. In particular, her work now focuses on novel strategies to deliver the insulin gene directly to the liver of diabetic animals, so far reversing diabetes with normal glucose tolerance in chemically diabetic rats, spontaneously diabetic mice, humanised mice, and a diabetic pig model by direct delivery of the insulin gene to the animal's livers using a viral vector.

Editorial to "Worker and Public Health and Safety: Current Views"

Health and safety in the occupational sector and the general public domain continue to be crucial areas of concern in our ever-advancing technological, demanding, and disease- and disaster-prone society. Pandemics, epidemics, public threats, and natural disasters continue to be on the rise. As we progress in the 21st century, worker and public health and safety concerns continue to escalate in many areas, including medical, transportation, security, defence, and multiple other industries and services. These issues have been exacerbated by the current 2020 COVID-19 (SARS-CoV-2) environment, with the pandemic detrimentally affecting health and safety not only in the work and public sectors, but in all domains of life globally. Therefore, understanding and advancing research into worker and public health and safety is a field that will continue to grow and evolve as mankind and society transitions through large-scale pandemics and natural disasters. The last few decades alone have seen epidemics and pandemics (with some continuing into the present-day) such as the HIV/AIDS, H1N1 Swine Flu, the deadly Ebola outbreak, and Zika Virus, and more recently the novel corona virus COVID-19. Geophysical and other natural disasters linked to global warming also corrode work and public health and safety, without even mentioning the immense financial and emotional burden associated with these catastrophes.

Fatigue and sleepiness, diabetes and metabolic disorders, cardiovascular diseases, mental disorders, cognitive decline, cancer, musculoskeletal disorders are only a few of the many major health issues and concerns inflicting the world, which add substantially to the socio-economic burden. For example, fatigue and sleep disorders are of major concern in the transportation, military, aviation, cleaning, mining, security, and medical sectors. Additionally, shift workers have added vulnerability to circadian rhythm disruption and multiple chronic diseases. The monotonous and demanding nature of many work environment is linked to excessive sleepiness, stress and mental disorders, cognitive decline, cardiovascular diseases, diabetes, etc., which contribute to detrimental human health, errors, accidents, and injuries. The probability of these hazards occurring increases rapidly over consecutive work hours, which can be catastrophic for the worker who may also be responsible for the safety and care of others. Furthermore, those engaged in the cleaning and security industries and work that requires physical exertion and lifting are also burdened with musculoskeletal disorder, pain, and other societal diseases. Moreover, environmental factors and infections also affect health and safety. For example, heat, noise, and pollutants/infections are detrimental for bodily, auditory, and normal respiratory function, respectively.

The compilation of papers in this book is targeted at research and reviews addressing all aspects of "Worker and Public Health and Safety: Current Views". The papers presented here from experts are widely representative of all fields of worker and public health and safety, and constitute original and experimental manuscripts and reviews, etc. The following worker types, work environment, and public sectors are represented, though this list is by no means exhaustive: nursing, the healthcare and medical sectors; video display operators; temporary workers, police officers, correction workers, Chinese public, agriculture, forestry employees; manual cultivation operation; public employees; low-skilled and low-income workers, industrial manufacturing, iron and steel workers, machine operators, work requiring motor skills, sheriffs and recruits, young workers, wind workers, university civil workers and army reserve soldiers, executives, coffee factory workers, and drivers. The topics included can be categorized as follows: sleepiness/fatigue, performance and coping, working hours, sick leave, burnout in the work environment and medical profession, nursing care, coping, job satisfaction, psychological and mental disorders, stress, anxiety, depression, emotion, driver behaviour, self-efficacy, therapy, exercise, fitness measures in first responders, physical work, musculoskeletal symptoms, spinal injuries, dietary links, obesity, oral health, chronic diseases, cerebrovascular diseases, cardiovascular diseases, metabolic diseases, occupational diseases, illness, job strain, job difficulty and risks, workload, work hazards and work safety, accidents, errors, injuries, risks and management, dust pollution and pesticides, lung function, lung infection, asbestos exposure, blood-borne pathogens, noise, hearing loss, employability and socio-economic and socio-demographic factors, and occupational health. The collection of papers presented in this book helps further the plethora of information available in the ever advancing field of health and safety.

Sara Lal
Editor

International Journal of
Environmental Research and Public Health

MDPI

Article

Prevalence, Related Factors, and Levels of Burnout Syndrome Among Nurses Working in Gynecology and Obstetrics Services: A Systematic Review and Meta-Analysis

Emilia I. De la Fuente-Solana [1], Nora Suleiman-Martos [2,*], Laura Pradas-Hernández [3], Jose L. Gomez-Urquiza [4], Guillermo A. Cañadas-De la Fuente [4] and Luis Albendín-García [3,4]

1 Brain, Mind and Behaviour Research Center (CIMCYC), University of Granada, Campus Universitario de Cartuja S.N., 18011 Granada, Spain
2 Faculty of Health Sciences, University of Granada, Calle Cortadura Del Valle S.N., 51001 Ceuta, Spain
3 Andalusian Health Service, Granada. Avenida del Sur N. 11, 18014 Granada, Spain
4 Faculty of Health Sciences, University of Granada, Avenida de la Ilustración N. 60, 18016 Granada, Spain
* Correspondence: norasm@ugr.es; Tel.: +34-958-248-047

Received: 6 June 2019; Accepted: 18 July 2019; Published: 19 July 2019

Abstract: Background: Although burnout levels and the corresponding risk factors have been studied in many nursing services, to date no meta-analytical studies have been undertaken of obstetrics and gynecology units to examine the heterogeneity of burnout in this environment and the variables associated with it. In the present paper, we aim to determine the prevalence, levels, and related factors of burnout syndrome among nurses working in gynecology and obstetrics services. Methods: A systematic review and meta-analysis of the literature were carried out using the following sources: CINAHL (Cumulative Index of Nursing and Allied Health Literature), LILACS (Latin American and Caribbean Health Sciences Literature), Medline, ProQuest (Proquest Health and Medical Complete), SciELO (Scientific Electronic Library Online), and Scopus. Results: Fourteen relevant studies were identified, including, for this meta-analysis, n = 464 nurses. The following prevalence values were obtained: emotional exhaustion 29% (95% CI: 11–52%), depersonalization 19% (95% CI: 6–38%), and low personal accomplishment 44% (95% CI: 18–71%). The burnout variables considered were sociodemographic (age, marital status, number of children, gender), work-related (duration of the workday, nurse-patient ratio, experience or number of miscarriages/abortions), and psychological (anxiety, stress, and verbal violence). Conclusion: Nurses working in obstetrics and gynecology units present high levels of burnout syndrome. In over 33% of the study sample, at least two of the burnout dimensions considered are apparent.

Keywords: burnout; gynecology; meta-analysis; nurses; obstetrics; prevalence

1. Introduction

Research has shown that occupational responsibilities may compromise workers' physical and mental health [1]. Among those affected are healthcare personnel, who are particularly vulnerable to disorders, such as anxiety [2], depression [3], and burnout syndrome [4].

Burnout occurs when the worker is exposed to a series of chronic stressors, which provoke a deterioration in one or more of the dimensions identified [5]. A commonly-used means of determining the magnitude of burnout is the Maslach Burnout Inventory (MBI) questionnaire, which considers three psychological dimensions of the syndrome: emotional exhaustion (EE), caused initially by the sensation of physical over-exertion, which, in turn, generates emotional weariness and loss of interest in the patient; depersonalization (D), characterized by detachment, coldness, cynicism, and indifference; low personal accomplishment (PA), i.e., a negative attitude towards the work, low self-esteem, and lack of job satisfaction, which, in turn, provoke a loss of interest and impaired professional performance [6,7].

The development of burnout syndrome is influenced by many factors, which can be analyzed to identify possible risk profiles. In this respect, relevant sociodemographic factors include the subject's age, gender, marital status, and the number of children [8,9]. Also, the psychological factors, such as personality type, anxiety, stress, or depression [10], and work-related factors, including a perceived lack of autonomy, the nature of the work environment, salary, and shift work obligation and duration [11–14], are important. Among the latter aspects, the specific characteristics of the workplace also exert an important influence. Thus, for nurses, the type of patient, family relationships, and the workload at the hospital unit may all contribute to the appearance of burnout [15].

In attempting to overcome the negative consequences of this syndrome, nurses may neglect their personal and occupational obligations, giving rise to negative attitudes towards their work. Given this consideration, systematic reviews and meta-analyses have examined the prevalence of burnout [16] and its associated risk factors [17–19] in different hospital units. However, some services, such as gynecology and obstetrics, have received little research attention in this respect.

The obstetrics and gynecology service, caring for women's sexual and reproductive health, is considered a particularly sensitive area. It requires a strong sense of vocation and considerable emotional control, as the nurses here are responsible for providing optimal comprehensive care throughout the female life cycle. Information and emotional support are essential to meet the needs of mothers, during pregnancy [20], in each stage of childbirth and post-partum [21].

As stated above, the gynecology and obstetrics unit has specific characteristics that distinguish it from all others, especially the close emotional contact between the nurses and their patients and the latter's extreme vulnerability. For this reason, the main aim of this study is to determine and analyze the prevalence, levels, and related factors of burnout syndrome among nurses working in the area of gynecology and obstetrics.

2. Material and Methods

2.1. Search Strategy

A systematic review with meta-analysis was carried out, following the guidelines of the Preferred Reporting Items for Systematic Reviews and Meta-Analyses (PRISMA) statement [22] (Table S1).

The search was carried out in May 2019 by applying the formula: "burnout AND nurs* AND (obstetrics OR gynaecology OR gynecology)" based on the Medical Subject Headings (MeSH) descriptors. The following sources were consulted: CINAHL (Cumulative Index of Nursing and Allied Health Literature), LILACS (Latin American and Caribbean Health Sciences Literature), Medline, Proquest Platform (Proquest Health and Medical Complete), SciELO (Scientific Electronic Library Online), and Scopus.

2.2. Study Selection, Critical Review, and Level of Evidence

In selecting the articles for analysis, the following inclusion criteria were followed: (a) original primary sources; (b) gynecology and obstetrics area; (c) exclusive sample of nurses; (d) published in English, Spanish, Portuguese, or French; (e) no restriction by year of publication; (f) assessment of the level of burnout; (g) outcome measures evaluated by an instrument measuring the level of burnout (MBI, which is based on the triad EE, D, and low PA, and PRoQOL (Professional Quality of Life), which evaluates the quality of working life, including one dimension, for burnout); (h) data on prevalence of burnout. Articles based on mixed samples with other healthcare categories and lacking independent data for gynecology and obstetrics nursing were excluded, as were those with insufficient statistical information.

Two authors selected the articles, according to the abstract and title provided. After removing duplicate articles, the full-text article was consulted. After ensuring compliance with the inclusion criteria, each study was assessed independently, and a consensus was reached between the same two authors regarding the quality of the article. In their evaluation, a checklist was applied to determine the presence/absence of methodological bias. If in any case, the two authors were unable to agree, a third author was consulted.

The methodological quality of each article was assessed using the critical reading checklist proposed by Ciapponi [23]. Specifically, the internal validity of each study was verified by reference to items 1 to 6 and 11 to 18.

The level of evidence was evaluated following the recommendations of the Oxford Centre for Evidence-Based Medicine (OCEBM) Levels of Evidence Working Group [24].

2.3. Data Coding

The following study variables were obtained:

Publication variables: (a) authors; (b) year of publication; (c) country; (d) gender distribution (male/female); (e) age; (f) language.

Methodological variables: (g) total sample; (h) type of study; (i) outcome measure (instruments used and measure); (j) original instrument or adapted version; (k) estimated reliability coefficient of the instrument.

Burnout measurement variables: (l) prevalence of high EE, high D, and low PA (the cut-off points for low and high levels of each dimension were applied by the authors of each study depending on the adaptation of the MBI); (m) average or percentage of each dimension; (n) related factors for each dimension.

The data were recorded in a data coding manual by two researchers working independently. Agreement between them was determined by reference to Cohen's kappa coefficient (mean value: 0.99; minimum: 0.97; maximum: 1) and to the intraclass correlation coefficient (mean value: 0.98; minimum: 0.96; maximum: 1).

2.4. Data Analysis

The data collected in the systematic review were examined by descriptive analysis, in which the information was classified into data tables and categorized accordingly. With the studies that included sufficient statistical information, three random-effects meta-analyses were performed, for the dimensions of high EE, high D, and low PA. The prevalence and the corresponding confidence intervals were analyzed for each dimension.

The publication bias, i.e., the probability of the study being published with statistically significant results, was evaluated by Egger's linear regression test. Data heterogeneity was assessed using the I^2 index. All data analysis was performed using the StatsDirect statistical software package (version 3, StatsDirect Ltd., Cambridge, UK).

3. Results

In total, fourteen articles were included in this systematic review and meta-analysis. Figure 1 shows the flow diagram of the study selection process. All the studies selected were cross-sectional. Twelve articles (85.71%) measured burnout according to the Maslach Burnout Inventory (MBI) scale, and two were adaptations of this questionnaire. Two articles (14.29%) used the Professional Quality of Life (PRoQOL) questionnaire.

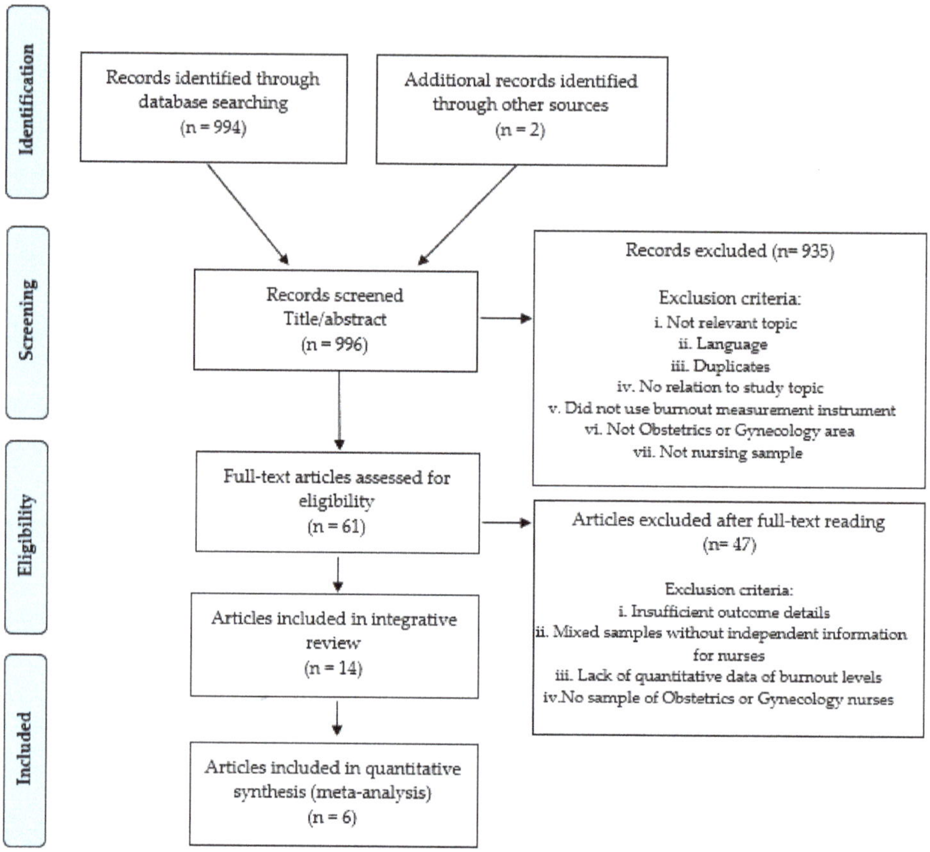

Figure 1. Study selection process to identify eligible articles for inclusion in the review and meta-analysis.

Nine of the studies (64.28%) were conducted in Asia (China, Japan, Korea, Pakistan, Turkey, Saudi Arabia), three (21.43%) in the Americas (Brazil, Mexico, USA), and the rest in Europe and South Africa. Most of the articles (80%) were published between 2012 and 2018. The reliability coefficient of the burnout questionnaire was only estimated in six articles, which reported values ranging from 0.60 to 0.90, considered in every case to be acceptable. Table 1 details these results.

Table 1. Characteristics of the studies included.

Author, Year, Country	Study Design	Sample (Gender and Mean Age)	Burnout Instrument (Reliability, Cronbach's α)	M (SD)/Percentage			Main Results	OCEBM GR/LE
				EE	D	PA		
Beaver et al., 1986, USA [25]	Cross-sectional	N = 98 O&G nurses 96.9% Female Age = 30–39: 55.2%	MBI (EE = 0.82, D = 0.60, PA = 0.80)	Low: 58.2% Moderate: 25.5% High: 16.3%	Low: 73.5% Moderate: 18.4% High: 8.2%	Low: 67.3% Moderate: 20.4% High: 12.2%	EE and D are negatively related to age and experience, and positively to the number of births and weekly work hours.	2c/B
Fontán and Dueñas, 2010, Spain [26]	Cross-sectional	N = 14 O&G nurses 78.57% Female Age = 46	MBI	12.2 (10.6) High: 14.2%	5.0 (5.5) High: 21.4%	45.1 (7.1) Low 7.1%	Highest levels are found in professionals who work more than 48 hours per week. Lower level of burnout at older age.	2c/B
Galindo et al., 2012, Brazil [27]	Cross-sectional	N = 64 O&G nurses 92.1% Female Age = 29	MBI (EE = 0.86, D = 0.69, PA = 0.76)	Low: 20.6% Moderate: 30.2% High: 49.2%	Low:14.3% Moderate: 58.7% High: 27%	Low: 4.8% Moderate: 11.1% High: 84.1%	Burnout correlates negatively with salary, experience, and age. A good organization of the service reduces the risk of burnout syndrome.	2c/B
Habadi et al., 2018, Saudi Arabia [28]	Cross-sectional	N = 14 O&G nurses	MBI	High: 50%	High: 14.28%	Low: 28.57%	O&G area is considered one of the lowest prevalences of burnout.	2c/B
Higashiguchi et al., 1999, Japan [29]	Cross-sectional	N = 28 O&G nurses	MBI (Japanese Version)	3.48 (1.29)	1.67 (0.72)	3.64 (1.10)	Low prevalence of burnout with high levels of PA in O&G unit nurses.	2c/B
Liu et al., 2018, China [30]	Cross-sectional	N = 93 O&G nurses	MBI (EE = 0.83, D = 0.83, PA = 0.81)	-	-	-	Low burnout score in O&G nurses (M: 6.19, SD: 2.71). Positive correlation between burnout and rotating shifts (r = 0.444).	2c/B
Mizuno et al., 2013, Japan [31]	Cross-sectional	N = 169 O&G nurses Age = 42.4	ProQOL FEWS	**Subscale** Compassion satisfaction = 33 (6.9) Burnout = 26.75 (5.4) Compassion fatigue = 20.75 (5.65)			High emotional burden on nurses in this area. Burnout correlates with the number of abortions, increasing stress, and reducing job satisfaction.	2c/B
Naz et al., 2016, Pakistan [32]	Cross-sectional	N = 28 O&G nurses	MBI	55.8 (6.7)	29.5 (3.4)	21.8 (4.9)	O&G service nurses have a higher burnout score compared to other services, such as medicine, surgery, neurology, or psychiatry.	2c/B
Nguyen et al., 2018, Korea [33]	Cross-sectional	N = 122 O&G nurses	MBI (Vietnamese version) (EE = 0.89, D = 0.77, PA = 0.80)	2.98 (1.00)	2.72 (0.88)	3.77 (0.77)	Higher EE scores in pediatric and medical area. Higher scores of D and lower in PA in pediatric and O&G area.	2c/B
Palmer-Morales et al., 2007, Mexico [34]	Cross-sectional	N=184 O&G nurses	MBI	Low: 78.8% Moderate: 16.3% High: 4.9%	Low: 91.85% Moderate: 4.35% High: 3.8%	Low: 75% Moderate: 14.7% High: 10.3%	There is no correlation between marital status and number of children and years of work experience with risk of burnout.	2c/B
Sun et al., 1996, China [35]	Cross-sectional	N = 273 O&G nurses	MBI (EE = 0.87, D = 0.81, PA = 0.84)	25.30 (2.99)	12.93 (1.75)	29.90 (2.65)	O&G units present high burnout. The main factor is stress and urgency related to the life of the mother or child.	2c/B

Table 1. *Cont.*

Author, Year, Country	Study Design	Sample (Gender and Mean Age)	Burnout Instrument (Reliability, Cronbach's α)	M (SD)/Percentage			Main Results	OCEBM GR/LE
				EE	D	PA		
Teffo et al., 2018, South Africa [36]	Cross-sectional	N = 73 O&G nurses	PRoQOL	**Subscale** Compassion satisfaction = 41 (5.7) Burnout = 33 (4.1) Secondary traumatic stress = 24 (7)			An adequate work environment increases motivation and job satisfaction. Burnout is related to years of experience.	2c/B
Yao et al., 2018, China [37]	Cross-sectional	N = 95 O&G nurses	MBI	12.0 (5.9)	7.0 (4.7)	10.9 (8.9)	Emergencies, mental health, and pediatrics are the areas with the highest burnout score. O&G area presents the lowest score in burnout.	2c/B
Yavuzşen and Vupa Çilengiroğlu, 2015, Turkey [38]	Cross-sectional	N = 90 O&G nurses 100% Female Age = 35.49	MBI (EE = 0.90, D = 0.77, PA = 0.74)	27.59 (7.27) High: 52%	10.00 (3.59) High: 50%	30.06 (4.41) Low 78%	D correlates negatively with age. Age, being a woman, and being single are considered related factors.	2c/B

Note: D = Depersonalization; EE = Emotional exhaustion; FEWS = Frankfurt Emotional Work Scale; GR = Grade of recommendation; LE = Level of evidence; MBI = Maslach Burnout Inventory; O&G = Obstetrics and Gynecology; OCEBM = Levels of evidence of the Oxford Centre for Evidence-Based Medicine; PA = Personal accomplishment; PRoQOL = Professional Quality of Life.

3.1. Dimensions of Burnout Syndrome in the Area of Gynecology and Obstetrics

High levels of EE were reported in two studies [32,38], with average scores of 27.59 and 55.8, respectively. Other authors, however, [26,35,37], had observed medium-low levels of EE, with mean scores ranging between 12 and 25.3. In a further three studies, half of the nurses (prevalence: 49.2–52%) presented high levels of EE [27,28,38]. In the final three studies for which these data are available [25,26,34], lower percentages were reported, ranging from 4.9% to 16.3% (Table 2).

For D, high levels were reported, with average scores between 10 and 29.5 [32,35,38]. Other authors had obtained lower mean scores, of five and seven [26,37]. High levels of D were found in 3.8% to 50% of the nurses sampled [25,27,34,38].

Several authors reported low levels of PA, with average scores of 10.9 to 30.06 [32,35,37,38]; only one author [26] reported high levels of PA, with a mean score of 45.1. The prevalence of low PA ranged from 4.8% to 78% of the nurses studied [25,27,38].

About the total score for burnout syndrome, one study [36] reported medium levels, but two others [30,37] recorded low levels among gynecology and obstetrics nurses, with total mean scores of 29.9 and 6.19, respectively. The prevalence of burnout reported in these studies was 0.55% [28], 6.52% [34], 13.1% [33], and 21.4% [25].

Table 2. Prevalence of high EE, high D, and low PA.

Study	Sample Size (n)	High EE (%)	High D (%)	Low PA (%)
Beaver et al., 1986 [25]	98	16.3	8.2	67.3
Fontán & Dueñas, 2010 [26]	14	14.2	21.4	7.1
Galindo et al., 2012 [27]	64	49.2	27	4.8
Habadi et al., 2018 [28]	14	50	14.28	28.57
Palmer-Morales et al., 2007 [34]	184	4.9	3.8	75
Yavuzşen & Vupa Çilengiroğlu, 2015 [38]	90	52	50	78

D = Depersonalization; EE = Emotional exhaustion; PA = Personal accomplishment.

3.2. Related Factors for Burnout in Gynecology and Obstetrics Services

Among the sociodemographic factors considered, age was found to be a factor related to burnout; thus, lower levels of EE and D were observed in older nurses [25–27,35,38]. With respect to gender, women showed higher levels of EE and D, and lower ones of PA than men [27,35,38]. Marital status is another significant factor; single nurses had lower scores for PA than those who are in a stable relationship [25,38]. According to one study, having children is related to higher EE and lower PA [25]. However, two authors found no statistical significance between marital status and number of children, in relation to the risk of burnout [29,34].

Among the work-related factors considered, a work schedule exceeding 48 hours per week was associated with higher levels of EE and D and lower ones of PA [25,26]. The same relationship was observed when the nurses work rotating and/or nocturnal shifts [30,32]. Levels of EE and D were higher with the increase in the patients per nurse ratio [25,33], with the decrease in the number of nurses working in the unit, and among less experienced nurses [25–27,29]. However, one study [34] observed no significant relationship between burnout syndrome, experience, and night-time work.

The poor organization was related to higher levels of EE and D [25,28]. Another study [29] concluded that this problem results, fundamentally, in lower PA, while another found that low job satisfaction [36] is a major problem in this respect. Moreover, the gynecology and obstetrics service was reported to be among the units presenting the highest dropout rate in the nursing profession [30]. Finally, low salary levels were also related to lower levels of PA [25].

Other work-related variables that were reported to be significant include working in rural or urban areas [25]; when nurses' work took place in both areas, the prevalence of burnout was lower. Within the gynecology and obstetrics service, the nurses who provide antenatal care presented lower levels of PA [25].

Some authors [25,32,36] studied the relationship between burnout and the intrinsic characteristics of the work performed in this unit, such as the high degree of involvement by the parents, death, perinatal grief, or participation in a large number of live births or abortions; in the latter respect, the greater the number of first-trimester abortions performed, the greater the risk of burnout, with falling levels of PA, in particular [31].

Finally, in terms of psychological factors, high levels of stress and anxiety were reported, with higher scores for all three dimensions [25,30,36]; on the other hand, the prevalence of depression was low (2.5%) [33]. A negative factor was that of verbal violence, which was associated with increased EE, related to a chronic state of stress [27]. However, 66.4% of the nurses considered their health status to be good [33]. Higher levels of post-traumatic stress were found among older nurses [36], with lower scores for PA.

3.3. Levels of Burnout in Comparison with Nurses Working in Other Hospital Services

Regarding the dimension of EE, the hospital areas presenting the highest prevalence and mean scores are those of dialysis, internal and general medicine [29], surgical medicine [33], emergencies and pediatrics [37].

Comparable findings have been reported for D [29]. In this respect, one study reported finding the highest scores for nurses working in pediatrics and obstetrics-gynecology [33], although other authors obtained the highest scores for the emergency, mental health, and surgical medicine areas [37].

Finally, for PA, the results obtained are conflicting. One paper reported that the nurses working in the areas of gynecology and obstetrics were less vulnerable to low PA [29]; others, however, recorded the lowest scores in these same areas, followed by internal medicine and surgery [33,37].

For the three dimensions of burnout as a whole, the intensive care, medical, surgical medicine, and emergency areas have the highest average scores [28], although one study [35] obtained the highest score in this respect for the obstetrics-gynecological area, followed by the surgical medicine, pediatric, and medical areas.

Other studies had observed a greater prevalence of burnout in the areas of pediatrics and surgical medicine [30] or in that of mental health [37].

3.4. Results of the Meta-Analysis

The I^2 index indicated a high level of heterogeneity, with values of 95.7% (95% CI = 93.6–96.9%) for EE, 94.6% (95% CI = 91.5–96.2%) for D, and 97% (95% CI) = 95.8–97.7%) for PA.

The application of Egger's test of publication bias produced results of 5.52 with $p = 0.07$ for EE, 4.05 with $p = 0.13$ for D, and 0.92 with $p = 0.92$ for PA. We conclude from this that there was no evident publication bias.

In total, 464 nurses working in the gynecology and obstetrics area were included in our meta-analysis. In this sample, the prevalence of high levels of EE was 29% (95% CI = 11–52%) (Figure 2); for D, the value was 19% (95% CI = 6–38%) (Figure 3), and for low PA, the prevalence was 44% (95% CI = 18–71%) (Figure 4).

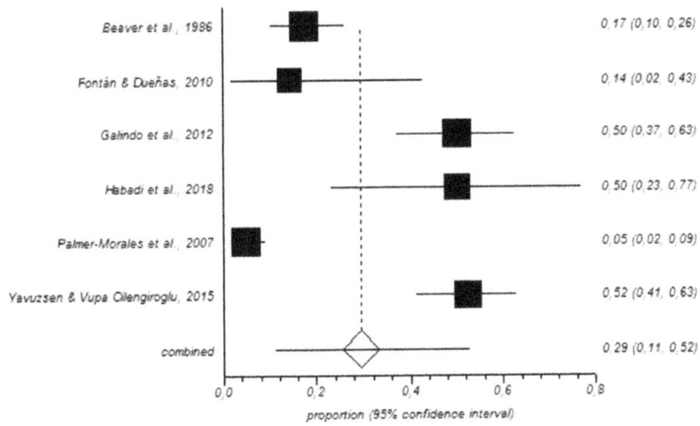

Figure 2. Forest plot for high emotional exhaustion.

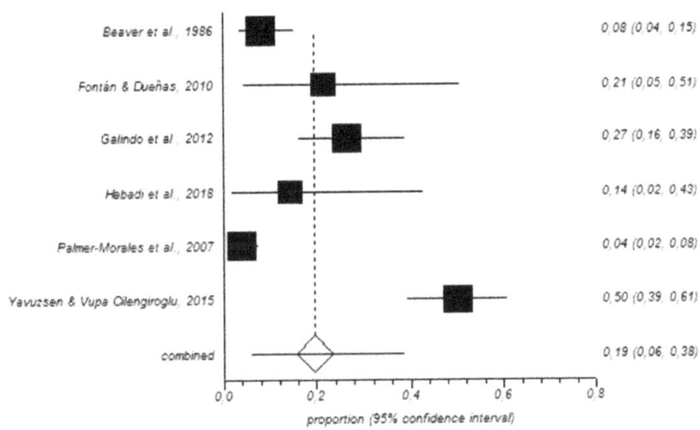

Figure 3. Forest plot for high depersonalization.

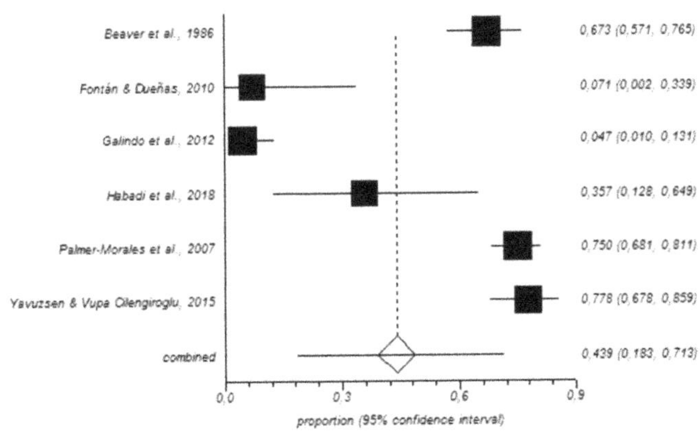

Figure 4. Forest plot for low personal accomplishment.

4. Discussion

This study aims to determine the prevalence, level of burnout, and the corresponding related factors in nurses who work in gynecology and obstetrics services, in the view that no previous meta-analyses have been conducted in this respect.

Burnout is commonly experienced by nurses working in these areas. Our analysis shows that the prevalence of high levels of EE is 29%, that of D is 19%, and that of low PA is 44%. These findings are similar to those for nurses working elsewhere, such as the medical area, with high levels of EE among 31% of nurses, of D among 24%, and low levels of PA among 38% [39]; in pediatrics, the corresponding scores are 31%, 21%, and 39% [40]; in primary care, the scores are 28%, 15%, and 31%, respectively [18]; in critical care and emergencies, the scores are 31%, 36%, and 29%, respectively [17].

However, study data reported for other occupational groups working in the same area, such as gynecologists, reflect higher levels of burnout, with 44–56.6% [41,42], among which the prevalence of high EE is 72%, that of high D is 43%, and that of low PA, 74%. Similarly, another study, of medical residents working in the gynecology service, reported high levels of EE and D in 50% of the sample, relating this to a low degree of professional satisfaction and even to regret at having opted for this area of specialization [43].

Regarding the relationship between burnout syndrome and the sociodemographic and work-related variables considered, studies have observed high levels of EE among young people, those who are single, and those with less experience [44] because these groups are less self-confident and are subject to greater tension when decisions must be taken [45]; on the other hand, one study reported that D is positively associated with the number of years spent in the profession [42]. Other researchers have concluded that women are more likely than men to experience burnout [8,46] and that the risk of D is aggravated by women's greater involvement in care, due to their dual roles, as mother and nurse [47]. Relative youth is also considered a risk factor [8,18] due to these nurses' greater uncertainty and low expectations of promotion [48]. Besides, it has been reported that PA is negatively correlated with the number of children in the nurse's family, due to occupational and personal overload [42,49]. On the other hand, more recent studies claim that having children is a protective factor, helping nurses live a fuller life [8].

In terms of organizational characteristics, factors, such as negative sensations regarding the work environment [50], low salaries [51], and lack of organization [52], despite (or in addition to) great responsibility, all contribute to reduced job satisfaction [53] and to nurses' abandoning the profession [54–56]. Also, falling staff numbers and the reorganization of services, due to low birth rates in developed countries [57], increase EE and reduce PA [58]. The lack of resources, concerning the demand for care, tends to make health care highly mechanized and medicalized, a situation in which nurses' competencies are limited [59], as is their freedom to exercise independent judgment [60]. Furthermore, rotating shifts and the imposition of a 70-hour week increase the risk of burnout, especially in terms of reduced PA [44], due to work overload and heightened levels of stress [61]. Some authors conclude that a lack of commitment, motivation, or time can be considered alarm signals and that the quality of care may be compromised [62,63].

Regarding the psychological variables considered, stress and verbal violence are major risk factors for burnout [64,65] and are related to the high demand for care, the need to attend a large number of patients, and the close link between the patients and the nursing staff [66]. Symptoms of depression are common among these professionals, with a prevalence of 64% [67], which is related to high EE and D and low PA. One of the main characteristics of this hospital area is exposure to traumatic situations. Thus, 25–35% of nurses assisting during births report suffering post-traumatic stress disorders [68,69]. Dealing with loss and alleviating grief is a fundamental aspect of these nurses' daily work [70], but helping mothers cope with perinatal death (whether natural or resulting from an abortion) increases their vulnerability and the risk of burnout. Possibly, for this reason, levels of PA are lower among nurses working in the antepartum area [71,72].

Finally, regarding the state of perceived health, high levels of EE are related to a high prevalence of physical alterations, such as musculoskeletal injuries [73]. Therefore, many authors show a series of effective interventions that can improve physical and mental health in nurses [74], reducing burnout levels by up to 30% [75]. These include training programs through multidisciplinary workshops, including communication skills, and presenting a positive impact on burnout levels, increasing job satisfaction and improving the level of confidence [76]. In the same way, physical exercise programs, such as yoga, show a reduction in the level of burnout and improve the quality of sleep [77]. Benefits have also been observed in residents of the gynecology and obstetrics area, reducing the blood pressure, as well as the levels of burnout and improvement in their nutritional habits [78]. Other types of interventions are those that increase self-awareness and promote acceptance and motivation towards a change in behavior, such as mindfulness [79], showing a negative correlation between EE, D and positive with PA. Brief 8-week interventions show a reduction in the prevalence of up to 31% in EE [80] and up to 17.60% in D [81], and there is even evidence of an increase in PA levels [82].

Limitations

Few papers have been published providing sufficient statistical data with which to analyze levels of burnout among gynecology and obstetrics nurses. In consequence, the number of studies included in our meta-analysis is, unfortunately, low. Moreover, the population samples studied are also restricted, and data are not supplied on the number of nurses who have left the profession. All the studies analyzed are cross-sectional; thus, it was not possible to study the long-term impact of burnout on these nurses. In short, only the associations between the variables are analyzed in our study, and the presence or absence of causality is not established. Also, some of the included studies have a small sample, and this must be taken into account before analyzing the related factors. Finally, it must be indicated that a new approach of burnout has established five personal profiles (burnout, engagement, overextended, disengaged, and ineffective) depending on the scores of each burnout dimension [83]. Because the included studies have not used these profiles, we have not been able to establish these profiles.

5. Conclusions

Nurses in gynecology and obstetrics services tend to have high levels of EE and D and low levels of PA, but it must be taken into account that due to the influence of occupational variables in each country, these levels may vary.

Some variables that may have a relation with burnout development in gynecological nurses, and that should be analyzed in the future, are being young, relatively inexperienced, single, and/or who have children. Other negative factors in this respect are long working days/weeks and the need to care for large numbers of patients.

Good leadership and appropriate organization of care duties, providing nurses with sufficient autonomy and appropriate staff numbers, are key factors in preventing the development of burnout.

Supplementary Materials: The following are available online at http://www.mdpi.com/1660-4601/16/14/2585/s1, Table S1: PRISMA 2009 Checklist.

Author Contributions: Conceptualization, E.I.D.l.F.-S., N.S.-M., L.P.-H., J.L.G.-U., G.A.C.-D.l.F., and L.A.-G.; Methodology, E.I.D.l.F.-S., N.S.-M., L.P.-H., J.L.G.-U., G.A.C.-D.l.F., and L.A.-G.; Software, J.L.G.-U. and L.A.-G.; Validation, E.I.D.l.F.-S., G.A.C.-D.l.F., and L.A.-G.; Formal analysis, N.S.-M., J.L.G.-U., G.A.C.-D.l.F., and L.A.-G.; Investigation, E.I.D.l.F.-S., N.S.-M., L.P.-H., J.L.G.-U., G.A.C.-D.l.F., and L.A.-G.; Resources, E.I.D.l.F.-S., N.S.-M., L.P.-H., J.L.G.-U., G.A.C.-D.l.F., and L.A.-G.; Data curation, N.S.-M. and J.L.G.-U.; Writing—Original Draft Preparation, E.I.D.l.F.-S., N.S.-M., and L.P.-H.; Writing—Review and Editing, E.I.D.l.F.-S., N.S.-M., L.P.-H., J.L.G.-U., G.A.C.-D.l.F., and L.A.-G.; Visualization, E.I.D.l.F.-S., N.S.-M., L.P.-H., J.L.G.-U., G.A.C.-D.l.F., and L.A.-G.; Supervision, E.I.D.l.F.-S., G.A.C.-D.l.F., and L.A.-G.; Project administration, E.I.D.l.F.-S., N.S.-M., L.P.-H., J.L.G.-U., G.A.C.-D.l.F., and L.A.-G.

Funding: This research was funded by the Excellence Research Project (P11HUM-7771) provided by the Andalusian Government (Spain).

Acknowledgments: This article forms part of the Doctoral Thesis of the corresponding author (Nora Suleiman-Martos) within the Psychology doctoral program offered at the University of Granada (Spain).

Conflicts of Interest: The authors declare no conflict of interest.

References

1. Salyers, M.P.; Bonfils, K.A.; Luther, L.; Firmin, R.L.; White, D.A.; Adams, E.L.; Rollins, A.L. The relationship between professional burnout and quality and safety in healthcare: A meta-analysis. *J. Gen. Intern. Med.* **2017**, *32*, 475–482. [CrossRef] [PubMed]
2. McVicar, A. Scoping the common antecedents of job stress and job satisfaction for nurses (2000–2013) using the job demands resources model of stress. *J. Nurs. Manag.* **2016**, *24*, E112–E136. [CrossRef] [PubMed]
3. Ruitenburg, M.M.; Frings-Dresen, M.H.; Sluiter, J.K. The prevalence of common mental disorders among hospital physicians and their association with self-reported work ability: A cross-sectional study. *BMC Health Serv. Res.* **2012**, *12*, 292–298. [CrossRef] [PubMed]
4. Hämmig, O. Explaining burnout and the intention to leave the profession among health professionals-A cross-sectional study in a hospital setting in Switzerland. *Bmc Health Serv. Res.* **2018**, *18*, 785. [CrossRef] [PubMed]
5. Maslach, C.; Schaufeli, W.B.; Leiter, M.P. Job burnout. *Annu. Rev. Psychol.* **2001**, *52*, 397–422. [CrossRef] [PubMed]
6. Maslach, C.; Jackson, S.E. The measurement of experienced burnout. *J. Organ. Behav.* **1981**, *2*, 99–113. [CrossRef]
7. Maslach, C.; Jackson, S.E.; Leiter, M.P.; Schaufeli, W.B.; Schwab, R.L. *MBI: The Maslach Burnout Inventory Manual*; Consulting Psychologists Press: Palo Alto, CA, USA, 1996.
8. Cañadas-De la Fuente, G.A.; Ortega, E.; Ramírez-Baena, L.; De la Fuente-Solana, E.I.; Vargas, C.; Gómez-Urquiza, J.L. Gender, marital Status, and children as risk factors for burnout in nurses: A Meta-Analytic Study. *Int. J. Environ. Res. Public Health* **2018**, *15*, 2102. [CrossRef] [PubMed]
9. Gómez-Urquiza, J.L.; Vargas, C.; De la Fuente, E.I.; Fernández-Castillo, R.; Cañadas-De la Fuente, G.A. Age as a risk factor for burnout syndrome in nursing professionals: A meta-analytic study. *Res. Nurs. Health* **2017**, *40*, 99–110. [CrossRef] [PubMed]
10. Emold, C.; Schneider, N.; Meller, I.; Yagil, Y. Communication skills, working environment and burnout among oncology nurses. *Eur. J. Oncol. Nurs.* **2011**, *15*, 358–363. [CrossRef] [PubMed]
11. Dos Santos Alves, D.F.; da Silva, D.; de Brito Guirardello, E. Nursing practice environment, job outcomes and safety climate: A structural equation modelling analysis. *J. Nurs. Manag.* **2017**, *25*, 46–55. [CrossRef]
12. Guo, Y.F.; Plummer, V.; Lam, L.; Wang, Y.; Cross, W.; Zhang, J.P. The effects of resilience and turnover intention on nurses burnout: Findings from a comparative cross-sectional study. *J. Clin. Nurs.* **2019**, *28*, 499–508. [CrossRef] [PubMed]
13. Lee, H.F.; Chiang, H.Y.; Kuo, H.T. Relationship between authentic leadership and nurses intent to leave: The mediating role of work environment and burnout. *J. Nurs. Manag.* **2019**, *27*, 52–65. [CrossRef] [PubMed]
14. Scanlan, J.N.; Still, M. Relationships between burnout, turnover intention, job satisfaction, job demands and job resources for mental health personnel in an Australian mental health service. *BMC Health Serv. Res.* **2019**, *19*, 62. [CrossRef] [PubMed]
15. Ahmadi, O.; Azizkhani, R.; Basravi, M. Correlation between workplace and occupational burnout syndrome in nurses. *Adv. Biomed. Res.* **2014**, *3*, 44. [CrossRef]
16. Cañadas-De la Fuente, G.A.; Vargas, C.; San Luis, C.; García, I.; Cañadas, G.R.; De La Fuente, E.I. Risk factors and prevalence of burnout syndrome in the nursing profession. *Int. J. Nurs. Stud.* **2015**, *52*, 240–249. [CrossRef] [PubMed]
17. Gómez-Urquiza, J.L.; De la Fuente-Solana, E.I.; Albendín-García, L.; Vargas-Pecino, C.; Ortega-Campos, E.M.; Cañadas-De la Fuente, G.A. Prevalence of burnout syndrome in emergency nurses: A Meta-Analysis. *Crit. Care Nurse* **2017**, *37*, e1–e9. [CrossRef] [PubMed]
18. Monsalve-Reyes, C.S.; San Luis-Costas, C.; Gómez-Urquiza, J.L.; Albendín-García, L.; Aguayo, R.; Cañadas-De la Fuente, G.A. Burnout syndrome and its prevalence in primary care nursing: A systematic review and meta-analysis. *BMC Fam. Pract.* **2018**, *19*, 59. [CrossRef] [PubMed]

19. Ramírez-Baena, L.; Ortega-Campos, E.; Gómez-Urquiza, J.L.; Cañadas-De la Fuente, G.R.; De la Fuente-Solana, E.I.; Cañadas-De la Fuente, G.A. A multicentre study of burnout prevalence and related psychological variables in medical area hospital nurses. *J. Clin. Med.* **2019**, *8*, 92. [CrossRef]
20. Noonan, M.; Jomeen, J.; Galvin, R.; Doody, O. Survey of midwives perinatal mental health knowledge, confidence, attitudes and learning needs. *Women Birth* **2018**, *31*, e358–e366. [CrossRef] [PubMed]
21. Wahlberg, A.; Högberg, U.; Emmelin, M. The erratic pathway to regaining a professional self-image after an obstetric work-related trauma: A grounded theory study. *Int. J. Nurs. Stud.* **2019**, *89*, 53–61. [CrossRef]
22. Moher, D.; Liberati, A.; Tetzlaff, J.; Altman, D.G.; The PRISMA Group. Preferred reporting items for systematic reviews and meta-analyses: The PRISMA statement. *PLoS Med.* **2009**, *6*, e1000097. [CrossRef] [PubMed]
23. Ciapponi, A. Critical appraisal guide of observational studies in epidemiology (first part). *Evidencia* **2010**, *13*, 135–140.
24. Howick, J.; Chalmers, I.; Glasziou, P.; Greenhalg, T.; Heneghan, C.; Liberati, A.; Moschetti, I.; Phillips, B.; Thornton, H. The Oxford 2011 Levels of Evidence. 2011. Available online: https://www.cebm.net/2016/05/ocebm-levels-of-evidence (accessed on 10 April 2019).
25. Beaver, R.C.; Sharp, E.S.; Cotsonis, G.A. Burnout experienced by nurse midwives. *J. Nurs. Midwifery* **1986**, *31*, 3–15. [CrossRef]
26. Fontán Atalaya, I.M.; Dueñas Díez, J.L. Burnout syndrome in an obstetrics and gynaecology management unit. *Rev. Calid. Asist.* **2010**, *25*, 260–267. [CrossRef] [PubMed]
27. Galindo, R.H.; Feliciano, K.V.; Lima, R.A.; de Souza, A.I. Burnout syndrome among general hospital nurses in Recife. *Rev. Esc. Enferm. USP* **2012**, *46*, 420–427. [CrossRef] [PubMed]
28. Habadi, A.I.; Alfaer, S.S.; Shilli, R.H.; Habadi, M.I.; Suliman, S.M.; Al-Aslany, S.J.; Habadi, M.I. The prevalence of burnout syndrome among nursing staff working at King Abdulaziz University Hospital, Jeddah, Saudi Arabia, 2017. *Divers. Equal. Health Care* **2018**, *15*, 122–126. [CrossRef]
29. Higashiguchi, K.; Morikawa, Y.; Miura, K.; Nishijo, M.; Tabata, M.; Ishizaki, M.; Nakagawa, H. Burnout and related factors among hospital Nurses. *J. Occup. Health* **1999**, *41*, 215–224. [CrossRef]
30. Liu, W.; Zhao, S.; Shi, L.; Zhang, Z.; Liu, X.; Li, L.; Duan, X.; Li, G.; Lou, F.; Jia, X.; et al. Workplace violence, job satisfaction, burnout, perceived organisational support and their effects on turnover intention among Chinese nurses in tertiary hospitals: A cross-sectional study. *BMJ Open* **2018**, *8*, e019525. [CrossRef]
31. Mizuno, M.; Kinefuchi, E.; Kimura, R.; Tsuda, A. Professional quality of life of Japanese nurses/midwives providing abortion/childbirth care. *Nurs. Ethics* **2013**, *20*, 539–550. [CrossRef]
32. Naz, S.; Hashmi, A.M.; Asif, A. Burnout and quality of life in nurses of a tertiary care hospital in Pakistan. *J. Pak. Med. Assoc.* **2016**, *66*, 532–536.
33. Nguyen, H.T.T.; Kitaoka, K.; Sukigara, M.; Thai, A.L. Burnout study of clinical nurses in Vietnam: Development of job burnout model based on Leiter and Maslachs Theory. *Asian Nurs. Res. (Korean Soc. Nurs. Sci.)* **2018**, *12*, 42–49. [CrossRef]
34. Palmer-Morales, Y.; Prince-Vélez, R.; Searcy-Bernal, R.; Compean-Saucedo, B. Prevalence of burnout syndrome in nurses in 2 Mexican hospitals. *Enferm. Clin.* **2007**, *17*, 256–260. [CrossRef]
35. Sun, W.Y.; Ling, G.P.; Chen, P.; Shan, L. Burnout among nurses in the peoples Republic of China. *Int. J. Occup. Environ. Health* **1996**, *2*, 274–279. [CrossRef]
36. Teffo, M.E.; Levin, J.; Rispel, L.C. Compassion satisfaction, burnout and secondary traumatic stress among termination of pregnancy providers in two South African provinces. *J. Obstet. Gynaecol. Res.* **2018**, *44*, 1202–1210. [CrossRef]
37. Yao, Y.; Zhao, S.; Gao, X.; An, Z.; Wang, S.; Li, H.; Li, Y.; Gao, L.; Lu, L.; Dong, Z. General self-efficacy modifies the effect of stress on burnout in nurses with different personality types. *BMC Health Serv. Res.* **2018**, *18*, 667. [CrossRef]
38. Yavuzşen, H.T.; Vupa Çilengiroğlu, O. Burnout in physicians and nurses working in Obstetrics/Gynecology clinics in Turkey. *Turkiye Klinikleri J. Gynecol. Obst.* **2015**, *25*, 160–167. [CrossRef]
39. Molina-Praena, J.; Ramírez-Baena, L.; Gómez-Urquiza, J.L.; Cañadas, G.R.; De la Fuente, E.I.; Cañadas-De la Fuente, G.A. Levels of burnout and risk factors in medical area nurses: A meta-analytic study. *Int. J. Environ. Res. Public Health* **2018**, *15*, 2800. [CrossRef]

40. Pradas-Hernández, L.; Ariza, T.; Gómez-Urquiza, J.L.; Albendín-García, L.; De la Fuente, E.I.; Cañadas-De la Fuente, G.A. Prevalence of burnout in paediatric nurses: A systematic review and meta-analysis. *PLoS ONE* **2018**, *13*, e0195039. [CrossRef]
41. Moradi, Y.; Baradaran, H.R.; Yazdandoost, M.; Atrak, S.; Kashanian, M. Prevalence of burnout in residents of obstetrics and gynecology: A systematic review and meta-analysis. *Med. J. Islam. Repub. Iran* **2015**, *29*, 235.
42. Thorsen, V.C.; Tharp, A.L.; Meguid, T. High rates of burnout among maternal health staff at a referral hospital in Malawi: A cross-sectional study. *BMC Nurs.* **2011**, *10*, 9. [CrossRef]
43. Govardhan, L.M.; Pinelli, V.; Schnatz, P.F. Burnout, depression and job satisfaction in obstetrics and gynecology residents. *Conn. Med.* **2012**, *76*, 389–395.
44. Gabbe, S.G.; Melville, J.; Mandel, L.; Walker, E. Burnout in chair of obstetrics and gynecology: Diagnosis, treatment, and prevention. *Am. J. Obstet. Gynecol.* **2002**, *186*, 601–612. [CrossRef]
45. De la Fuente-Solana, E.I.; Cañadas, G.R.; Ramirez-Baena, L.; Gómez-Urquiza, J.L.; Ariza, T.; Cañadas-De la Fuente, G.A. An explanatory model of potential changes in burnout diagnosis according to personality factors in oncology nurses. *Int. J. Environ. Res. Public Health* **2019**, *16*, 312. [CrossRef]
46. Iorga, M.; Socolov, V.; Muraru, D.; Dirtu, C.; Soponaru, C.; Ilea, C.; Socolov, D.M. Factors influencing burnout syndrome in obstetrics and gynecology physicians. *Biomed. Res. Int.* **2017**, *2017*, 1–10. [CrossRef]
47. Kavurmacı, M.; Cantekin, I.; Tan, M. Burnout levels of hemodialysis nurses. *Ren. Fail.* **2014**, *36*, 1038–1042. [CrossRef]
48. Flinkman, M.; Isopahkala-Bouret, U.; Salanterä, S. Young registered nurses intention to leave the profession and professional turnover in early career: A qualitative case study. *ISRN Nurs.* **2013**, *2013*, 1–12. [CrossRef]
49. França, S.P.; Martino, M.F.; Aniceto, E.V.; Silva, L.L. Preditores da síndrome de burnout emenfermeiros de serviços de urgencia pré-hospitalar. *Acta Paul. Enferm.* **2012**, *25*, 68–73. [CrossRef]
50. Hildingsson, I.; Westlund, K.; Wiklund, I. Burnout in Swedish midwives. *Sex. Reprod. Health* **2013**, *4*, 87–91. [CrossRef]
51. Rudman, A.; Gustavsson, P.; Hultell, D. A prospective study of nurses intentions to leave the profession during their first five years of practice in Sweden. *Int. J. Nurs. Stud.* **2014**, *51*, 612–662. [CrossRef]
52. McAuliffe, E.; Daly, M.; Kamwendo, F.; Masanja, H.; Sidat, M.; de Pinho, H. The critical role of supervision in retaining staff in obstetric services: A three country study. *PLoS ONE* **2013**, *8*, e58415. [CrossRef]
53. Hellyar, M.; Madani, C.; Yeaman, S.; O'Connor, K.; Kerr, K.M.; Davidson, J.E. Case study investigation decreases burnout while improving interprofessional teamwork, nurse satisfaction, and patient safety. *Crit Care Nurs Q.* **2019**, *42*, 96–105. [CrossRef]
54. Heinen, M.M.; van Achterberg, T.; Schwendimann, R.; Zander, B.; Matthews, A.; Kózka, M.; Ensio, A.; Sjetne, I.S.; Moreno Casbas, T.; Ball, J.; et al. Nurses intention to leave their profession: A cross sectional observational study in 10 European countries. *Int. J. Nurs. Stud.* **2013**, *50*, 174–184. [CrossRef]
55. Moloney, W.; Boxall, P.; Parsons, M.; Cheung, G. Factors predicting registered nurses intentions to leave their organization and profession: A job demands-resources framework. *J. Adv. Nurs.* **2018**, *74*, 864–875. [CrossRef]
56. Winkel, A.F.; Robinson, A.; Jones, A.A.; Squires, A.P. Physician resilience: A grounded theory study of obstetrics and gynaecology residents. *Med. Educ.* **2019**, *53*, 184–194. [CrossRef]
57. Kozhimannil, K.B.; Hung, P.; Henning-Smith, C.; Casey, M.M.; Prasad, S. Association between loss of hospital-based obstetric services and birth outcomes in rural counties in the United States. *JAMA* **2018**, *319*, 1239–1247. [CrossRef]
58. Nowrouzi, B.; Lightfoot, N.; Carter, L.; Larivière, M.; Rukholm, E.; Schinke, R.; Belanger-Gardner, D. The relationship between quality of work life and location of cross-training among obstetric nurses in urban northeastern Ontario, Canada: A population-based cross sectional study. *Int. J. Occup. Med. Environ. Health* **2015**, *28*, 571–586. [CrossRef]
59. Labrague, L.J.; McEnroe-Petitte, D.M.; Tsaras, K. Predictors and outcomes of nurse professional autonomy: A cross-sectional study. *Int. J. Nurs. Pract.* **2019**, *25*, 12711. [CrossRef]
60. Bermudez-Tamayo, C.; Fernández Ruiz, E.; Pastor Moreno, G.; Maroto-Navarro, G.; Garcia-Mochon, L.; Perez-Ramos, F.J.; Caño-Aguilar, A.; Velez, M.D.P. Barriers and enablers in the implementation of a program to reduce cesarean deliveries. *Reprod. Health* **2017**, *14*, 106. [CrossRef]

61. Cañadas-De la Fuente, G.A.; Albendín-García, L.; De la Fuente, E.I.; San Luis, C.; Gómez-Urquiza, J.L.; Cañadas, G.R. Síndrome de burnout en profesionales de enfermería que realizan jornada física complementaria en servicios de cuidados críticos y urgencias. *Rev. Esp. Salud Pública* **2016**, *90*, e1–e9.
62. Campanelli, S. The ties that bind-nurses, mothers, and antepartum care. *Nurs. Womens Health* **2019**, *23*, 181–182. [CrossRef]
63. Hall, L.H.; Johnson, J.; Watt, I.; Tsipa, A.; Daryl, B.O. Healthcare staff wellbeing, burnout, and patient safety: A systematic review. *PLoS ONE* **2016**, *11*, e0159015. [CrossRef]
64. Olsen, E.; Bjaalid, G.; Mikkelsen, A. Work climate and the mediating role of workplace bullying related to job performance, job satisfaction, and work ability: A study among hospital nurses. *J. Adv. Nurs.* **2017**, *73*, 2709–2719. [CrossRef]
65. Prentice, T.M.; Gillam, L.; Davis, P.G.; Janvier, A. Always a burden? Healthcare providers perspectives on moral distress. *Arch. Dis. Child. Fetal Neonatal. Ed.* **2018**, *103*, F441–F445. [CrossRef]
66. Elmir, R.; Pangas, J.; Dahlen, H.; Schmied, V. A meta-ethnographic synthesis of midwives and nurses experiences of adverse labour and birth events. *J. Clin. Nurs.* **2017**, *26*, 4184–4200. [CrossRef]
67. Gong, Y.; Han, T.; Yin, X.; Yang, G.; Zhuang, R.; Chen, Y.; Lu, Z. Prevalence of depressive symptoms and work-related risk factors among nurses in public hospitals in southern China: A cross-sectional study. *Sci. Rep.* **2014**, *4*, 7109. [CrossRef]
68. Beck, C.T.; Eaton, C.M.; Gable, R.K. Vicarious posttraumatic growth in labor and delivery nurses. *J. Obstet. Gynecol. Neonatal. Nurs.* **2016**, *45*, 801–812. [CrossRef]
69. Hamama-Raz, Y.; Walker, R.; Palgi, Y.; Mashiach, R.; Lee-Ovadia, K.; Manny, A.; Ben-Ezra, M. Comorbidity of post-traumatic stress symptoms and depressive symptoms among obstetric nurses with perinatal death exposure. *Isr. J. Psychiatry Relat. Sci.* **2016**, *53*, 58–62.
70. Ben-Ezra, M.; Palgi, Y.; Walker, R.; Many, A.; Hamam-Raz, Y. The impact of perinatal death on obstetrics nurses: A longitudinal and cross-sectional examination. *J. Perinat. Med.* **2014**, *42*, 75–81. [CrossRef]
71. Blackmore, E.R.; Côté-Arsenault, D.; Tang, W.; Glover, V.; Evans, J.; Golding, J.; O'Connor, T.G. Previous prenatal loss as a predictor of perinatal depression and anxiety. *Br. J. Psychiatry* **2011**, *198*, 373–378. [CrossRef]
72. Suplee, P.D.; Bingham, D.; Kleppel, L. Nurses knowledge and teaching of possible postpartum complications. *MCN Am. J. Matern. Child Nurs.* **2017**, *42*, 338–344. [CrossRef]
73. Wang, J.; Cui, Y.; He, L.; Xu, X.; Yuan, Z.; Jin, X.; Li, Z. Work-Related musculoskeletal disorders and risk factors among Chinese medical staff of obstetrics and gynecology. *Int. J. Environ. Res. Public Health* **2017**, *14*, 562. [CrossRef]
74. Ruotsalainen, J.H.; Verbeek, J.H.; Mariné, A.; Serra, C. Preventing occupational stress in healthcare workers. *Cochrane Database Syst. Rev.* **2014**, *13*, CD002892. [CrossRef]
75. Craigie, M.; Slatyer, S.; Hegney, D.; Osseiran-Moisson, R.; Gentry, E.; Davis, S.; Dolan, T.; Rees, C. A pilot evaluation of a Mindful Self-care and Resiliency (MSCR) intervention for nurses. *Mindfulness* **2016**, *7*, 764–774. [CrossRef]
76. Lupo, F.N.; Arnaboldi, P.; Santoro, L.; D'Anna, E.; Beltrami, C.; Mazzoleni, E.M.; Veronesi, P.; Maggioni, A.; Didier, F. The effects of a multimodal training program on burnout syndrome in gynecologic oncology nurses and on the multidisciplinary psychosocial care of gynecologic cancer patients: An Italian experience. *Palliat. Support Care* **2013**, *11*, 199–203. [CrossRef]
77. Cocchiara, R.A.; Peruzzo, M.; Mannocci, A.; Ottolenghi, L.; Villari, P.; Polimeni, A.; Guerra, F.; La Torre, G. The use of yoga to manage stress and burnout in healthcare workers: A systematic review. *J. Clin. Med.* **2019**, *8*, 284. [CrossRef]
78. Babbar, S.; Renner, K.; Williams, K. Addressing obstetrics and gynecology trainee burnout using a yoga-based wellness initiative during dedicated education time. *Obstet. Gynecol.* **2019**, *133*, 994–1001. [CrossRef]
79. Salvarani, V.; Rampoldi, G.; Ardenghi, S.; Bani, M.; Blasi, P.; Ausili, D.; Di Mauro, S.; Strepparava, M.G. Protecting emergency room nurses from burnout: The role of dispositional mindfulness, emotion regulation and empathy. *J. Nurs. Manag.* **2019**, *27*, 765–774. [CrossRef]
80. Montanari, K.M.; Bowe, C.; Chesak, S.S.; Cutshall, S.M. Assessing the feasibility of a pilot intervention to reduce stress and burnout. *J. Holist. Nurs.* **2019**, *37*, 175–188. [CrossRef]

81. Mealer, M.; Conrad, D.; Evans, J.; Jooste, K.; Solyntjes, J.; Rothbaum, B.; Moss, M. Feasibility and acceptability of a resilience training program for intensive care unit nurses. *Am. J. Crit. Care* **2014**, *23*, e97–e105. [CrossRef]
82. Mackenzie, C.S.; Poulin, P.A.; Seidman-Carlson, R. A brief mindfulness-based stress reduction intervention for nurses and nurse aides. *Appl. Nurs. Res.* **2006**, *19*, 105–109. [CrossRef]
83. Leiter, M.P.; Maslach, C. Latent burnout profiles: A new approach to understanding the burnout experience. *Burn. Res.* **2016**, *3*, 89–100. [CrossRef]

International Journal of
Environmental Research and Public Health

MDPI

Article

Video Display Operator Complaints: A 10-Year Follow-Up of Visual Fatigue and Refractive Disorders

Francesca Larese Filon *, Anna Drusian, Federico Ronchese and Corrado Negro

Unit of Occupational Medicine, University of Trieste, 34100 Trieste, Italy
* Correspondence: larese@units.it; Tel.: +39-040-399-2215

Received: 24 June 2019; Accepted: 6 July 2019; Published: 13 July 2019

Abstract: Visual fatigue and discomfort are very common complaints for video display operators (VDTs). The aim of our study was to study work-related visual symptoms in relation to refractive disorders and psychosocial factors in 3054 public employees by way of follow-ups for 10 years with periodic medical examinations with eye evaluation in the period 2000–2009. Factors related to visual fatigue were evaluated in the follow-up using generalized equation estimation. Visual fatigue was very common in VDT operators (64.03%). During the follow-up, no relationship between visual fatigue and age, sex, seniority of work, visual acuity and refractory disorders was found. Visual fatigue was significantly associated with anxiety perception in a dose-related matter (odds ratio (OR) 7.40, confidence interval (CI) 95% 1.77–31.3), psychosocial factors (OR 1.03, CI 95% 1.01–1.07), use of lenses (OR 1.34, CI 95% 1.09–1.64) and time of VDT usage (OR 1.27, CI 95% 1.04–1.53). This study confirmed that visual fatigue is common in VDT users and is related to anxiety perception, time of VDT usage, use of lenses and stress. No relationship was found between visual fatigue and refractory disorders or visual acuity.

Keywords: follow-up; video display terminal; visual fatigue; refractive disorders

---

1. Introduction

Workers that spend many hours on video display terminals (VDTs) can report visual fatigue and discomfort related to their work environment as well as vision defects, psychosocial stress and anxiety perception [1–4]. Many authors have studied musculoskeletal disorders in VDT operators that increased due to non-ergonomic workstations and postural demands [5,6], but there are, to our knowledge, no long-term follow-up studies that have analyzed visual fatigue and related factors.

Eye symptoms are very common in VDT users, and the American Optometric Association has started to refer to computer vision syndrome (CVS) as the combination of eye and vision problems associated with the use of computers. This derives from insufficient visual capabilities to perform the computer task comfortably. CVS is characterized by itching, redness, burning, eye tearing, headache, double vision, eye strain and blurred vision [1]. The prevalence of CVS increases significantly in individuals who spend more than 4 h daily working on VDT [4]. However, personal, environmental and ergonomic factors are also relevant as well as the long-term use of VDTs after work hours and mobile phones [7].

Visual fatigue is a major complaint in subjects with CVS and is characterized by weakness of the eyes, usually accompanied by headache and dimming of vision—symptoms that are transitory and recede with rest [4,8–13]. Eye fatigue appears because of the unconscious muscular effort of the eyes when preventive measures are not taken. Eye fatigue can be induced by repeated activation/deactivation of the ocular muscles [14] or by prolonged accommodative responses to similar focal distances [15]. The use of VDT leads to a reduction in the amplitude of accommodation with an increase in exophoria [16]; however, these alterations are temporary changes with no long-term permanent effect [1]. Close work can also induce transient myopia, and Luberto et al. [17] in 1989 suggested that the use of a temporary myopic shift can be a reliable objective assessment tool for VDT-related visual fatigue.

The subjective asthenopic symptoms, however, can also be related to environmental factors, such as lighting, screen resolution and work arrangements [18]. The surrounding illuminance causes greater changes in visual function with the reduction of amplitude of accommodation; also, the increase in illuminance has a negative effect on reaction time. Moreover, red and green-colored lights produced more visual fatigue compared to white and blue-colored lights. Janosik and Grzesik [19] in 2003 recommended illumination higher than 200 lux. The presence of reflections on the skin causes confusion, with multiple attempts required at focused reading on VDT and the need for additional accommodation responses. Working hours on VDTs without breaks can increase visual fatigue, and a relative humidity below 40% and high temperature can cause ocular discomfort and dry eye syndrome [10].

Visual fatigue prevalence ranges between 19.6% [20] and 72.1% [21] in office workers. The wide range of prevalence depends on the criteria used to define symptoms and methods used [20].

In addition to ergonomic and environmental factors [7,22,23], some research has focused on psychological factors as causative factors of CVS. Office work is sedentary and requires less physical energy than other jobs, but needs more mental attention and cognitive processes, sometimes with constant work pressure and at others with low levels of autonomy and few decision-making possibilities that can cause stress [24].

Visual fatigue and stress are common in VDT users [25–27] and are sometimes associated with musculoskeletal disorders [28], but research is lacking in terms of long-term follow-up. The aim of our study was to evaluate these symptoms in a large group of VDT users in 10-year follow-up, with the final aim of suggesting interventions which are useful to increase wellness in VDT workers.

2. Materials and Methods

We evaluated 3054 computer operators working with VDTs for more than 20 h per week in different public offices in Trieste (Italy) that underwent periodical health surveillance in the Clinical Unit of Occupational Medicine from 2000 to 2009. Two thousand two hundred and eight workers completed the follow-up with 3 or 4 medical examinations according to age: workers underwent a periodic medical evaluation with eye examination, as required by Italian law (every 5 years for workers <50 years-old and every 2 years for those ≥50 years-old). Lenses in use were defined using a lensmeter (Essilor Instruments CL60, Thornbury, Bristol, UK). Myopia was defined when >−0.25 dioptres (D). Hyperopia and presbyopia were defined when >0.25D and astigmatism was defined when >0.25D. Visual acuity using lenses was evaluated for far, near and intermediate distances (57 cm) using the Vision test (Essilor Instruments, Thornbury, Bristol, UK).

During the medical examinations, workers filled in a standardized questionnaire, divided into three sections. (1) The first part comprised 59 questions concerning personal data, years of use of a VDT, hours of use per day, computer programs used, screen size and type, work breaks, interruptions during VDT work, work environment in terms of lighting, glare on the screen, distance between the computer and operator, working desk, environmental noise and temperature; (2) the second part analyzed workers' life and health, marital status, schooling, sport, smoking habit, coffee consumption, eye illnesses, use of lenses, eye examinations, and joint diseases; (3) the third part investigated the frequency of eye-symptoms related to VDT use: fatigue, redness, burning, tearing, headache, photophobia, far and near blurred vision, myodesopsia, double vision, and eye drop application—defined as never, sometimes, and often in relation to VDTs or not related to VDTs; (4) anxiety perception was defined as never, sometimes, and often in relation to VDTs or not related to VDTs (the question asked was "do you feel anxious during work with VDTs? ", and possible answers were "never", "sometimes", "often" or "not related to VDT use"); (5) psychosocial factors were evaluated using a simplified questionnaire that investigated discomfort (1—yes or 0—no) during work at VDTs regarding the following aspects: overcrowding, relationship with users, relationship with colleagues, work condition, responsibility, repetitiveness, excessive concentration, excessive attention, low possibility of correcting errors, frequent interruption during work, computer slowness, excessive variability of work tasks, low control of work tasks, slow cadence of work tasks, and fast cadence of work tasks. Psychosocial factors were summarized as the sum of all answers. All subjects signed an informed consent, and data were analyzed anonymously. Periodical medical surveillance is compulsory in Italy under the law (81/2008) and, according to Italian rules, the Local Ethical Committee was informed about the study.

Data were collected using the program Excel for Windows, and statistical analyses were performed using the STATA program (StataCorp, 4905 Lakeway Drive, College Station, Texas, US). Continuous data were compared using the t-Student test and t-pair test for repeated measures; categorical data were compared with the chi-square test and with Mc Nemar test for repeated measures. Relationships between visual fatigue, occupational data and other symptoms were evaluated with Pearson correlation and univariate logistic regression. Significant findings were studied with multivariate logistic regression. The relationship between visual fatigue and potentially associated variables during follow-up was evaluated using generalized estimating equations (GEE) that permit the study of the same subject over time. Statistical significance was settled at $p < 0.05$.

3. Results

Figure 1 reports the study design: 3054 subjects underwent the first control, and 2208 completed the follow-up with 3 or 4 controls, as required by Italian law, depending on age.

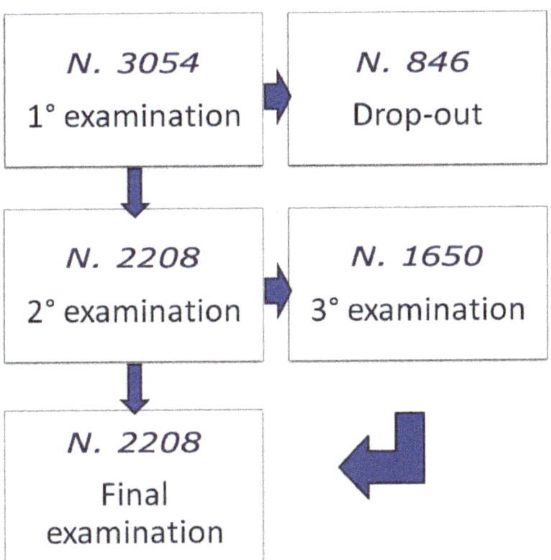

Figure 1. Design of the study.

The characteristics of the workers involved in the study are reported in Table 1. Gender is represented in similar proportions, and age increased obviously from the first control (36.7 ± 10.5 years) to the last one (46.5 ± 9.3 years) with $p < 0.005$. A similar trend was found for work seniority starting at 7.4 ± 6.7 years in the first control and reaching 14.5 ± 7.4 in the last follow-up ($p < 0.001$). The time of VDT use was around 5 h per day in the period considered. Refractive defects in workers over time are shown in the same table. Myopia was quite stable in terms of years; astigmatism ranged from 37.14% to 42.97%. Presbyopia increased according to the age of people (from 36.82% in the first examination to 52.26% in the last one ($p < 0.001$). Hyperopia grew from 7.5% in the first examination to 9.94% at the intermediate follow-up and to 11.59% at the last control ($p < 0.001$).

Table 1. Characteristics of participants, use of lenses and visual symptoms during the follow-up.

Characteristics	Description	1st Examination	2nd Examination	3rd Examination	Last Examination
Men (*n*)		1537	1032	841	1138
Women (*n*)		1558	1176	809	1070
Total (*n*)		3095	2208	1650	2208
Age Years (mean ± SD)		36.7 ± 10.5	41.1 ± 9.1	47.8 ± 8.2	46.5 * ± 9.3
Work seniority years (mean ± SD)		7.4 ±6.7	9.2 ±6.5	13.7 ±7.0	14.5 * ± 7.4
VDT per day hours (mean ± SD)		5.0 ± 2.5	4.8 ±2.1	5.4 ±2.0	5.4 ±1.9
Visual defects	Hyperopia % Myopia % Astigmatism % Presbyopia %	7.2 46.8 33.2 22.3	7.5 44.7 37.1 36.8	9.9 45.3 43.0 61.3	11.6 * 45.1 40.8 52.3 *
Use of lenses	%	80	82	84	82
Visual fatigue	Sometimes % Often %	46.3 12.1	48.8 13.8	48.4 17.3	50.3 13.7
Ocular redness	Sometimes % Often %	23.9 5.0	26.0 7.2	27.6 8.5	28.2 7.1
Ocular burning	Sometimes % Often %	20.9 4.5	22.1 6.6	21.9 7.6	23.7 5.82
Ocular tearing	Sometimes % Often %	11.2 2.5	12.4 3.4	14.5 4.4	15.6 4.2
Headache	Sometimes % Often %	9.5 2.5	12.2 3.5	10.8 3.6	11.2 2.8
Photophobia	Sometimes % Often %	8.2 2.0	10.9 2.8	11.4 3.4	9.0 3.1
Blurry vision far	Sometimes % Often %	10.6 2.7	10.5 3.0	9.8 3.1	9.9 3.2
Blurry vision near	Sometimes % Often %	6.8 1.9	10.0 3.1	11.2 3.8	9.8 3.1
Myodesmopsia	Sometimes % Often %	7.1 1.1	8.3 1.4	10.4 1.6	9.5 1.4
Double vision	Sometimes % Often %	6.2 1.5	7.9 1.4	9.2 2.1	7.0 2.1
Eye drop application	Sometimes % Often %	3.8 1.2	3.9 1.1	6.6 1.6	5.4 2.0
Anxiety	Sometimes % Often %	2.9 0.6	3.7 0.9	4.2 1.1	3.1 1.1

* $p < 0.005$.

The use of lenses was very common during the follow-up, with more than 80% of people using lenses.

The most common eye symptom was visual fatigue, followed by ocular redness, burning and tearing. In general, eye symptoms increased during follow up, reaching statistical significance for visual fatigue (58.4% to 64%, $p < 0.001$), ocular redness (28.9% to 35.2%, $p < 0.001$), and near blurred vision (8.7% to 12.9%, $p < 0.01$). Headache and anxiety were reported in similar figures during the follow-up (12% to 14% and 3.5% to 4.2%), respectively.

We evaluated visual fatigue in terms of years (Figure 2) to verify the improvement of symptoms in relation to the better quality of the screens; however, no difference was shown and no decrease in symptoms was reported.

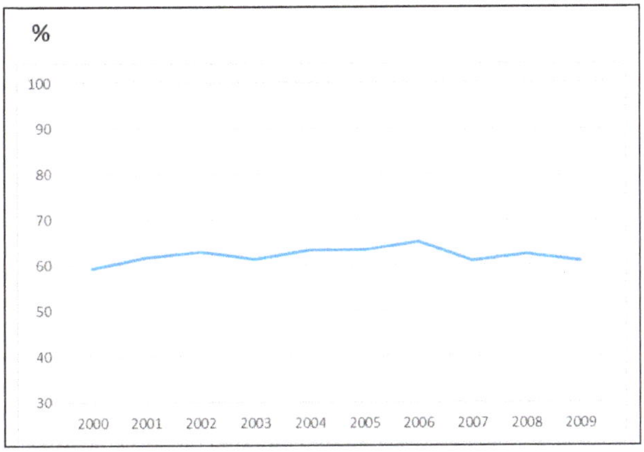

Figure 2. Percentages of visual fatigue in terms of years.

Visual fatigue, analyzed using Pearson's correlation, was not associated to far, near, or intermediate vision acuity. Univariate analysis confirmed this with values of OR = 1.1; 95% CI 0.98–1.24; OR = 1.02; 95%CI 0.97–1.07; OR = 1.06; CI95% 0.96–1.2, respectively. Visual fatigue was studied in relationship with environmental and ergonomic factors such as monitor characteristics, work place illumination, reflections on the screen, contrast, and incorrect distances from the computer using Pearson's correlation (Table 2).

Table 2. Pearson's correlation between visual fatigue and environmental variables.

Variables	Local Light	Natural Light	Contrast	Light Flickering	Reflections	Distance	Image
Local light	-						
Natural light	0.17 **	-					
Contrasts	0.22 **	0.31 *	-				
Light flickering	0.15 **	0.02	0.36 **	-			
Reflections	0.27 **	0.01	0.26 **	0.27 **	-		
Distance	0.33 **	0.02	0.25 **	0.19 **	0.24 **	-	
Image	0.29 **	0.02	0.26 **	0.27 **	0.25 **	0.33 **	-
Visual fatigue	0.06 **	0.01	0.05 **	0.03*	0.06 **	0.03 **	0.03 *

* $p < 0.05$; ** $p < 0.01$ (two tails).

All factors except natural light were significantly related with visual fatigue. The relationships between visual fatigue and psychosocial variables are reported in Table 3.

All psychosocial variables were significantly related each other. Factors associated to visual fatigue in the first and last examinations were evaluated using univariate logistic regression (Table 4).

Table 3. Relationships between visual fatigue and psychosocial variables, analyzed using Pearson's correlation.

Variables	1	2	3	4	5	6	7	8	9	10	11	12	13	14	15
1 Overcrowding	-														
2 Relationship with users	0.45 **	-													
3 Relationship with collegues	0.30 **	0.42 **	-												
4 Work condition	0.37 **	0.41 **	0.36 **	-											
5 Responsibility	0.26 **	0.39 **	0.39 **	0.33 **	-										
6 Repetitiveness	0.31 **	0.20 **	0.19 **	0.23 **	0.09 **	-									
7 Excessive concentration	0.24 **	0.27 **	0.27 **	0.29 **	0.43 **	0.11 **	-								
8 Excessive attention	0.19 **	0.24 **	0.24 **	0.24 **	0.41 **	0.09 **	0.66 **	-							
9 Low control of mistakes	0.37 **	0.31 **	0.31 **	0.36 **	0.32 **	0.33 **	0.26 **	0.22 **	-						
10 Frequent interruptions	0.34 **	0.29 **	0.26 **	0.28 **	0.27 **	0.27 **	0.22 **	0.19 **	0.40 **	-					
11 Computer slowness	0.28 **	0.25 **	0.19 **	0.25 **	0.14 **	0.30 **	0.16 **	0.10 **	0.36 **	0.45 **	-				
12 Variability	0.29 **	0.37 **	0.33 **	0.33 **	0.43 **	0.11 **	0.36 **	0.29 **	0.32 **	0.29 **	0.18 **	-			
13 Low control	0.35 **	0.33 **	0.32 **	0.34 **	0.31 **	0.32 **	0.24 **	0.23 **	0.38 **	0.32 **	0.24 **	0.30 **	-		
14 Slow cadence	0.28 **	0.25 **	0.21 **	0.22 **	0.12 **	0.43 **	0.09 **	0.05 **	0.31 **	0.28 **	0.34 **	0.14 **	0.28 **	-	
15 Fast cadence	0.28 **	0.22 **	0.21 **	0.24 **	0.33 **	0.14 **	0.40 **	0.41 **	0.22 **	0.24 **	0.12 **	0.36 **	0.31 **	0.04 **	-
16 Visual fatigue	0.04 **	0.02	0.03 **	0.03 *	0.02	0.01	0.05 **	0.04 **	0.01	0.02	0.01	0.03 *	0.04 **	0.00	0.04 **

* $p < 0.05$; ** $p < 0.01$ (two tails).

Table 4. Visual fatigue, visual acuity and refractive disorders in the first and in the last control evaluated with univariate logistic regression. Data are reported as odds ratios (OR) and 95% confidence intervals (CI).

Variables	1st Examination			Last Examination		
	OR	95% CI	*p*	OR	95% CI	*p*
Sex female	**1.3**	**1.1–1.56**	**0.005**	0.98	0.81–1.17	0.814
Age	**0.98**	**0.98–0.99**	**0.031**	**0.98**	**0.97–0.99**	**0.001**
Seniority of work	1.00	0.99-1.01	0.753	**0.98**	**0.97–0.99**	**0.022**
VDT working hours	**1.19**	**1.14–1.24**	**0.000**	**1.17**	**1.11–1.23**	**0.000**
Use of lenses	**1.42**	**1.1–1.85**	**0.011**	1.28	0.99–1.64	0.055
Presbyopia	**0.82**	**068–0.98**	**0.033**	0.89	0.74–1.05	0.186
Hyperopia	**1.52**	**1.1–2.2**	**0.020**	0.98	0.75–1.30	0.889
Astigmatism	**1.30**	**1.05–1.52**	**0.012**	1.05	0.88–1.25	0.582
Myopia	1.09	0.91–1.31	0.301	0.93	0.78–1.10	0.415
Visual acuity OO near	1.02	0.98–1.07	0.431	1.01	0.96–1.01	0.628
Visual acuity OO intermediate	1.06	0.96–1.17	0.213	1.02	0.98–1.12	0.137
Visual acuity OO far	1.02	0.92–1.13	0.734	1.10	0.98–1.24	0.112

VDT: video display operators; OO: both eyes; In bold, significant results.

In the first examination, females reported more visual symptoms, but no gender effect was shown in the last examination. Age was inversely related to visual fatigue, and seniority of work was also demonstrated to be a protective factor in the last control. Visual fatigue increased significantly in relation to VDT working hours and use of lenses. Visual acuity at near, intermediate and far distances was not related to ocular symptoms and, when analyzing refractive disorders, hyperopia increased ocular symptoms, but only in the first examination. To evaluate the role of different factors, we analyzed visual fatigue using the multivariate logistic regression in the first control (Table 5).

Table 5. Factors associated to visual fatigue in the first examination, evaluated with multivariate logistic regression (n = 3054 workers).

Variables	Odds Ratio	95% CI	Z Score	*p* Value
Female gender	1.09	0.94–1.28	1.18	0.239
Age	0.99	0.98–1.00	−1.52	0.128
Seniority of work	1.00	0.99–1.01	1.01	0.314
VDT working hours	**1.17**	**1.13–1.22**	**8.79**	**0.000**
Use of lenses	**1.30**	**1.08–1.58**	**2.71**	**0.007**
Presbyopia	0.87	0.67–1.13	−1.02	0.310
Hyperopia	**1.56**	**1.1–2.3**	**2.28**	**0.023**
Astigmatism	1.2	0.96–1.4	1.57	0.117
Environmental factors	1.10	0.99–1.30	1.78	0.078
Psychosocial factors	**1.03**	**1.00–1.06**	**2.25**	**0.025**
I feel anxious sometimes during VDT use	**2.62**	**1.56–4.4**	**3.65**	**0.000**
I feel anxious often during VDT use	**4.97**	**1.48–6.84**	**2.59**	**0.010**
I feel anxious not in relation with VDT use	**1.40**	**1.07–1.84**	**2.25**	**0.025**

CI: confidence interval; in bold, significant results.

Environmental factors were summarized in one variable that did not include natural light, which were not related with visual symptoms. Psychosocial factors were summarized in one item obtained by the sum of single items, and anxiety perception was analyzed alone as never, sometimes, and often both in relation with VDT use and not being work-related. In multivariate analysis, visual fatigue was not related to age, sex or work seniority, while symptoms increased with anxiety perception in a dose-related matter with OR 2.62 (CI 95% 1.56–4.4) and OR 4.97 (CI 95% 1.48–6.84) for "sometimes" or "often", respectively. VDT working hours, use of lenses, hyperopia and psychosocial factors were significantly related to visual fatigue.

To analyze factors related to visual fatigue in the follow-up, we used the generalized estimating equation (GEE) as shown in Table 6.

Table 6. Factors associated to visual fatigue during 10-year follow-up using the generalized estimating equation (2208 workers that repeated medical examinations 3 times were included in the analysis).

Variables	Odds Ratio	95% CI	Z Score	*p* Value
Female gender	1.05	0.90–1.24	0.66	0.508
Age	**0.98**	**0.97–0.99**	**−2.5**	**0.015**
Seniority of work	1.02	0.88–1.35	0.65	0.450
VDT work hours	**1.27**	**1.04–1.53**	**2.50**	**0.035**
Use of lenses	**1.34**	**1.09–1.64**	**2.80**	**0.005**
Environmental factors	**1.02**	**1.01–1.06**	**2.15**	**0.025**
Psychosocial factors	**1.03**	**1.01–1.07**	**2.23**	**0.026**
I sometimes feel anxious during VDT use	**2.69**	**1.57–4.61**	**3.60**	**0.000**
I often feel anxious during VDT use	**7.40**	**1.77–31.03**	**2.74**	**0.000**
I do not feel anxious in relation to VDT use	1.01	0.78–1.30	0.13	0.944

CI: confidence interval; in bold, significant results.

Age was inversely associated with visual fatigue, and no relationship was found with seniority of work and gender. Anxiety perception was strongly associated with visual fatigue in a dose-related matter with OR 2.69 (CI 95% 1.57–4.61) for "sometimes" feeling anxious during VDT use and OR 7.10 (CI 95% 1.77–31.03) for "often" feeling anxious during VDT use. A significant relationship was demonstrated also with hours of work with VDTs (OR 1.27; CI 95% 1.04–1.53), use of lenses (OR 1.34, CI 95% 1.09–1.64), environmental factors (OR 1.02; CI 95% 1.01–1.06) and psychosocial factors (OR 1.03; CI 95% 1.01–1.07).

4. Discussion

Many epidemiological studies on VDT users have reported the presence of computer vision syndrome [29], and our study confirmed this in a long-term follow-up. However, the longitudinal characteristics of our study permitted us to analyze factors related to visual symptoms in a more comprehensive way, finding that anxiety perception was the most important factor, followed by the time of VDT usage, the use of lenses, environmental and psychosocial factors. No associations were found with seniority of work and visual acuity. Age appeared to be inversely related to visual symptoms. Visual fatigue grew with increasing working hours in a poorly controlled environment with light disturbance [8,30,31], and VDT work could worsen visual problems [18,32–34] in the short term [35,36]. However, there was no relationship between refractive disorders and VDT use in a 4-year follow-up [37], and visual fatigue decreased significantly with age, as also shown in other studies [38], probably because older workers know better how to manage visual discomfort, despite the higher prevalence of presbyopia. Dry-eye syndrome can influence visual fatigue, and the use of contact lenses can increase ocular symptoms [39,40]. The wearing of contact lenses causes a reduction of blink amplitude and tear film instability with Meibomian gland atrophy with tear alteration with an increasing of dry-eye symptoms. The desiccation of the contact lens surfaces causes irregular refraction with visual discomfort [40].

Regarding refractive disorders, myopia prevalence did not increase in follow-up, while presbyopia and hyperopia were clearly age-related and astigmatism increased in small amounts during follow-up. We found visual defects to be higher than those in the literature [41] because we considered any view change starting from 0.25 dioptres—thus, with a lower cut-off—whereas in a European Eye Consortium study, myopia was defined as ≥ -0.75 dioptres, with hyperopia and presbyopia $\geq$ 1D. However, myopia prevalence did not increase during the follow-up, and we failed to find an association between myopia and work seniority. Overall, no relationship was found between visual fatigue, refractive disorders and visual acuity with lenses during the follow-up, while in the first examination, only hyperopia was significantly associated with visual complaints.

Visual fatigue was also related to environmental and ergonomic factors such as monitor characteristics and workplace illumination, in accordance with the literature [42–44]. Poor illumination, the presence of contrast, light flickering and reflections on the screen, poor-resolution images and an incorrect distance to the computer contributed to eye-symptom development. Environmental factors were associated with visual fatigue in our study as well, despite the fact that, in the last 10 years, the introduction of better flat video screens has resulted in an improvement of image quality.

Psychosocial factors were associated with visual fatigue. They are, in addiction to ergonomic factors, the basis of the occurrence of somatic disorders (such as headache and insomnia), generalized tension and stress [45–47]. All psychological variables were positively related to each other, confirming the fundamental role of perception of these factors in predicting the onset of symptoms in the workplace.

Some factors were more related to visual fatigue than others. Work in crowded places, having problems with colleagues, performing tasks that require too much attention and concentration, and having little control over decisions about work, intensity of work have relevant impacts on the occurrence of visual symptoms. Other important factors are job position and the repetitiveness of working duties.

Another important issue that must be considered in people using VDTs is motion sickness, which has been studied mainly in video game users [48] or in people watching 3D movies [49] but which can be present also in workers using mobile devices [50,51]. Visually-induced motion sickness experienced in a 3D immersive virtual environment is one of the crucial aspects that limits the widespread use of virtual reality [52] and can contribute to visual fatigue in VDT workers. However, in our study—a long-term follow-up—we did not consider this symptom, because the widespread use of mobile devices started after the start of our project. This can be considered a limitation of our study; however, we tried to focus on visual fatigue and stress, which were the most important symptoms in VDT users, together with musculoskeletal symptoms.

Our study is one of the largest and longest available in the literature, to our best knowledge, and demonstrated that visual fatigue did not increase with refractive disorders or with visual acuity with lenses, or in relation to work seniority and age, confirming that symptoms are not harmful for the eye. Visual symptoms are mainly caused by anxiety perception and psychosocial factors: this finding suggests the need to consider this and to suggest interventions to increase wellness in workplaces, but also the need to emphasize the safe characteristic of work with VDT, avoiding the overestimation of symptoms without signs of diseases. Moreover, visual symptoms in general are mild. To confirm this, the majority of workers reported "visual fatigue in relation to VDTs sometimes", while "visual fatigue in relation to VDTs often" was reported by a lower percentage of workers. Irritant symptoms such as "red eye" and "burning eye" were reported by less than 7% of subjects, meaning that important symptoms were rare, and acute and disabling symptoms were never reported [53]. Moreover, myopia did not increase during the follow-up, confirming what was already demonstrated by Rechichi et al. in 1996 [53] following 23,000 VDT users for 4 years. This author showed no relationship between refractive errors and VDT exposure [48], and a review of Mutti and Zandik [54] concluded that there is no evidence that VDT work causes myopia. Visual fatigue is a symptom and not a sign of eye disease, and Cole in 2003 [55] questioned the need for vision screening in VDT workers. He said that visual discomfort is common among workers even if they do not use VDTs and that visual screening would be better applied for workers when vision is critical for safety, such as professional drivers, air traffic controllers, etc.

5. Conclusions

Our study, in a long follow-up, failed to find an increase of refractory disorders in VDT users. Visual fatigue was common and symptoms were related to many factors, but not to refractive disorders and visual acuity with lenses. Anxiety perception was of paramount importance compared to environmental factors, use of lenses, time of VDT use and psychosocial factors. Visual fatigue did not increase in relation to age, and seniority of work and gender did not play any role in the occurrence of symptoms. In our 10-year follow-up, refractive disorders increased mainly in relation to age as presbyopia and hyperopia, while no increase in the prevalence of myopia was found, confirming that VDT use is not harmful for vision.

This study emphasizes the need to promote the wellness of workers, focusing on interventions to reduce anxiety, increasing good relationships between workers, and promoting a good psychosocial environment together with a good control of environmental variables and the correction of refractive disorders, which seems to be not relevant compared to other factors. Effort can be put into the good organization of the workplace, the environmental control of lights and a better evaluation of psychological factors.

Author Contributions: F.L.F. designed the study, contributed to the statistical analysis and wrote the final version of the paper, A.D. wrote the tables and contributed to the draft of the paper, F.R. collected the data, and C.N. did the statistical analysis.

Funding: This research received no external funding.

Acknowledgments: We thank Roberta Rosani for data input and vision test execution and workers for their participation in the study.

Conflicts of Interest: The authors declare no conflict of interest.

References

1. Blehm, C.; Vishnu, S.; Khattak, A.; Mitra, S.; Yee, R.W. Computer vision syndrome: A review. *Surv. Ophthalmol.* **2005**, *50*, 253–262. [CrossRef] [PubMed]
2. Bali, J.; Neeraj, N.; Bali, R.T. Computer vision syndrome: A review. *J. Clin. Ophtalmol. Res.* **2014**, *2*, 61–68. [CrossRef]
3. Porcar, E.; Pons, A.M.; Lorente, A. Visual and ocular effects from the use of flat-panel displays. *Int. J. Ophtalmol.* **2016**, *9*, 881–885.
4. Hayes, J.R.; Sheedy, J.E.; Stelmack, J.A.; Heaney, C.A. Computer use, symptoms, and quality of life. *Optom. Vis. Sci.* **2007**, *84*, 738–744. [CrossRef] [PubMed]
5. Basu, R.; Dasgupta, A.; Ghosal, G. Musculo-skeletal Disorders among Video Display Terminal Users: A Cross-Sectional Study in a Software Company, Kolkata. *J. Clin. Diagn. Res.* **2014**, *8*, JC01-4. [CrossRef] [PubMed]
6. Nakphet, N.; Chaikumarn, M.; Janwantanakul, P. Effect of different types of rest-break interventions on neck and shoulder muscle activity, perceived discomfort and productivity in symptomatic VDU operators: A randomized controlled trial. *Int. J. Occup. Saf. Ergon.* **2014**, *20*, 339–353. [CrossRef] [PubMed]
7. Parihar, J.K.; Jain, V.K.; Chaturvedi, P.; Kaushik, J.; Jain, G.; Parihar, A.K. Computer and visual display terminals (VDT) vision syndrome (CVDTS). *Med. J. Armed Forces India* **2016**, *72*, 270–276. [CrossRef]
8. Portello, J.K.; Rosenfield, M.; Bababekova, Y. Computer-related visual symptoms in office workers. *Ophthalmic Physiol. Opt.* **2012**, *32*, 375–382. [CrossRef]

9. Thorud, H.M.S.; Helland, M.; Aarås, A.; Kvikstad, T.M.; Lindberg, L.G.; Horgen, G. Eye-related pain induced by visually demanding computer work. *Optom. Vis. Sci.* **2012**, *89*, E452–E464. [CrossRef]
10. Uchino, M.; Yokoi, N.; Uchino, Y.; Dogru, M.; Kawashima, M.; Komuro, A.; Sonomura, Y.; Kato, H.; Kinoshita, S.; Schaumberg, D.A.; et al. Prevalence of dry eye disease and its risk factors in visual display terminal users: The Osaka study. *Am. J. Ophtalmol.* **2013**, *156*, 759–766. [CrossRef]
11. Agarwal, S.; Goel, D.; Sharma, A. Evaluation of the factors which contribute to the ocular complaints in computer users. *J. Clin. Diagn. Res.* **2013**, *7*, 331–335. [CrossRef] [PubMed]
12. Han, C.C.; Liu, R.; Liu, R.R.; Zhu, Z.H.; Yu, R.B.; Ma, L. Prevalence of asthenopia and its risk factors in Chinese collage students. *Int. J. Ophtalmol.* **2013**, *6*, 718–722.
13. Logaraj, M.; Madhupriya Hegde, S.K. Computer vision syndrome and associated factors among medical and engineering students in chennai. *Ann. Med. Helath Sci. Res.* **2014**, *4*, 179–185. [CrossRef] [PubMed]
14. Hsu, B.W.; Wang, M.J.J. Evaluating the effectiveness of using electroencephalogram power indices to measure visual fatigue. *Percept. Mot. Ski.* **2013**, *116*, 235–252. [CrossRef] [PubMed]
15. Eastman Kodak Company. *Kodak's Ergonomic Design for People at Work*; John Wiley & Sons: Hoboken, NJ, USA, 2009.
16. Qu, X.M. Effects of short-term VDT usage on visual functions. *Chin. J. Ophthalmol.* **2005**, *41*, 986–989.
17. Luberto, F.; Gobba, F.; Broglia, A. Temporary myopia and subjective symptoms in video display terminal operators. *Med. Lav.* **1989**, *80*, 155–163.
18. Sheedy, J.E.; Hayes, J.N.; Engle, J. Is all asthenopia the same? *Optom. Vis. Sci.* **2003**, *80*, 732–739. [CrossRef]
19. Janosik, E.; Grzesik, J. Influence of different lighting levels at workstations with video display terminals on operators' work efficiency. *Med. Pr.* **2003**, *54*, 123–132.
20. Ye, Z.; Honda, S.; Abe, Y.; Kusano, Y.; Takamura, N.; Imamura, Y.; Eida, K.; Takemoto, T.; Aoyagi, K. Influence of work duration or physical symptoms on mental health among Japanese visual display terminal users. *Ind. Health* **2007**, *45*, 328–333. [CrossRef]
21. Iwakiri, K.; Mori, I.; Sotoyama, M.; Horiguchi, K.; Ochiai, T.; Jonai, H.; Saito, S. Survey on visual and musculoskeletal symptoms in VDT workers. *J. Occup. Health* **2004**, *46*, 201–212.
22. Lodin, C.; Forsman, M.; Richter, H. Eye- and neck/shoulder-discomfort during visually demanding experimental near work. *Work* **2012**, *41*, 3388–3392. [PubMed]
23. Woods, V. Musculoskeletal disorders and visual strain in intensive data processing workers. *Occup. Med.* **2005**, *55*, 121–127. [CrossRef]
24. Mocci, F.; Serra, A.; Corrias, G.A. Psychological factors and visual fatigue in working with video display terminals. *Occup. Environ. Med.* **2001**, *58*, 267–271. [CrossRef] [PubMed]
25. Tomei, G.; Rosati, M.V.; Ciarrocca, M.; Capozzella, A.; Pimpinella, B.; Casale, T.; Monti, C.; Tomei, F. Assessment of subjective stress in video display terminal workers. *Ind. Health* **2006**, *44*, 291–295. [CrossRef] [PubMed]
26. Horgen, G.; Aarås, A.; Dainoff, M.J. A cross-country comparison of short- and long-term effects of an ergonomic intervention on musculoskeletal discomfort, eyestrain and psychosocial stress in VDT operators: Selected aspects of the international project. *Int. J. Occup. Saf. Ergon.* **2005**, *11*, 77–92. [CrossRef] [PubMed]
27. Balci, R.; Aghazadeh, F. The effect of work-rest schedules and type of task on the discomfort and performance of VDT users. *Ergonomics* **2003**, *46*, 455–465. [CrossRef] [PubMed]
28. Carayon, P.; Smith, M.J.; Haims, M.C. Work organization, job stress, and work-related musculoskeletal disorders. *Hum. Factors* **1999**, *41*, 644–663. [CrossRef] [PubMed]
29. Rosenfield, M. Computer vision syndrome: A review of ocular causes and potential treatments. *Ophtalmol. Physiol. Opt.* **2011**, *31*, 502–515. [CrossRef] [PubMed]
30. Ostrovsky, A.; Ribak, J.; Pereg, A.; Gaton, D. Effects of job-related stress and burnout on asthenopia among high-tech workers. *Ergonomics* **2012**, *55*, 854–862. [CrossRef]
31. Rossignol, A.M.; Morse, E.P.; Summers, V.M. Video display terminal use and reported health symptoms among Massachusetts clerical workers. *J. Occup. Med.* **1987**, *29*, 112–118.
32. Thomson, W.D. Eye problems and visual display terminals-the facts and the fallacies. *Ophthalmic Physiol. Opt.* **1998**, *18*, 111–119. [CrossRef]
33. Cole, B.L.; Maddocks, J.D.; Sharpe, K. Effect of VDUs on the eyes: Report of a 6-year epidemiological study. *Optom. Vis. Sci.* **1996**, *73*, 512–528. [CrossRef] [PubMed]

34. Bergqvist, U.O.; Knave, B.G. Eye discomfort and work with visual display terminals. *Scand. J. Work Environ. Health* **1994**, *20*, 27–33. [CrossRef] [PubMed]
35. Gratton, I.; Piccoli, B.; Zaniboni, A.; Meron, M.; Grieco, A. Change in visual function and viewing distance during work with VDTs. *Ergonomics* **1990**, *33*, 1433–1441. [CrossRef] [PubMed]
36. Culhane, H.M.; Winn, B. Dynamic accommodation and myopia. *Invest Ophthalmol. Vis. Sci.* **1999**, *40*, 1968–1974. [PubMed]
37. Rechichi, C.; Scullica, L. VDU work: Longitudinal survey on refractive defects. *Acta Ophthalmol. Scand.* **1996**, *74*, 629–631. [CrossRef] [PubMed]
38. Tarumi, K.; Nagami, M.; Kadowaki, I. An inquiry into the factors affecting the complaints of subjective symptoms in VDT operators. *Jpn. J. Ind. Health* **1990**, *32*, 77–88.
39. Tauste, A.; Ronda, E.; Molina, M.J.; Segui, M. Effect of contact lens use on computer vision syndrome. *Ophthalmic Physiol. Opt.* **2016**, *36*, 112–119. [CrossRef]
40. Tauste Frances, A.; Ronda-Perez, E.; Segui Crespo Mdle, M. Ocular and visual alterations in computer workers contact lens wearers: Scoping review. *Rev. Esp. Salud Publica* **2014**, *88*, 203–215.
41. Williams, K.M.; Verhoeven, V.J.; Cumberland, P.; Bertelsen, G.; Wolfram, C.; Buitendijk, G.H.; Hofman, A.; van Duijn, C.M.; Vingerling, J.R.; Kuijpers, R.W.; et al. Prevalence of refractive error in Europe: The European Eye Epidemiology (E(3)) Consortium. *Eur. J. Epidemiol.* **2015**, *30*, 305–315. [CrossRef]
42. Demure, B.; Luippold, R.S.; Bigelow, C.; Ali, D.; Mundt, K.; Liese, B. Video display terminal workstation improvement program: I. Baseline associations between musculoskeletal discomfort and ergonomic features of workstations. *J. Occup. Environ. Med.* **2000**, *42*, 783–791. [CrossRef] [PubMed]
43. Boyce, P.R.; Veitch, J.A.; Newsham, G.R.; Jones, C.C.; Heerwagen, J.; Myer, M.; Hunter, C.M. Lighting quality and office work: Two field simulation experiments. *Light. Res. Technol.* **2006**, *38*, 191–223. [CrossRef]
44. Jaschinski, W.; Heuer, H.; Kylian, H. Preferred position of visual displays relative to the eyes: A field study of visual strain and individual differences. *Ergonomics* **1998**, *41*, 1034–1049. [CrossRef] [PubMed]
45. Rocha, L.; Debert-Ribeiro, M.; Rocha, L.E. Working conditions, visual fatigue, and mental health among systems analysts in São Paulo, Brazil. *Occup. Environ. Med.* **2004**, *61*, 24–32. [PubMed]
46. Seppälä, P. Experience of stress, musculoskeletal discomfort, and eyestrain in computer-based office work: A study in municipal workplaces. *Int. J. Hum. Comput. Interact.* **2001**, *13*, 279–304. [CrossRef]
47. Travers, P.H.; Stanton, B.A. Office workers and video display terminals: Physical, psychological and ergonomic factors. *AAOHN J.* **2002**, *50*, 489–493. [CrossRef] [PubMed]
48. Keshavarz, B.; Novak, A.C.; Hettinger, L.J.; Stoffregen, T.A.; Campos, J.L. Passive restraint reduces visually induced motion sickness in older adults. *J. Exp. Psychol. Appl.* **2017**, *23*, 85–99. [CrossRef]
49. Solimini, A.G. Are there side effects to watching 3D movies? A prospective crossover observational study on visually induced motion sickness. *PLoS ONE* **2013**, *8*, e56160. [CrossRef]
50. Stanney, K.; Salvendy, G.; Deisinger, J.; DiZio, P.; Ellis, S.; Ellision, J.; Fogleman, G.; Gallimore, J.; Hettinger, L.; Kennedy, R.; et al. Aftereffects and sense of presence in virtual environments: Formulation of a research and development agenda. Report sponsored by the Life Sciences Division at NASA Headquarters. *Int. J. Hum. Comput. Interact.* **1998**, *10*, 135–187. [CrossRef]
51. Stoffregen, T.A.; Chen, Y.-C.; Koslucher, F.C. Motion control, motion sickness, and the postural dynamics of mobile devices. *Exp. Brain Res.* **2014**, *232*, 1389–1397. [CrossRef]
52. Nie, G.Y.; Duh, H.B.; Liu, Y.; Wang, Y. Analysis on Mitigation of Visually Induced Motion Sickness by Applying Dynamical Blurring on a User's Retina. *IEEE Trans. Vis. Comput. Graph.* **2019**, *18*, 1. [CrossRef] [PubMed]
53. Rechichi, C.; Scullica, M. Trends regarding myopia in video terminal operators. *Acta Ophthalmol. Scand.* **1996**, *74*, 493–496. [CrossRef] [PubMed]
54. Mutti, D.O.; Zadnik, K. Is computer use a risk factor for myopia? *J. Am. Optom. Assoc.* **1996**, *67*, 521–530. [PubMed]
55. Cole, L.C. Do video display units cause visual problems?—A bedsite story about the processes of public health decision-making. *Clin. Exp. Optom.* **2003**, *86*, 205–220. [CrossRef] [PubMed]

International Journal of
Environmental Research and Public Health

MDPI

Article

Psychosocial Risk Prevention in a Global Occupational Health Perspective. A Descriptive Analysis

Francesco Chirico [1,2], Tarja Heponiemi [3], Milena Pavlova [4], Salvatore Zaffina [5] and Nicola Magnavita [2,6,*]

1 Health Service Department, State Police, Ministry of Interior, Milan 20162, Italy
2 Post-graduate School of Occupational Medicine, Università Cattolica del Sacro Cuore, Rome 00168, Italy
3 Social and Health Systems Research Unit, National Institute for Health and Welfare, Helsinki FI-00271, Finland
4 Health Services Research (HSR), CAPHRI, Maastricht University Medical Center, Faculty of Health, Medicine and Life Sciences, Maastricht University, Maastricht 6202 AZ, The Netherlands
5 Occupational Health Unit, Ospedale Pediatrico Bambino Gesù, Rome 00165, Italy
6 Department of Woman/Child and Public Health, Fondazione Policlinico "A. Gemelli" IRCCS, Rome 00168, Italy
* Correspondence: nicolamagnavita@gmail.com; Tel.: +39-347-330-0367

Received: 30 May 2019; Accepted: 10 July 2019; Published: 11 July 2019

Abstract: This study aimed to find out which countries around the world require psychosocial hazards and workplace violence to be assessed by employers through a mandatory occupational risk assessment process and to compare the type of legislation between countries. We systematically searched the International Labour Office (ILO) "LEGOSH" database for documents published during the period between December 2017 and February 2018. The search included 132 countries, of which 23 were considered as developed and 109 as developing according to the United Nations. Our review showed that most countries (85, i.e., 64%) have not included mandatory psychosocial risk assessment and prevention in their national occupational safety and health legislation. Moreover, we found differences between developed and developing countries, showing that developed countries more frequently have legislative measures. Within developed countries, we also found differences between countries following the Scandinavian model of workplace health and safety culture and other countries. Moreover, in many countries, workplace violence was prohibited only if it involves an offence to moral or religious customs. In conclusion, the marked difference in psychosocial hazards and workplace violence regulations among countries leads to unequal levels of workers' protection, with adverse effects on global health.

Keywords: global health; health inequalities; legislation; mental health; psychosocial hazard; public health policy; workplace violence; job strain; psychosocial hazard; occupational health

1. Introduction

The existence of occupational diseases was first recognized nearly three centuries ago when Bernardino Ramazzini published "De Morbis Artificum Diatriba" [1]. Despite this, the global burden of occupational diseases is continuously growing around the world [2], and this requires a growing commitment on the part of all nations.

During the last century, many countries across the world have established laws for the prevention of occupational safety and health (OSH) risks. Generally, these legislative measures have especially taken into account traditional (chemical, physical or biological) risk factors. However, OSH legislation less frequently takes into consideration the so-called "fourth group", that is the psychosocial occupational risk factors. Psychosocial hazards (PSH) have been identified as one of the key emerging risks in OSH [3]. They are defined as "those aspects of work design and the organization and management of work, and their social and environmental context, which may have the potential to cause psychological or physical harm" [4]. They originate from "interactions between and among work environment, job content, work organization and workers' capacities, needs, culture, personal extra-job considerations that may, through perceptions and experience, influence health, work performance and job satisfaction" [5]. Such a broad definition includes countless possible stressors. Occupational or job-related stress is just one of them.

Despite its frequent use, no agreement upon the definition of job stress currently exists; it, however, refers to distinct job stressors, or stimuli in the workplace, leading to psychological strains or negative psychophysiological responses or reactions [6]. According to the WHO (World Health Organization), this negative response occurs when work demands and pressures do not match employees' abilities and instead challenge employees' ability to cope [7]. Job stress can be caused by poor work organization and work design, poor management, unsatisfactory working conditions, and lack of support from colleagues and supervisors [8]. Workplace violence (WV) can be included among the harmful psychosocial stress factors, both because sometimes it originates from inside of the work environment (assuming the character of bullying or mobbing), and because the attacked people often develop a condition of distress, which in turn makes them prone to violence, in a cyclical relationship [9,10]. According to the Occupational Safety and Health Administration (OSHA) (2002), WV can be defined as any "violence or the threat of violence against workers, which can range from threats and verbal abuse to physical assaults and homicide" [11].

The importance of PSH emerges from studies conducted in workplaces in many parts of the world. In Europe, where regional figures are available, stress/strain is the second most frequently reported work-related health problem. A European survey (EU-OSHA, 2009) showed that 50–60% of all lost working days are attributed to job strain, and the number of people suffering from stress-related conditions caused or made worse by work is likely to increase [12]. In the Asia-Pacific Region, one in five Australian employees reported to be mentally unwell in the past 12 months, and it was estimated that untreated mental health conditions cost Australian workplaces approximately $10.9 billion per year [13]. In Japan, a national report showed that almost every third worker reported suffering from job strain-related anxiety disorders during the previous year [14]. In the American nations, cross-sectional studies showed that more than 10% of respondents to the First Central American Survey on Working Conditions and Health (2012) reported various job strain-related symptoms, ranging from feeling depressed to sleep problems [15]. In the USA, more than 570,000 workers a year experience non-fatal WV [16,17]. Conversely, almost no information about prevalence or incidence rates of PSH- or WV-related diseases has been identified in African and other developing countries [14].

Due to their importance for health, safety and productivity, PSH and WV must be addressed and prevented in the workplace. However, the employer's decision to establish an Occupational Health and Safety (OHS) service, including measures for health surveillance of workers, health promotion, counselling and disability management, can only be established on the basis of a double legitimacy, being based on both scientific evidence (i.e., scientific legitimacy) and laws (i.e., legal legitimacy) [18]. Regulation of these topics is of importance, as it is well known that greater quality of healthcare systems' prevention efforts is linked with lower occupational fatality rates and higher levels of workers' health [19]. Reviewing the OSH regulatory framework is of great importance because the presence of differences in regulatory provisions could correspond to differences in the levels of safety and health in the workplace. By making these differences explicit in our review, we provide a base for further policy discussion and improvements.

Not all countries in the world utilize the same level of occupational risk prevention. The cultural and social differences that underlie the different regulatory situations are also the basis of different development models. In recent years, the process of globalization and liberalization have often increased health inequities [20]. For this reason, it is relevant to know whether or not the presence of laws or regulations in the countries around the world really promotes the development of effective OSH services for the prevention of PSH.

In this review, we aimed to evaluate the OSH regulatory frameworks developed by the countries worldwide, with a special focus on the differences between developing and developed countries and within developed countries, which have more resources to achieve occupational risk prevention. More specifically, our study aimed to clarify whether countries around the world require PSH and WV to be assessed by employers through the mandatory occupational risk assessment process. Such a legal requirement could inform policymakers and key stakeholders for improving occupational health and safety policy on PSH and WV in the workplace.

2. Materials and Methods

The International Labour Office (ILO) Global Database on Occupational Safety and Health Legislation (LEGOSH) is a database that compiles legislation in the OSH field [21]. The continuous updating of the collection of laws makes it one of the most suitable tools for evaluating the state of the main elements of OSH legislation, including OSH management and administration, employers' duties and obligations, workers' rights and duties, OSH inspection and enforcement, among others. We have systematically consulted the database, during the period between December 2017 and February 2018, to obtain information on the legislative provisions aimed at preventing PSH in different countries and to compare, from a global perspective, the different situations.

The LEGOSH classification structure is based on a comprehensive set of 11 themes, which follow and capture the main part of the key ILO standards. LEGOSH sub-divides the category of PSH into two sub-groups: (a) "psychosocial risks" and (b) "occupational violence". LEGOSH has a user-friendly interface, which allows, but is not limited to: a) access to the synthesis of OSH legislation in English; b) comparison of the legislation of several countries or regions on a particular subject (by using the function "Compare countries"); and (c) conducting customized searches. LEGOSH was independently screened and assessed by the authors of this study. We specifically analyzed the Subtheme 9.5 ("Psychosocial hazards") of Theme 9 ("Specific hazards or risks"), which provides an overview of the main pieces of legislation covering specific hazards or risks, including psychosocial ones.

Our search was limited to the 132 countries included in the LEGOSH database. Our search was firstly carried out for each country by using the function "Search". Then, we checked for each country ("Africa all", "Americas all", "Arab States all", "Asia all" and "Europe all") by using the function "Compare countries". Finally, we analyzed our findings drawn from all OSH legislation by comparing countries from developed continents (Europe, North America, Oceania) with countries from developing continents (Asia, Africa, Central and South America).

Criteria to include each country in "developed" or "developing" countries were based on the 2018 World Economic Situation Prospects report by the United Nations (United Nations, 2018), which arranges countries around the world into three classes: (a) developed economies, (b) economies in transition and (c) developing countries [22]. Economies in transition and developing countries were considered as one group in our study. In this study, we equated "no data available" about the mandatory assessment of PSH and WV with "no regulation". Moreover, we did not consider criminal law or laws against sexual violence that may be present in the codes of most countries but are not specifically referred to in the workplace.

We firstly performed a directed qualitative content analysis based on predefined themes (thematic analysis on PSH and WV), followed by a synthesis of the results and a narrative description, which is illustrated with tables.

3. Results

The characteristics of the legislation of the various countries are reported in Appendices A and B. The general characteristics of the OSH legislation reviewed are presented in Table 1. Explicit regulation on PSH is in force in 82.3% of the EU member states and in 16.6% of non-EU developed countries, but in less than 30% of the developing countries (Table 1). WV is regulated in three out of four developed countries, but roughly in one out of three developing countries. In many developing countries, OSH legislation includes only prevention of sexual harassment or protection of dignity and religion.

Table 1. Characteristics of occupational safety and health (OSH) legislation about psychosocial hazards and workplace violence in developed and developing countries.

Countries (n = 132)	Psychosocial Hazards		Workplace Violence	
	Yes	No/NDA	Yes/Partial *	No/NDA
Developed countries (n = 23)				
EU-countries (n = 17)	14 (82.3%)	3/0	14 (82.3%)	2/1
Non-EU countries (n = 6)	1 (16.6%)	2/3	3 (50%)	2/1
Total (n = 23)	15 (65.2%)	5/3	17 (73.9%)	4/2
Developing countries (n = 109)				
Europe (n = 14)	4 (28.5%)	1/9	2 (14.2%)	1/11
North America (n = 2)	0 (-)	0/2	0 (-)	0/2
Central and South America (n = 30)	5 (16%)	1/24	5/4 (30%)	0/20
Africa (n = 46)	15 (32.6%)	0/31	10/6 (34.7%)	0/30
The Middle East and Asia (n = 17)	8 (47%)	1/8	6/4 (58.8%)	0/7
Total (n = 109)	32 (29.3%)	3/74	33/15 (44%)	1/70

Note: NDA = No Data Available. * Partial: Including only sexual harassment or protection of dignity and religion.

3.1. Psychosocial Hazards and WV Regulation in Developed Countries

Most developed countries include some form of regulations on mental health and/or psychological hazards (psychosocial risks, occupational violence or both of them) in their OSH legislation. All of the EU member states available in LEGOSH (n = 17) explicitly or implicitly included PSH and WV in their OSH legislation. Most countries in Scandinavia, Continental Europe and the Mediterranean have a specific regulation for this topic. For instance, in Finland, workload factors, lone working, night work and work pauses, as well as harassment and occupational violence are specifically addressed. In Sweden, systematic work environment management includes provisions against the risk of violence or the threat of violence. In Latvia, there is a legal framework for harassment (both personal or through instructions to other people), direct (gender) and indirect discrimination and occupational violence, which can be in the form of physical abuse or sexual harassment. In the Netherlands, the employer is obliged to address psychosocial pressure of work and working conditions policy, which is aimed at preventing sexual intimidation, aggression, discrimination and violence. In France, the law provides protective measures against psychosocial risks and stipulates provisions against moral and sexual harassment. In Italy, all psychosocial hazards, including both psychosocial risk and occupational violence, must be assessed by employers. In Portugal, psychosocial risks including violence, discrimination and sexual harassment are covered under the general duties of the employers. In Spain, there is no data available on psychosocial risks; nevertheless, discrimination and harassment are considered by Spanish law as very serious infringements. In the United Kingdom, psychosocial risks and violence (including verbal abuse and the risk of reasonably foreseeable violence) are covered under general duties, however there is no specific OSH rule. In Ireland, despite the fact there is no data available about psychosocial hazards, employers are required to identify risks of violence at work to implement appropriate safeguards. In Greece, there is a framework agreement to tackle workplace "physical or psychological" violence exercised by co-workers or third parties, though this agreement has not yet been translated into law. In Croatia, any direct or indirect discrimination in the workplace is prohibited, and harassment or sexual harassment is regulated by special legislation, yet there is no explicit regulation for occupational violence. Occupational violence is explicitly included in the rules of prevention by almost all EU member states except for Bulgaria, Romania, and Poland. In Poland, however, the regulation of psychosocial risks includes mobbing that is considered as an unwanted behaviour aimed at or which has the effect of violating someone's dignity or creating an intimidating, hostile, demeaning or humiliating atmosphere towards an employee.

Developed European countries that are not part of the EU have an approach similar to those in the EU. In Norway, occupational law "foster inclusive working conditions and equality and facilitate adaptations to the employee's capabilities and circumstances of life". Moreover, employers must preserve the employees' integrity and dignity against harassment or other improper conduct (threats, undesirable strain and occupational violence). In Switzerland, law mandates the provision of information on occupational violence, including discrimination and sexual harassment, but not on other PSH.

The legislation of other developed countries outside Europe is less homogeneous than in the EU. Remarkably, we found "no data available" from the USA with regard to PSH. In Canada, the law provides prevention only for WV, not PSH, and in New Zealand, general duty provisions in principle address psychosocial risks and violence, however there are no OSH provisions that explicitly address PSH and WV. In Australia, even if the health of workers includes physical and mental aspects, neither psychosocial risk nor occupational violence are included in its legislation. A synthesis of the legislative framework of developed countries is reported in Table 2.

Table 2. Synthesis of differences among developed countries in Psychosocial Hazards (PSH) and Workplace Violence (WV) regulation.

Type of Regulation	Countries
Explicit provision of PSH and WV in OSH law	Croatia, Cyprus, Finland, France, Greece, Italy, Latvia, Netherlands, Norway, Portugal, Sweden, United Kingdom
Explicit provision of PSH (not WV)	Bulgaria, Poland, Romania
Explicit provision of WV (not PSH)	Canada, Denmark, Ireland, Spain, Switzerland
No provision	Australia, New Zealand, USA

3.2. Psychosocial Hazards and WV Regulation in Developing Countries

The legislation of developing and transition countries is less homogeneous than that of developed countries. In Europe, most of the non-EU developing countries have no specific regulation on this topic. Only Albania and the Former Yugoslav Republic of Macedonia explicitly included PSH in their legislation. In the Russian Federation, OSH legislation explicitly only covers physical health and there is no definition of PSH or WV.

In Dominica and Granada (North America), psychosocial risks and occupational violence are covered by their respective OSH legislation. In Central and South America, PSH is included by only 5 out of 30 countries (16.66%). More specifically, LEGOSH showed "no data available" on this topic for 24 countries. Finally, with regard to WV, out of 10 countries, 33.33% from Latin America consider this topic, and 5 of these countries (50%) focus only on "sexual harassment". In Colombia, there is a specific resolution on psychosocial risks in the workplace. The termination of the labour contract can be declared both by the employer or employee upon occupational violence. In Venezuela, employers have to ensure a safe and healthy working environment for the full enjoyment of physical and mental faculties of workers, preventing any harassment situations, including physical or psychological violence. In El Salvador, the law provides the institution of psychosocial risks preventive programmes, including training and the participation of an expert in the field and addressing violence against women and sexual harassment in the workplace. In Puerto Rico, the law does not explicitly refer to mental or psychological health, however there is a law indicating a general awareness about psychosocial risks and the importance of preventing them. In Haiti, although the pursuit of workers' well-being includes "physical, moral, spiritual and material matters", there is no data about PSH prevention in the workplace. In Saint Lucia, the regulation covers only sexual harassment. In Guatemala, the General Regulation on OSH does still contemplate the need to draft a specific regulation, but, to date, no legislation on the subject has been identified.

In Africa, PSH prevention is mandatory in 14 countries. WV is considered by the legislation of 16 African countries (34.78%), of which 6 exclusively deal with "sexual harassment". Only 10 countries have OHS regulations in their control of both PSH and WV. In Morocco, the employee may terminate the contract if the employer commits gross insult and incitement of corruption (PSH) or in case the employer commits any form of violence and sexual harassment (WV). In Burkina Faso, the Labour code requires the employer to include initiatives for the prevention of physical and mental violence, including sexual harassment. In Niger, stress is included among the emerging psychosocial risks to be considered by the employer in risk assessment; occupational violence is limited to sexual harassment. In Togo, no employee may be dismissed for having refused the acts of harassment of an employer; moreover, acts of coercion, violence against people and property are prosecuted and punished. According to Comoros' law, employers must take all necessary measures to prevent mental fatigue of workers, as well as sexual or moral harassment. In Zambia, the employer must adapt the working environment to the employee's physical, physiological and psychological ability. In Namibia, the law requires employers to consider discomfort, fatigue or psychological stress due to failure to apply ergonomic principles and regulates discrimination and sexual harassment in the workplace. In Uganda, both PSH and WV are regulated. In South Africa, physical assault from the employer, a fellow employee, client or customer is regarded as serious misconduct of the employer, since there is a constitutional obligation to respect and protect the dignity of the employees. Intimidation and sexual harassment are also regulated in Lesotho.

Other African countries only regulate PSH, without specifically considering WV. In Egypt, the employer must ascertain the workers' fitness from the point of view of their physical, mental and psychological abilities in order to ensure their fitness to work demands, however there is no regulation about WV. In the Central African Republic, regulations include PSH, but not WV. The same regulatory situation exists in other African countries: in Mozambique, Angola and Congo, there are rules for preventing psychosocial risks, but not occupational violence. Conversely, in other countries, the law provides specific rules against violence. In Mauritius, psychosocial risks are not specifically covered by the Labour Act, yet occupational violence, harassment, sexual and verbal abuse, the threat of violence and bullying are explicitly considered. In Tunisia, acts of violence or threats against any fellow worker or person not belonging to the enterprise are regulated. Occupational violence is also regulated in Kenya, Libya and Djibouti. In Rwanda, the law regulates the protection of workers against violence or harassment, however there is no data available on PSH.

In Asia, PSH is a specific topic of OSH in 8 countries, whereas occupational violence is included in the OSH legislation of 10 countries. In China, employers must take measures to protect the physical and mental health of employees and to prevent sexual harassment for female workers in the workplace. In India, psychosocial risks caused by economic pressure are recognized by certain statutes and employers are obliged to minimize instances of sexual harassment in the workplace. In Korea, the employer must evaluate some PSH, such as working for a long time, shift work including night duty, vehicles operation and precision machine control work; sexual harassment by a superior or co-workers is prohibited. In Singapore, despite the law covering both the physical and psychosocial health of persons at work, and WV is regulated, there is no legal provision that specifically addresses PSH in the workplace. The most frequent normative situation is the opposite one, in which PSH is regulated, however there are no laws on violence, or there are laws limited to conduct regarding sexual or religious customs. In the Philippines, the law provides that the workplace be supportive and enhancing of the psychological health of workers, however there is no provision about work-related violence. In Thailand, the legislation covers both physical and psychological health; however, there is currently no specific requirement about WV. Moreover, in China and the Republic of Korea, the concept of WV comprises only "sexual harassment", whereas, in Vietnam, the law mentions "sexual harassment and violence against domestic workers". In Qatar, psychological health has not specifically been addressed by OSH legislation. However, the law requires the employer to conduct pre-employment medical examinations to ensure that the worker is psychologically fit for the type of work required. In Oman, there is no rule on PSH, however violence is regulated. In Jordan, there is no data available on PSH; however, WV, i.e., using force, violence, threatening or illegal procedures in assaulting or attempting to violate the right of others, must be prevented. In Saudi Arabia and in Yemen, workplace sexual misconduct is regulated, however there is no legal provision against work-related stress (Table 3).

Table 3. Examples of differences in the regulation of workplace violence among developing and transition countries.

Type of Regulation	Countries
Any kind of violence	Albania, Burkina Faso, Colombia, Comoros, India, Jordan, Lebanon, Macedonia, Malaysia, Mauritius, Mexico, Morocco, Namibia, Paraguay, Rwanda, Singapore, South Africa, Togo, Tunisia, Uganda, Uruguay, Venezuela, Yemen, Zambia
Only infringement of sexual or religious custom	Belize, Chile, China, Djibouti, El Salvador, Kenya, Korea, Lesotho, Libya, Niger, Peru, Saint Lucia, Saudi Arabia, Vietnam
No specific provision on WV in OSH law	Angola, Central African Republic, Congo, Egypt, Mozambique, Philippines, Qatar, Russia, Thailand

4. Discussion

Our review showed that most countries around the world have not included mandatory PSH risk assessment and WV prevention in their own national OSH legislation. The lack of indications for employers is not justified in light of the scientific evidence that occupational stress causes cardiovascular [23,24] and psychiatric disorders [25–27], general health impairment and low levels of well-being [28], and influences the occurrence of injuries [29]. Similarly, WV has significant effects on workers' health and productivity [30–33]. We found a difference between developed and developing countries on this topic, showing a higher frequency of legislative measures in developed countries. This undoubtedly shows a shift towards a greater focus on the issues associated with work-related stress and WV by governments and civil societies of some developed countries. However, we found differences among developed countries, also showing that some of these countries fail to take measures that compel employers to prevent psychosocial risks. Moreover, in many countries, WV was prohibited only if it included an attack on sexual or religious customs.

Since the PSH and WV prevention policy may generate some costs for employers, a possible obstacle to its adoption may be of an economic nature. However, beyond the obvious distinction between developed and developing countries, we observed that some of the major world economies in the developing/transition area (China, Russia, India, Brasil) and countries with the highest per capita income (Qatar, Emirates, Singapore) have limited regulation on PSH or WV.

Moreover, it is remarkable that some developed countries do not have national laws that provide for the obligation to evaluate PSH or WV risk in the workplace. In particular, our research was incapable of finding any mandatory regulation in the USA, Australia and New Zealand, while Canada only had regulation for WV. Even if the LEGOSH database does not allow us to exclude that there may be some regional or local regulation, we must conclude that the situation in these countries is different from that of the other developed countries and, in particular, from the EU member states. A confirmation of the fact that these developed countries have no national mandating rules for the assessment of psychosocial risks or violence against workers is provided by training programs that are developed by the national safety and health agencies. In the USA, the Occupational Safety and Health Administration (OSHA) training courses do not include PSH or WV [34]. The opposite is the case for the equivalent EU administration (EU-OSHA) of which their current themes include stress and psychosocial risks [35] and where psychosocial occupational risks in different countries are constantly monitored [36]. The situation is similar for Safe Work Australia (SWA), the Australian government statutory body established in 2008 to develop national policy relating to OHS, which does not include PSH or WV in their model code of practices [37]. The Canadian Centre for Occupational Health and Safety (CCOHS) considers workplace violence and bullying in its health and safety programs, however it does not include stress or other psychosocial risks prevention into the action required under OHS legislation in Canadian jurisdictions [38].

The general framework, therefore, leads us to believe that a distinction among countries does exist, however it could be founded on different cultural and economic models for social development rather than on the availability of economic resources. Our findings show support for the Scandinavian model of workplace health and safety culture, which emerged during the 1970s and inspired the EU one, and is based on a "three-pillar" system of collective bargaining and extensive collaboration involving employers, employees and government [39–41], which undoubtedly facilitates the development of policies addressing PSH/WV prevention. On the contrary, many non-EU developed countries, such as the USA, Switzerland and others, leave these important aspects of occupational safety and health to be regulated by market forces rather than institutional actors [42].

With regard to WV, the observed differences may also derive from cultural, religious and socio-political roots. European countries generally recognize both psychosocial risks and occupational violence as important factors according to two European Framework Agreements (2004; 2007) [43,44]. However, the concept of "what" must be protected is substantially different in some non-European countries with respect to European states. For example, in some legislation of developing countries, protection from WV is limited to sexual harassment, consequently ignoring the health risk associated with all other forms of non-sexual violence [45–49].

Our search has the limitations that derive from the data source. Although LEGOSH is the most up-to-date database available, in some cases, the last update ranged between 2013 and 2015. We cannot, therefore, exclude that more recent legislation has been introduced. Moreover, we cannot even rule out the possibility that in some countries legislation exists, but that ILO-LEGOSH researchers have not been able to find it, even if this is unlikely.

The differences we identified among the national laws could roughly be related to differences in the health of workers. Health risk management in the workplace is a complex process that requires hazard identification, risk measurement and the adoption of preventive measures. When all this is not required by law but is entrusted to the will of individual entrepreneurs, this may lead to health problems among workers. Previous studies indeed observed that countries with well-established active labour market policies also have better working conditions and lower levels of work-related stress than unregulated countries [50–55]. Inequalities in preventive dispositions may favour inequalities in health between and among workers.

Naturally, the lack of national laws is only the first indication of reduced attention to the prevention of occupational risks. The lack of effective measures for the enforcement of the rules can be another important factor of inequality in the workplace and between workers. A systematic literature review showed that the introduction of regulatory policy levers is often effective in reducing injuries and/or increasing compliance with OHS legislation [56]. The lack of rules for the prevention of psychosocial risk in some developed countries may also reduce the effectiveness of programs for improving occupational health. Studies showed that integrated approaches to promoting and protecting worker health, addressing both environmental and psychosocial factors, are highly effective and responsive to specific productive needs [57,58].

The lack of health and safety laws for the prevention of occupational stress and violence in many areas with a high-income economy is worthy of consideration in relation to the presence of the migration phenomenon, which can greatly aggravate inequalities in workplaces. Migrating workers often have unrecognized mental health needs [53] because migration per se can be a very stress-inducing phenomenon [59]. Migrant workers are often engaged in what is known as 3-D jobs, i.e., dirty, dangerous and demanding [60]. This includes working in an isolated environment, with limited supervision and guidance, which makes them more prone to abuse and exploitation [61]. In cases where social and OSH policies are poor, the distress could lead to mental health consequences or other forms of health complications [62]. The remedy, typical of many authoritarian regimes, of countering or prohibiting migration has turned out to worsen the situation, favouring illegal migration with fewer safeguards [63].

In 2015, the migrant population represented nearly 4% of the total global population aged 15 years and over and cannot be neglected [64]. This leads, furthermore, to the need to homogenise the legislative tools to address psychosocial hazards in all countries. Policymakers should try to fill the existing gaps in national legislation on these topics. Making uniform interventions could also probably facilitate the achievement of the Sustainable Development Goal (SDG 3) established by the United Nations to achieve a better and more sustainable future for all, aiming at a reduction by one third of premature mortality from non-communicable diseases through prevention, treatment and promotion of mental health and wellbeing [65]. SDG 3 provides a rationale and a framework to address mental health from many perspectives with renewed urgency. A needed political action could boost actions to tackle the unequal psychosocial risk assessment policies in the workplace, giving decisive occupational health benefits.

5. Conclusions

Our study evidenced marked differences in the legislative framework of work-related psychosocial risks among countries. These differences may lead to unequal levels of worker protection in the workplace, which can be the subject of future research. Further studies should be focused on the relationship between social, economic and cultural factors and safety and health levels in the workplace. The legislation on PSH and WV is more frequently present in developed countries than in developing ones. In many cases, WV is prohibited only if it represents an attack on sexual or religious customs. There are also significant differences within the group of richer countries, where some fail to take measures that force employers to prevent psychosocial risks.

These inequalities in legislation could have adverse effects on global occupational health and health in general. We believe that the present situation is not acceptable, especially in a context of globalization and migrating workforce, thus legislative improvements are needed.

Author Contributions: Conceptualization, F.C.; methodology, F.C.; investigation, F.C. and N.M.; data curation, N.M, and S.Z.; writing—original draft preparation, F.C.; writing—review and editing, N.M.; supervision, T.H. and M.P.

Funding: This research received no external funding.

Conflicts of Interest: The authors declare no conflict of interest.

Appendix A

Table A1. Characteristics of OSH legislation concerning psychosocial hazards and workplace violence in developed countries. (EU = European Union).

Countries (n = 23)	Explicit Inclusion of Psychosocial Hazards into OSH Legislation		Last Update in the International Labour Office Global Database on Occupational Safety and Health Legislation (LEGOSH)
	Psychosocial Risks	Occupational Violence	
Bulgaria (EU)	Yes	No	February 2016
Croatia (EU)	Yes	Yes	March 2013
Cyprus (EU)	Yes	Yes	February 2013
Denmark (EU)	NDA	Yes	2014
Finland (EU)	Yes	Yes	October 2016
France (EU)	Yes	Yes	2015
Greece (EU)	Yes	Yes	January 2017
Ireland (EU)	NDA	Yes	March 2017
Italy (EU)	Yes	Yes	February 2016
Latvia (EU)	Yes	Yes	March 2017
Netherlands (EU)	Yes	Yes	March 2017
Poland (EU)	Yes	NDA	2016
Portugal (EU)	Yes	Yes	2014
Romania (EU)	Yes	NDA	2013
Spain (EU)	NDA	Yes	August 2015
Sweden (EU)	Yes	Yes	2014
United Kingdom (EU)	Yes	Yes	2013
Australia	No *	No *	2013
Canada	NDA	Yes	2013
New Zealand	No *	No *	2013
Switzerland	NDA	Yes	2013
Norway	Yes	Yes	January 2017
United States	NDA	NDA	2013

Note: NDA = No Data Available; * Only implicit provision.

Appendix B

Table A2. Characteristics of OSH legislation concerning psychosocial hazards and workplace violence in developing countries.

Countries (n = 109)	Explicit Inclusion of Psychosocial Hazards into OSH Legislation		Last Update in LEGOSH
	Psychosocial Risks	Occupational Violence	
	Europe (n = 14)		
Albania	Yes	Yes	March 2017
Armenia	NDA	NDA	2013
Azerbaijan	NDA	NDA	2013
Belarus	NDA	NDA	2013
Georgia	NDA	NDA	2013
Kazakhstan	NDA	NDA	2013
Kyrgyzstan	NDA	NDA	2013
Republic of Moldova	NDA	NDA	2013
Russian Federation	No	No	October 2016
Tajikistan	NDA	NDA	2013
The Former Yugoslav Republic of Macedonia	Yes	Yes	2013
Turkmenistan	Yes	NDA	2013
Ukraine	NDA	NDA	2013
Uzbekistan	Yes	NDA	2013
	North America (n = 2)		
Dominica	NDA	NDA	2015
Grenada	NDA	NDA	April 2015
	Central and South America (n = 30)		
Antigua and Barbuda	NDA	NDA	April 2015
Argentina	NDA	NDA	2013
Bahamas	NDA	NDA	February 2015
Barbados	NDA	NDA	2015
Belize	NDA	Yes *	April 2015
Bolivia	NDA	NDA	2013
Chile	NDA	Yes *	April 2015
Colombia	Yes	Yes	2013
Costa Rica	NDA	NDA	2013
Cuba	NDA	NDA	2013
Dominican Republic	NDA	NDA	2013
Ecuador	NDA	NDA	2013
El Salvador	Yes	Yes *	2013
Guatemala	No	NDA	2013
Guyana	NDA	NDA	March 2015
Haiti	NDA	NDA	2015
Honduras	NDA	NDA	2013
Jamaica	NDA	NDA	July 2015
Mexico	Yes	Yes	2013
Nicaragua	Yes	NDA	2013
Panama	NDA	NDA	2013
Paraguay	NDA	Yes	2013
Perù	Yes	Yes	2015
Puerto Rico	NDA	NDA	2013
Saint Lucia	NDA	Yes *	February 2015
Saint Vincent and the Grenadines	NDA	NDA	2015
Suriname	NDA	NDA	April 2015
Trinidad and Tobago	NDA	NDA	March 2015
Uruguay	NDA	Yes	2013
Bolivarian Republic of Venezuela	Yes	Yes	2013
	Africa (n = 46)		
Algeria	NDA	NDA	2013
Angola	Yes	NDA	2014
Benin	NDA	NDA	2013
Botswana	NDA	NDA	2013
Burkina Faso	Yes	Yes	2014
Burundi	NDA	NDA	2014
Cameroon	NDA	NDA	2014
Central African Republic	Yes	NDA	January 2015
Chad	NDA	NDA	January 2015
Comoros	Yes	Yes #	2013
Congo	Yes	NDA	February 2015
Cote d'Ivoire	NDA	NDA	2013
Democratic Republic of Congo	NDA	NDA	2014
Djibouti	NDA	Yes *	2013
Egypt	Yes	NDA	2013
Equatorial Guinea	NDA	NDA	2013
Eritrea	NDA	NDA	2013
eSwatini	NDA	NDA	2013

Table A2. *Cont.*

Countries (n = 109)	Explicit Inclusion of Psychosocial Hazards into OSH Legislation		Last Update in LEGOSH
	Psychosocial Risks	Occupational Violence	
Gabon	NDA	NDA	2015
Ghana	NDA	NDA	June 2015
Guinea	NDA	NDA	2015
Kenya	NDA	Yes *	July 2015
Lesotho	Yes	Yes *	2013
Libya	NDA	Yes *	2013
Madagascar	NDA	NDA	January 2015
Malawi	NDA	NDA	2013
Mali	NDA	NDA	2014
Mauritania	NDA	NDA	2013
Mauritius	NDA	Yes	2015
Morocco	Yes	Yes	2013
Mozambique	Yes	NDA	2014
Namibia	Yes	Yes	2013
Niger	Yes	Yes *	2013
Rwanda	NDA	Yes	February 2015
Senegal	NDA	NDA	2013
Seychelles	NDA	NDA	2013
Sierra Leone	NDA	NDA	June 2015
Somalia	NDA	NDA	2013
South Africa	Yes	Yes	2013
Sudan	NDA	NDA	2013
United Republic of Tanzania	NDA	NDA	2013
Togo	Yes	Yes	2014
Tunisia	NDA	Yes	2013
Uganda	Yes	Yes	2014
Zambia	Yes	Yes	2013
Zimbabwe	NDA	NDA	2013
Middle East and Asia (n = 17)			
Bahrain	NDA	NDA	2013
China	Yes	Yes *	2013
India	Yes	Yes	2013
Jordan	NDA	Yes	October 2015
Republic of Korea	Yes	Yes *	September 2015
Kuwait	NDA	NDA	October 2015
Lebanon	NDA	Yes	October 2015
Malaysia	Yes	Yes	2013
Oman	Yes	NDA	2013
Philippines	Yes	NDA	2013
Qatar	NDA	NDA	October 2015
Saudi Arabia	Yes	Yes $	October 2015
Singapore	No	Yes	October 2016
Thailand	Yes	NDA	2014
United Arab Emirates	NDA	NDA	2013
Vietnam	NDA	Yes &	August 2015
Yemen	NDA	Yes	2013

Notes: NDA = No Data Available; * Only sexual harassment; # Only sexual and moral harassment; $ Only protection of dignity and religion; & Only sexual harassment and violence against domestic workers.

References

1. Ramazzini, B. De Morbis Artificum Diatriba. Available online: https://archive.org/stream/bernramazzinide00porzgoog#page/n2/mode/2up (accessed on 14 August 2018).
2. GBD 2016 Risk Factors Collaborators. Global, regional, and national comparative risk assessment of 84 behavioural, environmental and occupational, and metabolic risks or clusters of risks, 1990–2016: A systematic analysis for the Global Burden of Disease Study 2016. *Lancet* **2017**, *390*, 1345–1422. [CrossRef]
3. Expert Forecast on Emerging Psychosocial Risks Related to Occupational Safety and Health. Available online: http://osha.europa.eu/en/publications/reports/7807118 (accessed on 14 August 2018).
4. Cox, T.; Griffiths, A.J. The nature and measurement of work stress: Theory and practice. In *The Evaluation of Human Work: A Practical Ergonomics Methodology*; Wilson, J.R., Corlett, E.N., Eds.; Taylor & Francis: London, UK, 1995.
5. Psychosocial Risk and Work-Related Stress. Available online: http://www.ilo.org/safework/areasofwork/workplace-health-promotion-and-well-being/WCMS_108557/lang--en/index.htm (accessed on 14 August 2018).
6. Siegrist, J.; Wahrendorf, M. *Work Stress and Health in a Globalized Economy. The Model of Effort-Reward Imbalance*; Springer International Publishing: Basel, Switzerland, 2016.

7. Stress at the Workplace. Available online: https://www.who.int/occupational_health/topics/stressatwp/en/ (accessed on 19 April 2019).
8. Chirico, F. Job stress models for predicting burnout syndrome: A review. *Ann. Ist. Super. Sanita* **2016**, *52*, 443–456. [CrossRef] [PubMed]
9. Magnavita, N. The exploding spark: Workplace violence in an infectious disease hospital—A longitudinal study. *Biomed. Res. Int.* **2013**. [CrossRef] [PubMed]
10. Magnavita, N. Workplace violence and occupational stress in healthcare workers: A chicken-and-egg situation-results of a 6-year follow-up study. *J. Nurs. Scholarsh.* **2014**, *46*, 366–376. [CrossRef] [PubMed]
11. Workplace Violence Fact Sheet. Available online: https://www.osha.gov/OshDoc/data_General_Facts/factsheet-workplace-violence.pdf (accessed on 14 August 2018).
12. OSH in Figures: Stress at Work—Facts and Figures. Available online: http://osha.europa.eu/en/publications/reports/TE-81-08-478-EN-C_OSH_in_figures_stress_at_work (accessed on 14 August 2018).
13. Psychosocial Hazards. Available online: https://www.comcare.gov.au/preventing/hazards/psychosocial_hazards (accessed on 14 August 2018).
14. International Labour Office (ILO/BIT). *Workplace Stress. A Collective Challenge*; ILO: Turin, Italy, 2016.
15. Benavides, F.G.; Wesseling, C.; Delclos, G.L.; Felknor, S.; Pinilla, J.; Rodrigo, F. Research Team of the First Central American Survey of Working Conditions and Health. Working conditions and health in Central America: A survey of 12,024 workers in six countries. *Occup. Environ. Med.* **2014**, *71*, 459–465. [CrossRef] [PubMed]
16. Homicide and Nonfatal Violent Crimes in the Workplace Declined. Available online: https://www.bjs.gov/content/pub/press/wv09pr.cfm (accessed on 15 April 2019).
17. Occupational Violence. Available online: https://www.cdc.gov/niosh/topics/violence/fastfacts.html (accessed on 14 August 2018).
18. Aw, T.C. Health surveillance. In *Occupational Health*; Sadhra, S., Rampal, K.C., Eds.; Risk Assessment and Management Blackwell: London, UK, 1999.
19. Stoffregen, S.A.; Giordano, F.B.; Lee, J. Psycho-socio-cultural factors and global occupational safety: Integrating micro- and macro-systems. *Soc. Sci. Med.* **2019**, *226*, 153–163. [CrossRef] [PubMed]
20. Baru, R.V.; Mohan, M. Globalisation and neoliberalism as structural drivers of health inequities. *Health Res. Policy Syst.* **2018**, *16*, 91. [CrossRef] [PubMed]
21. International Labour Office. Available online: http://www.ilo.org/dyn/legosh/en/f?p=14100:1000:0::NO:: (accessed on 14 August 2018).
22. World Economic Situation Prospects. 2018 Report. Available online: https://www.un.org/development/desa/dpad/wp-content/uploads/sites/45/publication/WESP2018_Full_Web-1.pdf (accessed on 14 August 2018).
23. Theorell, T. A long-term perspective on cardiovascular job stress research. *J. Occup. Health* **2019**, *61*, 3–9. [CrossRef] [PubMed]
24. Dragano, N.; Siegrist, J.; Nyberg, S.T.; Lunau, T.; Fransson, E.I.; Alfredsson, L.; Bjorner, J.B.; Borritz, M.; Burr, H.; Erbel, R.; et al. IPD-Work consortium. Effort-Reward Imbalance at Work and Incident Coronary Heart Disease: A Multicohort Study of 90,164 Individuals. *Epidemiology* **2017**, *28*, 619–626. [CrossRef] [PubMed]
25. Madsen, I.E.H.; Nyberg, S.T.; Magnusson Hanson, L.L.; Ferrie, J.E.; Ahola, K.; Alfredsson, L.; Batty, G.D.; Bjorner, J.B.; Borritz, M.; Burr, H.; et al. Job strain as a risk factor for clinical depression: Systematic review and meta-analysis with additional individual participant data. *Psychol. Med.* **2017**, *47*, 1342–1356. [CrossRef] [PubMed]
26. Stansfeld, S.; Candy, B. Psychosocial work environment and mental health—A meta-analytic review. *Scand. J. Work Environ. Health* **2006**, *32*, 443–462. [CrossRef] [PubMed]
27. Harvey, S.B.; Modini, M.; Joyce, S.; Milligan-Saville, J.S.; Tan, L.; Mykletun, A.; Bryant, R.A.; Christensen, H.; Mitchell, P.B. Can work make you mentally ill? A systematic meta-review of work-related risk factors for common mental health problems. *Occup. Environ. Med.* **2017**, *74*, 301–310. [CrossRef] [PubMed]
28. De Jonge, J.; Bosma, H.; Peter, R.; Siegrist, J. Job strain, effort-reward imbalance and employee well-being: A large-scale cross-sectional study. *Soc. Sci. Med.* **2000**, *50*, 1317–1327. [CrossRef]
29. Baidwan, N.K.; Gerberich, S.G.; Kim, H.; Ryan, A.; Church, T.; Capistrant, B. A longitudinal study of work-related psychosocial factors and injuries: Implications for the aging United States workforce. *Am. J. Ind. Med.* **2019**, *62*, 212–221. [CrossRef] [PubMed]

30. Magnavita, N.; Heponiemi, T. Workplace violence against nursing students and nurses. An Italian experience. *J. Nurs. Sch.* **2011**, *43*, 203–210. [CrossRef]
31. Phillips, J.P. Workplace Violence against Health Care Workers in the United States. *N. Engl. J. Med.* **2016**, *374*, 1661–1669. [CrossRef] [PubMed]
32. Lever, I.; Dyball, D.; Greenberg, N.; Stevelink, S.A.M. Health Consequences of Bullying in the Healthcare Workplace: A Systematic Review. *J. Adv. Nurs.* **2019**, *28*. [CrossRef]
33. Nielsen, M.B.; Indregard, A.M.; Øverland, S. Workplace bullying and sickness absence: A systematic review and meta-analysis of the research literature. *Scand. J. Work Environ. Health* **2016**, *42*, 359–370. [CrossRef]
34. OSHA Education Center. OSHA 30-Hour General Industry Training Online. Available online: https://www.oshaeducationcenter.com/osha-30-hour-general-industry/?lgr=34cf78ee-e5e1-4e2a-9bac-fb73843aa291 (accessed on 21 June 2019).
35. EU-OSHA. Themes. Available online: https://osha.europa.eu/en/themes (accessed on 21 June 2019).
36. Management of Psychosocial Risks in European Workplaces: Evidence from the Second European Survey of Enterprises on New and Emerging Risks (ESENER-2). Available online: https://osha.europa.eu/en/tools-and-publications/publications/management-psychosocial-risks-european-workplaces-evidence/view (accessed on 21 June 2019).
37. Safe Work Australia (SWA). Model Codes of Practice. Available online: https://www.safeworkaustralia.gov.au/resources_publications/model-codes-of-practice (accessed on 21 June 2019).
38. Canadian Centre for Occupational Health and Safety (CCOHS). Programs. Available online: https://www.ccohs.ca/topics/programs/ (accessed on 21 June 2019).
39. Kleinman, G.D. Occupational health and safety. The Swedish model. *J. Occup. Med.* **1984**, *26*, 901–905. [CrossRef]
40. Karlsen, J.E.; Lindøe, P. The Nordic Osh Model at a Turning Point? *Policy Pract. Health Saf.* **2006**, *4*, 17–30. [CrossRef]
41. Evolution of the Nordic Work Environment and Health Model: 60 Years Experience. Working Environment through the Work Life. Available online: https://www.vinnueftirlit.is/media/nordiskjubileumkonferens2014/RANTANEN_JORMA_2.pdf (accessed on 15 April 2019).
42. Schnall, P.L.; Dobson, M.; Rosskam, E. *Unhealthy Work: Causes, Consequences, Cures*; Baywood Publishing: Amityville, NY, USA, 2009.
43. Framework Agreement on Work-Related Stress. Available online: http://www.etuc.org/IMG/pdf_Framework_agreement_on_work-related_stress_EN.pdf (accessed on 14 August 2018).
44. European Social Partners. Framework Agreement on Harassment and Violence at Work. Available online: https://ueapme.com/docs/joint_position/2007_Framework_Agreement_Harassment_and_Violence_at_Work.pdf (accessed on 14 August 2018).
45. Chirico, F. The assessment of psychosocial risk: Only "work-related stress" or something else? *Med. Lav.* **2015**, *106*, 65–66. [PubMed]
46. Chirico, F. The forgotten realm of the new and emerging psychosocial risk factors. *J. Occup. Health* **2017**, *59*, 433–435. [CrossRef] [PubMed]
47. Chirico, F. Is burnout a syndrome or an occupational disease? Instructions for occupational physicians. *Epidemiol. Prev.* **2017**, *41*, 294–298. [CrossRef] [PubMed]
48. Workplace Violence and Harassment: A European Picture Workplace Violence and Harassment: A European Picture. Available online: https://osha.europa.eu/en/publications/reports/violence-harassmentTERO09010ENC/view?searchterm=Workplace%20violence%20and%20harassment:%20A%20European%20picture (accessed on 14 August 2018).
49. Eurofound. Violence and Harassment in European Workplaces: Causes, Impacts and Policies. Available online: https://www.eurofound.europa.eu/sites/default/files/ef_comparative_analytical_report/field_ef_documents/ef1473en.pdf (accessed on 14 August 2018).
50. Benach, J.; Muntaner, C.; Santana, V. Employment Conditions and Health Inequalities: Final Report to the WHO Commission on Social Determinants of Health (CSDH). Available online: https://www.who.int/social_determinants/resources/articles/emconet_who_report.pdf (accessed on 20 September 2007).
51. Siegrist, J.; Wahrendorf, M. Quality of work, health and early retirement: European comparisons. In *The Individual and the Welfare State: Life Histories in Europe*; Börsch-Supan, A., Brandt, M., Hank, K., Schröder, M., Eds.; Springer: Berlin, Heidelberg, 2011; pp. 169–177.

52. Final Scientific Report: Working Conditions and Health Inequalities, Evidence and Policy Implications. Available online: https://www.siis.net/documentos/ficha/499738.pdf (accessed on 14 August 2018).
53. Bhugra, D. Migration and mental health. *Acta Psychiatr. Scand.* **2004**, *109*, 243–258. [CrossRef] [PubMed]
54. Chopra, P. Mental health and the workplace: Issues for developing countries. *Int. J. Ment. Health Syst.* **2009**, *3*, 4. [CrossRef] [PubMed]
55. Health Impact of the Psychosocial Hazards of Work: An Overview. Available online: http://www.who.int/occupational_health/publications/hazardpsychosocial/en/ (accessed on 14 August 2018).
56. Tompa, E.; Kalcevich, C.; Foley, M.; McLeod, C.; Hogg-Johnson, S.; Cullen, K.; MacEachen, E.; Mahood, Q.; Irvin, E. A systematic literature review of the effectiveness of occupational health and safety regulatory enforcement. *Am. J. Ind. Med.* **2016**, *59*, 919–933. [CrossRef] [PubMed]
57. Sorensen, G.; McLellan, D.L.; Sabbath, E.L.; Dennerlein, J.T.; Nagler, E.M.; Hurtado, D.A.; Pronk, N.P.; Wagner, G.R. Integrating worksite health protection and health promotion: A conceptual model for intervention and research. *Prev. Med.* **2016**, *91*, 188–196. [CrossRef]
58. Magnavita, N. Obstacles and Future Prospects: Considerations on Health Promotion Activities for Older Workers in Europe. *Int. J. Environ. Res. Public Health* **2018**, *15*, 1096. [CrossRef]
59. Quandt, S.A.; Arcury-Quandt, A.E.; Lawlor, E.J.; Carrillo, L.; Marín, A.J.; Grzywacz, J.G.; Arcury, T.A. 3-D jobs and health disparities: The health implications of Latino chicken catchers' working conditions. *Am. J. Ind. Med.* **2013**, *56*, 206–215. [CrossRef]
60. Green, O.; Ayalon, L. Violations of workers' rights and exposure to work-related abuse of live-in migrant and live-out local home care workers—A preliminary study: Implications for health policy and practice. *Isr. J. Health Policy Res.* **2018**, *7*, 32. [CrossRef]
61. Virupaksha, H.G.; Kumar, A.; Nirmala, B.P. Migration and mental health: An interface. *J. Nat. Sci. Biol. Med.* **2014**, *5*, 233–239. [CrossRef] [PubMed]
62. Human Rights Watch. Kuwait/Philippines Protect Filipino Migrant Workers. Migration Ban Increases Abuse Risk. Available online: https://www.hrw.org/news/2018/02/21/kuwait/philippines-protect-filipino-migrant-workers (accessed on 19 April 2019).
63. International Labour Office. *ILO Global Estimates on Migrant Workers: Results and Methodology. Special Focus on Migrant Domestic Workers*; ILO: Geneva, Switzerland, 2015.
64. Vahabi, M.; Wong, J.P. Caught between a rock and a hard place: Mental health of migrant live-in caregivers in Canada. *BMC Public Health* **2017**, *17*, 498. [CrossRef] [PubMed]
65. United Nations. Sustainable Development Goal 3. Ensure Healthy Lives and Promote Well-Being for All at All Ages. Available online: https://sustainabledevelopment.un.org/sdg3 (accessed on 20 April 2019).

International Journal of
Environmental Research and Public Health

MDPI

Article

Temporary Workers' Skipping of Meals and Eating Alone in South Korea: The Korean National Health and Nutrition Examination Survey for 2013–2016

Ji-Sook Kong [1], Kyoung-Bok Min [2] and Jin-Young Min [3,*]

1 Department of Preventive Medicine, College of Medicine, Hanyang University, Seoul 04763, Korea
2 Department of Preventive Medicine, College of Medicine, Seoul National University, Seoul 03080, Korea
3 Institute of Health and Environment, Seoul National University, Seoul 08826, Korea
* Correspondence: yaemin00@snu.ac.kr

Received: 29 April 2019; Accepted: 26 June 2019; Published: 30 June 2019

Abstract: Available evidence suggests that social disadvantages are inextricably linked to unhealthy eating behaviors. Given that temporary workers face insecure employment and uncertainty in their work's terms and conditions, issues relevant to maintaining healthy eating behavior are likely to be affected. This study investigated the association between temporary employments and, specifically, the status and frequency of meal skipping and of eating alone among temporary and permanent Korean workers. We used data from the 2013–2016 Korean National Health and Nutrition Examination Survey. A total of 5912 working people were included as the study population. We classified them as temporary workers (n = 3036) and permanent workers (n = 2876). Eating behaviors included meal skipping and eating alone. The rate and frequency of meal skipping and eating alone were higher in temporary workers. After adjustment for potential confounders, the likelihoods for temporary workers' skipping lunch was twice as high (OR = 1.95, 95% CI 1.45–2.63) as for permanent workers. In particular, temporary workers had four-fold-increased odds (OR = 4.12, 95% CI 2.29–7.41) of eating alone three times per day relative to permanent workers. We found that temporary workers were more likely to skip meals and eat alone than were permanent workers.

Keywords: temporary worker; eating behaviors; meal skipping; eating alone; Korea

1. Introduction

Over the past three decades, globalization, financial crises, and the global economy's restructuring have promoted labor market 'flexibility' and entailed changes to work arrangements, especially in terms of the growth of temporary employment [1]. Temporary employment can be defined as wage employment relations other than those of unlimited duration, including fixed-term, subcontracted jobs, project or task-based contracts, as well as seasonal or casual work [2]. Although temporary jobs encompass a wide and diverse range of occupations and sectors, they tend to offer low wages and diverse poor working conditions (e.g., less access to paid vacations, sick leave, and unemployment insurance) relative to permanent jobs [3]. These detrimental aspects of temporary employment result in psychological morbidity and socioeconomic disadvantages for temporary workers [4,5].

Many studies have noted that temporary workers are more likely than standard workers to have poor health outcomes (e.g., cardiovascular disease, depression, anxiety, and suicide) [6–8], experience absenteeism caused by work-related injury or sickness [9], and choose unhealthy lifestyles (e.g., heavy smoking and alcohol dependence) [10]. In addition, temporary workers are more likely to have more difficulties accessing healthcare [11] and developing friendships in the workplace than are standard workers.

Eating is essential for survival, and healthy eating is essential for health and well-being [12–14]. Eating behavior is affected by individual perception (of health and nutrition benefits and of body weight) as well as the objective realities of socio-economic environments and physical access [15,16]. For example, lower education and lower occupation have been associated with fewer intakes of certain food products (i.e., vegetables, fish, and vitamins) [17], and skipping breakfast with low family socioeconomic status and sedentary lifestyle [18]. Employed parents' good working conditions positively affected the eating of more homemade meals, eating with the family, and less meal skipping, while employed parents' work conditions (e.g., long hours) were associated with missed breakfast, use of convenience entrees, and more restaurant meals [19]. The available evidence suggests that social disadvantages are inextricably linked to unhealthy eating behaviors. Since temporary workers face insecure employment and uncertainty in the terms and conditions of their work [20,21], all issues relevant to maintaining healthy eating behavior could be affected. However, not much is known about working arrangements' (i.e., contract types) effects on eating behaviors.

Therefore, the present study examined the association between temporary employments and eating behavior. Specifically, we compared the status and frequency of meal skipping and eating alone between temporary and permanent Korean adult workers.

2. Materials and Methods

2.1. Study Population

We used data from the 2013–2016 Korean National Health and Nutrition Examination Survey (KNHANES) conducted by the Centers for Disease Control and Prevention [22]. The KNHANES, was designed to assess Koreans' health and nutritional status by extracting representative samples via multistage, probability-cluster, and complex sampling design. The overall participation was 77.5% for the 4-year study period (KNHANES 2013–2016; 31,098 of 40,127). Of those 31,098 participants, we selected a population aged 19–64 years (n = 12,823). We initially included 7603 after excluding cases that were missing information on whether a wage worker was a permanent worker or not (n = 10,672). Among those, we excluded participants who did not complete questionnaire items on eating habits (n = 1113) such as meal skipping, meal frequency per week, and eating alone, or who were under dietary control (n = 578), for example starving or fasting for reasons such as disease or weight loss. Thus, the final sample was 5912 working people. All of the participants provided written informed consent. Also, because the KNHANES constitutes a publicly opened national statistical database without personally identifiable information, we performed a secondary analysis of the data without IRB approval.

2.2. Variable Definition

A waged worker is someone who is employed and paid by another person or company and has worked for more than one hour to earn pay for the past week (except for the self-employed). Identification of contract type was based on the following question: "What is your current job status?". Possible responses were "permanent job (guaranteed employment until retirement)" and "temporary job", according to which, respondents were classified as permanent workers and temporary workers, respectively.

Eating behaviors included meal skipping and eating alone. Skipping of breakfast, lunch, or dinner was determined by whether the respondent had eaten each meal on the day prior to the survey, via "yes or no" questions. Frequency of meal skipping was based on the question, "During the past year, how many days a week did you eat breakfast, lunch, or dinner?" Response included 5–7/week, 3–4/week, 1–2/week, and almost never. Frequencies were categorized into two groups: ≥5/week and <5/week. For eating alone, participants were asked, "When you have been eating breakfast, lunch, and dinner for the past year, have you usually eaten with someone else?" Responses were "yes" or "no." Participants also were asked to indicate how often they ate their daily meals (i.e., breakfast, lunch, or dinner) alone, as once, twice, or three times. Other variables included socio-demographic characteristics and health behaviors and conditions. The self-reported socio-demographic variables were age (19–29, 30–39, 40–49, or 50–64), gender, marital status (married, divorced/widowed, or never), number of family members (1 or ≥2), and household income (1st quartile, 2nd quartile, 3rd quartile, or 4th quartile). Jobs were classified into white collar (managerial, professional, or clerical), pink collar (services or sales), and blue collar (manual labor). Health behaviors included cigarette smoking (never, former, or current) and alcohol drinking (yes or no). Body mass index (BMI) was categorized into underweight ($0 < BMI < 18.5$), normal ($18.5 \leq BMI < 25$), and overweight/obesity ($BMI \geq 25.0$).

2.3. Statistical Analysis

Statistical differences in general characteristics between temporary and permanent workers were analyzed using the chi-square test. We compared eating behaviors such as meal skipping, meal frequency per week, and frequency of eating alone per day between temporary and permanent workers. To assess the association between temporary employment and eating behavior, we designated permanent workers as a reference group and conducted unadjusted and adjusted logistic regression models. The result provided odds ratios (OR) of temporary employment with 95% confidence intervals (CI). In the regression models, Model 1 was adjusted for demographic characteristics (i.e., age, gender, marital status, number of family members (1 or ≥2), and household income); Model 2 was adjusted for Model 1 + job types; and Model 3 was adjusted for Model 2 + health behavior and condition (i.e., cigarette smoking, alcohol drinking, and BMI). The KNHANES data was based on a complex survey design, survey non-response and post-stratification to represent the civilian, non-institutionalized Korean population. The sample weights were estimated by the inverse of selection probabilities and inverse of response rates by adjusting them to the sex- and age-specific Korean populations [23]. All of the statistics were based on sampling weights in order to take complex sampling into account and were performed with SAS 9.4 software (SAS Institute, Cary, NC, USA). Statistical significance was set at $p \leq 0.05$.

3. Results

3.1. General Characteristics of Study Population

Of the 5912 participants, 2876 workers were permanent and 3036 workers were temporary. Table 1 displays the general characteristics of the study's population, revealing significant differences in all demographic variables, health behaviors, and health conditions between the groups. Temporary workers were more likely to be younger or older, to be female, to be divorced/widowed, to live in one-person households, to have low income, and to be engaged in pink- or blue-collar jobs than permanent workers. They were more likely to be never smokers, non-drinkers, and underweight than permanent workers.

Table 1. Characteristics of permanent and temporary workers ($n = 5912$).

Variables	Total ($n = 5912$) [1]	Permanent ($n = 2876$)	Temporary Workers ($n = 3036$)	p-Value [2]
Age (years)				
19–29	948 (16.0)	349 (12.1)	599 (19.7)	<0.0001
30–39	1479 (25.0)	956 (33.2)	523 (17.2)	
40–49	1659 (28.1)	921 (32.0)	738 (24.3)	
50–64	1826 (30.9)	650 (22.6)	1176 (38.7)	
Gender				
Male	2893 (48.9)	1779 (61.9)	1114 (36.7)	<0.0001
Female	3019 (51.1)	1097 (38.1)	1922 (63.3)	
Marital status				
Married	4202 (71.2)	2258 (78.6)	1944 (64.1)	<0.0001
Divorced/widowed	411 (6.96)	90 (3.13)	321 (10.6)	
Never	1292 (21.9)	524 (18.3)	768 (25.3)	
Number of family members				
Single	416 (7.04)	147 (5.11)	269 (8.86)	<0.0001
≥two members	5496 (93.0)	2729 (94.9)	2767 (91.1)	

Table 1. *Cont.*

Variables	Total (n = 5912) [1]	Permanent (n = 2876)	Temporary Workers (n = 3036)	p-Value [2]
Household income				
1st quartile	373 (6.32)	51 (1.78)	322 (10.6)	<0.0001
2nd quartile	1337 (22.7)	435 (15.2)	902 (29.8)	
3rd quartile	1968 (33.4)	943 (32.9)	1025 (33.8)	
4th quartile	2222 (37.7)	1441 (50.2)	781 (25.8)	
Job type				
White-collar	2883 (49.0)	1867 (65.4)	1016 (33.5)	<0.0001
Pink-collar	1070 (18.2)	305 (10.7)	765 (25.2)	
Blue-collar	1937 (32.9)	685 (24.0)	1252 (41.3)	
Cigarette smoking				
Never	3388 (57.5)	1439 (50.1)	1949 (64.5)	<0.0001
Former	1129 (19.2)	677 (23.6)	452 (15.0)	
Current	1375 (23.3)	754 (26.3)	621 (20.6)	
Alcohol drinking				
Drinker	3769 (64.0)	1982 (69.1)	1787 (59.1)	<0.0001
Non-drinker	2123 (36.0)	888 (30.9)	1235 (40.9)	
Body weight status				
Underweight	284 (4.83)	118 (4.13)	166 (5.48)	0.0002
Normal	3804 (64.7)	1847 (64.7)	1957 (64.6)	
Obesity	1795 (30.5)	890 (31.2)	905 (29.9)	

[1] number (%). [2] p-value was calculated based on complex sample design and weights.

3.2. Comparisons of Eating Behaviors Between Temporary and Permanent Workers

We compared eating behaviors between the temporary and permanent workers (Table 2 and Figure 1). Except for breakfast, eating behaviors for each meal differed significantly between those groups. Temporary workers had relatively higher rates of meal skipping (lunch 7.52 vs. 5.50%; dinner 6.43 vs. 4.59%) and lower rates of meal frequency per week (≥5/week; lunch 90.4 vs. 95.1%; dinner 88.4 vs. 90.7%). The rate of eating alone was significantly higher in temporary workers than in their permanent counterparts (28.5 vs. 9.72% for lunch and 22.1 vs. 13.8% for dinner). The frequency of eating alone was higher in temporary workers: eating alone once per day, 60.4 vs. 49.4%; eating alone for two meals per day, 25.4 vs. 13.0%, and eating alone for three meals per day, 7.68 vs. 1.37%.

Table 2. Eating behaviors of participants by permanent and temporary worker status (n = 5912).

Variables		Total (n = 5912) [1]	Permanent (n = 2876)	Temporary Workers (n = 3036)	p-Value [2]
Meal skipping (on previous day)					
Skipping breakfast	Yes	1479 (25.0)	713 (24.8)	766 (25.3)	0.1132
	No	4429 (75.0)	2162 (75.2)	2267 (74.7)	
Skipping lunch	Yes	386 (6.53)	158 (5.50)	228 (7.52)	0.0002
	No	5522 (93.5)	2717 (94.5)	2805 (92.5)	
Skipping dinner	Yes	327 (5.53)	132 (4.59)	195 (6.43)	0.0021
	No	5581 (94.5)	2743 (95.4)	2838 (93.6)	
Meal frequency per week (in previous 1 year)					
Breakfast frequency per week	<5/week	2430 (41.3)	1218 (42.5)	1212 (40.2)	0.6898
	≥5/week	3458 (58.7)	1651 (57.6)	1807 (59.9)	
Lunch frequency per week	<5/week	432 (7.34)	142 (4.95)	290 (9.61)	<0.0001
	≥5/week	5456 (92.7)	2727 (95.1)	2729 (90.4)	
Dinner frequency per week	<5/week	615 (10.4)	266 (9.27)	349 (11.6)	0.0003
	≥5/week	5273 (89.6)	2603 (90.7)	2670 (88.4)	
Eating alone (in previous 1 year)					
Eating breakfast alone	Yes	1770 (41.9)	827 (40.9)	943 (42.8)	0.5183
	No	2459 (58.2)	1196 (59.1)	1263 (57.3)	
Eating lunch alone	Yes	1111 (19.3)	275 (9.72)	836 (28.5)	<0.0001
	No	4646 (80.7)	2553 (90.3)	2093 (71.5)	
Eating dinner alone	Yes	1037 (18.0)	389 (13.8)	648 (22.1)	<0.0001
	No	4717 (82.0)	2438 (86.2)	2279 (77.9)	
Frequency of eating alone per day (n = 4043) [3]					
Eating alone once or more per day	Yes	2225 (55.0)	975 (49.4)	1250 (60.4)	<0.0001
	No	1818 (45.0)	998 (50.6)	820 (39.6)	
Eating alone two or more times	Yes	783 (19.4)	257 (13.0)	526 (25.4)	<0.0001
	No	3260 (80.6)	1716 (87.0)	1544 (74.6)	
Eating alone three times per day	Yes	186 (4.60)	27 (1.37)	159 (7.68)	<0.0001
	No	3857 (95.4)	1946 (98.6)	1911 (92.3)	

[1] Results were reported as unweighted percentages (%). [2] p-value was calculated based on complex sample design and weights. [3] Frequency of eating alone was evaluated for participants who had three or more meals per day.

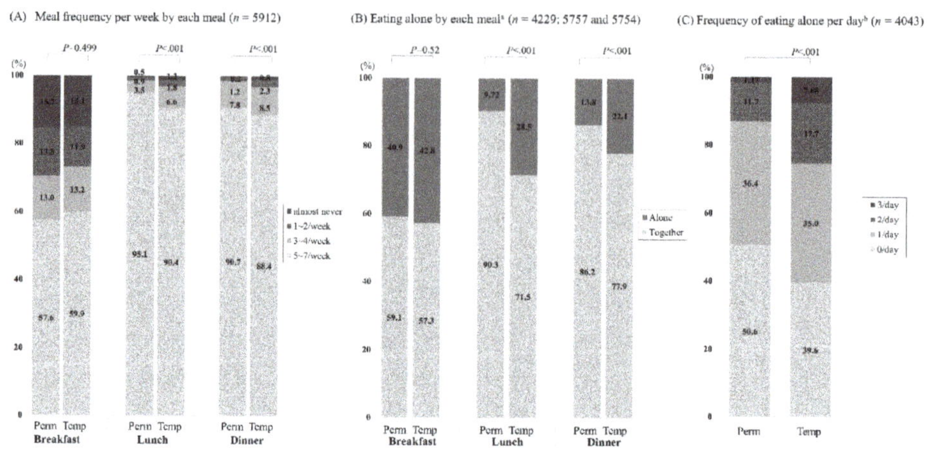

Figure 1. Percentage of eating behaviors by permanent and temporary worker status (2013–2016). Results were reported as unweighted percentages and the p-value was calculated based on the complex sample design and weights. Perm: permanent worker; Temp: temporary worker. [a] Frequency of eating alone was evaluated in participants who had three or more meals per week (breakfast, lunch, and dinner, respectively). [b] Frequency of eating alone was evaluated in participants who had three or more meals per day (breakfast, lunch, and dinner).

3.3. Association Between Temporary Employment and Eating Behaviors

Table 3 displays the ORs (95% CI) for temporary workers' eating behaviors. In the unadjusted regression model, temporary workers had a higher likelihood of skipping meals and eating alone, except for breakfast, than permanent workers. We then included confounding variables (i.e., age, sex, marital status, number of family members, household income, job type, cigarette smoking, alcohol drinking, and BMI) and gradually adjusted them in regression models 1–3. The adjusted ORs for skipping breakfast, lunch, and dinner were no longer significant in temporary workers relative to permanent workers. On the other hand, the likelihood of eating lunch less than five times a week was significantly higher in temporary workers than in permanent workers after adjustment for potential confounders (Model 3; OR = 1.95, 95% CI 1.45–2.63). The adjusted ORs for temporary workers' eating alone were significantly higher than for permanent workers, specifically, eating lunch alone (OR = 2.77, 95% CI 2.30–3.34), eating dinner alone (OR = 1.25, 95% CI 1.04–1.51), eating alone once per day (OR = 1.39, 95% CI 1.18–1.64), twice per day (OR = 1.67, 95% CI 1.33–2.11), and three times per day (OR = 4.12, 95% CI 2.29–7.41). We analyzed models 1–3 by adding confounders to the crude model. As has been reported of an association between demographic variables and dietary behavior, such as between meal skipping and eating alone [24,25], we found that the addition of demographic variables (age, sex, marital status, number of family members) to the crude model had the highest impact (odds ratio) on skipping meals and eating alone as covariates. In model 2, the variable of job type was added to model 1 and, in model 3, the variables of health behavior and conditions were added to model 2. The difference of result (odds ratio) between model 2 and model 3 was small.

Table 3. Odds ratios (95% CI) of eating behaviors for temporary workers (n = 5912).

Models	Permanent	Unadjusted	Model 1	Model 2	Model 3
Skipping breakfast (on previous day), yes	ref (1)	1.11 (0.98–1.25)	1.04 (0.90–1.21)	1.00 (0.85–1.17)	0.99 (0.85–1.16)
Skipping lunch (on previous day), yes	ref (1)	1.54 (1.22–1.95)	1.41 (1.09–1.82)	1.28 (0.98–1.67)	1.25 (0.96–1.64)
Skipping dinner (on previous day), yes	ref (1)	1.48 (1.15–1.91)	1.09 (0.83–1.43)	1.03 (0.78–1.35)	1.02 (0.78–1.34)
Breakfast frequency per week (in previous 1 year), <5/week	ref (1)	1.02 (0.91–1.15)	1.07 (0.92–1.23)	1.06 (0.91–1.23)	1.05 (0.91–1.23)
Lunch frequency per week (in previous 1 year), <5/week	ref (1)	2.29 (1.80–2.93)	2.07 (1.56–2.74)	1.93 (1.44–2.60)	1.95 (1.45–2.63)
Dinner frequency per week (in previous 1 year), <5/week	ref (1)	1.43 (1.18–1.74)	1.07 (0.87–1.32)	1.01 (0.81–1.26)	1.00 (0.81–1.25)
Eating breakfast alone (in previous 1 year), yes	ref (1)	1.05 (0.91–1.21)	1.00 (0.85–1.17)	1.02 (0.86–1.20)	1.03 (0.87–1.22)
Eating lunch alone (in previous 1 year), yes	ref (1)	3.65 (3.10–4.30)	2.88 (2.40–3.46)	2.76 (2.29–3.33)	2.77 (2.30–3.34)
Eating dinner alone (in previous 1 year), yes	ref (1)	1.73 (1.48–2.03)	1.24 (1.03–1.48)	1.24 (1.03–1.50)	1.25 (1.04–1.51)
Eating alone once or more per day (n = 4043), yes [1]	ref (1)	1.48 (1.28–1.71)	1.35 (1.15–1.59)	1.37 (1.16–1.61)	1.39 (1.18–1.64)
Eating alone two or more times (n = 4043), yes [1]	ref (1)	2.19 (1.81–2.65)	1.70 (1.36–2.11)	1.68 (1.34–2.11)	1.67 (1.33–2.11)
Eating alone three times per day (n = 4043), yes [1]	ref (1)	6.07 (3.73–9.87)	4.19 (2.37–7.42)	4.17 (2.32–7.52)	4.12 (2.29–7.41)

Model 1 (demographics) was adjusted for demographic characteristics (i.e., age, sex, marital status, number of family members (1 or ≥2) and household income); Model 2 was adjusted for Model 1 + job type; Model 3 was adjusted for Model 2 + health behavior and condition (i.e., cigarette smoking, alcohol drinking, and BMI). [1] Frequency of eating alone was evaluated in participants who had three or more meals per day.

4. Discussion

Using nationally representative sample data on South Koreans, this study examined whether temporary employment was associated with unhealthy eating behaviors. We found that temporary workers were more likely to skip lunch and eat alone than were permanent workers. The likelihood for temporary workers' skipping lunch was twice as high as for permanent workers. Eating alone was predominant among temporary workers and, particularly, their odds for eating alone three times per day were four-fold increased relative to permanent workers. Thus, our findings support prior evidence of poor eating behaviors among socially disadvantaged groups [26,27]; furthermore, our findings suggest that temporary employment contributes to inequalities in healthy eating behaviors.

Interest in the eating behaviors of skipping meals and eating alone has increased, because unhealthy behaviors alter the quantity and quality of food consumed, thereby affecting health outcomes [28]. People who skipped a meal were more likely to consume foods containing high level of cholesterol and carbohydrates and to have lower intakes of fruits, vegetables, vitamins, and minerals than those who never skipped a meal [29,30]. Further, those who skipped a meal faced increased risks to their cardio-metabolic health, notably of obesity and diabetes [31,32]. Additionally, eating alone has been associated with reduced energy intake [33], food diversity according to assessment of dietary quality using the 11-item scale [34], and inadequate intake through social interaction influence during mealtime [35]. In this way, eating alone can lead to detrimental effects on physical (metabolic syndrome) and mental health (depressive symptoms), even among those who live with family members [23,24].

Previous studies have focused on temporary workers' inferior health status [4,21]. The association between temporary employment and health is complex, though it has been explained by unhealthy behaviors (e.g., smoking, excess alcohol use, and sedentary leisure activity) in response to flexible employment [10]. In this context, temporary workers' unhealthy eating behaviors are not likely to differ significantly.

To our knowledge, this study is the first to show a significant association between temporary employment and unhealthy eating behaviors, i.e., skipping lunch and eating alone. Little evidence has been found on the effects of work types on eating behaviors [36]. Nevertheless, our findings are supported by prior results on the potential link between poor working conditions (e.g., job stress, long working hours, and shift work) and unhealthy diets [19]. In a study of Japanese male workers, negative psychological responses induced by job stress (e.g., fatigue, tension/anxiety, and depression) were significantly associated with eating behaviors causing obesity, namely with substitute eating and drinking and feelings of satiety, as well as motivations for eating [37]. In addition, observational studies have shown that workers engaged in rotating shift work exhibited more unbalanced diets (e.g., high fat intake and low intake of vegetables) and abnormal temporal eating patterns (e.g., skipping breakfast and/or late dinner) [38,39].

Based on the above research, the observed association between temporary employment and unhealthy eating behaviors is complex. Employment characteristics—specifically, greater job uncertainty, lower income, more limited workplace rights and social protection, and greater imbalance of power between employers and workers than in standard employment—could shape eating practices. Future studies are needed to confirm our findings and to examine potential mechanisms.

This study has several limitations. First, because of its cross-sectional design, we could not establish causal links between temporary employment and unhealthy eating habits. Confirming an association between them might require a prospective study or a longitudinal study, in which changes of employment status are accompanied by certain eating behaviors. Second, although this study was based on national representative data for the general population, our study sample was not truly representative of working people, due to possible bias arising from missing data on job status (contract type) and eating habits and due also to the exclusion of participants who were under dietary control (e.g., starving or fasting for reasons of disease or weight loss). However, this lack of representativeness was unlikely to have affected the association we observed between temporary employments and eating behaviors. Third, in the KNHANES survey, eating behaviors and confounding variables were investigated through retrospective, self-reports; thus, there remains a potential for recall and nonresponse biases. Finally, although we included many confounding variables including demographics and health behaviors, the effects of unmeasured confounders (e.g., job stress and work schedule) were not fully controlled in the statistical model.

5. Conclusions

In conclusion, we found that in Korea's working population, temporary workers skipped more meals and ate alone more than permanent workers. Despite this study's mentioned limitations, it provides preliminary evidence on unhealthy eating behaviors associated with contract type. Efforts to encourage temporary workers' healthy eating behaviors might be important in reducing health inequality due to employment status.

Author Contributions: J.-S.K. contributed to the design of the statistical analyses, the interpretation of the data, and the drafting of the manuscript for publication; K.-B.M. contributed to the design and interpretation of the data and the revising of the manuscript for publication; J.-Y.M. contributed to the conception and design of the study, the acquisition of data, the analysis and interpretation of data, and the drafting of the manuscript. All of the authors read and approved the final manuscript.

Funding: This research was funded by the Basic Science Research Program through the National Research Foundation of Korea (NRF) funded by the Ministry of Education, Science and Technology (grant no. 2017R1E1A1A01078235).

Conflicts of Interest: The authors declare no conflict of interest.

References

1. Caldbick, S.; Labonte, R.; Mohindra, K.; Ruckert, A. Globalization and the rise of precarious employment: The new frontier for workplace health promotion. *Glob. Health Promot.* **2014**, *21*, 23–31. [CrossRef] [PubMed]
2. *Non-Standard Forms of Employment–Report for Discussion at the Meeting of Experts on Non-Standard Forms of Employment*; International Labour Office (ILO): Geneva, Switzerland, 2015.
3. *Organisation for Economic Co-Operation and Development (OECD), Employment Outlook 2003: Towards More and Better Jobs*; OECD: Paris, France, 2003.
4. Virtanen, M.; Kivimäki, M.; Joensuu, M.; Virtanen, P.; Elovainio, M.; Vahtera, J. Temporary employment and health: A review. *Int. J. Epidemiol.* **2005**, *34*, 610–622. [CrossRef] [PubMed]
5. Virtanen, P.; Liukkonen, V.; Vahtera, J.; Kivimäki, M.; Koskenvuo, M. Health inequalities in the workforce: The labour market core–periphery structure. *Int. J. Epidemiol.* **2003**, *32*, 1015–1021. [CrossRef] [PubMed]
6. Kristensen, T.S. Challenges for research and prevention in relation to work and cardiovascular diseases. *Scand. J. Work. Environ. Health* **1999**, *25*, 550–557. [CrossRef] [PubMed]
7. Bonde, J.P.E. Psychosocial factors at work and risk of depression: A systematic review of the epidemiological evidence. *Occup. Environ. Med.* **2008**, *65*, 438–445. [CrossRef] [PubMed]
8. Min, K.B.; Park, S.G.; Hwang, S.H.; Min, J.Y. Precarious employment and the risk of suicidal ideation and suicide attempts. *Prev. Med.* **2015**, *71*, 72–76. [CrossRef]
9. Min, K.B.; Park, S.G.; Song, J.S.; Yi, K.H.; Jang, T.W.; Min, J.Y. Subcontractors and increased risk for work-related diseases and absenteeism. *Am. J. Ind. Med.* **2013**, *56*, 1296–1306. [CrossRef]
10. Jung, Y.; Oh, J.; Huh, S.; Kawachi, I. The effects of employment conditions on smoking status and smoking intensity: The analysis of Korean Labor & Income Panel 8th–10th wave. *PLoS ONE* **2013**, *8*, e57109.
11. Min, J.Y.; Park, S.G.; Hwang, S.H.; Min, K.B. Disparities in precarious workers' health care access in South Korea. *Am. J. Ind. Med.* **2016**, *59*, 1136–1144. [CrossRef]
12. Bauer, U.E.; Briss, P.A.; Goodman, R.A.; Bowman, B.A. Prevention of chronic disease in the 21st century: Elimination of the leading preventable causes of premature death and disability in the USA. *Lancet* **2014**, *384*, 45–52. [CrossRef]
13. Willett, W.C. Balancing life-style and genomics research for disease prevention. *Science* **2002**, *296*, 695–698. [CrossRef] [PubMed]
14. Mancini, P.; Marchini, A.; Simeone, M. Eating behaviour and well-being: An analysis on the aspects of Italian daily life. *Agric. Agric. Sci. Procedia* **2016**, *8*, 228–235. [CrossRef]
15. Darmon, N.; Drewnowski, A. Does social class predict diet quality? *Am. J. Clin. Nutr.* **2008**, *87*, 1107–1117. [CrossRef] [PubMed]

16. Belon, A.P.; Nieuwendyk, L.M.; Vallianatos, H.; Nykiforuk, C.I. Perceived community environmental influences on eating behaviors: A Photovoice analysis. *Soc. Sci. Med.* **2016**, *171*, 18–29. [CrossRef] [PubMed]
17. Galobardes, B.; Morabia, A.; Bernstein, M.S. Diet and socioeconomic position: does the use of different indicators matter? *Int. J. Epidemiol.* **2001**, *30*, 334–340. [CrossRef] [PubMed]
18. Keski-Rahkonen, A.; Kaprio, J.; Rissanen, A.; Virkkunen, M.; Rose, R.J. Breakfast skipping and health-compromising behaviors in adolescents and adults. *Eur. J. Clin. Nutr.* **2003**, *57*, 842. [CrossRef] [PubMed]
19. Devine, C.M.; Farrell, T.J.; Blake, C.E.; Jastran, M.; Wethington, E.; Bisogni, C.A. Work conditions and the food choice coping strategies of employed parents. *J. Nutr. Educ. Behav.* **2009**, *41*, 365–370. [CrossRef]
20. Benach, J.; Muntaner, C. Precarious employment and health: Developing a research agenda. *J. Epidemiol. Community Health* **2007**, *61*, 276–277. [CrossRef]
21. Lewchuk, W.; de Wolff, A.; King, A.; Polanyi, M. From job strain to employment strain: Health effects of precarious employment. *Just Labour* **2014**, *3*, 23–35. [CrossRef]
22. Kweon, S.; Kim, Y.; Jang, M.-j.; Kim, Y.; Kim, K.; Choi, S.; Chun, C.; Khang, Y.-H.; Oh, K. Data resource profile: The Korea National Health and Nutrition Examination Survey (KNHANES). *Int. J. Epidemiol.* **2014**, *43*, 69–77. [CrossRef]
23. Kuroda, A.; Tanaka, T.; Hirano, H.; Ohara, Y.; Kikutani, T.; Furuya, H.; Obuchi, S.P.; Kawai, H.; Ishii, S.; Akishita, M.; et al. Eating alone as social disengagement is strongly associated with depressive symptoms in Japanese community-dwelling older adults. *J. Am. Med. Dir. Assoc.* **2015**, *16*, 578–585. [CrossRef] [PubMed]
24. Kwon, A.R.; Yoon, Y.S.; Min, K.P.; Lee, Y.K.; Jeon, J.H. Eating alone and metabolic syndrome: A population-based Korean National Health and Nutrition Examination Survey 2013–2014. *Obes. Res. Clin. Pract.* **2018**, *12*, 146–157. [CrossRef] [PubMed]
25. Yokoyama, Y.; Onishi, K.; Hosoda, T.; Amano, H.; Otani, S.; Kurozawa, Y.; Tamakoshi, A. Skipping breakfast and risk of mortality from cancer, circulatory diseases and al causes: Findings from the Japan collaborative cohort study. *Yonago Acta Med.* **2016**, *59*, 55–60. [PubMed]
26. Drewnowski, A. Obesity, diets, and social inequalities. *Nutr. Res.* **2009**, *67*, S36–S39. [CrossRef] [PubMed]
27. De Irala-Estevez, J.; Groth, M.; Johansson, L.; Oltersdorf, U.; Prättälä, R.; Martínez-González, M.A. A systematic review of socio-economic differences in food habits in Europe: consumption of fruit and vegetables. *Eur. J. Clin. Nutr.* **2000**, *54*, 706. [CrossRef]
28. Smith, K.J.; Gall, S.L.; McNaughton, S.A.; Blizzard, L.; Dwyer, T.; Venn, A.J. Skipping breakfast: Longitudinal associations with cardiometabolic risk factors in the childhood determinants of adult health study. *Am. J. Clin. Nutr.* **2010**, *92*, 1316–1325. [CrossRef]
29. Pedersen, T.P.; Meilstrup, C.; Holstein, B.E.; Rasmussen, M. Fruit and vegetable intake is associated with frequency of breakfast, lunch and evening meal: cross-sectional study of 11-, 13-, and 15-year-olds. *Int. J. Behav. Nutr. Phys. Act.* **2012**, *9*, 9. [CrossRef]
30. Timlin, M.T.; Pereira, M.A. Breakfast frequency and quality in the etiology of adult obesity and chronic diseases. *Nutr. Res.* **2007**, *65*, 268–281. [CrossRef]
31. Ma, Y.; Bertone, E.R.; Stanek, E.J., 3rd; Reed, G.W.; Hebert, J.R.; Cohen, N.L.; Merriam, P.A.; Ockene, I.S. Association between eating patterns and obesity in a free-living US adult population. *Am. J. Epidemiol.* **2003**, *158*, 85–92. [CrossRef]
32. Bi, H.; Gan, Y.; Yang, C.; Chen, Y.; Tong, X.; Lu, Z. Breakfast skipping and the risk of type 2 diabetes: A meta-analysis of observational studies. *Public Health Nutr.* **2015**, *18*, 3013–3019. [CrossRef]
33. Hetherington, M.M.; Anderson, A.S.; Norton, G.N.; Newson, L. Situational effects on meal intake: A comparison of eating alone and eating with others. *Physiol. Behav.* **2006**, *88*, 498–505. [CrossRef] [PubMed]
34. Kimura, Y.; Wada, T.; Okumiya, K.; Ishimoto, Y.; Fukutomi, E.; Kasahara, Y.; Chen, W.; Sakamoto, R.; Fujisawa, M.; Otsuka, K.; et al. Eating alone among community-dwelling Japanese elderly: Association with depression and food diversity. *J. Nutr. Health Aging* **2012**, *16*, 728–731. [CrossRef] [PubMed]
35. Paquet, C.; St-Arnaud-McKenzie, D.; Ma, Z.; Kergoat, M.-J.; Ferland, G.; Dube, L. More than just not being alone: The number, nature, and complementarity of meal-time social interactions influence food intake in hospitalized elderly patients. *Gerontologist* **2008**, *48*, 603–611. [CrossRef] [PubMed]
36. Dixon, J.; Woodman, D.; Strazdins, L.; Banwell, C.; Broom, D.; Burgess, J. Flexible employment, flexible eating and health risks. *Crit Public Health* **2014**, *24*, 461–475. [CrossRef]
37. Nishitani, N.; Sakakibara, H.; Akiyama, I. Eating behavior related to obesity and job stress in male Japanese workers. *Nutrition* **2009**, *25*, 45–50. [CrossRef]

38. Hemiö, K.; Puttonen, S.; Viitasalo, K.; Härmä, M.; Peltonen, M.; Lindström, J. Food and nutrient intake among workers with different shift systems. *Occup. Environ. Med.* **2015**, *72*, 513–520. [CrossRef] [PubMed]
39. St-Onge, M.-P.; Ard, J.; Baskin, M.L.; Chiuve, S.E.; Johnson, H.M.; Kris-Etherton, P.; Varady, K. Meal timing and frequency: Implications for cardiovascular disease prevention: A scientific statement from the American Heart Association. *Circulation* **2017**, *135*, e96–e121. [CrossRef]

International Journal of
Environmental Research and Public Health

MDPI

Article

Sociodemographic Associations of Physical Activity in People of Working Age

Daniel Puciato

Faculty of Physical Education and Physiotherapy, Opole University of Technology, ul. Prószkowska 76, 45-758 Opole, Poland; d.puciato@po.edu.pl or d.puciato@po.opole.pl

Received: 29 April 2019; Accepted: 14 June 2019; Published: 17 June 2019

Abstract: The aim of this study was to identify relationships between the physical activity and sociodemographic status of respondents aged 18–64 years. The research was conducted in 2014 and 2015 in Wrocław, Poland. The study group comprised 4460 people. The sample selection was random and stratified. The research tool was the International Physical Activity Questionnaire—Short Form. Levels of physical activity declared by respondents were compared with the recommendations of the American College of Sports Medicine (ACSM). Data on respondents' sociodemographic status was also obtained. The Mann–Whitney *U* test for samples, Kruskal–Wallis test by ranks, and total and binary logistic regression were used in statistical analysis. Among the respondents, the ACSM health recommendations were met by 43.7% in total (43.2% women and 44.3% men). All analyzed sociodemographic variables differentiated respondents' physical activity. The youngest respondents were found to be the most physically active. Wrocław residents with a secondary education declared the highest level of physical activity. Among the respondents, manual workers revealed the highest, and the unemployed the lowest odds of meeting the ACSM standards of health-related physical activity. The level of physical activity of unmarried respondents was higher than that of married respondents. The highest percentage of respondents (50.9% women and 54.2% men) with sufficient physical activity levels was found among people living alone. Measures aimed at reducing hypokinesia should be addressed primarily in vulnerable groups, i.e., the unemployed and oldest men.

Keywords: physical activity; demographic factors; social factors; working age; city; population studies

---

1. Introduction

Reduced physical activity is associated with a growing incidence of lifestyle diseases and premature deaths [1,2]. The effects of hypokinesia are particularly acute for people of working age, as their ability to work depends, to a large extent, on their health status and fitness and performance endurance, which are determined and sustained by physical activity [3]. Therefore, physical exercise of the appropriate volume, frequency, and intensity plays a significant role in both disease prevention and rehabilitation. On the one hand, physical activity contributes to the maintenance or increase of performance capacity and general psychophysical fitness and, on the other hand, it enables the full recovery after diseases, injuries, and fatigue [4].

A low level of physical activity is indirectly related to the occurrence of a number of negative consequences for working-aged people and their families, workplaces, and the entire national economy. For employees, these consequences include, for example, longer working hours and lower work quality, more and longer absenteeism, lower income from work and pensions, and lower quality of life. Reduction of work efficiency, greater turnover of employees and related financial costs, problems with work organization, or declining economic efficiency are the main causes of employees' hypokinesia for the enterprises employing them. Potential negative effects on the national economy include a shorter life expectancy of physically inactive people, increased healthcare costs, increased spending on sickness benefits, rehabilitation and disability benefits, a lower number of economically active people, reduced state tax revenues and, ultimately, a low economic growth rate [5].

The above problems make it necessary to attach more and more importance to preventive measures aimed at improving people's lifestyles, including increasing the level of physical activity. However, the development of effective public health plans and strategies must be preceded by diagnostic activities aimed at identifying the main problem areas. With regard to physical activity, this is not only about its overall assessment, but also about its determinants. The results of previous studies show that physical activity is significantly differentiated among various social groups [6–8]. Such a diagnosis will make it possible to reach out to groups at particular risk of hypokinesia, and to plan activities aimed at increasing their level of physical activity.

An important group of determinants of physical activity are sociodemographic factors. Despite numerous studies on this issue, the results have been ambiguous and still indicate different directions and strengths of perceived associations [4,9–13]. So far, the number of people in the household has not been considered as a factor influencing the physical activity of working-aged individuals, especially during their professional work, at home, and in leisure time. Few studies have also been conducted on representative samples of local populations. Authors have also rarely examined associations between physical activity and socioeconomic status separately for men and women, while the impact of particular factors on physical activity can differ in respondents of both sexes.

Considering the above introductory remarks, the aim of this study is to identify relationships between the physical activity and sociodemographic status of respondents aged 18–64 years.

The study addresses the following research problems:

1. What percentage of respondents meets the criteria of health-related physical activity formulated by the American College of Sports Medicine?
2. Do such sociodemographic features as age, level of education, occupation, marital status, and the number of people in the household determine respondents' compliance with ACSM recommendations for health-related physical activity?
3. Are the strength and directions of relationships between physical activity and sociodemographic variables similar in both the studied women and men?

2. Methods

The study was conducted in March and November of both 2014 and 2015 in Wrocław, Poland. The research project had been given positive approval by the Commission of Bioethics of the University School of Physical Education in Wroclaw. The participants were 4460 people, including 2331 women and 2129 men aged 18–64 years. Their characteristics and selected sociodemographic variables are presented in Table 1. The sampling was random (three-stage group variant) and stratified (proportional variant). First, ten out of the alphabetically ranked housing estates of Wrocław were drawn using a random number table, then, following a similar mechanism, three streets were drawn in each housing estate, the inhabitants of which took part in the study. The number of respondents from each housing estate was proportional to the number of its inhabitants. Moreover, the planned sample was divided into layers in which the stratifying features included the respondents' sex and age. A proportional variant was adopted so that the number of respondents in each subpopulation was proportional to the size of the layers of the population of working aged people from Wrocław.

The minimum sample size was calculated following the formula [14]:

$$n = \frac{N}{1 + \frac{4d^2(N-1)}{z_\alpha^2}}$$

where n—minimum sample size; N—number of working-aged residents from Wrocław; d—standard error of estimate; z_α—critical value of normal distribution at assumed confidence interval.

Restrictive assumptions were made as to the acceptable error of estimate ($d = 0.02$) and confidence interval ($\alpha = 0.01$). Under these assumptions, the minimum sample size was estimated at 4122 people. During the survey about 10% more questionnaires were collected. After eliminating incomplete or incorrectly completed questionnaires, 4460 people remained in the sample. The number of respondents were taken into account and their random selection for the survey made the sample representative of the population of all Wrocław working-aged residents.

Table 1. Number and structure of respondents grouped according to sociodemographic characteristics.

Variable	Total (*n* = 4460)		Women (*n* = 2331)		Men (*n* = 2129)	
	n	%	*n*	%	*n*	%
Age (years)						
15–24	620	13.9	317	13.6	303	14.2
25–34	1189	26.7	609	26.1	580	27.2
35–44	882	19.8	444	19.0	438	20.6
45–54	756	17.0	396	17.0	360	16.9
55–64	1013	22.6	565	24.3	448	21.1
Education						
primary and basic vocational	1740	39.0	802	34.4	938	44.1
secondary	1617	36.3	996	42.7	621	29.2
higher	1103	24.7	533	22.9	570	26.7
Occupation						
manual worker	1165	26.1	424	18.2	741	34.8
white-collar worker	1356	30.4	764	32.8	592	27.8
self-employed	616	13.8	216	9.3	400	18.8
student	637	14.3	441	18.9	196	9.2
pensioner	283	6.3	240	10.3	43	2.0
unemployed	403	9.1	246	10.5	157	7.4
Marital status						
unmarried	1828	41.0	1000	42.9	828	38.9
married	2632	59.0	1331	57.1	1301	61.1
Number of people in the household						
1	561	12.6	218	9.4	343	16.1
2	1003	22.5	564	24.2	439	20.6
3	1264	28.3	675	29.0	589	27.7
4	1173	26.3	622	26.7	551	25.9
≥5	459	10.3	252	10.7	207	9.7

The main research method was a diagnostic questionnaire survey. The International Physical Activity Questionnaire—Short Form (IPAQ-SF) was used [15]. Consideration was given to total physical activity, including physical efforts at work, at home, while commuting, and during leisure time. Respondents' self-assessments of the volume (duration) and frequency of physical activity at two levels of intensity—high and moderate—were analyzed. The total volume of physical activity expressed in METmin/week was also determined. For this purpose, the MET (metabolic equivalent of task) value corresponding to a given level of physical activity intensity was multiplied by the number of days of physical activity per week and its duration in minutes per day. For example, the intensity of physical activity of an individual practicing jogging four times a week corresponding to 7 MET amounted to $4 \times 60 \times 7 = 1680$ (METmin/week).

The collected data permitted a comparison of the declared physical activity with the recommendations of the American College of Sports Medicine [16]. The ACSM recommendations were chosen because of the lack of Polish norms of physical activity for people in a wide age range and the authors' intention to compare the obtained results with the results of their previous research. [4,12]. According to the ACSM, it is recommended to undertake physical activity (1) with a high intensity—at least 3 times a week for 20 min a day, or (2) with a moderate intensity—at least 5 times a week for 30 min a day. In the opinion of the authors of the recommendations, this is the minimum level of physical activity, and the implementation of smaller physical efforts may contribute to deterioration of physical fitness and increase the risk of obesity, chronic diseases, and disabilities. Respondents meeting at least one of these criteria were considered to be following the ACSM recommendations. The questionnaire survey also provided information on selected sociodemographic factors, i.e., sex (male, female), age (15–24, 25–34, 35–44, 45–54, 55–64 years), education (primary and basic vocational, secondary, higher), occupation (manual workers, white-collar workers, self-employed, students, unemployed, pensioners), marital status, and the number of people in the household (1, 2, 3, 4, 5, and more).

The obtained data were ordered and subject to structured analysis. The main measures were the number and the percent, which were grouped according to different criteria and listed in tables. The study assessed the asymmetry of the distribution of variables using the asymmetry coefficient (S). Description of the data distribution structure was supplemented with the coefficient of aggregation, kurtosis (K). The test of compliance with the Kolmogorov–Smirnov normal distribution was also carried out. The analysis of test results indicated that the distribution significantly deviated from the standard normal distribution. As a consequence, medians and quartile deviations were calculated. The significance of differences between the total physical activity of male and female respondents in groups separated by age, education, occupation, and the number of people in the household was verified with the Mann–Whitney U test for samples of n and $m > 20$ while, for marital status, the Kruskal–Wallis test by ranks was used. The significance of differences between particular groups was determined with a post hoc test. The analysis of the relationships between the self-assessment of physical activity by the examined women and men and their sociodemographic characteristics was performed using binary logistic regression. All calculations were performed with the use of the SPSS Statistics 20 software (IBM, Armonk, NY, USA) package. The exante level of statistical significance was set at $\alpha = 0.05$.

3. Results

The total weekly physical activity of the studied women and men was significantly correlated with all sociodemographic variables ($p < 0.001$). The highest mean values of correlation were founded in respondents of both sexes aged 18–34 years, and in men aged 45–54 years. The median energy expenditure was the lowest in women aged 45–54 and in the oldest men. The fact that the average ranks of weekly physical activity in groups separated by age were significantly different was confirmed not only by the value of the Kruskal–Wallis test, but also by the p-values for multiple (post hoc) comparisons. The highest level of total physical activity was noted in respondents with a secondary education (2586.0 METmin/week in women, 2994 METmin/week in men), and the lowest in respondents with a primary education (1950.0 METmin/week and 2190.0 METmin/week). The comparison between the post hoc groups showed that statistically significant differences in average values of position measures were found between physical activity of women with a basic vocational education and either a secondary education or higher education, and between men with a basic vocational education and either a secondary and higher education. Considering the occupational status, the most physically active groups of women were students, manual workers, and self-employed, while the most physically active men included pensioners, students, and manual workers. The lowest level of physical activity in women (1752.0 METmin/week) and in men (2072.0 METmin/week) was found among the unemployed. The level of physical activity of women ($Z = 5.39$, $p < 0.001$) and men ($Z = 5.41$, $p < 0.001$) was also determined by their marital status. In both groups of respondents, unmarried individuals were more physically active (2550.0 METmin/week and 2910.0 METmin/week) than married people (2175.0 METmin/week and 2316.0 METmin/week). The median values of energy expenditure of weekly physical activity were the highest in women from one-member (2696.0 METmin/week), two-member (2670.0 METmin/week), and five-and-more-member households (2565.0 METmin/week), and in men from five-and-more (2925.0 METmin/week) and one-member households (2796.0 METmin/week). The least physically active were women from four-member (2034.0 METmin/week) and men from two-member households (2713.1 METmin/week). Statistically significant intragroup differentiation—post hoc test ($p = 0.02$)—was found in women from Wrocław from four- and five-and-more-member households, and between men from two- and three-member households, and from two- and five-and-more member households (Tables 2 and 3).

Table 2. Differences in energy expenditure of total weekly physical activity of women with regard to sociodemographic characteristics.

Variable	Category	Energy Expenditure of Physical Activity (METmin/week)				Test Post Hoc—*p*-Value					
		Me	Q	H (Z)	*p*	(1)	(2)	(3)	(4)	(5)	(6)
Age (years)	(1) 18–24	2430.0	1165.0			x	1.00	0.04	0.00	0.00	x
	(2) 25–34	2565.0	1404.2			1.00	x	0.00	0.00	0.00	x
	(3) 35–44	1980.0	1147.5	42.2	0.00	0.04	0.00	x	1.00	1.00	x
	(4) 45–54	1752.0	1042.5			0.00	0.00	1.00	x	1.00	x
	(5) 55–64	1880.0	1181.0			0.00	0.00	1.00	1.00	x	x
Education	(1) primary	1950.0	1200.0			x	0.00	0.00	x	x	x
	(2) secondary	2586.0	1392.3	47.1	0.00	0.00	x	1.00	x	x	x
	(3) higher	2556.0	1802.2			0.00	1.00	x	x	x	x
Occupation	(1) unemployed	1752.0	845.0			x	0.00	0.45	0.00	0.00	0.00
	(2) student	2748.0	1357.7			0.00	x	0.00	1.00	0.00	1.00
	(3) pensioner	1950.0	1520.5			0.45	0.00	x	0.00	1.00	0.06
	(4) worker	2785.0	1428.0	65.0	0.00	0.00	1.00	0.00	x	0.00	1.00
	(5) white collar	2100.0	1438.2			0.00	0.00	1.00	0.00	x	0.19
	(6) self-employed	2641.5	1227.0			0.00	1.00	0.06	1.00	0.19	x
Marital status	(1) unmarried	2550.0	1341.0	5.3	0.00	x	x	x	x	x	x
	(2) married	2175.0	1379.0			x	x	x	x	x	x
Number of people in the household	(1) 1	2696.0	1502.2			x	1.00	0.82	1.00	0.18	x
	(2) 2	2670.0	1210.0			1.00	x	1.00	0.38	1.00	x
	(3) 3	2455.0	1387.5	13.7	0.00	0.82	1.00	x	0.08	1.00	x
	(4) 4	2034.0	1174.0			1.00	0.38	0.08	x	0.02	x
	(5) ≥5	2565.0	1331.2			0.18	1.00	1.00	0.02	x	x

Abbreviations: Me—median, Q—quartile deviations, H—Kruskal–Wallis test, Z—Mann–Whitney test, *p*—test probability value, x—the item cannot be filled in due to the arrangement of the table, or it is not possible or intended to be filled in.

Table 3. Differences in energy expenditure of total weekly physical activity of men with regard to sociodemographic characteristics.

Variable	Category	Energy Expenditure of Physical Activity (METmin/week)				Test Post Hoc—*p*-Value					
		Me	Q	H (Z)	*p*	(1)	(2)	(3)	(4)	(5)	(6)
Age (years)	(1) 18–24	3386.0	1344.0			x	0.00	0.00	0.00	0.00	x
	(2) 25–34	3066.0	1653.3			0.00	x	0.00	1.00	0.00	x
	(3) 35–44	2316.0	1246.5	97.3	0.00	0.00	0.00	x	0.00	1.00	x
	(4) 45–54	3105.0	1713.3			0.00	1.00	0.00	x	0.05	x
	(5) 55–64	2031.0	1518.0			0.00	0.00	1.00	0.05	x	x
Education	(1) primary	2190.0	1680.0			x	0.00	0.11	x	xx	x
	(2) secondary	2994.0	1672.5	25.2	0.00	0.00	x	0.03	x	x	x
	(3) higher	2649.0	1555.7			0.11	0.03	x	x	x	x
Occupation	(1) unemployed	2072.0	720.0			x	0.00	0.00	0.00	0.47	1.00
	(2) student	3220.5	1248.3			0.00	x	1.00	0.05	0.00	0.00
	(3) pensioner	3390.0	1302.0			0.00	1.00	x	1.00	0.11	0.02
	(4) worker	2745.0	1776.0	58.0	0.00	0.00	0.05	1.00	x	0.03	0.00
	(5) white collar	2346.0	1404.3			0.47	0.00	0.11	0.03	x	1.00
	(6) self-employed	2316.0	1773.0			1.00	0.00	0.02	0.00	1.00	x
Marital status	(1) unmarried	2910.0	1528.8	5.41	0.00		x	x	x	x	x
	(2) married	2316.0	1584.0				x	x	x	x	x
Number of people in the household	(1) 1	2796.0	1885.5			x	0.05	1.00	1.00	1.00	x
	(2) 2	2072.0	1393.5			0.05	x	0.02	0.32	0.00	x
	(3) 3	2499.0	1588.0	16.6	0.00	1.00	0.02	x	1.00	1.00	x
	(4) 4	2613.0	1194.0			1.00	0.32	1.00	x	0.44	x
	(5) ≥5	2925.0	1687.5			1.00	0.00	1.00	0.44	x	x

Abbreviations: Me—median, Q—quartile deviations, H—Kruskal–Wallis test, Z—Mann–Whitney test, *p*—test probability value, x—the item cannot be filled in due to the arrangement of the table, or it is not possible or intended to be filled in.

Among the Wrocław residents aged 18–64 years, the ACSM health-related physical activity standards were met by 43.7% of respondents, 43.2% of whom were women and 44.3% were men. Tables 3 and 4 show the results of logistic regression, revealing associations between ACSM recommendations and respondents' sociodemographic characteristics. In the group of women, significant associations between physical activity and age were observed in women aged from 35 to 44 years. The odds of their meeting the ACSM recommendations were 33% lower than in the age group of 18 to 24 years. Considering the level of education, the women with a secondary education were almost 80% more likely to fulfill the health-related physical activity recommendations than women with a primary and vocational education. Statistically significant associations between physical activity and occupation were found among manual and white-collar workers, the self-employed, pensioners, and the unemployed. The highest percentage of sufficiently physically active respondents was observed among manual workers (54.2%), and the lowest among the unemployed (30.1%). The odds of meeting the health-related physical activity recommendations were almost three times higher among manual workers (OR = 0.36; CI: 0.26–0.51) than among the unemployed. Almost half of unmarried women and 38.5% of married women were sufficiently physically active. The odds of unmarried women meeting the ACSM standards were almost 40% higher than married women. The number of people in the household was a factor determining the physical activity of women living in one-, two-, and four-person households. Health-related physical activity recommendations were most frequently followed by respondents who lived alone, and the odds of their fulfilling the recommendations was about one-third higher than by women living in two- or four-person households (Table 4).

Table 4. Physical activity and selected sociodemographic associations in studied women from Wrocław (n = 2331).

Variable	ACSM				OR	CI	
	Yes		No				
	n	%	n	%		−95%	95%
Age (years)							
18–24	139	43.8	178	56.2	Ref.	-	
25–34	291	47.8	318	52.2	1.172	0.89	1.54
35–44	152	34.2	292	65.8	0.667	0.50	0.90
45–54	160	40.4	236	59.6	0.868	0.64	1.17
55–64	266	47.1	299	52.9	1.139	0.86	1.50
Education							
primary and basic vocational	293	36.5	509	63.5	Ref.	-	
secondary	503	50.5	493	49.5	1.772	1.47	2.14
higher	212	39.8	321	60.2	1.147	0.92	1.44
Occupation							
manual worker	230	54.2	194	45.8	Ref.	-	
white collar worker	292	38.2	472	61.8	0.522	0.41	0.66
self-employed	95	44.0	121	56.0	0.662	0.48	0.92
student	220	49.9	221	50.1	0.840	0.64	1.10
pensioner	97	40.4	143	59.6	0.572	0.42	0.79
unemployed	74	30.1	172	69.9	0.363	0.26	0.51
Marital status							
unmarried	496	49.6	504	50.4	Ref.	-	
married	512	38.5	819	61.5	0.635	0.54	0.75
Number of persons in the household							
1	111	50.9	107	49.1	Ref.	-	
2	223	39.5	341	60.5	0.630	0.46	0.86
3	309	45.8	366	54.2	0.814	0.60	1.10
4	249	40.0	373	60.0	0.644	0.47	0.88
≥ 5	116	46.0	136	54.0	0.822	0.57	1.18

Abbreviations: OR—odds ratio; CI—confidence interval; Ref.—reference groups; ACSM Yes—respondents meeting ACSM recommendations; ACSM No—respondents not meeting ACSM recommendations.

The highest percentage of sufficiently physically active men in terms of meeting ACSM recommendations was found among the representatives of the two youngest groups of respondents, 63.4% and 55.0%, respectively; and the lowest among the oldest respondents, i.e., 27.2%. The odds of meeting health-related physical activity standards were almost five times higher in the youngest men than in the oldest ones. In men with a secondary education, the odds of meeting the ACSM recommendations were nearly 50% higher than in respondents with a basic and vocational education (OR = 1.48; CI = 1.21–1.82). Statistically significant associations between physical activity and occupation were noted among manual and white-collar workers, the self-employed, and the unemployed. The odds of meeting ACSM standards in the manual workers was almost four times higher than in the unemployed respondents (OR = 0.28; CI = 0.20–0.42). In comparison with married men, the odds of meeting ACSM recommendations were more than twice as high as in single men. The lower limit of 95% confidence interval for odds ratio was 0.39, while the upper limit was 0.55. Among the unmarried men, the recommended physical activity was performed by 55.8%, while among married men, by 37.0%. Similarly to the group of women, this observation was confirmed by the high level of physical activity of men living alone, out of whom 54.2% met the ACSM standards. The odds of respondents from five-person households meeting these recommendations were almost twofold, and from two-person households almost threefold lower, compared to the reference group, i.e., men from one-person households (Table 5).

Table 5. Physical activity and selected sociodemographic associations in studied men from Wrocław (n = 2129).

Variable	ACSM				OR	CI	
	Yes		No				
	n	%	n	%		−95%	95%
Age (years)							
18–24	192	63.4	111	36.6	Ref.	-	
25–34	319	55.0	261	45.0	0.707	0.53	0.94
35–44	137	31.3	301	68.7	0.263	0.19	0.36
45–54	173	48.1	187	51.9	0.535	0.39	0.73
55–64	122	27.2	326	72.8	0.216	0.16	0.30
Education							
primary and basic vocational	396	42.2	542	57.8	Ref.	-	
secondary	323	52.0	298	48.0	1.484	1.21	1.82
higher	224	39.3	346	60.7	0.886	0.72	1.10
Occupation							
manual worker	402	54.3	339	45.7	Ref.	-	
white collar worker	215	36.3	377	63.7	0.481	0.39	0.60
self-employed	137	34.3	263	65.8	0.439	0.34	0.57
student	120	61.2	76	38.8	1.332	0.97	1.84
pensioner	29	67.4	14	32.6	1.747	0.91	3.36
unemployed	40	25.5	117	74.5	0.288	0.20	0.42
Marital status							
unmarried	462	55.8	366	44.2	Ref.	-	
married	481	37.0	820	63.0	0.465	0.39	0.55
Number of persons in the household							
1	186	54.2	157	45.8	Ref.	-	
2	131	29.8	308	70.2	0.359	0.27	0.48
3	280	47.5	309	52.5	0.765	0.59	1.00
4	263	47.7	288	52.3	0.771	0.59	1.01
≥ 5	83	40.1	124	59.9	0.565	0.40	0.80

Abbreviations: OR—odds ratio; CI—confidence interval; Ref.—reference groups; ACSM Yes—respondents meeting the ACSM recommendations; ACSM No—respondents not meeting the ACSM recommendations.

4. Discussion

During a typical week, the majority of respondents performed physical efforts that were insufficient to achieve positive health effects. In addition, an association between physical activity and sociodemographic factors was observed in the study, and groups of respondents with relatively high and particularly low levels of physical activity were identified. The most physically active were the youngest respondents, people with a secondary education, college students, manual workers, unmarried individuals, and respondents from one-member households. The groups of respondents with a particularly low level of physical activity were the unemployed and men from the oldest age group. As they are particularly threatened by hypokinesia, public health programs, including measures aimed at increasing physical activity, should be primarily addressed to them.

In terms of relationships between physical activity and age, it was noted that the most physically active were the youngest respondents of both sexes and the oldest women, while the least active were respondents aged 35–44 years and the oldest men. While the relatively high physical activity in young people and its decrease with age have been reported in the literature [4,8,12,17,18], the noted high level of physical activity in the oldest women and the low level in the age group of 35–44 year-olds have been rarely found. However, Moniruzzaman et al. [19] also observed relatively high levels of physical activity in urban women aged 55–64 years. This may be due to the fact that the workload and household duties of women at this age are often lower due to their retirement and their children living on their own. Still, good health and quite common participation of women in organized forms of leisure activities, e.g., universities of the third age, allow them to take part in relatively intensive physical activities [20]. It should be emphasized, however, that relatively high levels of physical activity of older people were not found in earlier studies. This may have been caused by the fact that in the group of women aged 55–64, there was an overrepresentation of people with normal body structure and good physical and health condition. Rocha et al. [21] also reported the lowest percentage of leisure time physical activity among 35–46-year-olds. However, Nawrocka et al. [7] found no significant correlations between physical activity and age. An attempt to explain this phenomenon could be that the fact that 30–50 years of age is often connected with the dynamic development of one's professional career, family life, and social activity. It may be connected with limited free time and decreasing motivation to undertake physical exercises. Moreover, in the current economic reality, it is also often a period of debt repayments resulting from the purchase of an apartment or a house, its furnishings, etc. This further intensifies the pressure to increase working time at the expense of reduced leisure time. This interpretation of low physical activity of people aged 35–44 years is also supported by the fact that only one in four respondents performed physical work. In most cases, an increase in working hours was not associated with an increase in physical activity. Not without significance may also be the health problems prevalent in people at this age, e.g., obesity, spinal pain, or emotional exhaustion, which are not conducive to undertaking physical activity [22–24].

Respondents' education level turned out to be a significant social factor determining physical activity. The respondents of both sexes with a secondary education were characterized by a higher level of total physical activity and fulfilled the ACSM standards more often than those with a primary and basic vocational education. Positive correlations between physical activity and the level of education had been found by Kwaśniewska et al. [8], Choi et al. [25], Msambichaka et al. [26], and Rocca et al. [27]. Our earlier research on the Katowice population [4,12] and studies by Biernat [9] and Gubelmann [28] indicated a decrease in physical activity with an increase in the level of education. The current study, however, revealed a rare phenomenon of the highest physical activity level in respondents with a secondary education. This may demonstrate that in today's urban environment, the secondary level of education has already been associated with sufficiently high cultural, social, and economic capital and its benefits, also in relation to health behaviors including health-related physical activity. Jurakic et al. [29] also showed that the amount of undertaken physical exercise was positively correlated with educational attainment. The education structure and labor market requirements may also significantly contribute to the fact that a large number of people with a secondary education perform physical work, which may affect the respondents' total physical activity analyzed in the present study.

In the Wrocław population, the highest probability of meeting physical activity standards among manual workers—as also previously noted among adult inhabitants of Katowice [4]—was confirmed. Similar results were obtained by Chen et al. [30]. Most likely, the high total physical activity of this occupational group is mainly due to their high physical activity levels unrelated to exercise. Mirecz et al. [31] also demonstrated that physical activity was one of the most important predictors of mental health and employees' ability to work in executive positions. This may also motivate manual workers to undertake physical efforts outside their occupational field. Low physical activity among non-working people was also documented in the literature [4,19,32], possibly determined by a lack of physical activity at work, limited financial resources, and the negative psychological and social consequences of unemployment. Higher physical activity levels were noted in unmarried than married persons. Similar observations were made by Basset et al. [32], according to whom one of the main reasons for this was mostly high physical activity associated with single people than in people in relationships. Individuals living alone, with no family life, have more free time, some of which they may use for physical exercise. This is confirmed by the relatively high percentage of male and female respondents from one-person households meeting the ACSM recommendations. Slightly surprising, however, is the noted lowest level of physical activity among respondents from four-member households (women) and two-member households (men). These groups were characterized by a lower level of physical activity than individuals living alone, as well as than respondents from three- or even five-or-more-member households. This factor has not been previously analyzed in studies of working-age populations. It was considered only by Peralta et al. [33] and only in relation to the elderly. These authors found the highest physical activity among people over 65 years living in households with five or more persons, and the lowest among people living alone. The high levels of physical activity of respondents from households with the largest number of people may be due to several reasons. The first one is the high intensity of physical activity in their professional work and house duties, which is probably necessary for the proper functioning of a large family. At present, well-paid jobs are also common in industrial labor posts which require significant physical contributions from employees. The second is the observation that large households are not always households with many children. Sometimes these are simply multigenerational families in which grandparents can financially support parents or help them carry out household duties or care for children. This offers them quite good prospects in terms of undertaking leisure time physical activity. On the other hand, two-person households are not only childless married couples or domestic partnerships, but also single parents with a child. While for childless couples, the possibilities of spending free time seem to be great, it can be quite different for single parents. For similar reasons, the low physical activity of women from four-person households can be observed.

The present study has its strengths and limitations. The strengths certainly include a research sample which is representative of Wrocław, and an analysis of physical activity among representatives of various sociodemographic groups. The analysis of occupational status as a modifier of physical activity should be considered particularly valuable, as previous studies have rarely compared manual workers, white-collar workers, entrepreneurs, school and college students, retired people, and the unemployed. The analysis of relations between the level of physical activity and the number of people in the household, which had not been carried out before among people in this age bracket, is also innovative in the context of obtained results. The relatively high physical activity in the oldest age group of women and the positive role of secondary education as a modifier of total physical activity are interesting observations that have not been accounted for in earlier research. On the other hand, limitations of the study included use of the short form of the physical activity questionnaire, and lack of data on respondents' body weight, physical fitness, and health status, the cross-sectional nature of research, and the limitation of the spatial scope to one city. The main drawbacks of the short version of the IPAQ questionnaire, as compared to objective methods of physical activity measurement, include difficulty in estimating the intensity and duration of physical activity, problems with remembering on which days of the week respondents engaged in physical activity, and a tendency to overestimate the level of their physical activity [34,35]. Future studies should use tools enabling not only a comprehensive but also a separate analysis of physical activity in different areas of human life, i.e., at work, at home, in leisure time, or while commuting. They should also include the measurement of somatic features and the assessment of respondents' physical fitness and health status. This will allow for an in-depth analysis of test results and an explanation of possible artefacts, e.g., the lack of a linear relationship between physical activity and the age of respondents. The continuity of such research and extending its spatial scope not only to other large cities but also to smaller towns and villages are definitely worth considering. This approach will allow researchers to create a specific map of spatial units and sociodemographic groups, especially those threatened by hypokinesia. Thanks to systematic research, it will also be possible to identify trends in physical activity which seem to be particularly important due to the dynamic and turbulent changes currently taking place in Central Europe and worldwide.

5. Conclusions

1. The level of physical activity of the majority of respondents was insufficient to obtain significant health benefits.
2. Age, level of education, occupation, marital status, and the number of people in the household significantly differentiated respondents' physical activity.
3. The highest physical activity was observed in persons aged up to 34 years, with a secondary education, manual workers, college students, single respondents, and respondents living in one-member households.
4. The unemployed respondents of both sexes and the oldest men are two groups at particular risk of hypokinesia. Consequently, programs aimed at physical activity improvement should be addressed primarily to these groups.
5. In the studied group, there were not many differences in the directions and strength of physical activity and sociodemographic characteristics in respondents of both sexes. The exceptions were the high physical activity of respondents aged 55–64 years, found only in the group of women, and the lowest level of physical activity among women from four-person households and men from two-person households.

Funding: This research received no external funding.

Conflicts of Interest: The authors declare no conflict of interests regarding the publication of this paper.

References

1. Li, J.; Siegrist, J. Physical Activity and Risk of Cardiovascular Disease-A Meta-Analysis of Prospective Cohort Studies. *Int. J. Environ. Res. Public Health* **2012**, *9*, 391–407. [CrossRef]
2. Śmigielski, J.; Ruszkowska, J.; Piotrowski, W.; Polakowska, M.; Bielecki, W.; Hanke, W.; Drygas, W. The relationship between physical activity level and selected cardiovascular risk factors and mortality of males ≥50 years in Poland—The results of follow-up of participants of National Multicentre Health Survey WOBASZ. *Int. J. Occup. Med. Environ. Health* **2016**, *29*, 633–648. [CrossRef] [PubMed]
3. Rożek-Piechura, K.; Ignasiak, Z.; Sławińska, T.; Piechura, R.; Ignasiak, T. Respiratory function. physical activity and body composition in adult rural population. *Ann. Agric. Environ. Med.* **2014**, *21*, 369–374. [CrossRef] [PubMed]
4. Puciato, D.; Rozpara, M.; Mynarski, W.; Łoś, A.; Królikowska, B. Physical activity of adult residents of Katowice and selected determinants of their occupational status and socio-economic characteristics. *Med. Pr.* **2013**, *64*, 649–657. [PubMed]
5. Puciato, D.; Rozpara, M.; Borysiuk, Z. Physical activity as a determinant of quality of life in working-age people in Wrocław. Poland. *Int. J. Environ. Res. Public Health* **2018**, *15*, 623. [CrossRef] [PubMed]
6. Mynarski, W.; Grabara, M.; Nawrocka, A.; Niestrój-Jaworska, M.; Wołkowycka, B.; Cholewa, J. Physical recreational activity and musculoskeletal disorders in nurses. *Med. Pr.* **2014**, *65*, 181–188. [PubMed]

7. Nawrocka, A.; Prończuk, A.; Mynarski, W.; Garbaciak, W. Physical activity of top level managers in the context of the public health recommendations. *Med. Pr.* **2012**, *63*, 271–279.
8. Kwaśniewska, M.; Pikała, M.; Bielecki, W.; Dziankowska-Zaborszczyk, E.; Rębowska, E.; Kozakiewicz, K.; Pająk, A.; Piwoński, J.; Tykarski, A.; Zdrojewski, T.; et al. Ten-year changes in the prevalence and socio-demographic determinants of physical activity among Polish adults aged 20 to 74 years. Results of the National Multicenter Health Surveys WOBASZ (2003–2005) and WOBASZ II (2013–2014). *PLoS ONE* **2016**, *11*, e0156766. [CrossRef]
9. Biernat, E. Factors increasing the risk of inactivity among administrative, technical and manual workers in Warszawa public institutions. *Int. J. Occup. Med. Environ. Health* **2015**, *28*, 283–294. [CrossRef]
10. Sallis, S.; Cervero, R.; Ascher, W.; Henderson, K.; Kraft, M.; Kerr, J. An ecological approach to creating more physically active communities. *Annu. Rev. Public Health* **2006**, *27*, 297–322. [CrossRef]
11. Biernat, E.; Krzepota, J.; Sadowska, D. Martial arts as a form of undertaking physical activity in leisure time analysis of factors determining participation of Poles. *Int. J. Environ. Res. Public Health* **2018**, *15*, 1989. [CrossRef] [PubMed]
12. Puciato, D.; Mynarski, W.; Rozpara, M.; Nawrocka, A. Physical activity of Katowice Urban Area residents with regard to selected physical traits and social factors. *Rocz. Panstw. Zakl. Hig.* **2018**, *69*, 273–280. [PubMed]
13. Drygas, W.; Sakłak, W.; Kwaśniewska, M.; Bandosz, P.; Rutkowski, M.; Bielecki, W.; Rębowska, E.; Prusik, K. Epidemiology of physical activity in adult Polish population in the second decade of the 21st century. Results of the NATPOL 2011 study. *Int. J. Occup. Med. Environ. Health* **2013**, *26*, 846–855. [CrossRef] [PubMed]
14. Brzeziński, J. *Methodology of Psychological Research*; PWN: Warsaw, Poland, 2011; pp. 246–247.
15. International Physical Activity Questionnaire. Available online: http://ipaq.ki.se/ipaq.htm (accessed on 17 October 2014).
16. American College of Sports Medicine. The recommended quantity and quality of exercise for developing and maintaining cardiorespiratory and muscular fitness in healthy adults. *Med. Sci. Sports Exerc.* **1990**, *22*, 265–274.
17. Hallal, P.; Andersen, L.; Bull, F.; Guthold, R.; Haskell, W.; Ekelund, U. Global physical activity levels: Surveillance progress pitfalls and prospects. *Lancet* **2012**, *380*, 247–257. [CrossRef]
18. Gerovasili, V.; Agaku, I.; Vardavas, C.; Filippidis, F. Levels of physical activity among adults 18–64 years old in 28 European countries. *Prev. Med.* **2015**, *81*, 87–91. [CrossRef] [PubMed]
19. Moniruzzaman, M.; Ahmed, M.; Zaman, M. Physical activity levels and associated socio-demographic factors in Bangladeshi adults: A cross-sectional study. *BMC Public Health* **2017**, *17*, 59. [CrossRef] [PubMed]
20. Krzepota, J.; Biernat, E.; Florkiewicz, B. The relationship between levels of physical activity and quality of life among students of the University of the Third Age. *Cent. Eur. J. Public Health* **2015**, *23*, 335–339.
21. Rocha, S.; Barbosa, A.; Araújo, T. Leisure-time physical inactivity among healthcare workers. *Int. J. Occup. Med. Environ. Health* **2018**, *31*, 251–260. [CrossRef]
22. Brienza, J.; Bobocel, D. Employee age alters the effects of justice on emotional exhaustion and organizational deviance. *Front. Psychol.* **2017**, *8*, 479. [CrossRef]
23. Cho, K.; Cho, E.; Hur, J.; Shin, D. Association of sleep duration and obesity according to gender and age in Korean adults: Results from the Korea National Health and Nutrition Examination Survey 2007–2015. *J. Korean Med. Sci.* **2018**, *33*, e345. [CrossRef] [PubMed]
24. Rottermund, J.; Knapik, A.; Saulicz, E.; Myśliwiec, A.; Saulicz, M.; Rygiel, K.; Linek, P. Back and neck pain among school teachers in Poland and its correlations with physical activity. *Med. Pr.* **2015**, *66*, 771–778. [CrossRef] [PubMed]
25. Choi, B.; Schnall, P.; Yang, H.; Dobson, M.; Landsbergis, P.; Israel, L.; Karasek, R.; Baker, D. Psychosocial working conditions and active leisure-time physical activity in middle-aged US workers. *Int. J. Occup. Med. Environ. Health* **2010**, *23*, 239–253. [CrossRef] [PubMed]
26. Msambichaka, B.; Abdul, R.; Abdulla, S.; Klatser, P.; Tanner, M.; Kaushik, R.; Bringolf-Isler, B.; Geubbels, E.; Eze, I. A cross-sectional examination of physical activity levels and their socio-demographic determinants in Southern Tanzania. *Int. J. Environ. Res. Public Health* **2018**, *15*, 1054. [CrossRef] [PubMed]
27. Rocca, P.; Beckman, A.; Hansson, E.; Ohlsson, H. Is the association between physical activity and healthcare utilization affected by self-rated health and socio-economic factors? *BMC Public Health* **2015**, *15*, 737. [CrossRef] [PubMed]

28. Gubelmann, C.; Vollenweider, P.; Marques-Vida, P. Of weekend warriors and couch potatoes: Socio-economic determinants of physical activity in Swiss middle-aged adults. *Prev. Med.* **2017**, *105*, 350–355. [CrossRef] [PubMed]
29. Jurakic, D.; Golubic, A.; Pedisic, Z.; Pori, M. Patterns and correlates of physical activity among middle-aged employees: A population-based cross-sectional study. *Int. J. Occup. Med. Environ. Health* **2014**, *27*, 487–497. [CrossRef]
30. Chen, M.; Wu, Y.; Narimatsu, H.; Li, X.; Wang, C.; Luo, J.; Zhao, G.; Chen, Z.; Xu, W. Socioeconomic status and physical activity in Chinese adults: A report from a community based survey in Jiaxing China. *PLoS ONE* **2015**, *10*, e0132. [CrossRef]
31. Merecz, D.; Mościcka, A.; Drabek, M.; Koniarek, J. Predictors of mental health status and work ability of blue-collar workers. *Med. Pr.* **2004**, *55*, 425–433.
32. Bassett, D.; Wyatt, H.; Thompson, H.; Peters, J.; Hill, J. Pedometer-measured physical activity and health behaviors in U.S. adults. *Med. Sci. Sports Exerc.* **2010**, *42*, 1819–1825. [CrossRef]
33. Peralta, M.; Martins, J.; Guedes, D.; Sarmento, H.; Marques, A. Socio-demographic correlates of physical activity among European older people. *Eur. J. Ageing* **2018**, *15*, 5–13. [CrossRef] [PubMed]
34. Craig, C.; Marshall, A.; Sjostrom, M.; Bauman, A.; Booth, M.; Ainsworth, B.; Pratt, M.; Ekelund, U.; Yngve, A.; Sallis, J.; et al. International physical activity questionnaire: 12-country reliability and validity. *Med. Sci. Sports Exerc.* **2003**, *35*, 1381–1395. [CrossRef] [PubMed]
35. Vuillemin, A.; Oppert, J.; Guillemin, F.; Essermeant, L.; Fontvieille, A.; Galan, P.; Kriska, A.; Hercberg, S. Self-administered questionnaire compared with interview to assess past-year physical activity. *Med. Sci. Sports Exerc.* **2000**, *32*, 1119–1124. [CrossRef] [PubMed]

International Journal of
Environmental Research and Public Health

MDPI

Article

Burnout and Metabolic Syndrome in Female Nurses: An Observational Study

Gabriela Chico-Barba [1,2], Karime Jiménez-Limas [2,*], Bernarda Sánchez-Jiménez [3], Reyna Sámano [1], Ana Lilia Rodríguez-Ventura [1], Rafael Castillo-Pérez [1] and Maricruz Tolentino [1]

1 Departmento de Nutrición y Bioprogramación, Instituto Nacional de Perinatología, Ciudad de México 11000, Mexico; gabyc3@gmail.com (G.C.-B.); ssmr0119@yahoo.com.mx (R.S.); rovalilia@hotmail.com (A.L.R.-V.); armando.castillo1958@gmail.com (R.C.-P.); cruz_tolentino@yahoo.com.mx (M.T.)

2 Escuela de Enfermería, Facultad de Ciencias de la Salud, Universidad Panamericana, Ciudad de México 03920, Mexico

3 Subdirección de Investigación en Intervenciones Comunitarias, Instituto Nacional de Perinatología, Ciudad de México 11000, Mexico; emiberna20@yahoo.com.mx

* Correspondence: 0192342@up.edu.mx or kari_jilk@hotmail.com

Received: 25 April 2019; Accepted: 28 May 2019; Published: 5 June 2019

Abstract: Nurses are at risk of having burnout due to workload and job stress—studies have reported that chronic stress is associated with metabolic syndrome. This study aimed to assess the association between burnout and metabolic syndrome in a sample of female nurses. Data were collected from a cross-sectional study from 2016 to 2018 in a tertiary hospital in Mexico City. All nurses that work in the hospital were invited to participate. Information pertaining to sociodemographic (age, education level), work (labor seniority, service area, shift work), anthropometric (weight, waist circumference, blood pressure) and biochemical (glucose, serum lipids) variables were collected. Burnout was assessed using the Maslach Burnout Inventory test, and metabolic syndrome was defined according to the International Diabetes Federation criteria. A total of 168 nurses participated with a median age of 44 years. The prevalence of burnout and metabolic syndrome was 19.6% and 38.7%, respectively. There was no association between burnout and metabolic syndrome ($p = 0.373$). However, associations of emotional exhaustion (aOR: 14.95; 95% CI: 1.5–148.7), personal accomplishment (aOR: 0.13; 95% CI: 0.01–0.99), and night shift (aOR: 12.39; 95% CI: 1.02–150.5) with increased waist circumference were found. Strategies are needed to prevent burnout and metabolic syndrome in nurses, especially in those who work at night shift.

Keywords: nurses; burnout; metabolic syndrome; waist circumference; emotional exhaustion; personal accomplishment; Mexico

1. Introduction

Burnout is a syndrome of emotional exhaustion, depersonalization, and low personal accomplishment, which is acquired by workers who have direct contact with customers and users [1]. Among the healthcare professionals, nurses are especially at risk of developing burnout due to the high workload and job stress that is mostly caused by working proximity to patients and taking care of them [2].

Some studies have shown that chronic stress is associated with metabolic syndrome in animal models [3] and clinical settings [4–6], but little is known about the relationship between burnout and metabolic syndrome.

There is evidence that burnout has an impact not only to the emotional status [7] and self-esteem [8] but also on metabolic profile. Cross-sectional studies have shown an association between cardiovascular risk factors and burnout [9,10]. On the other hand, a longitudinal study found an association between the risk factors for arteriosclerotic disease and the presence of burnout in healthy, middle-aged men [11]—burned out men had significant increases in their waist circumference and body weight at 4–5 years of follow-up.

The possible pathway between burnout and metabolic syndrome could be explained by the hypothalamic–pituitary–adrenal (HPA) axis. The HPA axis remains hyperactive in the presence of burnout due to exposure to chronic stress, resulting in fat accumulation [12,13]. Body fat mass is a risk factor for cardiometabolic diseases [14,15].

As health professionals, nurses should have good health to take care of the patients and also to be a health promoter, as they are role models, advocates, and educators. Nurses are exposed to different risk factors for non-chronic diseases, for instance, stress and anxiety as a result of their workload and daily interaction with sick people, low physical activity, and long working hours [16–18]. Their job characteristics make it difficult for nurses to have healthy habits, as studies have reported low self-care in nurses [16–18]. There is also a high prevalence of metabolic syndrome [19]. For the reasons mentioned above, the aim of this study was to assess the association between burnout and metabolic syndrome in a sample of female nurses.

2. Materials and Methods

2.1. Study Design

This observational, cross-sectional study included nurses who work at the Instituto Nacional de Perinatología (National Perinatology Institute, INPer) in Mexico City. Sampling was convenience, non-probabilistic, and based on consecutive cases that met the following inclusion criteria: to be a formal institutional employee, any age, any shift, and area of service. Nursing students, practitioners, and rotating personnel were excluded from the study, as well as pregnant women. Participants were enrolled from 2016 to 2018, with 509 nurses invited to participate, but only 171 (33%) joined the study. As only three men participated, they have been eliminated from the final sample, in addition to participants with incomplete questionnaires. The total sample consisted of 168 female nurses.

2.2. Sociodemographic Data and Working Information

The information regarding age, educational level, socioeconomic status, marital status, working shift, the area of service, labor seniority, having children, and having more than one job was obtained through a questionnaire.

2.3. Anthropometric Assessment

The method of measurement was standardized and performed by fixed personnel. Weight was obtained using a digital scale (Tanita Terraillon, 100 g of precision) and height was assessed using a stadiometer (SECA 231, 0.1 cm of precision). Body mass index (BMI) was calculated by dividing weight in kilograms by the height in square meters and was categorized according to the World Health Organization cutoff points [20]. Waist circumference was measured using a non-extensible tape (SECA 201, 1 mm of precision); the participants were asked to stand with their arms raised and abdomen uncovered, the tape was set at the midpoint between the last rib and the iliac crest, and after a normal exhalation, the measurement was taken. Blood pressure was obtained using a mercury sphygmomanometer in the non-dominant arm in the seated position after 5 min of resting, according to international standards [21]. Two measurements were made and the average was recorded.

2.4. Biochemical Analyses

Blood samples were obtained from 7:00 to 8:00 in the morning, after fasting for 12 h. Serum samples were frozen at −70 °C until the determination of glucose, glycated hemoglobin (HbA1c), total cholesterol, high-density lipoprotein (HDL) cholesterol, and triglycerides. Participants with an HbA1c >5.7% were given an oral glucose tolerance test (OGTT), as this cutoff point is an indicator of increased risk for diabetes, according to the American Diabetes Association guidelines [22]. For the OGTT, an amount of 75 g of glucose was used, and the reading was taken 2h post-test.

2.5. Burnout Assessment

Burnout was assessed using the Maslach Burnout Inventory—Human Services Survey test [23]. The questionnaire consists of 22 items, which evaluates three domains: emotional exhaustion (9 items), depersonalization (5 items), and personal accomplishment (8 items). Each item is assessed on a Likert scale, scoring from 0 to 6. A score was calculated by the sum of points of the items of each domain. Emotional exhaustion and depersonalization have a direct relationship with burnout while, contrarily, personal accomplishment has a negative relation. Even though Maslach proposed to classify each domain as low, mild, or high, it does not give a cutoff point to determine burnout as present or absent. For this study, the total points of each domain were divided into tertiles, and burnout was defined as tertile 3 of emotional exhaustion plus tertile 3 of depersonalization and/or tertile 1 of personal accomplishment, according to Kitaoka-Higashiguchi [11].

2.6. Metabolic Syndrome Definition

Metabolic syndrome was defined according to the International Diabetes Federation (IDF) [24]. The criteria are central obesity plus any two of the following: (1) triglycerides ≥150 mg/dL (1.7 mmol/L) or specific treatment for this lipid abnormality; (2) HDL cholesterol <50 mg/dL (1.29 mmol/L) in females or specific treatment for this lipid abnormality; (3) systolic blood pressure ≥130 mmHg or diastolic blood pressure ≥85 mm Hg or treatment of previously diagnosed hypertension; and (4) fasting plasma glucose ≥100 mg/dL or previously diagnosed type 2 diabetes. Central obesity was defined as waist circumference ≥80 cm.

2.7. Ethics

The Institutional Review Boards and Ethics Committees from Instituto Nacional de Perinatología (Reg. 212250-3300-11402-01-15) and Facultad de Ciencias de la Salud Universidad Panamericana (Reg. CIEE-001-2017-01) approved the study. Data gathering was confidential, taking into account ethical issues such as autonomy and respect for persons. The guidelines of the Helsinki Declaration were followed. The identification information of the patients was replaced by a folio number, to ensure the confidentiality of the data. All participants received nutritional attention at INPer. If necessary, they also received psychological and medical attention.

2.8. Statistical Analysis

We performed a descriptive analysis of the characteristics of the study population. Metabolic syndrome factors were categorized into two categories, according to IDF cutoff points (e.g., triglycerides ≥150 mg/dL), and frequencies and percentages were calculated for each factor. A Chi-square test was used to determine the association between burnout and metabolic syndrome. Logistic regression models were performed using the metabolic syndrome factors separately as dependent variables and burnout domains in tertiles as independent variables. The reference categories were tertile 1 for emotional exhaustion and depersonalization, and tertile 3 of personal accomplishment. The models were adjusted for sociodemographic, anthropometric and working variables. All statistical analyses were carried out using IBM SPSS Statistics for Windows, Version 20.0 (IBM Corp, Armonk, NY, USA). Statistical significance was considered at $p < 0.05$.

3. Results

A total of 168 nurses participated in the study. Table 1 shows that the median age of the participants was 44 years. Most of them were married (61.3%) and had children (74.4%). The most frequent education level was college (37.5%), followed by technician (28.6%). It was found that 60.7% of the nurses worked in intensive care units. More than half of our sample belonged to the day shift (61.9%) and had only one job (89.9%).

Table 1. General characteristics of the total sample of nurses.

Category	Variable		n (%)
Sociodemographics	Age (years) [1]		44 (38–50)
	Marital status		
		Single	65 (39)
		Married	103 (61)
	Educational level		
		Technician	57 (34)
		College	63 (38)
		Graduate	48 (28)
	Having children		
		Yes	125 (74)
		No	43 (26)
Working related variables	Labor senority (years) [2]		24 (16–28)
	Working years in current service		4 (2–13)
	Service area		
		Intensive care units	102 (61)
		Inpatients	20 (12)
		Outpatients	22 (13)
		No contact with patients	24 (14)
	Shift work		
		Day (8-hour length)	104 (62)
		Mid-day (7-hour length)	14 (8)
		Night(12-hour length)	50 (30)
	More than one job		
		Yes	17 (10)
		No	151 (90)

[1] Median (P25–P75). [2] Service area according to the type of patients attended.

The prevalence of burnout and metabolic syndrome in the sample were 19.6% and 38.7%, respectively. Regarding metabolic syndrome criteria, 82.1% of the nurses had increased waist circumference (82.1%), followed by low HDL cholesterol (60.1%). Only 4.2% had high blood pressure (Figure 1).

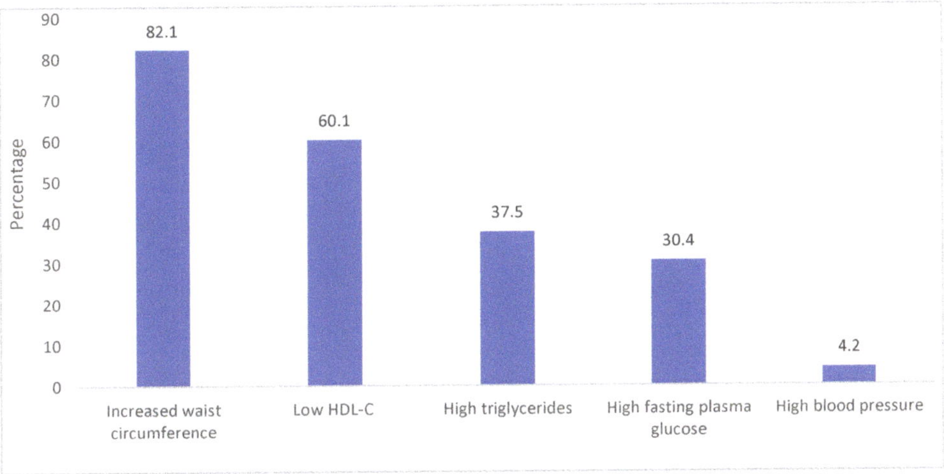

Figure 1. Prevalence of metabolic syndrome criteria in the total sample of nurses. HDL-C: high-density lipoprotein cholesterol.

There was no association between burnout and metabolic syndrome ($p = 0.373$). However, an association between the burnout domains and components of the metabolic syndrome factors was found (Table 2).

Nurses in tertile 2 of emotional exhaustion had a higher risk of having increased waist circumference (adjusted OR: 14.95; 95% CI: 1.5–148.7; $p = 0.021$), compared to tertile 1. Contrarily, nurses in tertile 2 of personal accomplishment had a lower risk of having increased waist circumference (aOR: 0.13; 95% CI: 0.01–0.99; $p = 0.049$), compared to tertile 1. Also, nurses who work in the night shift had a higher risk of having increased waist circumference (aOR: 12.39; 95% CI: 1.02–150.5; $p = 0.048$). The service area did not show an association with increased waist circumference. There was no association between the burnout domains and the other metabolic syndrome criteria (Table 2).

Table 2. Association of burnout domains with metabolic syndrome factors.

Independent Variables	Increased Waist Circumference			Low HDL-C			High Triglycerides			High Fasting Plasma Glucose			High Blood Pressure		
	aOR	95% CI	*p*	aOR	95% CI	*p*	aOR	95% CI	*p*	aOR	95% CI	*p*	aOR	95% CI	*p*
Emotional exhaustion															
T1		Reference			Reference			Reference			Reference			Reference	
T2	**14.95**	**1.50–148.71**	**0.021**	0.84	0.35–2.01	0.710	1.26	0.53–3.01	0.593	0.54	0.21–1.38	0.199	0.43	0.03–5.33	0.513
T3	3.57	0.70–18.15	0.125	0.66	0.28–1.57	0.356	1.24	0.52–2.95	0.613	0.40	0.15–1.06	0.067	2.35	0.25–21.7	0.450
Depersonalization															
T1		Reference			Reference			Reference			Reference			Reference	
T2	4.28	0.62–29.65	0.140	1.45	0.63–3.35	0.380	1.17	0.51–2.65	0.706	1.11	0.44–2.76	0.816	0.42	0.05–3.52	0.425
T3	1.60	0.25–10.24	0.615	1.10	0.47–2.54	0.822	0.91	0.39–2.14	0.838	1.60	0.63–4.04	0.316	0.23	0.01–3.80	0.308
Personal accomplishment															
T1	0.26	0.03–2.36	0.234	1.20	0.50–2.84	0.673	0.61	0.25–1.46	0.271	0.80	0.30–2.08	0.653	0	0–0	0.997
T2	**0.13**	**0.01–0.99**	**0.049**	0.77	0.33–1.80	0.551	0.77	0.33–1.78	0.546	2.10	0.86–5.15	0.103	1.60	0.25–9.98	0.611
T3		Reference			Reference			Reference			Reference			Reference	
Shift															
Day		Reference			Reference			Reference			Reference			Reference	
Mid-day	13.93	0.52–369.9	0.115	2.58	0.59–11.2	0.206	0.61	0.13–2.84	0.534	1.19	0.28–5.09	0.810	0.82	0.3–18.71	0.904
Night	**12.39**	**1.02–150.5**	**0.048**	0.55	0.24–1.25	0.156	1.08	0.47–2.46	0.846	0.97	0.39–2.38	0.948	0.75	0.08–6.97	0.805

aOR: adjusted odds ratio, CI: confidence interval, HDL-c: high density lipoprotein cholesterol. Logistic regression models adjusted by age, service area, and body mass index. Bold numbers show statistically significant associations.

4. Discussion

In this sample of Mexican female nurses, the prevalence of burnout (19.6%) was lower than that reported in other studies. Miranda-Lara et al. found a 33.8% rate of burnout in a similar sample of Mexican nurses [25]. We have considered different possible explanations for this difference. The first one is that the Maslach Burnout Inventory classifies the level to which the syndrome domains are found (low, mild, or high) but it does not give a cutoff point to determine burnout [23]. The second explanation is that the study performed by Miranda-Lara et al. does not mention the cutoff points used to define the presence of burnout, so the figures cannot be comparable. Finally, more than half of our sample (66%) had a high education level—it has been demonstrated in other studies that women with high burnout scores were more likely to have lower education levels [26].

Regarding the metabolic syndrome, the prevalence in our study was lower than the reported for Mexican female adults [27] (38.7% vs. 52.7%), but similar when compared to nurses from other countries. In a sample of Brazilian nurses, the prevalence of metabolic syndrome was 38.1% [9]. Again, we consider the presence of a high education level as a possible explanation, as it has been reported that the lower the education, the higher the frequencies of metabolic syndrome [27,28]. The reason may be because a low education level could cause differences in opportunities for workers to access health services and affect health-related behaviors. In particular, the lower the socioeconomic status of female workers (which usually may depend on education level), the less they care about healthcare and, hence, the higher the risk of metabolic syndrome [28].

When analyzing the metabolic syndrome criteria separately, we found that the prevalence of increased waist circumference in our study (82.1%) was close to the 87.8% reported for Mexican adult women, described in the 2016 Halfway National Health and Nutrition Survey (Ensanut MC 2016) [29]. Moreover, waist circumference was higher in those who worked night shifts. Other studies report similar findings, as working at night is associated with an increased risk of obesity [30], cardiovascular diseases [31], and cancer [32].

On the other hand, the low prevalence of hypertension found in this study (4%) was surprisingly low compared to the 25.5% [29] and 32% reported for the Mexican population and Brazilian nurses, respectively [33]. The reasons behind this low prevalence are still being studied. We consider that the nurses that already had hypertension did not want to participate in the study because they wanted their health information to remain confidential. We came to this assumption after having informal and confidential interviews with some nurses after their participation in the study—they said that they prefer to hide their hypertension diagnosis. There is little evidence regarding this issue. The World Medical Association, in their statement on physician well-being, says that physicians hide their diseases because of denial, confidentiality issues, aversion to the patient role, fear of disciplinary action, and loss of performance-based payment, among others [34]. We believe that the same phenomenon occurs with nurses, as they act as role models in healthcare.

As for the association between burnout domains and metabolic syndrome criteria separately, we found that low emotional exhaustion was associated with increased waist circumference. There is no study that has ever tried to associate these variables. Other articles have related the burnout syndrome with an increase in abdominal adiposity [35], waist circumference, body weight, and BMI [11], but no one has ever reported associations with a specific dimension of burnout. An explanation for this finding is that emotional exhaustion is associated with stress [36,37], and stress increases the risk of metabolic syndrome [4].

Regarding the association of mild personal accomplishment and lower odds of having high waist circumference, other studies reported similar findings by showing that low personal accomplishment was associated with sedentarism in adults [38]. Sedentarism may lead to increased waist circumference and overweight. Another study found that low self-esteem was associated with unhealthy lifestyle (less of 3 days per week and/or less of 30 min per session of physical activity and poor dietary habits) and, therefore, with increased adiposity [39].

Strategies are needed to prevent burnout and metabolic syndrome, and an exercise program may improve both. A previous interventional study explored the impact of an exercise program in banking and insurance workers. The study showed that the workers in the high-intensity exercise program had decreased burnout indicators and their systolic blood pressure was reduced, compared to the control group. In addition, systolic blood pressure was independently associated with burnout and exercise intensity in the crude model, but this was not significant in the adjusted model [40]. Nevertheless, strategies like this should be adapted to nurses' job and lifestyle, especially in those who work at night shift. Another intervention that has shown beneficial effects in health is yoga, with evidence from randomized control trials and systematic reviews showing that yoga reduced burnout, specifically emotional exhaustion and depersonalization [41,42], and improved cardiometabolic parameters, like fasting blood glucose, triglycerides, and blood pressure [43–45].

Regarding the pathway between burnout and metabolic syndrome, future studies should adequately assess biomarkers involved in the activation of the HPA axis, like serum cortisol. Even though cortisol levels increase when the HPA axis is activated in chronic stress [12], there is inconsistent evidence about the levels of cortisol and burnout. The evidence from different systematic reviews and meta-analysis showed that the comparability of the studies is limited due to poor quality assessments of cortisol and burnout [46,47].

One of the strengths of this study is that, to our knowledge, it is one of the few studies that assess the association of burnout and metabolic syndrome. Also, for the assessment of burnout, we used the Maslach Burnout Inventory, which continues to be the most widely used instrument and is considered to be the gold standard. Moreover, we had a high percentage of participation (33%) from nurses, since a 15% participation has been reported in other studies [40]. However, it is likely that non-participants may have had pre-existing cardiovascular diseases and, thus, did not wish to participate in the study. Another possible reason for not participating is that often the number of nurses in each service is inadequate, so they cannot leave their service to participate in our study assessments.

The sample size is one of the limitations of our study, as it is likely that a greater sample size would result in narrower confidence intervals and burnout domains to be associated with other metabolic syndrome criteria. Also, our sample is not representative of all Mexican nurses as it consists only of female nurses of a tertiary hospital. Regarding the cross-sectional design, we cannot assume causality in the associations that we found.

5. Conclusions

Amongst female nurses working in a tertiary hospital, there was no association between burnout and metabolic syndrome. Nevertheless, nurses in tertile 2 of emotional exhaustion had a higher risk of having increased waist circumference, and nurses in tertile 2 of personal accomplishment had a lower risk of having increased waist circumference. Strategies are needed to prevent burnout and metabolic syndrome in female nurses, especially in those who work at night shift.

Author Contributions: Conceptualization: B.S.-J., G.C.-B., and K.J.-L.; formal analysis: G.C.-B., and K.J.-L.; funding acquisition: B.S.-J., and A.L.R.-V.; investigation: B.S.-J., K.J.-L., R.S., M.T., R.C.-P., and A.L.R.-V.; methodology: K.J.-L., B.S.-J., A.L.R.-V., M.T., R.C.-P., and R.S.; project administration: G.C.-B.; supervision: G.C.-B.; writing—original draft: K.J.-L., and G.C.-B.; writing—review and editing: K.J.-L., G.C.-B., B.S.-J., and R.S.

Funding: This research was funded by Instituto Nacional de Perinatología, grant number 212250-3300-11402-01-15.

Acknowledgments: We thank Natalie Ávila-González, Antonio Villa and Ximena Rubilar for their contribution to this research.

Conflicts of Interest: The authors declare no conflict of interest.

References

1. Maslach, C.; Jackson, S.; Leiter, M. *Maslach Burnout Inventory*, 3rd ed.; Consulting Psychologists Press: Palo Alto, CA, USA, 1996.
2. Gómez-Urquiza, J.L.; De la Fuente-Solana, E.I.; Albendín-García, L. Prevalence of Burnout Syndrome in Emergency Nurses: A Meta-Analysis. *Crit. Care Nurse* **2017**, *37*, e1–e9. [CrossRef] [PubMed]
3. Branyan, K.W.; Devallance, E.R.; Lemaster, K.A.; Skinner, R.C.; Bryner, R.W.; Olfert, I.M.; Kelley, E.E.; Frisbee, J.C.; Chantler, P.D. Role of Chronic Stress and Exercise on Microvascular Function in Metabolic Syndrome. *Med. Sci. Sports Exerc.* **2018**, *50*, 957–966. [CrossRef] [PubMed]
4. Ortiz, M.S.; Sapunar, J. Longitudinal association between chronic psychological stress and metabolic syndrome. *Rev. Med. Chile* **2018**, *146*, 1278–1285. [CrossRef] [PubMed]
5. Chandola, T.; Brunner, E.; Marmot, M. Chronic stress at work and the metabolic syndrome: Prospective study. *Br. Med. J.* **2006**, *332*, 521–525. [CrossRef] [PubMed]
6. Bergmann, N.; Ballegaard, S.; Krogh, J.; Bech, P.; Hjalmarson, Å.; Gyntelberg, F.; Faber, J. Chronic psychological stress seems associated with elements of the metabolic syndrome in patients with ischaemic heart disease. *Scand. J. Clin. Lab. Investig.* **2017**, *77*, 513–519. [CrossRef] [PubMed]
7. Sánchez-Jiménez, B.; Flores-Ramos, M.; Sámano, R.; Rodíguez-Ventura, A.L.; Chinchilla Ochoa, D. Factores relacionados a la presencia del síndrome de burnout en una muestra de enfermeras del sector salud, Ciudad de México. *Rev. Salud Pública y Nutr.* **2018**, *17*, 1–8.
8. Chakraborty, R.; Chatterjee, A.; Chaudhury, S. Internal predictors of burnout in psychiatric nurses: An Indian study. *Ind. Psychiatry J.* **2012**, *21*, 119–124. [PubMed]
9. Ribeiro, P.R.; Marziale, H.M.P.; Martins, J.T.; Ribeiro, P.H.V.; Robazzi, M.L.D.C.C.; Dalmas, J.C. Prevalence of Metabolic Syndrome among nursing personnel and its association with occupational stress, anxiety and depression. *Rev. Lat.-Am. Enferm.* **2015**, *23*, 435–440. [CrossRef] [PubMed]
10. Das Merces, M.C.; Gomes, A.M.T.; Guimarães, E.L.P.; Santana, A.I.C.; De Souza e Silva, D.; Machado, Y.Y.; Couto, P.L.S.; França, L.C.M.; De Figueiredo, V.P.; D'Oliveira Júnior, A. Burnout and metabolic conditions are professionals of nursing: A pilot study. *Enfermagem Brasil.* **2018**, *17*, 90–98. [CrossRef]
11. Kitaoka-Higashiguchi, K.; Morikawa, Y.; Miura, K.; Sakurai, M.; Ishizaki, M.; Kido, T.; Naruse, Y.; Nakagawa, H. Burnout and risk factors for arteriosclerotic disease: Follow-up study. *J. Occup. Health* **2009**, *51*, 123–131. [CrossRef]
12. Melamed, S.; Shirom, A.; Toker, S.; Berliner, S.; Shapira, I. Burnout and risk of cardiovascular disease: Evidence, possible causal paths, and promising research directions. *Psychol. Bull.* **2006**, *132*, 327–353. [CrossRef] [PubMed]
13. Brunner, E.; Marmot, M. Social organization, stress, and health. In *Social Determinants of Health*; Marmot, M., Wilkinson, R., Eds.; Oxford University Press: New York, NY, USA, 2006; pp. 6–30.
14. Bastien, M.; Poirier, P.; Lemieux, I.; Després, J.P. Overview of epidemiology and contribution of obesity to cardiovascular disease. *Prog. Cardiovasc. Dis.* **2014**, *56*, 369–381. [CrossRef] [PubMed]
15. Ortega-Loubon, C.; Fernández-Molina, M.; Singh, G.; Correa, R. Obesity and its cardiovascular effects. *Diabetes Metab. Res. Rev.* **2019**, *35*, e3135. [CrossRef] [PubMed]
16. Priano, S.; Hong, O.; Chen, J. Lifestyles and Health-Related Outcomes of U.S. Hospital Nurses: A Systematic Review. *Nurs. Outlook* **2018**, *66*, 66–76. [CrossRef] [PubMed]
17. Blake, H.; Stanulewicz, N.; Griffiths, K. Healthy Lifestyle Behaviors and Health Promotion Attitudes in Preregistered Nurses: A Questionnaire Study. *J. Nurs. Educ.* **2017**, *56*, 94–103. [CrossRef] [PubMed]
18. Mustafaei Najaf-Abadi, H.; Rezaei, B. Health-promoting behaviours of Iranian nurses and its relationship with some occupational factors: A cross sectional study. *J. Nurs. Manag.* **2018**, *26*, 717–725. [CrossRef] [PubMed]
19. Shin, D.; Kongpakpaisarn, K.; Bohra, C. Trends in the prevalence of metabolic syndrome and its components in the United States 2007–2014. *Int. J. Cardiol.* **2018**, *259*, 216–219. [CrossRef] [PubMed]
20. World Health Organization. Obesity and Overweight. Fact Sheets. Available online: https://www.who.int/news-room/fact-sheets/detail/obesity-and-overweight (accessed on 20 April 2019).
21. Pickering, T.G.; Hall, J.E.; Appel, L.J.; Falkner, B.E.; Graves, J.; Hill, M.N.; Jones, D.W.; Kurtz, T.; Sheps, S.G.; Roccella, E.J. Recommendations for Blood Pressure Measurement in Humans and Experimental Animals. *Hypertension* **2004**, *45*, 142–161. [CrossRef]

22. American Diabetes Association. Classification and Diagnosis of Diabetes: Standards of Medical Care in Diabetes—2019. *Diabetes Care* **2019**, *42*, S13–S28. [CrossRef]
23. Maslach, C.; Leiter, M.P.; Schaufeli, W. Measuring Burnout. In *The Oxford Handbook of Organizational Well Being*; Cartwright, S., Cooper, C.L., Eds.; Oxford University Press: Oxford, UK, 2008; pp. 86–108. ISBN 9780199211913.
24. International Diabetes Federation. *IDF Diabetes Atlas*, 8th ed.; International Diabetes Federation: Brussels, Belgium, 2017; ISBN 9782930229874.
25. Miranda-Lara, V.R.; Monzalvo-Herrera, G.; Hernández-Caballero, B.; Ocampo-Torres, M. Prevalence of burnout syndrome in nursing staff of two health institutions. *Rev. Enferm Inst. Mex. Seguro Soc.* **2016**, *24*, 115–122.
26. Soares, J.J.F.; Grossi, G.; Sundin, Ö. Burnout among women: Associations with demographic/socio-economic, work, life-style and health factors. *Arch. Women's Ment. Health* **2007**, *10*, 61–71. [CrossRef]
27. Rojas, R.; Aguilar-Salinas, C.A.; Jiménez-Corona, A.; Shamah-Levy, T.; Rauda, J.; Ávila-Burgos, L.; Villalpando, S.; Lazcano Ponce, E. Metabolic syndrome in Mexican adults. Results from the National Health and Nutrition Survey 2006. *Salud Publica Mex.* **2010**, *52*, s11–s18. [CrossRef]
28. Cho, D.Y.; Koo, J.W. Differences in metabolic syndrome prevalence by employment type and sex. *Int. J. Environ. Res. Public Health* **2018**, *15*, 1798. [CrossRef]
29. Secretaría de Salud. *Encuesta Nacional de Salud y Nutrición de Medio Camino 2016*; Instituto Nacional de Salud Pública: Cuernavaca, Mexico, 2016.
30. Saulle, R.; Bernardi, M.; Chiarini, M.; Backhaus, I.; La Torre, G. Shift work, overweight and obesity in health professionals: A systematic review and meta-analysis. *Clin. Ter.* **2018**, *169*, e189–e197.
31. Peplonska, B.; Bukowska, A.; Sobala, W. Association of rotating night shift work with BMI and abdominal obesity among nurses and midwives. *PLoS ONE* **2015**, *10*, e0133761. [CrossRef]
32. Straif, K.; Baan, R.; Grosse, Y.; El Ghissassi, F.; Altieri, A.; Cogliano, V.; Group, W. Carcinogenicity of shift-work, painting, and fire-fighting. *Lancet Oncol.* **2007**, *8*, 1065–1066. [CrossRef]
33. Urbanetto, J.D.S.; Prado Lima Figuereido, A.E.; da Silva Gustavo, A.; Bosi de Souza Magnago, T.S.; Pinheiro da Costa, B.E.; Poli-de-Figueiredo, C.E. Arterial hypertension in nursing personnel of an emergency hospital. *Int. J. Nurs. Pract.* **2015**, *21*, 433–442. [CrossRef]
34. World Medical Association General Assembly. WMA Statement on Physicians Well-being. In Proceedings of the 66th WMA General Assembly, Moscow, Russia, 14–17 October 2015.
35. das Merces, M.C.; de Souza e Silva, D.; Lua, I.; Oliveira, D.S.; de Souza, M.C.; Júnior, A.D.O. Burnout syndrome and abdominal adiposity among Primary Health Care nursing professionals. *Psicol. Reflexão E Crítica* **2016**, *29*, 44. [CrossRef]
36. Halm, M.; Peterson, M.; Kandels, M.; Sabo, J.; Blalock, M.; Braden, R.; Gryczman, A.; Krisko-Hagel, K.; Larson, D.; Lemay, D.; et al. Hospital nurse staffing and patient mortality, emotional exhaustion, and job dissatisfaction. *Clin. Nurse Spec.* **2005**, *19*, 241–251. [CrossRef]
37. Friganović, A.; Selič, P.; Ilić, B.; Sedić, B. Stress and burnout syndrome and their associations with coping and job satisfaction in critical care nurses: A literature review. *Psychiatr. Danub.* **2019**, *31*, 21–31.
38. Agüero, S.D.; Sánchez, H.; Valladares, M.; López, A.; Badilla, P.V.; Herrera, T. Physical activity and style profile of life health promoters in older Chilean adults. *Rev. Med. Chile* **2017**, *145*, 1535–1540.
39. Sánchez-Jiménez, B.; Sámano, R.; Chinchilla-Ochoa, D.; Morales-Hernández, R.; Rodríguez-Ventura, A. Demographics and psychological factors associated with adiposity in nurses. *Int. J. Environ. Res. Public Health* **2018**, *15*, 634. [CrossRef]
40. Tsai, H.H.; Yeh, C.Y.; Su, C.T.; Chen, C.J.; Peng, S.M.; Chen, R.Y. The Effects of Exercise Program on Burnout and Metabolic Syndrome Components in Banking and Insurance Workers. *Ind. Health* **2013**, *51*, 336–346. [CrossRef]
41. Alexander, G.K.; Rollins, K.; Walker, D.; Wong, L.; Pennings, J. Yoga for Self-Care and Burnout Prevention among Nurses. *Workplace Health Saf.* **2015**, *63*, 462–470. [CrossRef]
42. Cocchiara, R.; Peruzzo, M.; Mannocci, A.; Ottolenghi, L.; Villari, P.; Polimeni, A.; Guerra, F.; La Torre, G. The Use of Yoga to Manage Stress and Burnout in Healthcare Workers: A Systematic Review. *J. Clin. Med.* **2019**, *8*, 284. [CrossRef]
43. Cramer, H.; Lauche, R.; Haller, H.; Steckhan, N.; Michalsen, A.; Dobos, G. Effects of yoga on cardiovascular disease risk factors: A systematic review and meta-analysis. *Int. J. Cardiol.* **2014**, *173*, 170–183. [CrossRef]

44. Cramer, H.; Langhorst, J.; Dobos, G.; Lauche, R. Yoga for metabolic syndrome: A systematic review and meta-analysis. *Eur. J. Prev. Cardiol.* **2016**, *23*, 1982–1993. [CrossRef]
45. Chu, P.; Gotink, R.A.; Yeh, G.Y.; Goldie, S.J.; Hunink, M.G.M. The effectiveness of yoga in modifying risk factors for cardiovascular disease and metabolic syndrome: A systematic review and meta-analysis of randomized controlled trials. *Eur. J. Prev. Cardiol.* **2016**, *23*, 291–307. [CrossRef]
46. Danhof-Pont, M.B.; van Veen, T.; Zitman, F.G. Biomarkers in burnout: A systematic review. *J. Psychosom. Res.* **2011**, *70*, 505–524. [CrossRef]
47. Cadegiani, F.A.; Kater, C.E. Adrenal fatigue does not exist: A systematic review. *BMC Endocr. Disord.* **2016**, *16*, 48.

International Journal of
Environmental Research and Public Health

MDPI

Article

Association between Occupational and Radiological Factors and Nontuberculous Mycobacteria Lung Infection in Workers with Prior Dust Exposure

Ji-Won Lee [1] and Jun-Pyo Myong [2,*]

[1] Department of Research for Occupational Health, Institute of Occupation and Environment, Incheon 21417, Korea; celest2120@gmail.com

[2] Department of Occupational and Environmental Medicine, Seoul St. Mary's Hospital, College of Medicine, The Catholic University of Korea, Seoul 06591, Korea

* Correspondence: dr_mjp@naver.com; Tel.: +82-2258-6267; Fax: +82-2258-6691

Received: 29 March 2019; Accepted: 30 May 2019; Published: 3 June 2019

Abstract: This retrospective cross-sectional study was conducted to identify the factors that promote the risk of nontuberculous mycobacteria (NTM) lung infection in subjects with prior occupational dust exposure. All consecutive patients with a history of occupational dust exposure whose expectorated sputum, bronchial wash, or bronchial lavage was subjected to acid-fast Bacilli culture in a tertiary hospital between 2011 and 2016 were identified. The patients who were infected with NTM were identified according to the bacteriological criteria of the American Thoracic Society (ATS) and The Infectious Diseases Society of America (IDSA) statement. Pneumoconiosis-associated radiological findings were graded according to the International Labor Organization guidelines. Of the 1392 patients with prior dust exposure, NTM was isolated from 82. Logistic regression analysis showed that risk factors for NTM lung infection were a history of pulmonary tuberculosis (adjusted odds ratio [aOR] = 1.82, 95% confidence intervals [CI] = 1.03–3.16). Moreover, the unadjusted odds ratios (ORs) were higher when both small-opacity profusion and the large-opacity grades increased. Even after adjustment, the ORs for the A, B, and C large-opacity grades were 2.32 (95% CI = 1.01–4.99), 2.68 (95% CI = 1.35–5.24), and 7.58 (95% CI = 3.02–17.95). Previous tuberculosis, bronchiectasis, and especially extensive small-opacity profusion, and high large-opacity grade associated significantly with NTM lung infection in dust-exposed workers.

Keywords: nontuberculous mycobacteria; occupational exposure; pneumoconiosis

---

1. Introduction

The nontuberculous mycobacteria (NTM) consist of all mycobacteria species except for *Mycobacterium tuberculosis* complex and *Mycobacterium leprae*. The most frequent target organ in NTM infections is the lung; more than 90% of NTM infections are in the lung [1,2]. Since untreated NTM lung disease can progress into extensive lung parenchymal destruction and death within years [1], there is an increasing interest in the diagnosis and treatment of NTM lung disease.

Risk factors for NTM lung disease include pulmonary conditions that associate with structural lung changes. These conditions include chronic obstructive pulmonary disease (COPD), bronchiectasis, previous tuberculosis (TB), and pneumoconiosis [3,4]. The latter disease, pneumoconiosis, is a restrictive lung disease that is caused by working for prolonged periods in dusty conditions (e.g., mining). Indeed, the Korean government considers NTM lung disease to be a complication of pneumoconiosis that deserves financial compensation.

While a history of silica exposure is a well-known risk factor for mycobacterial pulmonary infection in general [5], only a few clinical studies have addressed NTM infection in dust-exposed workers [6–11].

Moreover, none of these studies assessed the relationship between NTM infection and large opacities, which are a characteristic radiological feature of pneumoconiosis along with small opacities.

This retrospective cross-sectional study was conducted to identify the risk factors for NTM lung infection in patients who had a history of occupational dust exposure.

2. Methods

2.1. Patient Selection

This was a retrospective cross-sectional study that was conducted in a single hospital. The study cohort consisted of all consecutive inpatients and outpatients who had a history of occupational dust exposure and whose expectorated sputum, bronchial wash, or bronchial lavage was subjected to acid-fast Bacilli (AFB) culture in the Department of Occupational and Environmental Medicine of Seoul St. Mary's Hospital between 1 May 2011 and 28 February 2016. Patients with respiratory symptoms were recruited, but those with respiratory symptoms and other diseases such as stroke and musculoskeletal diseases were excluded. If the patient had a history of exposure to cotton dust or asbestos, which causes diseases other than coal worker's pneumoconiosis and silicosis, the patient was also excluded.

The study patients were considered to have an NTM lung infection on the basis of the diagnostic criteria for NTM lung disease that were established in 2007 by the American Thoracic Society (ATS) and The Infectious Diseases Society of America (IDSA) [3]. All subjects who had a dust-exposure history also had respiratory symptoms; therefore, it was hard to make a differential diagnosis based on the clinical criteria alone. Therefore, bacteriologic criteria alone were used to justify the case, and the term "NTM lung infection" was used instead of "NTM lung disease". This study was reviewed and approved by the Institutional Review Board of Seoul St. Mary's Hospital (KC17RESI0713).

2.2. Extraction of the General and Occupational Characteristics of the Patients

The age, medical history, and smoking status of each subject were extracted from the medical records. The patients were classified as a non-smoker (smoked ≤100 cigarettes in their lifetime and then stopped), ex-smoker (smoked >100 cigarettes in their lifetime and then quit), or current smoker (smoked >100 cigarettes in their lifetime and were currently smoking). The occupational characteristics, namely, type of job, duration of work, and type of dust to which the subjects had been exposed, were also determined. The type of job was classified as coal worker's pneumoconiosis or another job involving dust exposure. If the patients had several jobs, the job that had the longest duration was selected.

2.3. Radiological Findings

All patients underwent standard chest radiographs around the time of their AFB culture. These radiographs were assessed for the characteristic radiological findings of pneumoconiosis, and the opacities were classified according to their concentration into the four profusion categories (0, 1, 2, or 3) of the International Labor Organization (ILO) classification system. '0' profusion means that small opacities are absent, '1' profusion indicates the presence of a few small opacities, '2' profusion indicates the presence of partially obliterating vascular markings, and '3' profusion signifies the presence of totally obliterating vascular markings. In addition, the large opacities (i.e., those whose longest dimension exceeded 10 mm) were graded as A, B, or C opacities on the basis of the ILO classification system. 'A' indicates one (or more) large opacities whose (combined) longest dimension is 10–50 mm. 'B' indicates one (or more) large opacities whose (combined) longest dimension exceeds 50 mm but does not exceed the equivalent area of the right upper lung zone. 'C' indicates one (or more) large opacities whose (combined) longest dimension exceeds the equivalent area of the right upper lung zone [12].

Whether the patients had pulmonary comorbid radiological findings, namely, pneumoconiosis with emphysema, bronchitis, bronchiectasis, or cavitary lesion, was also assessed. These assessments were preferentially made on the basis of computed tomography (CT) chest images around the time that the AFB cultures were being performed. However, if the subjects did not undergo chest CT, the chest x-rays were used to assess comorbidity with emphysema, bronchitis, and bronchiectasis. The presence of a cavitary lesion was confirmed on the basis of chest CT only because some records did not mention the existence of a cavity.

2.4. Statistical Analysis

The patients with and without NTM were compared in terms of demographic, radiological, and clinical variables. Wilcoxon rank sum test was used to compare the two groups in terms of age and work duration because these continuous variables did not have normal distributions. The Chi-squared test and Fisher's exact test were used to compare the two groups. Multiple logistic regression analysis was performed to identify risk factors for NTM. Adjustments were made for age, work duration, smoking status, small-opacity profusion category, large-opacity grade, presence of bronchiectasis, and presence of a pulmonary cavity. The data were expressed as Odds ratios (OR) and 95% confidence intervals (CI). p-values of <0.05 were considered to indicate statistical significance. All analyses were performed using the Statistical Analysis System (SAS) version 9.4 (SAS Institute, Cary, NC, USA).

3. Results

In total, 1438 patients underwent an AFB culture of their sputum, bronchial wash, or lavage sample(s) during the study period. Of these, 46 were excluded because they had other diseases or were exposed to other dust such as asbestos. Therefore, the study cohort consisted of 1392 patients.

Of the 1392 subjects, 82 received a microbiological diagnosis of pulmonary NTM infection. The mean age of all subjects was 67.8 ± 8.1 years, and the mean duration of dusty work was 21.7 ± 10.7 years. Compared with the patients without NTM lung infection, the patients with NTM lung infection were significantly more likely to be in their 60 s and 70 s, to have diabetes and hypertension, to have a history of pulmonary TB, and to have been a coal worker. In terms of radiological features, the patients with lung NTM infection were significantly more likely than the patients without this infection to have category 2 and 3 small-opacity profusion and higher large-opacity grades (Table 1). They were also significantly more likely to have bronchiectasis and especially emphysema (Table 2).

Table 1. Differences between patients with and without NTM lung infection in terms of demographic, occupational, and radiological characteristics.

Total		No Recovery of Lung NTM, *n* (%)	Recovery of Lung NTM, *n* (%)	*p*-Value [a]
		1310 (94.1)	82 (5.9)	
Age, years				
	40–49	11 (0.8)	3 (3.6)	0.0052 *
	50–59	216 (16.5)	4 (4.9)	
	60–69	495 (37.8)	33 (40.3)	
	70–79	513 (39.2)	39 (47.6)	
	≥80	75 (5.7)	3 (3.6)	
Work duration, years				
	<10	273 (20.8)	7 (8.5)	0.0550
	10–19	354 (27.0)	30 (36.6)	
	20–29	338 (25.8)	25 (30.5)	
	30–39	238 (18.2)	13 (15.9)	
	≥40	107 (8.2)	7 (8.5)	
Gender				
	Male	1258 (96.0)	82 (100)	0.0659
	Female	52 (4.0)	0 (0)	

Table 1. *Cont.*

Total	No Recovery of Lung NTM, *n* (%)	Recovery of Lung NTM, *n* (%)	*p*-Value [a]
	1310 (94.1)	82 (5.9)	
Diabetes †			
No	749 (78.8)	39 (72.2)	0.2495
Yes	201 (21.2)	15 (27.8)	
Hypertension ‡			
No	552 (56.2)	30 (50)	0. 3514
Yes	431 (43.8)	30 (50)	
History of pulmonary tuberculosis §			
No	905 (77.7)	38 (60.3)	0.0015 *
Yes	260 (22.3)	25 (39.7)	
Smoking status			
Non-smoker	191 (21.3)	17 (22.4)	0.0644
Ex-smoker	571 (63.7)	55 (72.4)	
Current smoker	134 (15.0)	4 (5.2)	
Type of job			
Coal worker	932 (71.2)	68 (82.9)	0.0214 *
Other	378 (28.9)	14 (17.1)	
Pneumoconiosis characteristics			
Profusion of small opacities			
0	319 (24.4)	9 (11.0)	<0.0001 *
1	456 (34.8)	19 (23.2)	
2	438 (33.4)	43 (52.4)	
3	97 (7.4)	11 (13.4)	
Grade of large opacities			
No	926 (70.7)	35 (42.7)	<0.0001 *
A	154 (11.8)	17 (20.7)	
B	193 (14.7)	20 (24.4)	
C	37 (2.8)	10 (12.2)	

[a] *p*-values were obtained by comparing the groups using the Chi-squared test or Fisher's exact test. * Statistically significant values ($p < 0.05$). † 388 missing data on diabetes. A total of 1004 subjects were included. ‡ 349 missing data on hypertension. A total of 1043 subjects were included. § 164 missing data on tuberculosis. A total of 1228 subjects were included. 420 missing data on smoking status. A total of 972 subjects were included. NTM, nontuberculous mycobacteria.

Table 2. Differences between patients with and without NTM lung infection in terms of selected radiological features.

	No Recovery of Lung NTM, *n* (%)	Recovery of Lung NTM, *n* (%)	*p*-Value [a]
Pulmonary cavity on chest CT †			0.1954
No	764 (88.3)	65 (83.3)	
Yes	101 (11.7)	13 (16.7)	
Bronchitis			1.0000
No	1289 (98.4)	81 (98.8)	
Yes	21 (1.6)	1 (1.2)	
Bronchiectasis			0.0341 *
No	1182 (90.2)	68 (82.9)	
Yes	128 (9.8)	14 (17.1)	
Emphysema			<0.0001 *
No	811 (61.9)	22 (26.8)	
Yes	499 (38.1)	60 (73.2)	

[a] *p*-values were obtained by comparing the groups using the Chi-squared test or Fisher's exact test. * Statistically significant values ($p < 0.05$). † 449 missing data on pulmonary cavity on chest CT. A total of 943 subjects were included. CT, computed tomography; NTM, nontuberculous mycobacteria.

Multiple logistic regression analysis showed that, before adjustment, a history of pulmonary TB (OR = 2.29, 95% CI = 1.34–3.84) and the presence of bronchiectasis (OR = 1.90, 95% CI = 1.00–3.38) were risk factors for NTM lung infection (Table 3). Moreover, the risk of NTM lung infection rose with the degree of small-opacity profusion: category 1, 2, and 3 small-opacity profusion associated with crude ORs of 1.48 (95% CI = 0.68–3.47), 3.48 (95% CI = 1.75–7.72), and 4.02 (95% CI = 1.62–10.24), respectively. The risk of NTM lung infection also rose as the large-opacity grade rose: grades A, B, and C associated with crude ORs of 2.92 (95% CI = 1.56–5.27), 2.74 (95% CI = 1.53–4.81), and 7.15 (95% CI = 3.15–15.11), respectively.

Table 3. Multiple logistic regression analysis of the relationship between nontuberculous mycobacteria infection and occupational, clinical, and radiological characteristics.

	Unadjusted Model		Model 1 †		Model 2 ‡	
	OR	95% CI	OR	95% CI	OR	95% CI
Age (per year)	1.02	0.99–1.05	1.01	0.98–1.05	1.01	0.98–1.05
Work duration, years						
<20	1.00		1.00		1.00	
≥20	1.12	0.71–1.76	0.92	0.53–1.59	0.89	0.51–1.55
History of pulmonary tuberculosis						
No	1.00		1.00		1.00	
Yes	2.29 *	1.34–3.84	1.82 *	1.03–3.16	1.71	0.95–3.01
Bronchiectasis						
No	1.00		1.00		1.00	
Yes	1.90 *	1.00–3.38	0.99	0.43–2.03	1.01	0.44–2.09
Pulmonary cavity on chest CT						
No	1.00		1.00		1.00	
Yes	1.51	0.77–2.76	1.47	0.69–2.90	1.34	0.62–2.70
Profusion of small opacities						
0	1.00		1.00			
1	1.48	0.68–3.47	1.22	0.47–3.36		
2	3.48 *	1.75–7.72	2.79 *	1.25–7.10		
3	4.02 *	1.62–10.24	3.76 *	1.36–10.94		
Grade of large opacities						
No	1.00				1.00	
A	2.92	1.56–5.27			2.32 *	1.01–4.99
B	2.74	1.53–4.81			2.68 *	1.35–5.24
C	7.15 *	3.15–15.11			7.58 *	3.02–17.95

* Statistically significant values ($p < 0.05$). † Model 1: Adjusted for age, work duration, history of pulmonary tuberculosis, bronchiectasis, pulmonary cavity, and profusion of small opacities. ‡ Model 2: Adjusted for age, work duration, history of pulmonary tuberculosis, bronchiectasis, pulmonary cavity, and grade of large opacities. OR, odds ratio; CI, confidence interval.

When adjustments were made for age, work duration, history of pulmonary TB, bronchiectasis, pulmonary cavity, and small-opacity profusion (Model 1), history of pulmonary TB (OR = 1.82, 95% CI = 1.03–3.16) and category 2 (OR = 2.79, 95% CI = 1.25–7.10), and 3 (OR = 3.76, 95% CI = 1.36–10.94) small-opacity profusion remained risk factors for NTM lung infection. When the same adjustments were made except that small-opacity profusion was substituted by the large-opacity grade (Model 2), grade A (OR = 2.32, 95% CI = 1.01–4.99), B (OR = 2.68, 95% CI = 1.35–5.24), and C (OR = 7.58, 95% CI = 3.02–17.95), large opacities were risk factors for NTM lung infection.

The NTM species in 43 of 82 NTM lung infected patients were identified. A total of 61 outcomes were identified, including the isolation of multiple species from the same patient. Identified NTM species are shown in Table 4. Some species from respiratory specimens were considered not pathogenic and to be contaminants. *M. gordonae* in seven patients and *M. terrae* complex in one patient were also considered contaminants.

Table 4. NTM infected patients with species identification.

Species	Number of Patients	Number of Patients with Other Species	Other Species
M. avium	13	3	*M. kansasii, M. abscessus, M. fortuitum, M. gordonae*
M. intracellulare	13	5	*M. fortuitum, M. gordonae*
M. fortuitum	10	8	*M. avium, M. intracellulare, M. gordonae, M. abscessus, M. peregrinum, M. lentiflavum, M. celatum*
M. gordonae *	7	5	*M. avium, M. intracellulare, M. fortuitum, M. abscessus, M. smegmatis, M. lentiflavum*
M. abscessus	4	3	*M. avium, M. fortuitum, M. gordonae*
M. peregrinum	3	2	*M. fortuitum, M. lentiflavum*
M. smegmatis	3	2	*M. gordonae, M. lentiflavum*
M. lentiflavum	3	3	*M. fortuitum, M. gordonae, M. peregrinum, M. smegmatis*
M. kansasii	1	1	*M. avium*
M. chelonae	1	0	
M. celatum	1	0	
M. terrae complex *	1	0	
Other type	1	0	
Total	61		

* Species generally considered as environmental contamination. Three patients were identified with more than three species.

4. Discussion

Immunocompromised patients and patients with a pre-existing pulmonary disease often develop NTM infections, of which the *Mycobacterium avium* complex (MAC) are the most common agents. This study showed that the risk factors for a diagnosis of NTM lung infection in patients with prior occupational dust exposure were previous TB, bronchiectasis, extensive small-opacity profusion, and higher large-opacity grades. Even after adjustment, extensive small-opacity profusion and higher grade large opacities remained significant risk factors for NTM lung infection in dust-exposed workers.

While prior TB infection was a significant risk factor for NTM lung infection in the unadjusted model and Model 1, it had an increased OR without statistical significance in Model 2. This finding is consistent with the case-control study of Corbett et al., who showed that prior TB infection was also a risk factor for NTM lung disease in South African gold miners [13]. Corbett et al. suggested a post-tuberculous structure distortion and poor immunologic response to Mycobacterium antigen after TB infection to explain the association between prior TB and susceptibility to NTM lung disease. It is also largely accepted that bronchiectasis associates with NTM lung disease [14–17]. However, the statistical significance of the association was not observed after adjusting for other factors such as the type of dust exposure and pneumoconiosis. Pneumoconiosis, the immune reaction induced by macrophages that remove deposited dust in the lung, and the epithelial fibrosis induced by inflammatory cells, such as polymorphonuclear leukocytes (PMN), are likely to cause structural changes [18]. All patients in this study had pneumoconiosis, which distorts lung structure as a result of the immunologic reaction to inhaled dust. Since patients are vulnerable to NTM pulmonary infection, the history of tuberculosis may have lost its significance after adjustment for the profusion of small opacity perfusion or large opacity grades. Also, prior TB is merely a marker of the poor ability of the individual to respond immunologically to mycobacterial antigens.

Although the results of univariate analyses showed that emphysema also associated significantly with NTM lung disease, emphysema was excluded from the analysis because it correlated with large-opacity grade (Data not shown). Note that, because the large opacities, which indicate progressive massive fibrosis (PMF) caused by pneumoconiosis, are commonly accompanied by paracicatricial emphysema [19], which can be seen next to areas of scarring, emphysema was not included in the multivariate analysis.

In addition, Corbett et al. found that a dust-exposed job at diagnosis was a risk factor for NTM lung disease in the South African gold miners, even after adjustment for silicosis [13]. This is consistent with the study of Sonnenberg et al., which showed that the miners who had spent more than 20 years underground were more likely to have NTM lung disease than those who had spent less than 10 years underground [6]. Silica exposure may promote NTM lung disease via two mechanisms. First, people who work in a dusty environment may have a higher risk of TB lung disease and chronic bronchitis, both of which promote susceptibility to NTM lung disease [6,20]. This possibility is consistent with the study by Beamer et al. on mice that were instilled intranasally with silica. They found that silica exposure altered the phenotype of the alveolar macrophages, which in turn impaired their ability to take up and respond protectively to bacterial lipoproteins [21]. Second, not only is dust a common source of NTM, wet processes in association with a dusty job environment have the potential to increase the incidence of pathogenic mycobacterial exposure in the workplace [13,22,23].

Corbett et al. also reported that the gold miners with NTM were significantly more likely to have early/high-grade silicosis than the control patients, who were gold miners who attended hospital for trauma or human immunodeficiency virus (HIV)-unrelated surgery [13]. However, it was not clear how they graded silicosis. Consequently, whether their early/high-grade silicosis category reflects the higher ILO grades of large opacities in complicated pneumoconiosis or only greater small profusion opacities in simple pneumoconiosis is unclear. However, another, more recent, study by Sonnenberg et al. reported that South African gold miners with NTM lung disease were significantly more likely than gold miners with TB to exhibit silicosis, as defined by ILO categories of the small-opacity profusion of 1/1 or higher. This relationship between NTM lung disease and silicosis remained significant even after adjusting for age, alcohol consumption, HIV status, years spent working underground, prior TB treatment, and silicosis [10]. Similarly, we found that NTM-infected patients with previous dust exposure were significantly more likely than uninfected dust-exposed patients to have category 2 and 3 small-opacity profusion. These findings suggest that pneumoconiosis promotes NTM lung disease.

To the best of our knowledge, the association between large-opacity grade (as shown by chest X-rays) and the risk of NTM lung infection has not been studied. We found that patients with NTM lung infection were significantly more likely to have large-opacity grade A, B, and C radiological findings and that the association between severe large opacity and NTM lung infection remained significant after adjustment. Alternatively, it may be that large opacities lead to lung distortion, which could cause ventilatory disturbances. Emphysema is the result of lung parenchymal destruction and is a type of COPD that restricts airflow. Ringshausen et al. showed that diagnosed COPD (either the chronic bronchitis-predominant type or the emphysema-predominant type) associated with NTM lung disease [24]. Chan et al. suggested that the low blood supply of emphysematous lesions encourages the colonization of NTMs in these areas [25].

This study has several limitations. First, its cross-sectional design made it difficult to assess the causal relationship between NTM lung infection and radiological factors. However, given the natural course of pneumoconiosis and the fact that the radiological charts were obtained around the time NTM was isolated, it is likely that there is a causal relationship, namely, that the structural lung changes in pneumoconiosis promote NTM lung infection. Second, the subjects were enrolled in a single center, which may reduce the generalizability of the study observations to other settings. However, this limitation may be mitigated by the fact that the subjects worked in heterogeneous workplaces and varied in their occupational history. Third, we did not analyze the pulmonary function test data. Further studies on the relationship between NTM lung infection and lung function are warranted. Fourth, the NTM species could not be identified in many cases; as a result, we could not assess their relationship with NTM lung infection in pneumoconiosis. However, all NTM lung infections were confirmed according to the American Thoracic Society (ATS) and The Infectious Diseases Society of America (IDSA) guidelines. Fifth, some of the subjects who had decreased FEV1 (Forced expiratory volume in one second) might have used inhaled corticosteroids, and most patients under medication might have used acid-suppressive drugs as part of a clinical regimen. Unfortunately, it was difficult to evaluate the medication history data in the analysis because of the retrospective design of the study. Additionally, although slender body habitus has been reported to be associated with NTM, infections, we did not evaluate individual anthropometric data such as height, weight, body mass index, mainly because the main focus of our study was the association between radiologic findings of pneumoconiosis and NTM lung infection. Considering that some of them needed medical treatment including inhaled corticosteroids to relieve their respiratory symptoms and most patients with a history of dust exposure who complain of chronic respiratory symptoms have slender body habitus, the present study suggests that occupational history of respiratory dust and its complex health effect are a risk factor for NTM pulmonary infection.

Despite these limitations, this study also has a number of methodologically robust elements. First, the NTM-infected patients satisfied the bacteriological criteria of the ATS/IDSA statement about NTM diagnosis. Second, there were 82 patients with NTM lung infection, which is markedly larger than the sample sizes in other studies on NTM in pneumoconiosis. Third, the occupational history data included the work duration. Consequently, we could examine the relationship between dust exposure duration and NTM infection. Fourth, this is the first study that evaluates the relationship between the large opacities of pneumoconiosis and NTM lung infection.

5. Conclusions

The diagnosis of NTM lung infection in dust-exposed workers was significantly associated with previous TB, bronchiectasis, marked profusion of small opacities, and high-grade large opacities, as assessed using the ILO classification system. Even after adjustment, extensive small-opacity profusion and high-grade large opacities remained significant risk factors for NTM lung infection in dust-exposed workers. The relationship between pneumoconiosis features and NTM species, and the relationship between lung function and NTM lung infection remain to be studied.

Author Contributions: The research was designed and conducted by J.M. J.L. participated in the data collection. J.L. and J.M. reviewed the radiology. Statistical analysis was performed by J.L. All authors edited and revised the final submission and signed off on the final version.

Funding: This research received no specific grant from any funding agency in the public, commercial, or not-for-profit sectors.

Conflicts of Interest: The authors declare no conflict of interest.

References

1. Koh, W.-J. Diagnosis and treatment of nontuberculous mycobacterial lung disease. *J. Korean Med. Assoc.* **2011**, *54*, 1053–1058. [CrossRef]
2. Park, Y.S.; Lee, C.H.; Lee, S.M.; Yang, S.C.; Yoo, C.G.; Kim, Y.W.; Han, S.K.; Shim, Y.S.; Yim, J.J. Rapid increase of non-tuberculous mycobacterial lung diseases at a tertiary referral hospital in South Korea. *Int. J. Tuberc. Lung Dis.* **2010**, *14*, 1069–1071. [PubMed]
3. Griffith, D.E.; Aksamit, T.; Brown-Elliott, B.A.; Catanzaro, A.; Daley, C.; Gordin, F.; Holland, S.M.; Horsburgh, R.; Huitt, G.; Iademarco, M.F.; et al. An official ATS/IDSA statement: Diagnosis, treatment, and prevention of nontuberculous mycobacterial diseases. *Am. J. Respir. Crit. Care Med.* **2007**, *175*, 367–416. [CrossRef] [PubMed]
4. Huang, C.T.; Tsai, Y.J.; Wu, H.D.; Wang, J.Y.; Yu, C.J.; Lee, L.N.; Yang, P.C. Impact of non-tuberculous mycobacteria on pulmonary function decline in chronic obstructive pulmonary disease. *Int. J. Tuberc. Lung Dis.* **2012**, *16*, 539–545. [CrossRef] [PubMed]
5. Pasula, R.; Britigan, B.E.; Turner, J.; Martin, W.J. Airway delivery of silica increases susceptibility to mycobacterial infection in mice: Potential role of repopulating macrophages. *J. Immunol.* **2009**, *182*, 7102–7109. [CrossRef] [PubMed]
6. Sonnenberg, P.; Murray, J.; Glynn, J.R.; Thomas, R.G.; Godfrey-Faussett, P.; Shearer, S. Risk factors for pulmonary disease due to culture-positive *M. tuberculosis* or nontuberculous mycobacteria in South African gold miners. *Eur. Respir. J.* **2000**, *15*, 291–296. [CrossRef] [PubMed]
7. Kim, Y.M.; Kim, M.; Kim, S.K.; Park, K.; Jin, S.H.; Lee, U.S.; Kim, Y.; Chae, G.T.; Lee, S.B. Mycobacterial infections in coal workers' pneumoconiosis patients in South Korea. *Scand. J. Infect. Dis.* **2009**, *41*, 656–662. [CrossRef]

8. British Thoracic and Tuberculosis Association. Opportunist mycobacterial pulmonary infection and occupational dust exposure: An investigation in England and Wales. *Tubercle* **1975**, *56*, 295–313. [CrossRef]
9. Corbett, E.L.; Hay, M.; Churchyard, G.J.; Herselman, P.; Clayton, T.; Williams, B.G.; Hayes, R.; Mulder, D.; De Cock, K.M. Mycobacterium kansasii and *M. scrofulaceum* isolates from HIV-negative South African gold miners: Incidence, clinical significance and radiology. *Int. J. Tuberc. Lung Dis.* **1999**, *3*, 501–507.
10. Sonnenberg, P.; Thomas, R.G.; Glynn, J.R.; Shearer, S.; Godfrey-Faussett, P.; Murray, J. Clinical and radiological features of pulmonary disease due to culture-positive *M. tuberculosis* or nontuberculous mycobacteria in South African gold miners. *S. Afr. J. Epidemiol. Infect.* **2005**, *20*, 130–135. [CrossRef]
11. Van Halsema, C.L.; Chihota, V.N.; Gey van Pittius, N.C.; Fielding, K.L.; Lewis, J.J.; van Helden, P.D.; Churchyard, G.J.; Grant, A.D. Clinical Relevance of Nontuberculous Mycobacteria Isolated from Sputum in a Gold Mining Workforce in South Africa: An Observational, Clinical Study. *Biomed. Res. Int.* **2015**. [CrossRef] [PubMed]
12. Jo, B.S.; Lee, J.; Cho, Y.; Byun, J.; Kim, H.R.; Koo, J.W.; Myong, J.P. Risk factors associated with mortality from pneumonia among patients with pneumoconiosis. *Ann. Occup. Environ. Med.* **2016**, *28*, 19. [CrossRef]
13. Corbett, E.L.; Churchyard, G.J.; Clayton, T.; Herselman, P.; Williams, B.; Hayes, R.; Mulder, D.; De Cock, K.M. Risk factors for pulmonary mycobacterial disease in South African gold miners. A case-control study. *Am. J. Respir. Crit. Care Med.* **1999**, *159*, 94–99. [CrossRef] [PubMed]
14. Griffith, D.E.; Aksamit, T.R. Bronchiectasis and nontuberculous mycobacterial disease. *Clin. Chest Med.* **2012**, *33*, 283–295. [CrossRef]
15. McShane, P.J.; Glassroth, J. Pulmonary Disease Due to Nontuberculous Mycobacteria: Current State and New Insights. *Chest* **2015**, *148*, 1517–1527. [CrossRef] [PubMed]
16. Weiss, C.H.; Glassroth, J. Pulmonary disease caused by nontuberculous mycobacteria. *Expert Rev. Respir. Med.* **2012**, *6*, 597–612. [CrossRef] [PubMed]
17. Aksamit, T.R.; Philley, J.V.; Griffith, D.E. Nontuberculous mycobacterial (NTM) lung disease: The top ten essentials. *Respir. Med.* **2014**, *108*, 417–425. [CrossRef]
18. Rom, W.N. *Environmental and Occupational Medicine*; Wolters Kluwer: Philadelphia, PR, USA, 2015.
19. Cockcroft, A.E.; Wagner, J.C.; Seal, E.M.; Lyons, J.P.; Campbell, M.J. Irregular opacities in coalworkers' pneumoconiosis—Correlation with pulmonary function and pathology. *Ann. Occup. Hyg.* **1982**, *26*, 767–787.
20. Hnizdo, E.; Murray, J. Risk of pulmonary tuberculosis relative to silicosis and exposure to silica dust in South African gold miners. *Occup. Environ. Med.* **1998**, *55*, 496–502. [CrossRef]
21. Beamer, G.L.; Seaver, B.P.; Jessop, F.; Shepherd, D.M.; Beamer, C.A. Acute Exposure to Crystalline Silica Reduces Macrophage Activation in Response to Bacterial Lipoproteins. *Front. Immunol.* **2016**, *7*, 49. [CrossRef]
22. Primm, T.P.; Lucero, C.A.; Falkinham, J.O. Health impacts of environmental mycobacteria. *Clin. Microbiol. Rev.* **2004**, *17*, 98–106. [CrossRef] [PubMed]
23. Ulmann, V.; Kracalikova, A.; Dziedzinska, R. Mycobacteria in Water Used for Personal Hygiene in Heavy Industry and Collieries: A Potential Risk for Employees. *Int. J. Environ. Res. Public Health* **2015**, *12*, 2870–2877. [CrossRef] [PubMed]
24. Ringshausen, F.C.; Wagner, D.; de Roux, A.; Diel, R.; Hohmann, D.; Hickstein, L.; Welte, T.; Rademacher, J. Prevalence of Nontuberculous Mycobacterial Pulmonary Disease, Germany, 2009–2014. *Emerg. Infect. Dis.* **2016**, *22*, 1102–1105. [CrossRef] [PubMed]
25. Chan, E.D.; Iseman, M.D. Underlying host risk factors for nontuberculous mycobacterial lung disease. *Semin. Respir. Crit. Care Med.* **2013**, *34*, 110–123. [PubMed]

International Journal of
Environmental Research and Public Health

MDPI

Article

Associations between Fitness Measures and Change of Direction Speeds with and without Occupational Loads in Female Police Officers

Robin M. Orr [1,2,*], Filip Kukić [3], Aleksandar Čvorović [3], Nenad Koropanovski [4], Radivoje Janković [4], Jay Dawes [5] and Robert Lockie [6]

1. Faculty of Health Sciences and Medicine, Bond Institute of Health and Sport, Bond University, Gold Coast QLD 4229, Australia
2. Tactical Research Unit, Bond University, Gold Coast QLD 4229, Australia
3. Police Sports Education Center, Abu Dhabi Police 253, UAE; filip.kukic@gmail.com (F.K.); cvorovic77@yahoo.com (A.Č.)
4. Specialized Physical Education at the department of Criminalistics, University of Criminal Investigation and Police Studies, 11080 Belgrade, Serbia; korpan82@gmail.com (N.K.); radejankovic@yahoo.com (R.J.)
5. Department of Helath and Human Performance, Oklahoma State University, Stillwater, OK 74074, USA; jdawes@uccs.edu
6. Department of Kinesiology, California State Fullerton, Fullerton, CA 92831, USA; rlockie@Fullerton.edu

* Correspondence: rorr@bond.edu.au; Tel.: +61-0468-646-027

Received: 17 April 2019; Accepted: 28 May 2019; Published: 1 June 2019

Abstract: Female police officers may be required to pursue offenders on foot while wearing occupational loads. The aim of this study was to determine relationships between fitness measures and change of direction speed (CODS) in female police officers and the influence of their occupational loads. Retrospective data were provided for 27 female police officers (age = 32.19 ± 5.09 y, height = 162.78 ± 5.01 cm, and mass = 71.31 ± 13.42 kg) and included fitness measures of: lower-body power (standing long jump (SLJ)), upper-body and trunk muscle endurance (push-up (PU) and sit-up (SU)), aerobic power (estimated VO_{2max}), and CODS (Illinois agility test). The CODS test was performed without and with occupational load (10 kg). Paired sample *t*-tests (between-load conditions) and Pearson's correlations (relationships between measures) were performed with linear regression analysis used to account for the contribution of measures to unloaded and loaded CODS performance. CODS was significantly slower when loaded (unloaded = ~23.17 s, loaded = ~24.14 s, $p < 0.001$) with a strong, significant relationship between load conditions ($r = 0.956$, $p < 0.001$). Moderate to strong, significant relationships were found between all fitness measures ranging from estimated VO_{2max} ($r = -0.448$) to SU ($r = -0.673$) in the unloaded condition, with the strength of these relationships increasing in the loaded condition accounting for 61% to 67% of the variance, respectively. While unloaded agility test performance was strongly associated with loaded performance, female police officer CODS was significantly reduced when carrying occupational loads. A variety of fitness measures that influence officer CODS performances become increasingly important when occupational loads are carried.

Keywords: law enforcement; foot pursuit; load carriage; chase; body armor

1. Introduction

Police officers are required to carry out a variety of physical tasks that can range from attending a domestic disturbance and verifying a person's identity [1] to chasing offenders on foot across varying distances [2,3]. Often these foot pursuits can occur while the officer is wearing their daily occupational load. Occupational loads for police officers can vary depending on job type, but they are typically around 10 kg for general duties officers [4] and over 20 kg [5], or even 40 kg [6], for specialist response police. For the general duties officer, these loads typically comprise essential equipment like a baton, radio, handcuffs, flashlight, etc. [4], and they often include body armor [7]. Specialist police loads are made heavier by the specialist equipment they must carry, which can include gas masks, riot or ballistic shields, and breaching equipment. Of note however, given that the average female officer is lighter than the average male officer [5], the relative load carried by female officers may be significantly heavier than those carried by male officers [4].

The impacts of occupational loads on mobility of the carrier are well reported in the literature, whereby measures of short-distance sprints [8–10], prone-start sprints [10–12], and agility runs [13] have been found to significantly decrease the mobility of tactically loaded participants. However, these studies were all conducted in military populations, who are known to generally carry heavier loads than law enforcement [4]. The findings of three studies on law enforcement that compared the impacts of body armor on police officer mobility were mixed with two studies [5,14] that found significant decreases in performance with added load and one study that did not [15]. Carlton et al. [5] found a significant decrease in time to complete an 80 kg dummy drag task when specialist tactical officers were loaded with 22 kg as opposed to their unloaded condition. Similarly, a study by Dempsey et al. [14] found that participants wearing stab-resistant body armor (7.65 ± 0.73 kg) significantly increased time to complete a simulated vehicle exit and sprint (mean time = 1.95 s loaded, 1.67 s unloaded, $p < 0.001$) and time to complete a mobility battery (mean time = 18.16 s loaded, 15.85 s unloaded, $p < 0.001$). Conversely, research by Schram et al. [15] found that there were no significant differences in completion time for the Illinois agility run performance between officers wearing duty loads, which included body armor (10.8–11.5 kg) when compared to station loads (no body armor).

Various fitness measures have been found to relate to occupational load carriage ability [4,16]. For example, Robinson, et al. [17] conducted a study of specialist tactical response police carrying 20 kg of load as fast as possible over a 5 km distance at three different time intervals (several months apart). In their study it was found that strength measures of repetition maximum (RM) (bench press, squat, and pull-up), lower-body power (vertical jump (VJ)), and aerobic (multistage fitness, progressive shuttle run, or 'beep', test) performances were significantly correlated with all three load carriage performance events. As such, it is not surprising that research has found the combination of resistance and aerobic training as best associated with improvements in load carriage ability [18,19], and as such, they form the recommendations for physically conditioning tactical personnel to carry loads [20,21]. However, the majority of this research has focused on time to complete a distance march with loads above those required of general duties police, as opposed to shorter distances with the lighter loads utilized by general duties police.

Female police officers may have to pursue offenders on foot, while wearing occupational loads that are relatively heavier than those carried by male officers. These occupational loads reduce mobility and are associated with measures of fitness. Therefore, understanding the relationships between fitness measures and load carriage during a change of direction speed (CODS) task may help inform physical conditioning requirements to optimize their ability to pursue offenders on foot whilst wearing occupational loads. On this basis, the aims of this research were to investigate the impacts of the occupational loads carried by female general duties police officers on a short explosive CODS task and determine which measures of fitness were related to this occupational load carriage requirement.

2. Materials and Methods

Retrospective data were provided for 27 healthy female police officers (age = 32.19 ± 5.09 y, height = 162.78 ± 5.01 cm, and mass = 71.31 ± 13.42 kg) from the Abu Dhabi Police and included fitness measures of lower-body power (SLJ), upper-body and trunk muscle endurance (push-up (PU), sit-up (SU), aerobic power (estimated VO_{2max}), and CODS (Illinois agility test). The female officers who applied to take part in sports activities as part of the competition and teams section of the Abu Dhabi Police were recruited for this study. Only the participants with no history of injuries or cardiovascular illness underwent testing procedures. Research was carried out in accordance with the conditions of the Declaration of Helsinki, recommendations guiding physicians in biomedical research involving human subjects [22], and with the ethical approval (number 484-2) from the ethical board of the Faculty of Sport and Physical Education, University of Belgrade.

2.1. Procedures

The explosive power of leg extensors was assessed by the SLJ test. Markovic [23] reported a high intratrial reliability for this test (Intraclass Correlation Coefficient = 0.95). The participants were instructed to jump as far as possible by performing a standing jump from a standard standing position. The distance from the starting line to the landing point at the heel contact was used for further analysis. The precision of the measurement was to the nearest 1 cm.

The Illinois agility test was used as the measure of CODS [24]. Hachana [25] reported a high intratrial reliability of this test (ICC = 0.96). In addition to a standard Illinois agility test, the participants in this research also wore a 10 kg vest (Illinois agility loaded). A Star Fitness™ (Tortola, British Virgin Islands) adjustable weighted vest was firmly tightened to the upper body with two side straps that overlapped about the waistline in the front. The weight of the west was equally distributed at the front and back of the trunk. This load alone, without a sidearm or accoutrements, provided the 10 kg load. Following a 10 min respite from the SLJ, Illinois agility tests were performed with outcomes of both tests recorded using electronic timing gates (Fitro Light Gates, Fitronic, Bratislava, Slovakia). Measurement precision was to the nearest 0.01 s. The test course was used as previously reported in literature [24,26]. Two cones were used to mark the turning points, while four center cones were placed down the middle of the square grid and spaced 3.3 m apart for the weaving component (see Figure 1). The participants began the test lying prone on the floor behind the starting line. The timing gate was positioned 1 m above the starting line so the participants triggered the signal when they had already commenced the push up off the ground and started to move forward. On command, the participants stood and ran forward to the first turning cone in a straight line as fast as possible. The participants were required to turn around the first turning cone and moved back to the first center cone, where they weaved up and back around the four center cones. The participants then ran to the second turning cone. After turning around this cone, the participants were required to run in a straight line past the finish line. Following a slow then slightly faster (but submaximal) completion of the course as a warmup, participants were instructed to complete the test as quickly as possible. Participants were familiar with the course and repeated the course twice, firstly without load and then, after a short period of respite of 10 min, with load.

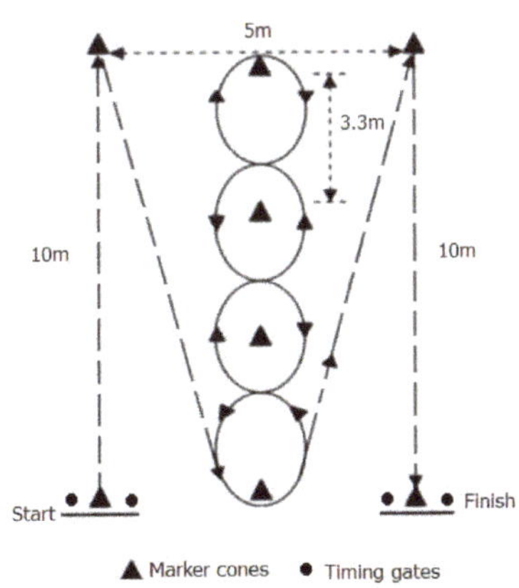

Figure 1. Schematic of the Illinois agility test.

The 1 min PU and SU tests were conducted 10 min after the Illinois agility test following the procedures previously described in the literature [27], with the exception of the PU, which was completed on the knees rather than the toes. In short, each participant was positioned so that only a maximum of four points contacted the ground (knees and hands) while the body was straight from heels to head. The participants were advised that the between-hand width should be approximately one palm wider than their shoulder width. The starting position had the arms fully extended with one PU counted when the elbow joint bent to at least 90 degrees and then extended back to the starting position. After the PU test, participants rested for 15 min before completing the SU test. Participants started the test from a laying position with hands crossed at chest height, palms on the opposing shoulders, and knees bent at an angle of 90°. The feet were placed flat on the ground and secured by the tester. One repetition was counted when the participant completed an SU by raising the upper body and touching the knees with elbows. Hips had to maintain contact with the ground, and hands had to remain on the chest during the full range of movement throughout the test. The only permissible resting position was the 'start' position. Every SU that did not meet these standards were not counted. For both the PU and SU, participants were required to complete as many repetitions as possible in the time or until volition fatigue. Results were measured in single repetitions.

Female police officer VO_{2max} values were estimated using an incremental, multistage 20 m shuttle-run test on an indoor rubber matt, according to previously reported procedures [28]. This test was conducted 10 min after the SU test. Shuttle run levels were controlled using the mobile app beep test, 'police military multistage assessment' connected to a loudspeaker so each change of the level was clearly and loudly announced. After the test was finished, results were written down in forms of levels and shuttles attained by each participant. To further estimate VO_{2max}, results were typed into a Microsoft Excel file (Microsoft Corporation™, Redmond, Washington, DC, USA) and calculated using the formula developed by Ramsbottom et al. [29], which was based on age and completed number of levels and shuttles.

2.2. Statistics

Data were transferred from a Microsoft Excel spreadsheet, on which the data were recorded, into Statistical Package for the Social Sciences (SPSS version 25, Chicago, IL, USA) for analysis. Following descriptive analysis and tests for normality and homogeneity, paired sample *t*-tests were used to determine differences between loaded and unloaded conditions. Pearson's product correlations were performed to investigate relationships between load conditions and fitness variables. A regression analysis was performed with all significantly correlated variables to determine how much of the CODS task could be attributed to these variables. The regressions were conducted both including and excluding the opposing CODS task (i.e., loaded/unloaded CODS task). Alpha levels were set at 0.05 a priori.

3. Results

Descriptive data are provided in Table 1. The results of the paired sample *t*-test indicated that female officers were significantly slower ($t(26) = -6.001$, $p < 0.001$) when performing the CODS task while wearing occupational loads.

Table 1. Demographic and fitness measure results.

	Mean ± SD (Range)
Age (y)	32.19 ± 5.09 (22.00–42.00)
Height (cm)	162.78 ± 5.01 (155.00–173.00)
Mass (kg)	71.31 ± 13.42 (50.50–109.50)
Body mass index (kg/m^2)	26.86 ± 4.57 (20.80–36.60)
Push-Ups (repetitions)	24.04 ± 11.77 (7.00–49.00)
Sit-Ups (repetitions)	28.48 ± 10.79 (13.00–53.00)
Standing Long Jump (cm)	166.00 ± 25.81 (116.00–210.00)
Estimated VO_{2max} (mL/kg/min)	24.32 ± 4.32 (19.55–35.06)
Illinois agility (s)	23.17 ± 2.75 (18.58–28.21)
Illinois agility loaded with 10 kg (s)	24.14 ± 2.78 (18.96–29.86)

SD: Standard Deviation.

All fitness measures were significantly correlated with both the unloaded and loaded Illinois agility run, with the strength of the correlations [30] ranging from moderate (estimated VO_{2max}) to strong (SU) (Table 2). In all cases, the strength of the correlations between the fitness measures and the Illinois agility run increased when load was added. As would be expected, the unloaded Illinois agility test was very strongly correlated with the Illinois agility when loaded ($r = 0.956$, $p < 0.001$).

Table 2. Correlations between fitness measures and Illinois agility test in both the unloaded and loaded conditions.

	SLJ	SU	PU	Estimated VO_{2max}	Illinois Agility	Illinois Agility Loaded (10 kg)
Illinois agility	−0.649 **	−0.673 **	−0.605 **	−0.448 *	1	0.956 **
Illinois agility loaded (10 kg)	−0.686 **	−0.707 **	−0.624 **	−0.514 **	0.956 **	1

Correlation is significant at: * $p < 0.05$, ** $p < 0.01$. SLJ = standing long jump; SU = sit-up; and PU = push-up.

When all measures that correlated to the unloaded CODS were entered into the regression, the variables equated to 92% of the variance, dropping to 61% of the variance when the loaded CODS was removed from the regression. Subsequently, when all measures that correlated to the loaded CODS were entered into the regression, the variables equated to 93% of the variance, dropping to 67% of the variance when the unloaded CODS was removed from the regression.

4. Discussion

The aims of this research were to investigate the impacts of the occupational loads carried by female general duties police officers of the Abu Dhabi Police on a CODS task and determine which measures of fitness were related to this occupational load carriage requirement. The study found that when female police officers wore a 10 kg duty load their CODS was significantly slower. Furthermore, while moderate-to-strong significant relationships were found between all fitness measures and CODS, the strength of these relationships increased in the loaded condition.

The results of this study suggested that lower-body power, upper-body and trunk endurance, and aerobic fitness are associated with police officer CODS, especially when the officer was wearing occupational load. Previous research has found that measures of fitness are associated with mobility-styled activities in law enforcement personnel [31]. Lockie et al. [31] found that SU ($r = -0.208$), pull-ups ($r = -0.272$) and 2.4 km run ($r = 0.253$) performances were all associated with a 99-yard (90.53 m) obstacle course run, which was designed to simulate a foot pursuit and required police recruits to step over simulated curbs and high obstacles over the course. Similarly, Dawes et al. [32] found a moderate to strong relationship between VJ and sprint performance (5–20 m) in specialist police officers—findings that were supported by Marques et al. [33,34] and Wisløff, et al. [35]. Thus,

VJ was strongly associated with short distance sprints, which was a performance measure known to be reduced by the wearing of body armor in police [36,37].

In a military population, soldiers wearing and carrying a total load of approximately 42 kg completed an anaerobic based task, which included a 27 m zigzag run, and they were significantly slower when carrying their additional loads [38]. Of note, and in support of aforementioned research, the initial 5 m start, in particular, was found to be significantly slower when the soldiers were loaded [38]. However, the zigzag component (while slower) was not shown to be significantly different between load conditions. Considering this, the study found significant, strong correlations between overall course performance times in both the unloaded and loaded conditions with lower body strength (1 RM squat), lower-body power (peak power), and upper-body strength (1 RM bench press). PU, SU, and a 2 mi run were not significantly correlated with performance on the course (in either load condition) [38]. Of note, the study found PUs were significantly correlated with time to rise from the prone position to begin the initial 5 m sprint of the course. This coincided with other research, which suggested that PU ability was related to other military-styled tasks that required the load carrier to rise from a prone position [12,39]. This also coincided with this current study, whereby female police officers were required to rise from a prone position to commence the initial forward sprint.

The CODS time to completion was between 23.17 ± 2.75 s (unloaded) to 24.14 ± 2.78 s (loaded) and was an anaerobic task [40]. As such, correlation with aerobic performance measures was not expected. For example, in the aforementioned research by Mala et al. [38], there was no correlation between two-mile run times and performance on a short, explosive anaerobic task (from 25.4 ± 1.8 s unloaded to 38.7 ± 4.8 s when loaded). However, Lockie et al. [31] did likewise find that 2.4 km run times were associated with several work sample test battery tasks ranging from a solid wall fence climb (7.75 ± 1.37 s) to a longer 500-yard run (89.20 ± 7.99 s). A potential reason for the findings of this study may lie in the fact that the officers may have been more likely to be more physically active (as the testing occurred at the end of a 22 week academy) and would have completed more physical activity (and hence be more fit in general).

The findings of this study, whereby measures of fitness were correlated to CODS (more so when the officers were loaded), and whereby unloaded CODS was very strongly correlated to loaded CODS, provide some guidance for the conditioning of female police officers who are required to wear occupational loads and pursue a suspect on foot. Poor CODS performance can be improved by increasing general fitness, more specifically PU, SU, and SLJ ability. Likewise, unloaded CODS ability can be used to inform loaded CODS potential and allow for this progression when a suitable unloaded CODS has been achieved.

Limitations

Key limitations to this study were the inability to change assessment order or to randomize the unloaded and loaded conditions. While these restrictions are common in retrospective cohort studies, familiarization of the course is expected to minimize any potential learning effect induced by the assessment order. Furthermore, long breaks of over 10 min between each condition, a period exceeding the recommended recovery period of power-based activities [41], should mitigate any fatigue concerns. It should also be noted that female police officer participants were from a group which may have been more physically active, and as such, the influence of fitness measures on CODS performance may not be reflective of less physically active female police officers.

5. Conclusions

While unloaded agility performance was strongly associated with loaded performance, female police officer CODS was reduced when officers carried occupational loads. All fitness measures were correlated with unloaded CODS performance, with this relationship increasing when occupational loads were worn. As such, upper-body and trunk endurance, lower-body power, and aerobic fitness become increasingly important when preparing female police officers to carry occupational loads.

Furthermore, unloaded CODS performance (as measured by the Illinois agility test) can be used to gauge readiness to perform loaded CODS.

Author Contributions: Contribution by the authors included: Conceptualization, R.M.O., F.K., A.Č., and J.D.; methodology, F.K., A.Č., N.K., and R.J.; formal analysis, R.M.O., J.D., and R.L.; investigation, R.M.O., F.K., A.Č., J.D., and R.L.; resources, F.K., A.Č., N.K., and R.J.; data curation, R.M.O., F.K., A.Č., and J.D.; writing—original draft preparation, R.M.O., F.K.; writing—review and editing, A.Č., N.K., R.J., J.D., and R.L.; project administration, F.K., A.Č., N.K., and R.J.

Funding: This research received no external funding.

Conflicts of Interest: The authors declare no conflict of interest.

References

1. Orr, R.M.; Wilson, A.F.; Pope, R.; Hinton, B. Profiling the routine tasks of police officers. In Proceedings of the ASCA National Conference on Applied Strength and Conditioning, Melbourne, Australia, 4–6 November 2016.
2. Anderson, G.S.; Plecas, D.; Segger, T. Police officer physical ability testing—Re-validating a selection criterion. *Policing* **2001**, *24*, 8–31. [CrossRef]
3. Maupin, D.; Wills, T.; Orr, R.; Schram, B.E.N. Fitness Profiles in Elite Tactical Units: A Critical Review. *Int. J. Exerc. Sci.* **2018**, *11*, 1041–1062.
4. Baran, K.; Dulla, J.; Orr, R.; Dawes, J.; Pope, R. Duty loads carried by the LA sheriff's department deputies. *J. Aust. Strength Cond.* **2018**, *26*, 34–38.
5. Carlton, S.D.; Carbone, P.D.; Stierli, M.; Orr, R.M. The Impact of Occupational Load Carriage on the Mobility of the Tactical Police Officer. *J. Aust. Strength Cond.* **2014**, *22*, 32–37.
6. Keeler, J.M. The Effect of Tactical Tasks and Gear on Muscle Activation of SWAT Officers. Master's Thesis, University of Kentucky, Kentucky, UK, 2014.
7. Schram, B.; Hinton, B.; Orr, R.; Pope, R.; Norris, G. The perceived effects and comfort of various body armour systems on police officers while performing occupational tasks. *Ann. Occup. Environ. Med.* **2018**, *30*, 15. [CrossRef] [PubMed]
8. Hunt, A.P.; Tofari, P.J.; Billing, D.C.; Silk, A.J. Tactical Combat Movements: Inter-individual Variation in Performance due to the Effects of Load Carriage. *Ergonomics* **2016**, *59*, 1232–1241. [CrossRef]
9. Hasselquist, L.; Bensel, C.K.; Corner, B.; Gregorczyk, K.N.; Schiffman, J.M. Understanding the Physiological, Biomechanical, and Performance Effects of Body Armor Use. Available online: https://www.researchgate.net/profile/Carolyn_Bensel/publication/235200699_Understanding_the_Physiological_Biomechanical_and_Performance_Effects_of_Body_Armor_Use/links/00b7d52cd65e423786000000/Understanding-the-Physiological-Biomechanical-and-Performance-Effects-of-Body-Armor-Use.pdf (accessed on 17 April 2019).
10. Taylor, N.A.S.; Burdon, C.A.; Van Den Heuvel, A.M.J.; Fogarty, A.L.; Notley, S.R.; Hunt, A.P.; Billing, D.C.; Drain, J.R.; Silk, A.J.; Patterson, M.J.; et al. Balancing Ballistic Protection against Physiological Strain: Evidence from Laboratory and Field Trials. *Appl. Physiol. Nutr. Metab.* **2015**, *41*, 117–124. [CrossRef]
11. Loverro, K.L.; Brown, T.N.; Coyne, M.E.; Schiffman, J.M. Use of Body Armor Protection with Fighting Load Impacts Soldier Performance and Kinematics. *Appl. Ergon.* **2015**, *46*, 168–175. [CrossRef]
12. Laing Treloar, A.K.; Billing, D.C. Effect of Load Carriage on Performance of an Explosive, Anaerobic Military Task. *Mil. Med.* **2011**, *176*, 1027–1031. [CrossRef]
13. Martin, P.E.; Nelson, R.C. The Effect of Carried Loads on the Combative Movement Performance of Men and Women. *Mil. Med.* **1985**, *150*, 357–362. [CrossRef]
14. Dempsey, P.C.; Handcock, P.J.; Rehrer, N.J. Impact of police body armour and equipment on mobility. *Appl. Ergon.* **2013**, *44*, 957–961. [CrossRef]
15. Schram, B.; Orr, R.; Pope, R. The Effects of Body Armour on the Power Development and Agility of Police Officers. *Ergonomics* **2019**. post review.
16. Lyons, J.; Allsopp, A.; Bilzon, J. Influences of body composition upon the relative metabolic and cardiovascular demands of load-carriage. *Occup. Med.* **2005**, *55*, 380–384. [CrossRef]

17. Robinson, J.; Roberts, A.; Irving, S.; Orr, R. Aerobic Fitness is of Greater Importance Than Strength and Power in the Load Carriage Performance of Specialist Police. *Int. J. Exerc. Sci.* **2018**, *11*, 987–998.
18. Harman, E.; Gutekunst, D.J.; Frykman, P.N.; Nindl, B.C.; Alemany, J.A.; Mello, R.P.; Sharp, M. Effects of two different eight-week training programs on military physical performance. *J. Strength Cond. Res.* **2008**, *22*, 524–534. [CrossRef] [PubMed]
19. Kraemer, W.; Vescovi, J.D.; Volek, J.S.; Nindl, B.C.; Newton, R.U.; Patton, J.F.; Dziados, J.E.; French, D.N.; Hakkinen, K. Effects of concurrent resistance and aerobic training on load-bearing performance and the army physical fitness test. *Mil. Med.* **2004**, *169*, 994–999. [CrossRef]
20. Orr, R.; Pope, R.; Johnston, V.; Coyle, J. Load carriage: Minimising soldier injuries through physical conditioning—A narrative review. *J. Mil. Veterans Health* **2010**, *18*, 31–38.
21. Knapik, J.J.; Harman, E.A.; Steelman, R.A.; Graham, B.S. A systematic review of the effects of physical training on load carriage performance. *J. Strength Cond. Res.* **2012**, *26*, 585–597. [CrossRef] [PubMed]
22. Christie, B. Doctors revise declaration of Helsinki. *Br. Med. J.* **2000**, *321*, 913. [CrossRef]
23. Markovic, G.; Dizdar, D.; Jukic, I.; Cardinale, M. Reliability and factorial validity of squat and countermovement jump tests. *J. Strength Cond. Res.* **2004**, *18*, 551–555.
24. Miller, M.G.; Herniman, J.J.; Ricard, M.D.; Cheatham, C.C.; Michael, T.J. The effects of a 6-week plyometric training program on agility. *J. Sports Sci. Med.* **2006**, *5*, 459–465. [PubMed]
25. Hachana, Y.; Chaabène, H.; Nabli, M.A.; Attia, A.; Moualhi, J.; Farhat, N.; Elloumi, M. Test-retest reliability, criterion-related validity, and minimal detectable change of the Illinois agility test in male team sport athletes. *J. Strength Cond. Res.* **2013**, *27*, 2752–2759. [CrossRef] [PubMed]
26. Beck, A.Q.; Clasey, J.L.; Yates, J.W.; Koebke, N.C.; Palmer, T.G.; Abel, M.G. Relationship of physical fitness measures vs. occupational physical ability in campus law enforcement officers. *J. Strength Cond. Res.* **2015**, *29*, 2340–2350. [CrossRef] [PubMed]
27. Čvorović, A.; Kukić, F.; Orr, R.M.; Dawes, J.J.; Jeknić, V.; Stojković, M. Impact of a 12-Week Postgraduate Training Course on the Body Composition and Physical Abilities of Police Trainees. *J. Strength Cond. Res.* **2018**. [CrossRef] [PubMed]
28. Kukić, F.; Dopsaj, M.; Dawes, J.; Prcic, D. Effects of a 4-week training intervention on estimated VO_{2max} and body composition among female police officers: Pilot study. In Proceedings of the International Scientific Conference Archibald Reiss Days, Belgrade, Serbia, 2–3 October 2018; Belgrade Academy of Criminalistic and Police Studies: Zemun, Belgrade, 2018.
29. Ramsbottom, R.; Brewer, J.; Williams, C. A progressive shuttle run test to estimate maximal oxygen uptake. *Br. J. Sports Med.* **1988**, *22*, 141–144. [CrossRef] [PubMed]
30. Evans, J.D. *Straightforward Statistics for the Behavioral Sciences*; Brooks Cole Publishers: Belmont, CA, USA, 1996.
31. Lockie, R.; Dawes, J.; Balfany, K.; Gonzales, C.; Beitzel, M.; Dulla, J.; Orr, R. Physical Fitness Characteristics that Relate to Work Sample Test Battery Performance in Law Enforcement Recruits. *Int. J. Environ. Res. Public Health* **2018**, *15*, 2477. [CrossRef]
32. Dawes, J.J.; Orr, R.M.; Elder, C.L.; Krall, K.; Stierli, M.; Schilling, B. Relationship between selected measures of power and strength and linear running speed amongst Special Weapons and Tactics police officers. *J. Aust. Strength Cond.* **2015**, *23*, 23–28.
33. Marques, M.; Gil, H.; Ramos, R.; Costa, A.; Marinho, D. Relationships between vertical jump strength metrics and 5 meters sprint time. *J. Hum. Kinet.* **2011**, *29*, 115–122. [CrossRef]
34. Marques, M.C.; Izquierdo, M.; Ferraz, R.; Carneiro, A.L.; Gonzalez-Badillo, J.J. Force plate vertical jump measurements and 30 meters sprint performance in trained athletes: A short report. *Int. Sportmed J.* **2014**, *15*, 77–83.
35. Wisløff, U.; Castagna, C.; Helgerud, J.; Jones, R.; Hoff, J. Strong correlation of maximal squat strength with sprint performance and vertical jump height in elite soccer players. *Br. J. Sports Med.* **2004**, *38*, 285–288. [CrossRef]
36. Joseph, A.; Wiley, A.; Orr, R.; Schram, B.; Dawes, J.J. The Impact of Load Carriage on Measures of Power and Agility in Tactical Occupations: A Critical Review. *Int. J. Environ. Res. Public Health* **2018**, *15*, 88. [CrossRef] [PubMed]

37. Wiley, A.; Joseph, A.; Orr, R.; Schram, B.; Kornhauser, C.; Holmes, R.; Dawes, J.J. The impact of external loads carried by police officers on vertical jump performance. In Proceedings of the 3rd International Conference on Physical Employments Standards, Portsmouth, UK, 17–19 July 2018; University of Portsmouth: Portsmouth, UK, 2018.
38. Mala, J.; Szivak, T.K.; Flanagan, S.D.; Comstock, B.A.; Laferrier, J.Z.; Maresh, C.M.; Kraemer, W.J. The Role of Strength and Power during Performance of High Intensity Military Tasks under Heavy Load Carriage. Available online: https://pdfs.semanticscholar.org/68c1/e86ba81a1312ae21075d8d5f10292baddbd5.pdf#page=5 (accessed on 17 April 2019).
39. Harman, E.; Gutekunst, D.J.; Frykman, P.N.; Sharp, M.; Nindl, B.C.; Alemany, J.A.; Mello, R.P. Prediction of Simulated Battlefield physical performance from Field-Expedient Tests. *Mil. Med.* **2008**, *173*, 36–41. [CrossRef] [PubMed]
40. Wilmore, J.H.; Costill, D.L.; Kenney, L. *Physiology of Sport and Exercise*, 4th ed.; Human Kinetics Publisher: Champaign, IL, USA, 2007.
41. Baechle, T.R.; Earle, R.W. *Essentials of Strength Training and Conditioning*, 3rd ed.; Baechle, T.R., Earle, R.W., Eds.; Human Kinetics Publisher: Champaign, IL, USA, 2008.

International Journal of
Environmental Research and Public Health

MDPI

Article

Chinese Public Response to Occupational Safety and Health Problems—A Study Based on Psychological Distance

Shanshan Li †, Hong Chen *,†, Xinru Huang, Congmei Hou and Feiyu Chen

School of Management, China University of Mining and Technology, Xuzhou 221116, China; shanshanli0809@163.com (S.L.); hxr881003@163.com (X.H.); houcongmei333@163.com (C.H.); chenfeiyu@cumt.edu.cn (F.C.)

* Correspondence: hongchenxz@cumt.edu.cn; Tel.: +86-133-722-10769

† These authors contributed equally to this work.

Received: 25 April 2019; Accepted: 28 May 2019; Published: 31 May 2019

Abstract: *Background:* The effective governance of occupational safety and health problems is inseparable from public participation and response. *Methods:* Based on the perspective of psychological distance, this paper adopted a quadratic response surface regression analysis method to investigate cognitive, emotional, expected and behavioral distances to occupational safety and health topics and their corresponding responses. *Results:* As demonstrated by the data statistics and response surface regression analysis results for 2386 valid samples, the relatively close psychological distance dimensions of the public with regard to occupational safety and health problems indicated the high endogenous tendency of the public to pay attention to occupational safety and health problems. The consistency between public cognitive and emotional distance with regard to occupational safety and health presented a "progressive decrease" in response towards behavioral distance, whereas the consistency between cognitive and expected distance reflected "convex" changes towards behavioral distance. Finally, the consistency between emotional and expected distance generally presented a "progressive increase" response towards behavioral distance. *Conclusions:* This research provides information regarding the public awareness of and response to occupational safety and health issues and how to promote occupational safety and health issues in order to improve them.

Keywords: occupational safety and health; psychological distance; public response; response gap

1. Introduction

The acceleration of global economic integration, liberalization of worldwide trade and investment in and application of new technologies, new materials, and new crafts in modern industry are causing the categories and number of occupational accidents and occupational diseases to increase continually in numerous developing countries. According to the statistics of the International Labor Organization (ILO), there are around 250 million production casualty accidents per year worldwide, with 475.6 accidents per minute on average. Among these, the death toll for production accidents and labor diseases totals about 1.1 million. In addition, the ILO estimates that by 2020, the incidence of labor diseases in the world will double and the global occupational safety and health situation will present an obvious tendency to deteriorate. The occupational safety and health situation in China will become increasingly austere—200 million workers are already currently suffering from the hazards of occupational diseases in varying degrees according to 2018 State Administration of Work Safety data. Statistics from the Ministry of Human Resources and Social Security indicate that the working-age (16–59) population in China exceeded 900 million in 2017 and this number may stabilize at around 800 million up to 2035. Occupational safety and health problems involve the core rights and interests of every worker. They not only affect the production activities in the working world, but also closely connect with the happiness of every family throughout society.

Occupational safety and health has typical attributes of public health concern. According to Spijkers and Honniball [1], public participation is conducive to the handling of public health concerns. As a result, the development of the occupational safety and health cause is inseparable from the public society, because public concern and support directly determine the social atmosphere which confronts occupational safety and health problems. However, the public tend to ignore occupational safety and health problems. In particular, in comparison with industrial accidents, occupational diseases and relevant symptoms are usually invisible to a large extent. In this sense, it is necessary to probe into public attitudes and the response to occupational safety and health problems. By introducing psychological distance, this research was systematically and comprehensively designed to investigate public awareness of and attitudes to occupational safety and health problems.

Occupational health psychology has been preceded by over a century of inquiry in psychology, sociology, philosophy, and other disciplines regarding the conditions of work and the welfare of workers, organizations, and society [2]. In 1912, Bullough proposed the concept of psychological distance, and its scope of application gradually expanded from aesthetic principles to the social group field of study for the measurement of social attitudes [3], and later to the trade sector for the description of individual perception [4] and to the domain of social relations [5]. With growing attention from researchers, studies of psychological distance have gradually but continually expanded to other fields. Agnew et al. defined psychological distance as "individuals' subjective perception about others and self-relation distance and resulting emotional experience after integrating all sorts of social information" [6]. Trope and Liberman deemed psychological distance to be "individuals' perception about different time contexts, space contexts, social relations and possible event occurrence contexts at this very moment" [7]. Both of these explanations regard psychological distance as a kind of perception, and a kind of psychological construction made by individuals based on the interpretation and processing of objective information. Psychological distance is used to explain people's response mechanisms for object perception and assessment decisions. With regard to occupational safety and health problems, the public also perceive and make assessment decisions with a self-centered perspective. For this reason, it is appropriate to start from psychological distance in order to discuss public intimacy with occupational safety and health problems.

In combination with relevant knowledge of psychological distance, this research builds up a four-dimensional structure for occupational safety and health psychological distance, starting from the dimensions of cognitive, emotional, expected and behavioral distance to explore public attitudes and responses to occupational safety and health problems. Cognitive distance refers to public occupational safety and health knowledge status and degree of cognition; emotional distance refers to public emotional perception of the intimacy and degree of integration of occupational safety and health problems; expected distance refers to public perception of the future expectation of occupational safety and health problems based on existing tendencies or judgment experience; and behavioral distance refers to the public perception of participatory behavior in occupational safety and health governance. Against this backdrop, residents in six cities from eastern, middle and western regions of China were selected for investigation and acquiring information on public psychological distance intimacy with regard to occupational safety and health problems. Furthermore, by analyzing the relationships and mechanisms of influence among cognitive, emotional, expected and behavioral distance, our research was designed to provide information for the further study of occupational safety and health problems in China. This research is significant for the promotion of occupational safety and health governance.

2. Theoretical Analysis

2.1. Implication Analysis of Public Psychological Distance towards Occupational Safety and Health Problems

Existing studies on occupational safety and health mostly concentrate on the structural aspects of the occupational safety and health system [8] and start from the perspective of state policy to prevent and solve occupational safety and health problems. Although policy efficacy itself plays a vital role in the solution of occupational safety and health problems, the public has a more important status as the executor of policy. On the other hand, occupational safety and health problems may also be governed from the perspective of occupational safety and health supervision. Relevant studies list the establishment of state occupational safety and health supervision agencies and the enforcement of effective supervision as an important move to ensure occupational safety and health [9]. It cannot be denied that supervision may be useful in urging practitioners to reduce unsafe actions and to normalize employee operation, but public attention on occupational safety and health problems is probably more persistent and stable because of endogenous factors (such as health, civic and responsibility awareness). As demonstrated by academic studies, the public have a stronger sense of identity towards garbage regulation policies as a result of endogenous factors [10,11]. Existing studies do not start from the public perspective in order to observe their attitudes and response towards occupational safety and health. Therefore, no solutions have been made for the governance of occupational safety and health in essence.

Distance in natural science generally means the interval length of objects in space or time, while psychological distance emphasizes the importance of individual perceptions and comprehension of the environment as a kind of social cognitive theory. One of the core tenets is that people's responses towards social events depends upon their psychological representation [12]. Individuals' psychological distance towards objects reflects their intimacy with, and emphasis on, the objects and directly determines individual behaviors. Consequently, this research incorporates psychological distance into the study of occupational safety and health problems. Psychological distance manifests individuals' intrinsic perceptions about intimacy. In this sense, public psychological distance towards occupational safety and health explicitly reflects their concern with occupational safety and health.

In the study of psychological distance, different researchers give interpretations from different perspectives. From the perspective of trade, psychological distance is defined as the factor which hinders or disturbs suppliers and consumers [4]. From an interpersonal relations angle, psychological distance is defined as individual subjective feelings towards intimacy or alienation generated from the sense of uncertainty about surrounding relations, subject to the discrepancy in status, values and cultural backgrounds. In the field of organization management, psychological distance is defined as employees' subjective judgments about distance intimacy, which predict and evaluate their behavior within the organization based on their degree of acceptance and actual degree of contribution. It is also used to describe the degree of conformity or integration between subjects and perception objects [13]. In all research fields, psychological distance in nature is a kind of subjective judgment. Likewise, in the field of public health, the public also makes subjective judgments about intimacy with or alienation from occupational safety and health. Accordingly, this research defines psychological distance as a subjective, public intimacy perception with a resulting promotion of action and inclination based on the comprehension and degree of perception of occupational safety and health problems.

2.2. Structural Analysis of Public Psychological Distance towards Occupational Safety and Health Problems

At present, studies concerning psychological distance primarily exhibit the following four dimensions: spatial distance, temporal distance, social distance and hypotheticality. Spatial distance is defined as the distance between stimulant and individual in the spatial dimension; temporal distance is defined as the time between individual and present and target events in the past or future; social distance is defined as the intimacy or specificity of the relation between social objects and individual; hypotheticality is defined as the occurrence possibility of event, existence possibility of thing, or closeness degree to individual real life [7]. In their study of employee-organization psychological distance, Chen and Li grouped psychological distance into six dimensions: experiential, behavioral, emotional, cognitive, time-space and objective social distance [13]. For example, if employees felt close to organization time-space distance, they would like to stay in the organization (voluntary overtime). Otherwise, they might get out of the organization immediately after work. If employees felt close to organization emotional distance, they would have sense of happiness in the organization or otherwise suffer from pains and depression. If employees felt close to organization behavioral distance, they might sacrifice their own interests to safeguard the interests of the organization. On the contrary, they would pursue their own best interests in the organization. This research proposes that public perceptions regarding psychological distance towards occupational safety and health also vary at different levels.

As demonstrated by research, public perceptions about objects reveal their focus on those objects. Li recruited urban citizens as research objects and deemed public perception to be the comprehension and degree of perception of public and social affairs [14]. In a study on residents' focus on health knowledge, Dai et al. observed that the health knowledge aspects that concerned individuals the most were, in order of importance, food safety, chronic disease, infectious disease and psychological health, and that they accordingly developed pertinent health promotion strategies [15]. Given that public perceptions of occupational safety and health embody public psychological distance intimacy in occupational safety and health, this research illustrates public cognitive distance towards occupational safety and health as a measurement dimension of psychological distance, and highlights the assessment of the degree of public comprehension of relevant occupational safety and health knowledge.

Emotions are individuals' attitudes and experiences regarding whether objective things have satisfied personal demands, and include love, pleasure, happiness, detestation, anger, or contempt. Emotion is the immediate reflection of relation intimacy. As found by relevant studies, establishing psychological contacts can induce individuals to maintain similar emotional and even physiological states to others [16]. This implies that when individuals keep emotional intimacy with others (or other objects), their focus on those objects can be inferred to some extent. While studying the employee-organization relationship, Chen and Li used emotional distance to express employees' emotional intimacy and integration perceptions about their organization [13]. In the same way, public perceptions of occupational safety and health problems also involve a certain degree of emotional integration. Such emotions may include a sense of depression or anger towards occupational safety and health problems that have occurred, or a sense of happiness and comfort resulting from the progress made with regard to existing occupational safety and health problems. Hence, this research chose public emotional distance towards occupational safety and health as a measurement dimension of psychological distance, and emphasized the measurement of public emotional integration in occupational safety and health problems.

The term "expectancy" refers to an estimation regarding future events. From the perspective of realistic behaviors, expectancy is a process whereby subjects make specific behavioral decisions pursuant to a judgment made with collected information about the future. At present, available studies about public expectancy mainly emphasize the macroeconomic expectancy management field. Bernanke held the opinion that currency policy is essentially about the problem of expectancy [17]. Public expectancy management has become the key content and core of the currency policy of central bank macro-control work [18]. To describe the employee-organization relationship, Chen and Li put forward the concept of experiential distance to represent employees' perceptions about future expectancies based on existing tendencies or experiences [13]. From this view, the public would also form some explicit perception about the future direction of occupational safety and health on account of acquired information related to occupational safety and health problems. This is known as the expected distance.

Behavior includes all purposeful activities of organizations or individuals, namely the conduct and actions of subjects. Qin and Jing started from the perspective of behavioral distance to explore behavioral difficulties in management, and their study provided a new channel for investigation of the harmonious development of organizations [19]. Chen and Li put forward behavioral distance to represent employees' perceptions about organizational intimacy in terms of "favor-organization" behavior [13]. Actions here specifically mean organizational citizenship behaviors, namely employees' out-of-duty behaviors in favor of the organization, including personal initiative, helping behaviors and organization loyalty [20]. Similarly, this means that the public needs to have a relatively close psychological distance towards occupational safety and health in order to solve related issues. As a consequence, public behavioral willingness and responses towards occupational safety and health problems reflect their focus on occupational safety and health. Public behavioral distance towards occupational safety and health is a key indicator of psychological distance.

2.3. Structural Relation Analysis of Psychological Distance

Cognition determines the way that individuals perceive objects and has a significant influence on individual behavioral patterns. Researchers have conducted many studies on the relation between cognition and behavior. In the environmental studies field, Vringer et al. proposed that recognition of environmental problems and diverse insights about the role of environmental behaviors strongly influenced residents' energy consumption behaviors [21]. According to Groot and Steg [22], environmental cognition, environmental knowledge and concern for the environment could significantly affect residents' choice of travel mode. In education, Li and Liu explored the relation between left-behind middle school students' cognitive emotion regulation and characteristics of dangerous behaviors, finding that passive cognitive emotion regulation was a risk factor for dangerous behaviors, while positive cognitive emotion regulation was a protective factor for dangerous behaviors [23]. Shao used the example of an emergency incident to probe into the rhetoric strategies and communication paths of news releases under the perspective of public cognition [24]. Given that this research concentrates on public familiarity with occupational safety and health-related knowledge with regard to public cognitive distance towards occupational safety and health, the relation between knowledge and behavior is also a key concern of our study. As demonstrated by research findings, knowledge has a significant impact on behavior, and related knowledge concerning specific behaviors is an important predictive variable for those specific behaviors [25]. Duerden and Witt also pointed out the significant correlation between environmental knowledge and individuals' environment-related behaviors [26]. As a result, this research speculates that there exists a certain relationship between public cognitive distance towards occupational safety and health and behavioral distance.

Research has also shown the significant influence of emotion on behavior [27,28]. Specifically, in their study of green purchasing behaviors, Kanchanapibul et al. restricted influential factors to emotional variables, concluding that the standardization path coefficient of emotion against green purchasing behaviors was as high as 0.489 [29]. Wang and Wu observed that positive emotion had a stronger influence on green purchasing behaviors than negative emotion, through further exploration of the correlation and inherent laws of emotion and behavior [30]. Cheng et al. discussed the relation between college students' cognition and procrastination behavior and eventually demonstrated a positive correlation between passive emotion and procrastination behavior, and a negative correlation between positive emotion and procrastination behavior [31]. Accordingly, this research tests the hypothesis that there exists a certain relationship between public emotional distance towards occupational safety and health and behavioral distance.

As a psychological phenomenon, expectancy is another key factor that affects individuals' behaviors. Hussain stressed that changes in future information lead to changes in economic agents' expectations and further manipulates their specific investment, consumption, labor supply and other behavioral decisions in the current period [32]. The study of public expectancy has been widely applied in all fields. In the field of consumption, Zhai analyzed multiple forms of expression of residents' negative consumption expectancies, including a reduction in income, growing expenditure in the future, and a rise in product price [33]. Subsequently, pertinent measures were proposed to regulate these negative expectancies so as to promote consumption behaviors. Consumption expectancy had a direct influence on consumption demand as the prerequisite for consumers to formulate and implement consumption behaviors. In the domain of macroeconomics, Lu demonstrated the influence of public expectancy on the macroeconomy in a study of publically expected monetary policy effects [34]. Therefore, this research speculates that a certain relationship exists between public expected distance towards occupational safety and health and behavioral distance.

In summary, there exists certain relation among the four dimensions of public occupational safety and health psychological distance. Public occupational safety and health cognitive distance as the basis can adjust emotional distance and expected distance, and play a decisive role in behavioral distance. Furthermore, emotional distance can promote expected distance. If the public have closer occupational safety and health emotional distance, they probably have closer expected distance and vice versa. Simultaneously, emotional distance can directly trigger behavioral distance, which means that if the public have closer occupational safety and health emotional distance, they probably show high willingness of concern, willingness of implementing, willingness of dissemination and willingness of donations to occupational safety and health problems and vice versa. Expected distance can intensify behavioral distance. If the public have closer occupational safety and health expected distance, they probably have closer behavioral distance. The analysis of public psychological distance structural relationships with regard to occupational safety and health behaviors is shown in Figure 1.

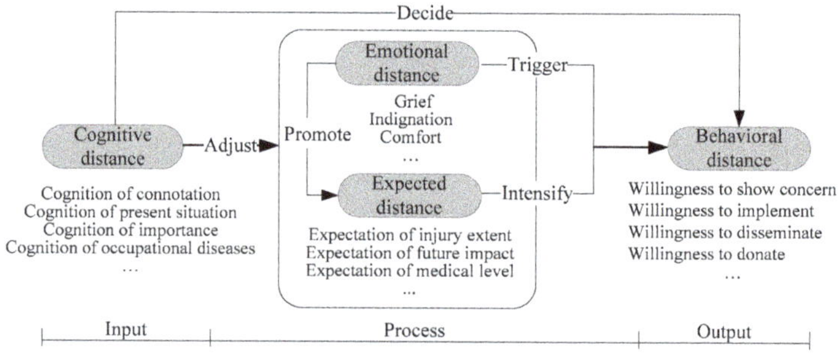

Figure 1. Profile chart of public psychological distance structural relationships in occupational safety and health behaviors.

3. Research Method

3.1. *Quadratic Response Surface Regression Analysis*

Based on our literature review, there exists a certain relation between the four dimensions in public occupational safety and health psychological distance (Figure 1), but until now few scholars have studied the influence of matching degree between cognition and emotion, cognition and expectation, emotion and expectation on behaviors. Public intimacy with occupational safety and health behavioral distance should not be simply ascribed to single factor like cognitive distance, emotional distance, behavioral distance, but should be the joint effect caused by the interaction of cognitive, emotional and expected distances. Therefore, discussion about the influence of matching degree between cognitive, emotional and expected distances on behavioral distance has very important theoretical and practical values. This research plans to conduct the research with quadratic response surface regression analysis method.

Response surface methodology utilizes integrated experimental technologies in statistics to solve the correlation between complicated system input (variable) and output (response). Mathematical expression of response methodology involves multiple linear regression (MLR) analysis, as shown in Equation (1):

$$y = \alpha_0 + \sum_{j=1}^{n} \alpha_j x_j + \sum_{j-n+1}^{2n} \alpha_j x_{j-k}^2 + \sum_{i=1}^{n-1} \sum_{j=i+1}^{n} a_{ij} x_i x_j \quad (1)$$

whereby n is the design variable, α_0 is a constant term for an undetermined coefficient, α_j is a one-degree term for an undetermined coefficient and α_{ij} is a quadratic term for an undetermined coefficient.

Quadratic response surface regression analysis combines quadratic polynomial regression with response surface methodology. This method has been primarily applied in the study of individual-organization matching theory [35,36]. Subsequently, Chen et al. applied this method in the field of urban household garbage regulation policy to investigate the relationships between the degree of public policy understanding, support willingness, performance willingness, and promotion willingness [37]. In matching measurement research, there often include two measurement methods. The first one is direct matching measurement method which requires the respondent to directly determine the degree of matching between the two [38]. Though the method is rather simple, but the independent effects cannot be examined. Another method is indirect matching measurement which requests the respondent to respectively assess the features of the two, and then compare the consistency or similarity of their grading scores [39]. Indirect measurement usually adopts difference scores, Q classification method, product term indicator method, etc. However, these indirect matching measurement statistical strategies are defective in theory and methodology. For instance, difference scores can result in decreased measurement reliability and mutual confusion between the two effects [40]. Quadratic response surface regression analysis method belongs to a matching measurement and statistical analysis strategy developed to overcome above-mentioned defects [35]. It possesses the following advantages: Firstly, it provides an entire statistical analysis and explanation framework for matching measurement research that can not only well explain the secondary coefficient of polynomial regression equation, but also test the response surface features and shape formed by these coefficients. Secondly, it is not only limited to measuring the matching relation of representatives, but also can examine the influence caused by mismatching relation, thus providing a more robust evaluation method for the theoretical model related to matching research. Thirdly, compared with the traditional indirect matching method, it has higher predictive validity. Admittedly, the method also has limitations. Firstly, as quadratic response surface regression analysis adopts a series of statistical tests to judge the slope and curvature significance of all target lines on the response surface, it greatly increases statistical mistakes due to repeated examination [35]. Secondly, quadratic response surface regression analysis has the same problem with general regression analysis application. All of these methods assume measured indicator variables have no error, but this is not up to the real measurement conditions. Though quadratic response surface regression analysis does not totally jump out of traditional statistical analysis framework, available statistical analysis technology indicates that quadratic response surface regression analysis has extensive application prospects in matching or consistency research.

In our study, there was also a relationship between cognitive, emotional, expected and behavioral distance, which indicates a degree of "consistency" among all of these public distances towards occupational safety and health. This accords with the "matching" implied in individual-organization matching theory. Consequently, this research used quadratic response surface regression analysis to thoroughly investigate the response relationship between public cognitive, emotional, expected and behavioral distance in occupational safety and health. It defines consistency as the situation in which the score of cognitive distance equals that of emotional distance, cognitive distance equals expected distance, and emotional distance equals expected distance. The score is divided into five points according to a scale grade. Higher grades indicate a higher degree of consistency. In addition, this research calculates inconsistency (gaps) by comparing in pairs from the score of cognitive, emotional and expected distance, and separately calculating difference value in each pair.

3.2. Scale and Investigation

There is a lack of a mature scale for the study of public occupational safety and health psychological distance. Therefore, this research included an exploratory qualitative study to determine scale questions and collected material during interviews with 67 citizens associated with different industries, and of different age groups and characteristics. The interview material was sorted in strict accordance with open coding, axial coding and selective coding. In addition, six professionals (two professors, two associate professors and two lecturers) were invited to negotiate and determine question accuracy, scale feasibility and expression readability. Eventually, 16 questions were developed for the measurement of occupational safety and health psychological distance, on the dimensions of cognitive, emotional, expected and behavioral distance (see Table A1). Among these dimensions, cognitive distance primarily includes public cognition of occupational safety and health implications, the present situation, importance and occupational diseases. Emotional distance highlights the focus on occupational safety and health accidents, or state and corporate occupational safety and health problems, and public emotions such as grief, indignation and comfort. Expected distance is concerned with whether public perceptions of occupational safety accidents and the extent of injury are exaggerated, whether the quality of occupational safety and health problem governance has any influence on the future perceptions of the public, and whether the development of medical treatments and techniques ensures that occupational safety and health problems will not severely threaten the public. Behavioral distance deals with public understanding and willingness to concentrate on occupational safety and health problems, to commit to occupational safety and health problem governance, to popularize occupational safety and health knowledge to surrounding people, and to make donations to those injured in occupational accidents and occupational disease patients. Responses were on a Lickert five-point scale whereby 1 signified "totally incongruent", 2 meant "not too congruent", 3 meant "noncommittal", 4 meant "relatively congruent", and 5 meant "totally congruent". A higher score indicated greater occupational safety and health psychological distance.

The pilot investigation took place in Jiangsu and Anhui Provinces in March 2018. Altogether 550 questionnaires for anonymous completion were distributed and 478 completed questionnaires were collected, with an effective response rate of 86.91%. As indicated by the descriptive statistical analysis of the test samples, the gender ratio of the samples was basically balanced, with males accounting for 59.7% and females accounting for 40.3%. Age distribution was relatively even, with participants aged below 20 years accounting for 1.3%, those aged 21–30 accounting for 25.1%, those aged 31–40 accounting for 29.6%, those aged 41–50 accounting for 23.4%, those aged 50–60 accounting for 14.8% and those aged above 60 accounting for 5.8%. The investigation targeted a variety of participants including government staff, coal mine enterprise leaders, and common social groups. The questionnaire was finally designed after reliability and validity analysis and correction of questions.

The formal investigation was composed of two parts. The first part collected individual socio-demographic information and the second part investigated public occupational safety and health psychological distance. The formal investigation started in April–July 2018. Altogether 3000 questionnaires were distributed and 2386 completed questionnaires were collected, with an effective response rate of 79.53%. Before distributing the questionnaires, regional respondents were selected via stratified sampling. Due to the diverse economic and regional features in the eastern, middle and western regions, the research screened two cities from each of the three regions: Hebei and Jiangsu Province in the eastern region, Anhui and Hunan Province in the middle region, and Sichuan and Xinjiang Province in the western region. Simultaneously, in consideration of the wide variety of potential respondents concerned with occupational safety and health problems, including government staff, coal mine enterprise leaders, coal mine safety supervisors, coal mine front-line workers, third-party social organization staff (including those working for occupational disease hospitals, occupational disease relief funds, and industrial association organization staffs), and patients with diseases such as pneumoconiosis as well as ordinary people, seven types of respondents were selected for the investigation to provide a sample including people from all walks of life and of both genders and different educational backgrounds, ages, and marital and political status. To be specific, the research chose three samples from 45 state-owned large and medium coal mine enterprises in China, and selected six types of coal mine front-line workers in ventilation and fire prevention, coal mining, tunneling, mechatronics, transportation, and ground work and leaders with different positions. Moreover, the research chose coal mine safety supervisors according to age and position discrepancy. For ensuring the rationality of third-party social organization staff samples, the research chose staff and volunteers from Chinese Occupational Safety and Health Association, China Coal Miner Pneumoconiosis Prevention Foundation, and Love Save Pneumoconiosis. The sample selection conformed to the practical distribution situation. The subject and purpose of the investigation were explained in detail to the participants. The researchers sent gifts to participants to express their gratitude and to improve the response rate and effectiveness of the questionnaire survey. Please refer to Table 1 for the specific sample structure.

Table 1. Sample structure.

Social-Demographic Variable		Frequency (N)	Proportion (%)	Social-Demographic Variable		Frequency (N)	Proportion (%)
Gender	Male	1782	74.69	Age	<20	8	0.34
	Female	604	25.31		21–30	671	28.12
Education	Primary school and below	61	2.56		31–40	775	32.48
	Junior middle school	403	16.89		41–50	556	23.30
	Senior middle school	635	26.61		51–60	273	11.44
	Junior college	600	25.15		>60	103	4.32
	Undergraduate	469	19.66	Marital status	Single	306	12.82
	Master and higher	218	9.14		Married	1978	82.90
Identity	Government staff	109	4.57		Divorced	69	2.89
	Coal mine enterprise leader	106	4.44		Widowed	33	1.38
	Coal mine safety supervisor	155	6.50	Political status	CPC member	660	27.66
	Coal mine front-line worker	887	37.18		Democratic party	48	2.01
	Third-party social staff	210	8.80		Non-Party personage	169	7.08
	Pneumoconiosis patient	207	8.68		The mass	1509	63.24
	Ordinary people	712	29.84				

Note: CPC = Communist Party of China, N = number.

3.3. Ethical Approval

This study was carried out in accordance with the recommendations of the Ethical Codes of Consulting and Clinical Psychology of Chinese Psychological Society, Chinese Psychological Society. The protocol was approved by the China Occupational Safety and Health Association—Occupational Mental Health Professional Committee. All subjects gave written informed consent in accordance with the Declaration of Helsinki. It is the duty of researchers who are involved in psychological research to protect the life, health, dignity, integrity, right to self-determination, privacy, and confidentiality of personal information of the research subjects. The responsibility for the protection of research subjects always rested with our research team and the China Occupational Safety and Health Association—Occupational Mental Health Professional Committee, and never with the research subjects, even though they had given consent.

4. Data Analysis

4.1. Factor Analysis

Formal questionnaire validity and reliability test results indicated that the Cronbach's α value for public psychological distance towards occupational safety and health, at 0.830, was above 0.8. This implied that the scale had relatively high reliability in general. The Cronbach's α values of all latent variables were 0.743, 0.661, 0.702 and 0.823 respectively and the corresponding CR values were 0.859, 0.805, 0.825 and 0.871. Given that both statistics exceeded the acceptability criteria, the scale passed the reliability test.

We then rigorously developed the program in line with the scale. Based on considerable literature research, the scale finally exhibited a favorable content validity after being repeatedly negotiated and corrected by five experts in the field of management. Moreover, the standardization load of 16 scale questions with corresponding latent variables, ranging between 0.584 and 0.815, was far above 0.5 and attained significance. The corresponding average variance extracted (AVE) were 0.604, 0.509, 0.545 and 0.629 respectively. Given the criterion of AVE > 0.5, the scale had good convergent validity. In addition, the AVE square root of the latent variables being above the correlation coefficient of the latent variables implied a favorable degree of latent variable structural discrimination. The scale accordingly passed the validity test.

AMOS 17.0 (SPSS Inc., Chicago, IL, USA) was adopted to carry out confirmatory factor analysis on the structural validity of the questionnaire. After two attempts at model regulation, the final fitting indicators were chi-square (χ^2) = 3055, degree of freedom (df) = 887, χ^2/df = 3.444, root mean square error of approximation (RMSEA) = 0.047, goodness of fit index (GFI) = 0.903, normed fit index (NFI) = 0.906, comparative fit index (CFI) = 0.915, incremental fit index (IFI) = 0.904, and Tacker-Lewis index (TLI) = 0.898. All indicators attained an ideal scope. In summary, the research verified the four-dimensional structure of public occupational safety and health psychological distance comprising cognitive, emotional, expected and behavioral distance.

4.2. Statistical Analysis

Descriptive statistical analysis was conducted for public occupational safety and health psychological distance and its four corresponding dimensions. Given that closer psychological distance indicates a higher public focus on occupational safety and health problems, the overall questions were marked in reverse. Lower scores showed closer public occupational safety and health psychological distance, while higher scores indicated farther public occupational safety and health psychological distance. (1–2) points indicated intimate distance, (2–3) points indicated relatively close distance, (3–4) points indicated relatively far distance and (4–5) points indicated far distance. The specific analysis results are shown in Table 2.

Table 2. Descriptive statistical analysis of psychological distance (N = 2386).

Variable	M	SD	(1–2)	(2–3)	(3–4)	(4–5)
PD	2.5520	0.53745	454, 19.04%	1434, 60.15%	495, 20.76%	1, 0.04%
CD	3.2791	0.90552	316, 13.24%	580, 24.31%	1111, 46.56%	379, 15.88%
ED	2.1954	0.68459	1194, 50.08%	929, 38.97%	243, 10.19%	18, 0.76%
ExD	2.5624	0.96773	900, 37.72%	797, 33.40%	535, 22.42%	154, 6.45%
BD	2.1698	0.89793	1286, 53.90%	792, 33.19%	250, 10.48%	58, 2.43%

Note: PD = Psychological distance, CD = cognitive distance, ED = emotional distance, ExD = expected distance, BD = behavioral distance, N = number, M = mean value, SD = standard deviation.

Table 2 shows that the mean value of public occupational safety and health psychological distance was 2.552. Over 60% of respondents and nearly 20% of respondents respectively showed a relatively close and intimate psychological distance to occupational safety and health. This implies that the public pays great attention to occupational safety and health problems. Specific analysis of these dimensions revealed that around 50% of respondents exhibited relatively far cognitive distance for occupational safety and health problems (in the range of 3–4 points), and that most respondents' emotional, expected and behavioral distance towards occupational safety and health problems was relatively close, in the range of 1–3 points.

4.3. Quadratic Response Surface Regression Analysis

Analysis of the four dimensions of occupational safety and health, as shown in Figure 2, demonstrated that public cognitive, emotional, expected and behavioral distance all exhibit a gap. The group that had congruent cognitive, emotional, expected and behavioral distance (≥3 or <3) accounted for only 18.75%, while the group that was incongruent (i.e., had gaps) accounted for 81.25%.

Additionally, the group with the scores of cognitive distance (≥3), emotional distance (<3), expected distance (<3) and behavioral distance (<3) accounted for 26.51% (highest occupation). In contrast, the group with the scores of cognitive distance (<3), emotional distance (≥3), expected distance (≥3) and behavioral distance (≥3) accounted for 0.17% (lowest occupation).

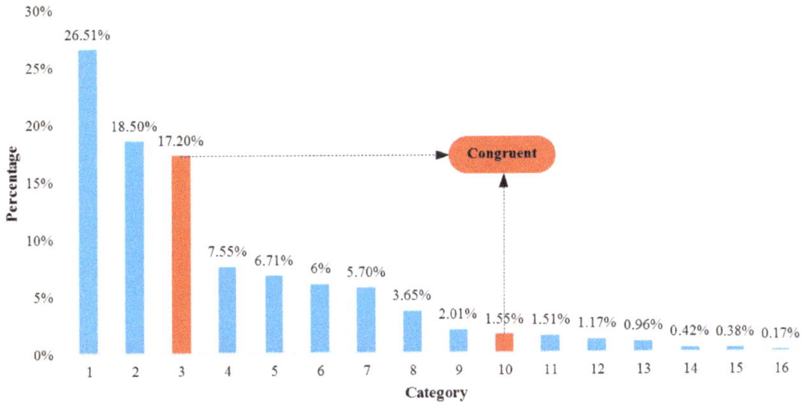

Figure 2. Public occupational safety and health psychological distance four-dimension gap analysis. Note: 1: cognitive distance (CD) ≥ 3, emotional distance (ED) < 3, expected distance (ExD) < 3, behavioral distance (BD) < 3; 2: CD ≥ 3, ED < 3, ExD ≥ 3, BD < 3; 3: CD < 3, ED < 3, ExD < 3, BD < 3; 4: CD ≥ 3, ED ≥ 3, ExD < 3, BD ≥ 3; 5: CD < 3, ED < 3, ExD ≥ 3, BD < 3; 6: CD ≥ 3, ED < 3, ExD ≥ 3, BD ≥ 3; 7: CD ≥ 3, ED < 3, ExD < 3, BD ≥ 3; 8: CD ≥ 3, ED ≥ 3, ExD < 3, BD < 3; 9: CD ≥ 3, ED ≥ 3, ExD ≥ 3, BD < 3; 10: CD ≥ 3, ED ≥ 3, ExD ≥ 3, BD ≥ 3; 11: CD < 3, ED < 3, ExD ≥ 3, BD ≥ 3; 12: CD < 3, ED < 3, ExD < 3, BD ≥ 3; 13: CD < 3, ED ≥ 3, ExD < 3, BD < 3; 14: CD < 3, ED ≥ 3, ExD ≥ 3, BD < 3; 15: CD < 3, ED ≥ 3, ExD < 3, BD ≥ 3; 16: CD < 3, ED ≥ 3, ExD ≥ 3, BD ≥ 3. The bold indicates congruence.

In combination with the above analysis, quadratic response surface regression analysis was used in a conceptual model to investigate the gaps in cognitive, emotional, expected and behavioral distance. From the perspective of behavioral distance, the following three models were constructed: cognitive distance/emotional distance model 1 (equations (2) and (3)), cognitive distance/expected distance model 2 (equations (4) and (5)), and emotional distance/expected distance model 3 (Equations (6) and (7)). In order to prevent multi-collinearity, centralization processing was applied to public cognitive distance (X), emotional distance (Y), expected distance (Z) and behavioral distance (M) towards occupational safety and health, and subsequently the quadratic components of X, Y and Z (X2, Y2, Z2) and the product terms X × Y, X × Z and Y × Z were calculated. The calculations were then completed using the SPSS 21.0 statistical software (International Business Machines Corporation, New York, NY, USA).

$$\text{Cognitive/emotional distance M1}: \ M1 = \alpha_0 + \alpha_1 x + \alpha_2 y + e \tag{2}$$

$$\text{Cognitive/emotional distance M2}: \ M2 = \alpha_0 + \alpha_1 x + \alpha_2 y + \alpha_3 x^2 + \alpha_4 y^2 + \alpha_5 x \cdot y + e \tag{3}$$

$$\text{Cognitive/expected distance M1}: \ M1 = \alpha_0 + \alpha_1 x + \alpha_2 z + e \tag{4}$$

$$\text{Cognitive/expected distance M2}: \ M2 = \alpha_0 + \alpha_1 x + \alpha_2 z + \alpha_3 x^2 + \alpha_4 z^2 + \alpha_5 x \cdot z + e \tag{5}$$

$$\text{Emotional/expected distance M1}: \ M1 = \alpha_0 + \alpha_1 y + \alpha_2 z + e \tag{6}$$

$$\text{Emotional/expected distance M2}: \ M2 = \alpha_0 + \alpha_1 y + \alpha_2 z + \alpha_3 y^2 + \alpha_4 z^2 + \alpha_5 y \cdot z + e \tag{7}$$

Correlation analysis (Table 3) demonstrated the significantly positive correlation among public cognitive, emotional, expected and behavioral distance towards occupational safety and health problems. In further regression analysis results (Table 4), both behavior M1 and behavior M2 showed significant linear correlation with cognitive, emotional, expected and behavioral distance. Moreover, the regulation R2 of three-group behavior M2's comparative behavior M1 was on a rising trend, which showed that behavior M2, with relatively strong explanatory power, was a more accurate representation of the correlation between the independent and dependent variable.

Table 3. Correlation analysis of public cognitive/emotional/expected/behavioral distance towards occupational safety and health.

Variable	Observed Value	Cognitive Distance	Emotional Distance	Expected Distance	Behavioral Distance
Cognitive distance	Pearson correlation Sig. (2-tailed)	1			
Emotional distance	Pearson correlation Sig. (2-tailed)	0.280 ** 0.000	1		
Expected distance	Pearson correlation Sig. (2-tailed)	0.129 * 0.044	0.05 1* 0.012	1	
Behavioral distance	Pearson correlation Sig. (2-tailed)	0.180 ** 0.000	0.564 ** 0.000	0.079 ** 0.000	1

Note: Sig. = significance. * indicates significant correlation at 0.05 level (bilateral). ** indicates significant correlation at 0.01 level (bilateral).

Table 4. Regression analysis on public occupational safety and health psychological distance.

Variable	Behavior M1	Behavior M2	Variable	Behavior M1	Behavior M2	Variable	Behavior M1	Behavior M2
Constant	0.001	−0.024	Constant	0.000	0.239 ***	Constant	0.001	0.147 ***
Cognition	0.023	0.047 *	Cognition	0.180 ***	0.190 ***	Emotion	0.428 ***	0.359 ***
Emotion	0.425 ***	0.416 ***	Expectation	0.080 ***	0.166 ***	Expectation	0.055 **	0.084 ***
Cognition ^{2}		0.011	Cognition ^{2}		0.045 **	Emotion ^{2}		0.016 *
Emotion ^{2}		−0.007	Expectation ^{2}		−0.272 ***	Expectation ^{2}		−0.162 ***
Cognition × Emotion		0.058 ***	Cognition × Expectation		−0.088 ***	Emotion × Expectation		−0.088 ***
Adjustment R^2	0.318	0.323		0.037	0.125		0.320	0.352

Note: M1: model 1, M2: model 2. R^2: R^2 is the ratio of the sum of the squares of the regression to the sum of the squares used to measure the goodness of fit of the model. * indicates significant correlation at 0.05 level (bilateral). ** indicates significant correlation at 0.01 level (bilateral). *** indicates significant correlation at 0.001 level (bilateral). Cognition ^{2}: Cognition distance square, Emotion ^{2}: Emotion distance square, Cognition × Emotion: Interaction item of cognition distance and emotion distance.

Edward points out the necessity to draw up a three-dimensional diagram to express the relation between independent variables and the dependent variable in case of any significance in a polynomial regression model with multiple quadratic terms. Consequently, response surface analysis was conducted on the regression model. The MatLab R2008a software (MathWorks, Natick, MA, USA) was used for programming and presentation of the three-dimensional diagram of public cognitive, emotional, expected and behavioral distance towards occupational safety and health. The Y = X transverse line indicates the line of congruence. On the X–Y plane, the two measurement indicators have equal value and orientation. A larger abscissa indicates higher congruence between the two indicators, while a larger ordinate indicates farther behavioral distance. To summarize, the response diagram of public cognitive, emotional, expected and behavioral distance towards occupational safety and health follows the Y = X transverse line (Figures 3b, 4b and 5b).

Next, the public response towards occupational safety and health cognitive, emotional and behavioral distance were analyzed. As suggested by the regression analysis results (Table 4), public emotional distance towards occupational safety and health problems in behavior M1 could significantly predict behavioral distance, but cognitive distance did not significantly predict behavioral distance. Public cognitive and emotional distance towards occupational safety and health problems in behavior M2 could significantly predict behavioral distance. The rising trend of behavior M2's comparative behavior to M1 regulation R2 demonstrates the relatively strong exploratory power of behavior M2, and reflects the non-linear relation between independent variables and the dependent variable. To exhibit directly the response of public cognitive distance and emotional distance in occupational safety and health problems to behavioral distance and the influence of cognitive and emotional distance congruence (or incongruence) on behavioral distance, response surface analysis was carried out on the three-dimensional diagram of the regression model. Figure 3b reveals the "progressively decreasing" response of cognitive and emotional distance congruence towards behavioral distance, which means that higher congruence between cognitive and emotional distance leads to closer public behavioral distance towards occupational safety and health. In other words, a larger gap between cognitive and emotional distance indicates farther behavioral distance of the public towards occupational safety and health.

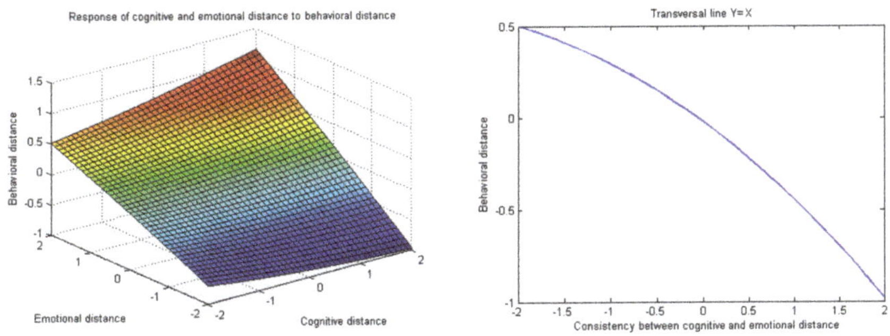

(a) Response surface (b) Congruence line

Figure 3. Response diagram of public cognitive and emotional distance towards occupational safety and health against behavioral distance.

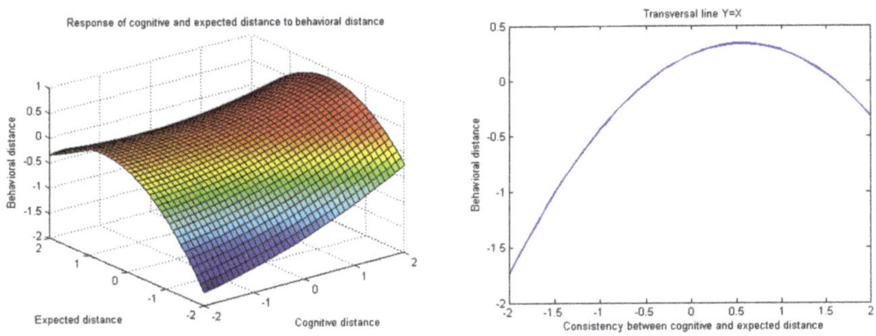

(a) Response surface (b) Congruence line

Figure 4. Response diagram of public cognitive and expected distance towards occupational safety and health against behavioral distance.

A similar method was adopted to analyze the response of public cognitive distance and expected distance towards behavioral distance in occupational safety and health. The regression analysis results indicated (Table 4) that public cognitive and expected distance towards occupational safety and health problems in behavior M2 could significantly predict behavioral distance. The significant rising trend of behavior M2's comparative behavior to M1 regulation R2 demonstrated the relatively strong exploratory power of behavior M2 and reflected the non-linear relation between independent variables and the dependent variable. Figure 4b shows that the response surface congruence line Y = X "convex" throughout the response surface analysis on the three-dimensional diagram of the regression model. This implies that when cognitive and expected distance become congruent, public behavioral distance towards occupational safety and health first increases and later declines. The ultimate trend signaled that a smaller gap between cognitive and expected distance for public occupational safety and health leads to closer behavioral distance. The calculation result derived an inflection point coordinate on the response surface of (0.53, 0.38).

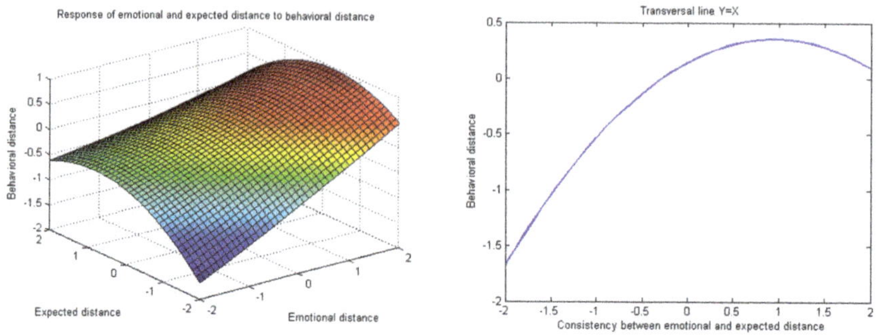

(a) Response surface (b) Congruence line

Figure 5. Response diagram of public emotional and expected distance towards occupational safety and health against behavioral distance.

A similar method was also applied to the analysis of the response of public emotional distance and expected distance towards behavioral distance in occupational safety and health. The regression analysis results indicated (Table 4) that public cognitive distance and expected distance towards occupational safety and health problems in behavior M2 could significantly predict behavioral distance. The rising trend of behavior M2's comparative behavior to M1 regulation R2 demonstrated the relatively strong exploratory power of behavior M2 and reflected the non-linear relation between independent variables and the dependent variable. Throughout the response surface analysis on the three-dimensional diagram of the regression model, Figure 5b displays the congruence calculation formula for emotional and expected distance. The congruence line Y = X shows that when cognitive and expected distance become congruent, public behavioral distance towards occupational safety and health problems first increases and later declines, and the general incongruence between emotional and expected distance presented the negative correlation with behavioral distance. In other words, although behavioral distance is at a relatively low level when cognitive and expected distance become incongruent, the final trend signals that a very small gap between cognitive and expected distance in public occupational safety and health perceptions leads to close behavioral distance. The calculation shows that the inflection point coordinate on the response surface was (0.76, 0.39).

5. Discussion

The descriptive statistical analysis of the sample demonstrated that approximately 80% of respondents had intimate or relatively close psychological distance towards occupational safety and health. Until 2017, the number of all types of workers in China totaled 776 million (National Bureau of Statistics of China 2017 data). Occupational safety and health problems concerned with the core rights and interests of workers are closely related to the survival and development of every single worker and their family. In this sense, public psychological distance towards occupational safety and health is relatively close overall. However, 62.44% of respondents presented a relatively remote cognitive distance towards occupational safety and health, or perhaps had insufficient understanding or knowledge of occupational safety and health. The research findings imply that this phenomenon is primarily attributable to two causes. First, the government or enterprise does not emphasize the publicity of occupational safety and health-related knowledge. Although they may have formulated many policies or regulations concerning occupational safety and health, inadequate publicity will result in the relatively far cognitive distance of the public. Second, the public lacks willingness to learn about occupational safety and health-related matters. Research shows that individuals encounter various barriers in the knowledge learning process [41,42]. Alternatively, individuals generally may not actively want to acquire such knowledge. Consequently, the government and relevant enterprises should optimize occupational safety and health-related knowledge publicity and overcome learning obstacles to the maximum extent possible.

The research demonstrated a gap among public cognitive, emotional, expected and behavioral distance towards occupational safety and health. This can be divided into two situations: a "weak attitude–strong behavior" situation (typical example: cognitive distance ≥3, emotional distance ≥3, expected distance ≥ 3 and behavioral distance < 3) and a "strong attitude–weak behavior" situation (typical example: cognitive distance < 3, emotional distance < 3, expected distance < 3 and behavioral distance ≥ 3). Research suggests that the cause of the "weak attitude–strong behavior" mismatch might be ascribed to an individual ability [43] and situational dilemma [44], with the former mainly including economic [45] and time restrictions [46]. However, in practice, there may be all kinds of restrictive situations in which the public cannot manage behavioral processing of public occupational safety and health issues. The cause of "strong attitude–weak behavior" is probably related to individuals' self-presentation behaviors in the process of solving occupational safety and health problems. For instance, based on competitive altruism theory, Griskevicius et al. proposed that individual altruistic behaviors could be guided by stimulating individual momentum to seek status and identity [47]. Antonetti's research also showed that the purpose of conspicuous green consumption was to pursue social status and reputation, and that it was also a type of altruistic behavior [48]. All of these are possible causes of the gap among cognitive, emotional, expected and behavioral distance.

The quadratic response surface regression analysis demonstrated that higher congruence between cognitive and emotional distance led to closer public behavioral distance towards occupational safety and health, which meant that congruence between of cognitive and emotional distance had a "driving effect" on behavioral distance. The Cognitive-Affective Personality System (CAPS) states that individual stable personality system structure is constituted by cognitive-affective units (CAUs) in some stable organizational relationship which may reflect individual peculiarities of personality. In addition, the events encountered by individuals interact with complex CAUs in the personality system and eventually determine an individual's behavior [49]. Existing studies generally verify the close connection between personal internal congruence and behavior [50]. This also means that, on account of the understanding and relevant knowledge of occupational safety and health, the public will have much closer behavioral distance under emotional support.

It has been shown that congruence between public cognitive and emotional distance towards occupational safety and health and behavioral distance presents "convex" changes. When cognitive and expected distance become congruent, public behavioral distance towards occupational safety and health will first increase and later decline. When cognitive and expected distance become incongruent, two situations will emerge, namely "positive sequence" incongruence and "reversed sequence" incongruence. In "positive sequence" incongruence, the public still have noncommittal attitudes towards the expected effects of future occupational safety and health governance and this will further positively influence their behavioral distance. In "reversed sequence" incongruence, although the public has great confidence in future occupational safety and health governance, their expectations might be blindly optimistic. Expectancy based on insufficient cognition is unstable and lacking basis. Therefore, the behavioral distance is naturally very great. However, when the congruence between public cognitive and expected distance reaches a high level, public behavioral distance towards occupational safety and health will show a declining trend. In a study of cognition and expectancy, Zhang and Zhao also suggested that the interactive function among different cognitive biases that takes expectancy as the medium is the underlying cause which affects individual risk assets pricing [51].

It is worth noticing that the congruence between public cognitive and emotional distance towards occupational safety and health presents a "progressive increase" response towards behavioral distance. This phenomenon deviates from psychology and behavior. In combination with the congruence between public cognitive and expected distance, behavioral distance should also increase. Accordingly, it can be predicted that expectancy has a hysteresis effect [52]. In management psychology, a hysteresis effect is used to describe the phenomenon in which decision, management and many other factors fall behind situation development and trigger adverse consequences [53]. Expectancy is a kind of psychological representation. Expectancy hysteresis results in the primary rising and subsequent declining trend of behavioral distance, even though public cognitive and emotional distance towards occupational safety and health become closer. Simultaneously, the deviation between the congruence of public emotional and expected distance towards occupational safety and health and behavioral distance is a phenomenon of "incongruent speech and behavior". The fundamental reason behind this may be the influence of a social commendatory effect [54]. When catering for social norms or management of impressions, the self-report bias tends to manifest itself in the form of positive attitudes (shown here as positive emotions and positive expectancy) and further deviate from following practical behaviors [55].

6. Conclusions

6.1. Conclusions

This study describes the connotations of the psychological distance of occupational safety and health for the public. Through literature and qualitative analysis, it has been shown that the psychological distance of the public with regard to occupational safety and health can be measured from four aspects: cognitive distance, emotional distance, expected distance and behavioral distance. The following conclusions were obtained from the data analysis.

Firstly, the public's psychological distance to occupational safety and health is at a relatively close level, which indicates that the public has a high endogenous tendency to be concerned about occupational safety and health problems. On the specific dimensions, nearly half of the public investigated had a far cognitive distance with regard to occupational safety and health. The public's distances to occupational safety and health, from near to far, are behavioral distance, emotional distance, expected distance and cognitive distance respectively. In general, the cognitive and expected distance are large, while the emotional and behavioral distance are small.

Second, a "gap" was demonstrated for the public's cognitive, emotional, expected and behavioral distance with regard to occupational safety and health problems; the proportion of the group with a "gap" was up to 81.25%.

Third, there was a significant positive correlation between the cognitive, emotional, expected and behavioral distance for problems related to occupational safety and health, with cognitive, emotional and expected distance all able to significantly predict behavioral distance.

Fourth, further analysis showed that the consistency in the public's cognitive and emotional distance for occupational safety and health had a progressively decreasing response to behavioral distance. That is, the higher the consistency existing in the public's cognitive and emotional distance for occupational safety and health, the shorter the behavioral distance and the larger the gap between cognitive and emotional distance, the farther the behavioral distance. The consistency existing in the public's cognitive and expected distance for occupational safety and health shows a "convex" change with behavioral distance. That is, when the cognitive and expected distance are consistent, the public's behavioral distance to occupational safety and health first increases and then decreases. Generally, the consistency existing in the public's emotional and expected distance for occupational safety and health shows a progressively increasing response to behavioral distance. However, the final trend is that the public's behavioral distance for occupational safety and health will be shorter when the gap between emotional and expected distance is very small.

6.2. Policy Implications

In order to improve the public's response to occupational safety and health, and effectively deal with, control and reduce the risk of occupational safety and health problems, the following policy recommendations are put forward according to the results of this study.

Firstly, the shortfall in the public's psychological distances for occupational safety and health should be filled, especially to decrease the public's cognitive distance to occupational safety and health. Cognitive distance is the basis of emotional, expected and behavioral distance, and the emotions, expectations and behaviors formed without the cognition of occupational safety and health are currently unstable. Therefore, it is necessary to improve the education of the public regarding occupational safety and health. On the one hand, the government should strengthen the popularization of knowledge related to occupational safety and health through innovative approaches to propaganda, broadening channels and intensifying publicity. On the other hand, occupational safety and health management is an activity that must be participated in by all, and the government should adopt a simple and interesting format when formulating pertinent policies or taking relevant measures, so as to maximize the public's enthusiasm for knowledge related to occupational safety and health.

Second, the public should be guided to progress from the gap-type of psychological distance to a consistent psychological distance. From the previous analysis, we could see that the causes of the "strong attitude–weak behavior" gap were individual ability and situational dilemma. The government should strengthen the public to improve their individual abilities, eliminate constraints and create an environment for behaviors that are beneficial to occupational safety and health. With regard to "weak attitude–strong behavior", it is known that individuals hope to express themselves and gain face through certain behaviors in view of the promotional effect of occupational safety and health governance on personal status, such as donating to patients who have suffered occupational injury. According to the theory of self-perception, people judge their own attitude to any particular occurrence on the basis of their own behavior and, to a certain extent, the situation. Based on theories of compensatory psychological mechanisms, the kind of behavior that is beneficial to occupational safety and health will also enhance the self-perception of the individual's occupational safety and health, including cognitive, emotional and expected distance. The theory of behavioral learning level also advocates changing attitudes through behavior. It can be seen that the psychological compensation effect can not only be directly beneficial to professional safety and health behavior, but also further promote the public's positive attitude towards occupational safety and health. This will, finally, repair the "gaps" of cognitive, emotional, expected and behavioral distance.

Thirdly, it is necessary to distinguish between the public's behavioral distance values for various kinds of occupational safety and health. The mechanisms for forming different types of behavior distance are distinct, so that the gaps for cognitive, emotional, expected and behavioral distance are also different. Understanding these processes is a prerequisite for policy formulation, and neglect of gaps by the government and related enterprises will lead to mismatches between policy and implementation. In the future, we should further explore the process by which the public forms different types of behavior distance to occupational safety and health, and investigate the causes of the gaps generated between behavioral distance and cognitive, emotional, and expected distance. Further deepening the public's motives for certain behaviors that are beneficial to occupational safety and health, constantly strengthening the public's cognition of, cultivating the public's affection for, and raising the public's expectations of occupational safety and health will fundamentally alter the contradiction between "different knowing and doing" and promote the public's level of response to occupational safety and health.

6.3. Study Limitations

This research also has some study limitations. The first one is limited research sample. Restricted by survey conditions and time, the research just recollects 2386 valid questionnaires. Though they can well represent public distribution condition, and meet basic sampling requirements under the statistical research method, the chosen samples are still limited in regional distribution. Even though the research has chosen samples from two provinces in eastern, two in middle and two in western regions, it still fails to totally reflect public occupational safety and health psychological distance conditions. Therefore, further research should enlarge the sample size. Secondly, as all data of items come from the retrospective answers of respondents, memory bias is inevitable. Thirdly, as psychological distance is perceived by individuals, corresponding theoretical construction is very sophisticated. Therefore, it is essential to further revise and modify public occupational safety and health psychological distance scale.

Author Contributions: Conceptualization, S.L. and H.C.; Methodology, S.L.; Software, S.L. and F.C.; Validation, H.C., X.H., C.H. and F.C.; Formal Analysis, S.L.; Investigation, S.L. and X.H.; Resources, H.C.; Data Curation, H.C.; Writing—Original Draft Preparation, S.L.; Writing—Review & Editing, H.C. and F.C.; Visualization, H.C.; Supervision, H.C.; Project Administration, S.L. and H.C.; Funding Acquisition, H.C.

Funding: This research was supported by the [Future Scientists Program of "Double First Rate" of China University of Mining and Technology] grant number [2019WLKXJ041].

Conflicts of Interest: The authors declare no conflict of interest.

Appendix A

Table A1. The scale items for public occupational safety and health psychological distance.

Dimensions	Items Descriptions
Cognitive distance	I am very familiar with occupational safety and health implications
	I am very familiar with occupational safety and health present situation
	I am very familiar with the importance of occupational safety and health
	I am very familiar with occupational disease-related knowledge in occupational safety and health
Emotional distance	I feel grief about domestic security incidents and occupational diseases in my mind
	I feel indignation about the frequent occurrence condition of domestic security incidents and occupational diseases in my mind
	I feel comfort about the high attention paid by the country and enterprises to occupational safety and health problems
	I always focus on the development of occupational safety and health in my mind
Expected distance	I think that the public perceptions of occupational safety accidents and the extent of injury are exaggerated
	I think that the development of medical treatments and techniques ensures that occupational safety and health problems will not severely threaten the public
	I think that the quality of occupational safety and health problem governance has influence on the future perceptions of the public
	I think that occupational safety and health problems will be controlled within a rational scope if everyone stresses them
Behavioral distance	I am willing to concentrate on occupational safety and health problems in response to the call of the country
	I am willing to commit to occupational safety and health problem governance
	I am willing to popularize occupational safety and health knowledge to surrounding people
	I am willing to make donations to those injured in occupational accidents and occupational disease patients

References

1. Spijkers, O.; Honniball, A. Developing Global Public Participation. *Int. Community Law Rev.* **2015**, *17*, 251–296. [CrossRef]
2. Casey, T.; Griffin, M.A.; Harrison, H.F.; Neal, A. Safety climate and culture: Integrating psychological and systems perspectives. *J. Occup. Health Psychol.* **2017**, *22*, 341–353. [CrossRef] [PubMed]
3. Harth, R. Attitudes towards minority groups as a construct in assessing attitudes towards the mentally retarded. *Educ. Train. Ment. Retard.* **1971**, *6*, 142–147.
4. Håkanson, L. The role of psychic distance in international trade: A longitudinal analysis. *Int. Market. Rev.* **2014**, *31*, 210–236. [CrossRef]
5. Huang, Y.N. Research of psychological distance in interpersonal relationship. *J. Chifeng Coll.* **2015**, *31*, 114–116.
6. Agnew, C.R.; Loving, T.J.; Le, B.; Goodfriend, W. Thinking close: Measuring relational closeness as perceived self-other inclusion. In *Handbook of Closeness and Intimacy*; Mashek, D.J., Aron, A.P., Eds.; Lawrence Erlbaum Associates Publishers: Mahwah, NJ, USA, 2004; pp. 103–115.
7. Trope, Y.; Liberman, N. Construal-level theory of psychological distance. *Psychol. Rev.* **2010**, *117*, 440–463. [CrossRef]
8. Njeru, D.K. Factors that influence implementation of occupational safety and health management system at public universities in kenya—A case study of Egerton university. *Int. J. Curr. Res.* **2017**, *6*, 6602–6609.

9. Niskanen, T.; Louhelainen, K.; Hirvonen, M.L. An evaluation of the effects of the occupational safety and health inspectors' supervision in workplaces. *Accid. Anal. Prev.* **2014**, *68*, 139–155. [CrossRef]
10. Asensio, O.I.; Delmas, M.A. Nonprice incentives and energy conservation. *Proc. Natl. Acad. Sci. USA* **2015**, *112*, 510–515. [CrossRef]
11. McKinley, E.; Fletcher, S. Improving marine environmental health through marine citizenship: A call for debate. *Mar. Policy* **2012**, *36*, 839–843. [CrossRef]
12. Bar-Anan, Y.; Liberman, N.; Trope, Y.; Algom, D. Automatic processing of psychological distance: Evidence from a Stroop task. *J. Exp. Psychol. Gen.* **2007**, *136*, 610–622. [CrossRef]
13. Chen, H.; Li, S. Measuring the Psychological distance between an organization and its members—The construction and validation of a new scale. *Front. Psychol.* **2018**, *8*, 2296. [CrossRef] [PubMed]
14. Li, L.L. The study on the influencing mechanism of films and TV dramas on the travel intention of urban residents—Taking films and TV dramas shot in Qingdao as an example. *J. Qingdao Tech. Coll.* **2013**, *26*, 19–23.
15. Dai, L.; Tian, D.; Luo, J.Y.; Liu, X.T.; Chen, Y.L. Analysis of public health knowledge access mode and the attention degree in Xiamen. *Chin. J. Health Educ.* **2013**, *29*, 348–351. (In Chinese)
16. Cwir, D.; Carr, P.B.; Walton, G.M.; Spencer, S.J. Your heart makes my heart move: Cues of social connectedness cause shared emotions and physiological states among strangers. *J. Exp. Soc. Psychol.* **2011**, *47*, 661–664. [CrossRef]
17. Bernanke, B.S. The federal reserve and the financial crisis. *Econ. Record* **2013**, *89*, 271–273.
18. Woodford, M. Central bank communication and policy effectiveness. *Soc. Sci. Electron. Publ.* **2005**, *8*, 1–65.
19. Qin, Z.; Jing, R.Z. Study on the model of assessing organization behavior distance based on functional analysis. *J. Syst. Manag.* **2006**, *15*, 90–92.
20. Podsakoff, P.M.; MacKenzie, S.B.; Paine, J.B.; Bachrach, D.G. Organizational Citizenship Behaviors: A Critical Review of the Theoretical and Empirical Literature and Suggestions for Future Research. *J. Manag.* **2000**, *26*, 513–563. [CrossRef]
21. Vringer, K.; Aalbers, T.; Blok, K. Household energy requirement and value patterns. *Energy Policy* **2007**, *35*, 553–566. [CrossRef]
22. Groot, J.D.; Steg, L. General Beliefs and the Theory of Planned Behavior: The Role of Environmental Concerns in the TPB. *J. Appl. Soc. Psychol.* **2007**, *37*, 1817–1836. [CrossRef]
23. Li, S.T.; Liu, J.H. A study on the status of risk behavior and its relationship with cognitive emotion regulation in left-behind students in junior high school. *Adv. Psychol.* **2017**, *7*, 21–26. [CrossRef]
24. Shao, Y. Research on rhetorical strategies and communication paths of news broadcast under the perception of public. Ph.D. Thesis, Sichuan International Studies University, Chongqing, China, 6 April 2015.
25. Sia, A.P.; Hungerford, H.R.; Tomera, A.N. Selected predictors of responsible environmental behavior: An analysis. *J. Environ. Educ.* **1986**, *17*, 31–40. [CrossRef]
26. Duerden, M.D.; Witt, P.A. The impact of direct and indirect experiences on the development of environmental knowledge, attitudes, and behavior. *J. Environ. Psychol.* **2010**, *30*, 379–392. [CrossRef]
27. Koenig-Lewis, N.; Palmer, A.; Dermody, J.; Urbye, A. Consumers' evaluations of ecological packaging—Rational and emotional approaches. *J. Environ. Psychol.* **2014**, *37*, 94–105. [CrossRef]
28. Chen, M.F.; Lee, C.L. The impacts of green claims on coffee consumers' purchase intention. *Br. Food J.* **2015**, *117*, 195–209. [CrossRef]
29. Kanchanapibul, M.; Lacka, E.; Wang, X.; Chan, H.K. An empirical investigation of green purchase behaviour among the young generation. *J. Clean. Prod.* **2014**, *66*, 528–536. [CrossRef]
30. Wang, J.M.; Wu, L.C. Two-factor model of affection-behavior in green purchase: Hypotheses and test. *J. Manag. Sci.* **2015**, *28*, 80–94.
31. Cheng, S.P.; Li, M.; Zhang, W. A survey on undergraduates' procrastination behavior and its relationship with meta-cognitive and emotion. *Chin. J. Clin. Psychol.* **2010**, *18*, 238–240.
32. Hussain, S.M. Simultaneous monetary policy announcements and international stock markets response: An intraday analysis. *J. Bank. Financ.* **2011**, *35*, 752–764. [CrossRef]
33. Zhai, Z.H. Strategies for adjusting negative consumption expectations. *Pop. Stand.* **2005**, *3*, 31–33.
34. Lu, Z. A research on the monetary policy effect of the public expectation. *Macroecon. Res.* **2016**, *9*, 72–79.
35. Edwards, J.R. Person–Environment fit in organizations: An assessment of theoretical progress. *Acad. Manag. Ann.* **2008**, *2*, 167–230. [CrossRef]
36. Zhang, S.S.; Zhang, J.X.; Zhou, M.J. The quadratic polynomial regression with response surface analysis and its use in person-environment fit research. *Adv. Psychol. Sci.* **2012**, *20*, 825–833. [CrossRef]

37. Chen, F.; Chen, H.; Huang, X.; Long, R.; Lu, H.; Yue, T. Public response to the regulation policy of urban household waste: Evidence from a survey of Jiangsu province in China. *Sustainability* **2017**, *9*, 1034. [CrossRef]
38. Resick, C.J.; Baltes, B.B.; Shantz, C.W. Person-organization fit and work-related attitudes and decisions: Examining interactive effects with job fit and conscientiousness. *J. Appl. Psychol.* **2007**, *92*, 1446–1455. [CrossRef]
39. Tang, Y.H.; Lu, X.F.; Li, K. The concept, measuring strategy and applying of person-organization fit: Based on the reflection of interactivity and flexibility. *Adv. Psychol. Sci.* **2010**, *18*, 1762–1770.
40. Edwards, J.R. Problems with the use of profile similarity indices in the study of congruence in organizational research. *Pers. Psychol.* **1993**, *46*, 641–665. [CrossRef]
41. Aydogan, A.F.; Gonsalkorale, K. Breaking down a barrier: Increasing perceived out-group knowledge reduces negative expectancies about intergroup interaction. *Eur. J. Soc. Psychol.* **2015**, *45*, 401–408. [CrossRef]
42. Si, Z.H. The impact of knowledge preparation on learning disabilities of Tibetan college students in Tibet. *J. Changsha Aeronaut. Vocat. Tech. Coll.* **2017**, *17*, 44–46. (In Chinese)
43. Sun, J.; Li, J.J.; Yang, X.R. Why consumer's word is not in agreement with their deed: Study on factors impeding green consumption behavior. *J. Huazhong Agric. Univ. Soc. Sci. Ed.* **2015**, *5*, 72–81.
44. Chen, K.; Peng, X. Green consumption attitude—A study on the influencing factors of behavior disparity. *Enterp. Econ.* **2014**, *8*, 25–30.
45. Gleim, M.R.; Smith, J.S.; Andrews, D.; Cronin, J.J. Against the Green: A Multi-method Examination of the Barriers to Green Consumption. *J. Retail.* **2013**, *89*, 44–61. [CrossRef]
46. Meyer, D.; Newton, P. Exploring the attitudes-action gap in household resource consumption: Does "environmental lifestyle" segmentation align with consumer behavior. *Sustainability* **2013**, *5*, 1211–1233.
47. Griskevicius, V.; Tybur, J.M.; Van den Bergh, B. Going green to be seen: Status, reputation, and conspicuous conservation. *J. Pers. Soc. Psychol.* **2010**, *98*, 392–404. [CrossRef] [PubMed]
48. Antonetti, P.; Maklan, S. How categorisation shapes the attitude–behaviour gap in responsible consumption. *Int. J. Mark. Res.* **2015**, *57*, 51–72. [CrossRef]
49. Mischel, W.; Shoda, Y. A cognitive-affective system theory of personality: Reconceptualizing situations, dispositions, dynamics, and invariance in personality structure. *Psychol. Rev.* **1995**, *102*, 246–268. [CrossRef] [PubMed]
50. Sherman, R.A.; Nave, C.S.; Funder, D.C. Properties of persons and situations related to overall and distinctive personality-behavior congruence. *J. Res. Pers.* **2012**, *46*, 87–101. [CrossRef]
51. Zhang, W.; Zhao, S.T. Cognitive biases, heterogeneous expectation and asset pricing. *J. Manag. Sci. China* **2010**, *13*, 52–59.
52. He, X.; Zhang, W.; Hao, Y. The conformity of the expected publication time-lag by the author and the real publication time-lag of domestic core journals on library and information science. *J. Intell.* **2014**, *33*, 99–102.
53. Jin, H.Y.; Jian, L.R. China's regional innovation efficiency and its influencing factors considering the lag effect. *Syst. Eng.* **2013**, *9*, 98–106.
54. Carrigan, M.; Attalla, A. The myth of the ethical consumer—Do ethics matter in purchase behavior. *J. Consum. Mark.* **2001**, *18*, 560–578. [CrossRef]
55. Auger, P.; Devinney, T.M. Do what consumers say matter? The misalignment of preferences with unconstrained ethical intentions. *J. Bus. Ethics* **2007**, *76*, 361–383. [CrossRef]

International Journal of
Environmental Research and Public Health

MDPI

Article

Manual Cultivation Operations in Poplar Stands: A Characterization of Job Difficulty and Risks of Health Impairment

Tiberiu Marogel-Popa [1], Marius Cheţa [1], Marina Viorela Marcu [1], Cristian Ionuţ Duţă [1], Florin Ioraş [2] and Stelian Alexandru Borz [1,*]

1 Department of Forest Engineering, Forest Management Planning and Terrestrial Measurements, Faculty of Silviculture and Forest Engineering, Transilvania University of Braşov, Şirul Beethoven No. 1, 500123 Braşov, Romania; marogel_tibi@yahoo.com (T.M.-P.); marius.cheta@unitbv.ro (M.C.); viorela.marcu@unitbv.ro (M.V.M.); duta_cristianionut@yahoo.com (C.I.D.)

2 Buckinghamshire New University, Queen Alexandra Road, High Wycombe, Buckinghamshire HP11 2JZ, UK; florin.ioras@bucks.ac.uk

* Correspondence: stelian.borz@unitbv.ro; Tel.: +40-742-042-455

Received: 4 May 2019; Accepted: 28 May 2019; Published: 30 May 2019

Abstract: Short rotation poplar forests are a viable alternative in producing high quality wood for industrial applications. Their success depends on timely and high-quality implementation of a series of operations. Weed control operations are implemented to favor the trees in their competition for soil resources, and cultivation is an option typically used in many European countries. For the moment, a complete mechanization of such operations is virtually impossible, and they still require an intensive use of manual labor. Since information on work difficulty and risks in manual cultivation operations is limited, this study aimed to characterize this job. Evaluation was made in terms of work efficiency, cardiovascular workload, work intensity and postural risks by implementing a time and motion study combined with heart rate measurements, accelerometry and whole-body postural analysis. Work efficiency was particularly low even if the share of effective work time was high (70% of the observation time). Job was characterized as moderate to high intensity, which resulted into a moderate to high cardiovascular strain. While the postural analysis indicated rather small risks, the main problem was found for the back postures assumed during the work. Improvements should aim to extend mechanization, train the workers and appropriately design rest breaks.

Keywords: manual cultivation; job characterization; ergonomics; efficiency; cardiovascular workload; work intensity; risk of musculoskeletal disorders

1. Introduction

Short rotation cultivated forests are considered to be a valuable alternative for wood provisioning, enabling the possibility to reduce the anthropogenic disturbance on natural forests and to conserve them. To enable a timely provisioning of wood to industry, such forests need to be cultivated using fast-growing trees able to provide high-quality wood. Among the existing fast-growing species, poplars are intensively used in many countries for such outcomes [1]. Their cultivation supposes a sequence of operations including fertilization, irrigation and weed control [2], with the last one aiming to balance the competition for soil resources and being carried out, in many regions, by herbicide application, cultivation or a combination of the two [1]. Some of these practices (i.e., in Romania) are used even in regular poplar forests that could be easily assimilated to short rotation cultures due to the propagation techniques and geometrical plantation schemes that are used, types of implemented operations and rotation length. In such conditions, the typical way of carrying on the weed control is by cultivation.

The level of mechanization in forest operations depends on many factors such as the forest type, wood species, management methods, terrain and climatic conditions [3], with many of the Eastern European countries using operational systems that are partly mechanized [4]. This is particularly the case of forest establishment [5] and cultivation operations [6] that are still requiring manual labor to a great extent. In addition, many of the forest work places are characterized by difficult operational conditions and the work in forest itself is seen to be amongst the most difficult and hazardous jobs [7]. Since many of forest operations still require manual work, their engineering and management requires, at least in a first stage, their understanding in terms of difficulty and hazards. Based on such knowledge, work (re)design may be employed to ensure that work tasks are aligned to human capability, by measures designed to prevent adverse health effects [8] that should be further related to several key areas of the general work system such as the risk assessment, accountability awareness, physical and mental workload, quality of work environment and work technology [9].

Manual cultivation operations have received less attention in ergonomic assessments of forest operations which are dominated by research on harvesting operations [10]. As a fact, only one study [11] was found in the available literature dealing with similar problems; it concluded that manual weed control is a highly demanding job from a physiological point of view, exposing the workers to increased cardiovascular workloads [11]. In the Romanian practice, manual cultivation operations of poplar forests are typically coupled with mechanized ones, in a double-pass system in which the mechanized equipment is operating on the space available between the rows of trees in such a manner that enables the protection of aerial tree parts; the rest of area is approached by workers equipped with hoes [6].

Given the limited information availability on the difficulty and risks of such jobs, the main aim of this study was to describe, document and characterize manual cultivation operations from an ergonomic point of view, to be able to draw conclusions and implications for the public health associated with this occupation. Since the ergonomics and public health cover many key sub-disciplines, it was virtually impossible to approach all the inter-relations between the workers, their job tasks and the operational environment.

To this end, musculoskeletal disorders (MSDs) are the most common cause of severe long-term pain and physical disability, and they affect hundreds of millions of people around the world. The role of psychosocial factors and work-related stress in the development of MSDs has received increased attention. Indeed, a number of epidemiological studies have been conducted in different sectors (from office work to manual work), repeatedly showing linkages between work-related psychosocial factors and MSDs. Overall, it is evident that the incidence of MSDs is associated with high perceived work-related stress levels, high workload and demands, and monotonous work [12], that may lead to public health problems related to different kinds of occupations, highlighting serious problems associated with the forest operations industry [13] which, in turn, may lead to significant temporary or permanent disability of workers [14].

In regard to manual cultivation operations, the initial assumptions of this study were that the work productivity would be particularly low and the workplace time would be characterized by an increased proportion of the time spent in rest pauses and delays, the experienced work difficulty would be particularly high given the characteristics of the tasks, the job itself would be characterized by a high intensity of dynamic work, as well as the assumed postures would generate risks for the upper limbs of the body, in particular for the back. For this reason, the study focused on: (i) characterizing the work performance by a typical time and motion study, (ii) describing the physiological workload in terms of cardiovascular activity, (iii) evaluating the intensity of work by body movement benchmarking techniques and (iv) assessing the risks of musculoskeletal disorders by a postural assessment method.

2. Materials and Methods

2.1. Study Locations, Forest Condition and Study Subjects

Three study locations (Table 1) were chosen in the southeastern part of Romania, close to the Danube river, in the forests managed by three forest districts. The first study location (L1) was selected in the Management Unit II Ciuperceni, compartment no. 88D managed by Forest District of Calafat where the observations were carried out in two days: 13rd and 22nd of June 2018. The second location (L2) was selected from the forests managed by Forest District of Segarcea (Management Unit I, compartment no. 6C) and the third location (L3) was selected from the forests managed by Forest District of Poiana Mare (Management Unit IV Rast, compartment no. 70A). In L2, field observations were carried out in 18th of June 2018, while in L3 they were extended on 3 days (19th to 21st of June 2018). Location selection in the field was based on criteria such as the current practices used to establish the forests, job availability in given areas and the dimensional variability of weed to be removed by manual cultivation.

In all of the selected locations, hybrid poplar (*Populus × euroamericana* (Dode) Guinier) [15] forests were established by artificial regeneration (plantation). The forest in L1 was established in 2013 by a 4 × 4 m plantation scheme, while the forests from L2 and L3 were established in 2015 and 2017 respectively, using a 5 × 4 m plantation scheme. Both, plantation and cultivation operations of poplar forests in the area are carried out using locally available workers who are quite experienced in such operations given their background in similar agricultural practices. A number of 14 male workers (hereafter subjects) having an extended experience in regular farming, including cultivation operations, were selected from the local population based on their verbal and informed consent to participate as anonymous subjects in the study. The goal of the study, the intended use of data as well as the procedures required by the study were detailly explained to each of them in advance and they were instructed to carry on their jobs as they are used to. Given the limited availability of monitoring devices (3 sets of devices), form these workers, three subjects were randomly sampled each day and for each location for a detailed monitoring of work.

Table 1. Locations taken into study, study dates and weather condition during the study.

Forest District	Geographical Location	Forest Compartment and Area (Ha)	Observation Day	Weather Condition During the Study	Weed Height (M)	Abbreviation Used in This Study
Calafat	43°58′31.27″ N 22°54′04.42″ E	88D 0.76	13rd of June	T^1 = 25.9 °C RH^2 = 69.75%	0.7	L1 × 13
Segarcea	43°47′59.81″ N 23°36′01.88″ E	6C 2.00	18th of June	T^1 = 22.0 °C RH^2 = 76.75%	1.3	L2 × 18
Poiana Mare	43°50′50.12″ N 23°14′17.45″ E	70A 2.92	19th of June	T^1 = 23.4 °C RH^2 = 71.85%	0.5	L3 × 19
Poiana Mare	43°50′50.12″ N 23°14′17.45″ E	70A 2.92	20th of June	T^1 = 23.6 °C RH^2 = 69.33%	0.5	L3 × 20
Poiana Mare	43°50′50.12″ N 23°14′17.45″ E	70A 2.92	21st of June	T^1 = 23.8 °C RH^2 = 75.83%	0.5	L3 × 21
Calafat	43°58′31.27″ N 22°54′04.42″ E	88D 0.76	22nd of June	T^1 = 19.8 °C RH^2 = 85.00%	0.7	L1 × 22

[1] T—air temperature. [2] RH—air relative humidity.

The sample of workers taken into study was characterized by an age of 46.4 ± 14.0 years, a body weight of 82.94 ± 15.43 kg and a height of 174.5 ± 5.9 cm (Table 2), being representative for the population of workers from the study area which, in many cases is quite aged.

Table 2. Characteristics of the study group.

Subject	Abbreviation in This Study	Age (years)	Body Weight (kg)	Body Height (cm)	Body Mass Index
Subject 1	S1	36	100	186	28.91
Subject 2	S2	31	105	175	34.29
Subject 3	S3	40	110	180	33.95
Subject 4	S4	50	100	180	30.86
Subject 5	S5	47	71	176	22.92 [1]
Subject 6	S6	40	70	165	25.71
Subject 7	S7	18	70	169	24.51 [1]
Subject 8	S8	49	70	175	22.86 [1]
Subject 9	S9	57	85	170	29.41
Subject 10	S10	50	68	165	24.98 [1]
Subject 11	S11	67	67	170	23.18 [1]
Subject 12	S12	62	75	179	24.41 [1]
Subject 13	S13	45	70	173	23.39 [1]
Subject 14	S14	57	102	180	30.79

[1] Denotes normal weight according to Body Mass Index.

2.2. Work Layout

In the Romanian practice related to hybrid poplar forests, cultivation operations are typically implemented using a two-pass operational system. In a first step, machines such as tractors equipped with mowers, ploughs or harrows are used for cultivation operations on a single direction of the operated plots to mobilize the soil and to remove the weed between rows (Figure 1). The remaining strips which contain the trees are manually operated in a second pass, by teams of manual workers using hoes. In this operational configuration, the local practice makes use of mechanization for approximately 80% of the area while the rest is operated by manual means.

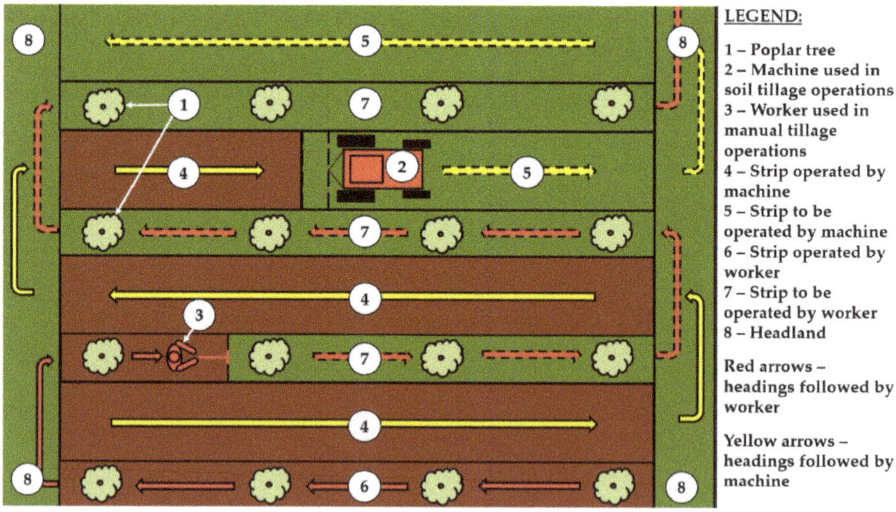

Figure 1. Operational layout (concept) used for cultivation operations in the area taken into study.

Nevertheless, depending on the plantation scheme and spaces existing between the tree rows, on one hand, and on the width of equipment attached to tractors, on the other hand, some cases require more than one inter-row tractor pass. It was the case of this study, where the inter-row area was covered by more than one mechanized pass, following that, on each tree row, the area to be operated by manual means to account for approximately one meter in width. For the manual operations, which made the scope of this study, the work organization was rather simple: each worker entered one row at the headland, operated the row and reentered a new row at the opposite headland. Therefore, the work was divided for further analysis based on the tasks observed in the field such as the effective work (EW) consisting of manual cultivation, rest pauses (RP) consisting of all the breaks taken by subjects in the field to rest, meal pauses (MP) and delays (D) which included the delays caused by the study itself and some minor technical delays. During the study, the sky was partly clouded and the air temperature (Table 1) was considered to be low enough to exclude the thermal stress effects on the subjects (e.g., [16]), given the fact that the locations were partly shaded by the surrounding mature forests.

2.3. Data Collection Procedures

In each study location and for each day, the operations were monitored by video recording using a digital camera placed on a tripod at the closest headland and set to continuously record video files of 20 min in length each. The camera was placed is such a manner that enabled the best field of view on the collected files and covered all the three workers monitored in a given day. As the work progressed on the rows, the location of the camera was changed accordingly to be able to keep the needed details visible in its field of view. Data collected this way was used to document the observed work tasks, to extract the time consumption on tasks and to evaluate the cardiovascular workload and the risks of musculoskeletal disorders by a postural analysis implemented in the office phase of the study. The height and the width of the weed stratum was visually evaluated and noted into a field book along with the main anthropometric characteristics of the observed subjects such as the age (A, years), body weight (W, kilograms) and height (H, centimeters), with the last two being used to compute the body mass index (BMI, Table 2) using its specific formula.

Polar ® V800 dataloggers (Polar, Kempele, Finland) including their H7 heart monitoring sensors mounted on straps were used to monitor the subjects' cardiovascular activity during the undertaken tasks in terms of heart rate (HR, beats per minute). Procedures used to estimate the heart rate at rest (HRr, beats per minute), setup, collect, download and pre-process the data including that referring to location, were similar to those described in [17]. Data needed to evaluate the intensity of work (WI) was collected by the means of new, factory-calibrated, tri-axial accelerometers—Extech ® VB300 (Extech Instruments, FLIR Commercial Systems Inc., Nashua, NH, USA) attached to the pericardial strap of the heart rate datalogger. The devices were placed on the back of each subject in between scapulae, as close as possible to the middle of spine's thoracic vertebrae section. The choice of this body part was based on the assumption that most of the changes in the acceleration signal, therefore changes in work intensity, will be caused by movements of the subjects' back, given the characteristics of monitored operations. Procedures used to setup, collect, download and pre-process the raw acceleration data were similar to those described in [18]. Both dataloggers were setup to collect data at one second rate.

The main weather characteristics during the study (air temperature—T, °C and relative humidity—RH, %) were documented as average values for the study periods specific to each observation day. This data was procured from the closest weather station (Calafat, 62 m a.s.l., 43°59′06″ N–22°56′46″ E, distance range from study locations of 4 to 56 km).

2.4. Data Processing Procedures

Data processing procedures consisted of several steps that were required to obtain the initial databases needed for statistical analysis. Video data was downloaded from digital cameras at the end of each observation day. An initial processing task consisted of a detailed time and motion study that was framed around the concepts used in forest operations [19,20] and which supposed the analysis of video files in their real sequence of observation, followed by data extraction into a Microsoft Excel (Microsoft Excel 2013, Microsoft, Redmond, WA, USA) sheet per time consumption categories, subjects and tasks. To this end, the unit of production (P) in this study was considered to be the manually operated area of one hectare, while the time consumption (t_{EW}, t_{RP}, t_{MP} and t_D, seconds) was assumed to belong to the previously identified tasks (EW, RP, MP, D). Given the specificity of this study, only the efficiency metrics were computed (GWER - gross work efficiency rate and NWER - net work efficiency rate, hours/hectare) after time conversion from seconds to hours. The supporting calculation relations are given in Equations (1)–(5):

$$GWT_i \text{ (hours)} = t_{EWi} \text{ (hours)} + t_{RPi} \text{ (hours)} + t_{MPi} \text{ (hours)} + t_{Di} \text{ (hours)}, \quad (1)$$

$$NWT_i \text{ (hours)} = t_{EWi} \text{ (hours)} + t_{RPi} \text{ (hours)}, \quad (2)$$

$$GWER_i \text{ (hours/ha)} = GWT_i \text{ (hours)}/P_i \text{ (ha)}, \quad (3)$$

$$NWER_i \text{ (hours/ha)} = NWT_i \text{ (hours)}/P_i \text{ (ha)}, \quad (4)$$

$$P_i \text{ (ha)} = ARW \text{ (m)} \times TRL_i \text{ (m)}/10{,}000, \quad (5)$$

where: i stands for a given monitored subject, GWT_i—gross time of subject i, t_{EWi}—effective work time of subject i, t_{RPi}—rest pauses time of subject i, t_{MPi}—meal pause time of subject i, t_{Di}—delay time of subject i, NWT_i—net time of subject i, $GWER_i$—gross work efficiency rate of subject i, P_i—production of subject i, $NWER_i$—net work efficiency rate to subject i, ARW—average row width based on field observation (1 m), TRL_i—total row length operated by subject i.

The cardiovascular workload of each subject was evaluated at the task, day and location level using the heart rate reserve (%HRR) metric as defined, for instance, in [21]. Acknowledging the usefulness of several other metrics in evaluating the physiological workload in terms of heart activity, the choice of %HRR was based on the limited applicability of average heart rate per tasks to different age groups [22], as well as on the fact that it is expected to be a good predictor of workload only in the range of 100 to 140 beats per minute [16]. Since it was virtually impossible to test the subjects by a preestablished protocol aiming to determine their maximum heart rate (HRmax), the formula HRmax = 220 – age (years) was used to estimate this metric [21]. Procedurally, for each heart rate sample collected in the field, codes were used to document the belonging of each 1-s observation to a given task using as a reference the time labels from heart rate samples and video files respectively.

Tri-axial raw acceleration data was processed in a different way. Assuming that for the same task the intensity of work could vary in a given range, this data was not further documented by codes. Instead, the vector magnitudes for each 1-s observation (Equation (6)) were further processed to exclude the gravity component from the signal using the Euclidian Norm Minus One (ENMO, g) metric (Equation (7)) [23]; then, the resulting, otherwise few and small negative values were converted to zero by a logical function of Microsoft Excel:

$$vm_j \text{ (g)} = \sqrt{x_j^2 + y_j^2 + z_j^2}, \quad (6)$$

$$ENMO_j \text{ (g)} = vm_j \text{ (g)} - 1, \quad (7)$$

where j stands for a given observation, vm_j - vector magnitude for observation j, x_j - raw response on axis x for observation j, y_j - raw response on axis y for observation j, z_j - raw response on axis z for observation j, $ENMO_j$ - Euclidian Norm Minus One of observation j.

Two work intensity thresholds (WIT) were designed based on the literature documentation to separate the time spent in different work intensities. An ENMO value of less than 0.25 g was used to separate the light intensity work (LIW) and a value of more than 1.00 g was used to separate the high intensity work (HIW) from the datasets collected for each subject. These assumptions were based on the work of [24,25]. Observations falling in the range of 0.25–1.00 g were categorized as moderate intensity work (MIW). Separation and categorization were implemented by simple logical functions applied to the corrected ENMO data in Microsoft Excel (Figure 2).

Risks of musculoskeletal disorders (MSD) were evaluated for each subject, work day and location by the means of Ovako Working posture Analysis System (OWAS) as introduced by Karhu et al. [26], then detailed e.g., [16] and discussed for its applicability in forest operations [7]. The choice of this postural analysis method was based on its history in use in forest operations [17,27,28] capability to analyze the whole body [26,29], simplicity in use [7,26], and possibility to compare the results e.g., [30] including comparisons to those coming from other industries. To this end, each video file collected in the field was broken in frames extracted at 1-s rate. Then, random numbers produced by simple functions in Microsoft Excel were used to extract exactly 100 frames from each video file and for each worker and location of study (Table 3).

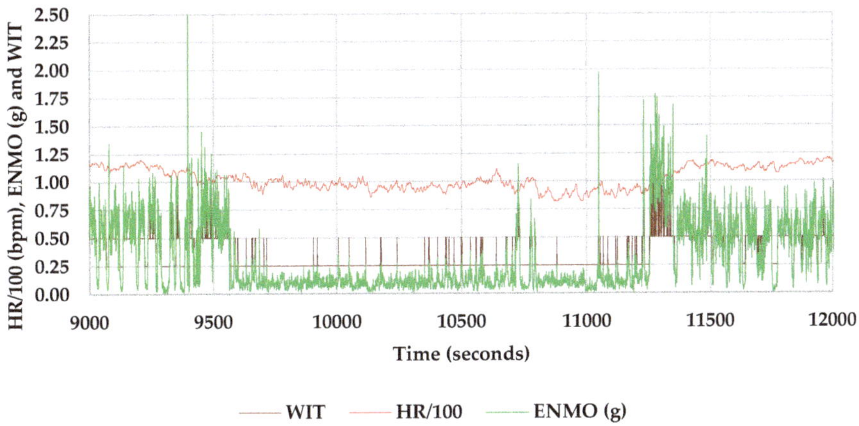

Figure 2. Concept used to separate time epochs for light intensity work (LIW), moderate intensity work (MIW) and high intensity work (HIW). Legend: WIT - work intensity threshold (0.00 to 0.25 for LIW, 0.25 to 1.00 for MIW and more than 1.00 for HIW), HR/100 - heart rate divided by 100 (only for concept demonstration), ENMO—Euclidian Norm Minus One corrected for negative values.

Table 3. Number of analyzed video files and frames.

Location and Observation Day	Number of Collected Video Files	Number of Frames Extracted for Postural Analysis of Each Worker	Number of Analyzed Frames	Number of Valid Frames
L2 × 18	13	1300	3900	1433
L3 × 19	18	1800	5400	2918
L3 × 20	16	1600	4800	3643
L3 × 21	17	1700	5100	2616
L1 × 13	8	800	2400	1657
L1 × 22	7	700	2100	946
Overall	79	7900	23,700	13,213

This approach resulted in the analysis of 23,700 still images. Those images failing to give in their field of view all the information needed to analyze the whole-body posture of a given subject were considered to be non-valid. Approximately 56% (13,123) of the initial frames were retained as valid and used in statistical analysis (Table 3). Postural analysis was implemented as a detailed analysis of back, arms and legs according to the OWAS method, followed by data coding into Microsoft Excel sheets. Since the force exertion was difficult to evaluate, this component was assumed to be less than 10 kg for each frame, based on the subjective evaluation of researchers that carried out this data processing task. Nevertheless, this approach was consistent with the type and weight of the tools used during the work. Each frame was documented by coding the task to which it belonged, a fact that supposed in some cases some revisions of video files. A Visual Basic for Applications (VBA) logical code was designed to attribute action category (AC) codes for each valid frame. Then, for each worker, day and location, a postural risk index (PRI) was calculated based on the approach described in [28,30]. As an aggregated metric, PRI was used to judge the exposure to risks of developing MSDs. It can take values in between 100 and 400%, where 100% corresponds to AC1, 200% to AC2, 300% to AC3 and 400% to AC4 while the intermediate values need to be judged to choose the appropriate action category.

To enable the characterization of work, data on time consumption, work efficiency, cardiovascular workload, work intensity and postural analysis was aggregated at study level following the statistical analysis.

2.5. Statistical Analysis

Right at the beginning of statistical analysis it was evident that the aggregated data coming from each subject working in a given day and location was quite heterogeneous. For this reason, no comparison tests were undertaken to check if there are any differences in terms of work performance outcomes and input resources between subjects, work days and locations. Instead, the statistical techniques used were aligned to the goal of this study that was to characterize the manual cultivation operations as a job. Obviously, this approach needs to include the variability produced by different types of factors [20] such as that given by changes in anthropometric features and human capability, tools used and operational environment conditions. For that, descriptive statistics specific to central tendency were computed and reported. Operational performance in terms of time consumption and efficiency was reported as total time, time shares per work tasks and efficiency rates. Mean values of heart rate reserve were used to characterize the cardiovascular workload per tasks and at the study level while the share of time spent per categories of work intensity was used for similar characterizations. Postural data was computed as shares per action categories at subject and study level, then this data was used to compute the postural risk indexes at subject and study level. Then, a more detailed analysis of back, arms and legs postures was implemented to see what approaches should be taken for work redesign and improvement. To this end, shares of back, arms and legs postures per specific codes were analyzed for all the data taken into study. All of the statistical analyses were carried out in Microsoft Excel.

3. Results

3.1. Estimates on Time Consumption per Tasks and Operational Performance Metrics

Table 4 shows a breakdown of time consumption and efficiency rates per subjects, days of observations and locations. At study level, field observations were carried out for roughly 85 h. In average, almost 70% of that time was spent as effective work time and approximately 22% was used as rest time. Having meals accounted for approximately 9% of the study time but it was not specific to all the subjects and all the study locations. Other delays, including those caused by the study itself were only minor in the time consumption structure, accounting for less than 1%.

Given the overall distribution of time consumption, net work efficiency rate was estimated at 34.31 h per hectare which was close to gross work efficiency rate (36.35 h per hectare). Since these figures apply to the effective operated area, under real circumstances in which approximately 75–80% of the area is mechanically operated, they will translate into average gross and net efficiency rates in the range of 9.09 to 8.58 h per hectare respectively.

At subject, observation day and location level, on the other hand, time consumption and efficiency rates figures were rather heterogeneous. The effective work time, for instance, accounted for 45.20 to 83.89% of the observed time, while the rest time varied widely between 13.04 and 54.80%. In general, meal pauses were taken only in those situations in which the total observation time exceeded four hours. Accordingly, the net efficiency rates varied between 14.98 and 69.15 h per hectare while the gross work efficiency rates varied between 16.92 and 62.29 h per hectare.

Given the fact that operational conditions in the three locations were quite different, one could have been expected to find some differences related to that. However, expectations were not entirely met as, for instance, the work performance in L2 was, in average, higher compared to L1, while the height of the weed to be removed was lower in the latter. In this last case, however, the subjects taken into study were characterized by the greatest ages of the sample taken into study (over 45-year-old, most of them over 50).

Table 4. Statistics of time consumption and estimates of work performance.

Subject, Location and Observation Day	Observation Time (h)	Effective Work Time (%)	Rest Time (%)	Meal Pause Time (%)	Delays (%)	Net Work Efficiency Rate (h/Ha)	Gross Work Efficiency Rate (h/Ha)
S1 × L2 × 18	4.8	61.80	26.91	9.86	1.43	26.295	29.599
S2 × L2 × 18	4.7	71.97	17.11	9.03	1.89	22.925	25.692
S3 × L2 × 18	4.5	74.84	13.04	11.66	0.46	23.159	26.352
S4 × L3 × 19	6.3	73.94	14.43	11.63	-	25.922	29.322
S5 × L3 × 19	6.2	57.36	28.44	11.61	2.59	25.074	29.234
S6 × L3 × 19	6.3	64.59	15.60	19.81	-	25.859	29.733
S7 × L3 × 20	5.7	75.18	14.49	10.20	0.13	21.695	24.163
S8 × L3 × 20	5.6	73.48	14.30	12.22	-	22.220	24.875
S9 × L3 × 20	5.5	74.44	14.60	10.96	-	22.044	24.754
S9 × L3 × 21	5.8	70.47	19.83	9.56	0.14	15.250	16.920
S4 × L3 × 21	5.8	52.77	37.18	9.92	0.13	14.981	17.497
S7 × L3 × 21	5.7	83.60	16.40	-	-	16.013	17.739
S10 × L1 × 13	3.4	73.85	24.65	-	1.50	69.148	69.711
S11 × L1 × 13	3.3	71.86	27.72	-	0.42	59.298	59.298
S12 × L1 × 13	3.4	77.54	22.46	-	-	59.438	59.438
S13 × L1 × 22	2.6	51.64	46.44	-	1.92	61.104	62.289
S12 × L1 × 22	2.5	83.89	15.58	-	0.53	50.118	50.699
S14 × L1 × 22	2.5	45.20	54.80	-	-	57.046	57.046
Overall	84.6	68.33	22.34	8.69	0.64	34.310	36.353

When comparing the work performance between L2 and L3, one could find that, in average, it was higher in L3, probably due to the better operational conditions but, in general, the work performance was correlated and related to the subject's age ($R = 0.5$, $R^2 = 0.26$, $\alpha = 0.05$, $p < 0.05$).

3.2. Cardiovascular Workload

In average, the heart rate of the observed subjects varied between 95 (S6) and 126 (S14) beats per minute (Table 5). From this point of view, it seems that S14, in particular, experienced a very heavy work. This may be supported by the greatest share of time spent in rest pauses (Table 4) and by the increased overall heart rate (Table 5).

At the observed sample level, manual cultivation operation seems to be rather a heavy job, taking almost 37% of the heart rate reserve. Rest pauses have not led to a full recovery and to a normal cardiovascular activity (%HRR = 33.6) which is likely not to be reached also during the meal pauses (%HRR = 21.42). Overall, the heart rate reserve was particularly high (%HRR = 35.2) at the observed sample level.

At subject, work day and location level, there was a certain variability in terms of average heart rate, heart rate at rest and heart rate reserve per tasks and per days of observation. Even for the same subject, the average heart rate varied from day to day and from one location to other. Heart rate reserve during the effective work varied between 21.98 and 52.68%, and it was clearly correlated and related to the age of the subjects ($R = 0.63$, $R^2 = 0.40$, $\alpha = 0.05$, $p < 0.05$). This was true also in the case of the overall heart rate reserve ($R = 0.64$, $R^2 = 0.40$, $\alpha = 0.05$, $p < 0.05$) which was calculated by taking into account all of the observation time.

In particular, subjects S1, S5, S8, and S10 to S14, accounting for almost 60% of the sample, were those that spent the greatest effort in the observed operations during the effective work. For most of the subjects the effort spent was probably related to their age and less related to the local operational conditions. This was even more so evident as the air temperature of the last observational day was the closest to the thermal comfort (Table 1), the operational conditions were averaged compared to the other two locations (Table 1), while the subjects working there were amongst the oldest in the studied sample (Table 2).

Table 5. Statistics of cardiovascular activity.

Subject, Location and Observation Day	Average Heart Rate (Bpm)	Heart Rate at Rest (Bpm)	Heart Rate Reserve for Effective Work	Heart Rate Reserve for Rest Pauses	Heart Rate Reserve for Meal Pauses	Overall Heart Rate Reserve
S1 × L2 × 18	108	50	44.00	42.98	37.19	42.95
S2 × L2 × 18	106	81	23.94	23.28	11.70	22.76
S3 × L2 × 18	104	69	32.06	33.24	23.37	31.25
S4 × L3 × 19	108	82	31.31	27.25	17.59	29.13
S5 × L3 × 19	117	87	38.95	33.77	13.89	34.56
S6 × L3 × 19	95	70	25.85	25.27	12.28	23.07
S7 × L3 × 20	105	67	30.64	25.23	16.53	28.40
S8 × L3 × 20	107	66	41.87	34.19	28.92	39.19
S9 × L3 × 20	102	71	32.99	35.70	35.10	33.62
S9 × L3 × 21	97	63	34.88	32.40	26.14	33.57
S4 × L3 × 21	100	78	25.08	23.94	12.86	23.45
S7 × L3 × 21	99	72	21.98	16.49	-	21.08
S10 × L1 × 13	114	80	39.26	31.42	-	37.24
S11 × L1 × 13	109	74	46.32	38.44	-	44.12
S12 × L1 × 13	112	67	51.23	45.67	-	49.98
S13 × L1 × 22	111	61	45.44	41.77	-	43.56
S12 × L1 × 22	109	70	44.17	42.38	-	43.85
S14 × L1 × 22	126	86	52.68	52.05	-	52.33
Overall	-	-	36.81	33.64	21.42	35.23

3.3. *Work Intensity*

Tri-axial acceleration dataloggers performed well during the field observation excepting two cases—S10 and S11 working in L1 (Table 6)—where they failed to collect data covering all the observed time. For that reason, data coming from these dataloggers in case of L1 was excluded when characterizing the work intensity at the sample level. Also, some minor differences between the total observed time and the work intensity related survey time were unavoidable since the dataloggers were placed on the workers after starting the camera for video recording. Nevertheless, these differences were only minor.

Table 6. Statistics of work intensity.

Subject, Location and Observation Day	Work Intensity Survey Time (h)	Share of Light Intensity Work (%)	Share of Moderate Intensity Work (%)	Share of High Intensity Work (%)
S1 × L2 × 18	4.7	38.96	55.93	5.11
S2 × L2 × 18	4.7	30.45	61.80	7.74
S3 × L2 × 18	4.5	33.25	59.71	7.05
S4 × L3 × 19	6.2	31.19	64.38	4.43
S5 × L3 × 19	6.2	54.01	43.76	2.22
S6 × L3 × 19	6.3	37.89	58.76	3.34
S7 × L3 × 20	5.7	33.00	62.43	4.57
S8 × L3 × 20	5.6	36.29	57.03	6.68
S9 × L3 × 20	5.5	23.64	74.05	2.31
S9 × L3 × 21	5.8	23.73	74.69	1.58
S4 × L3 × 21	5.8	44.44	53.43	2.12
S7 × L3 × 21	5.7	31.28	60.08	8.64
S10 × L1 × 13 [1]	2.7 [1]	15.80 [1]	81.61 [1]	2.59 [1]
S11 × L1 × 13 [1]	2.3 [1]	96.24 [1]	0.74 [1]	3.02 [1]
S12 × L1 × 13	3.3	18.61	71.67	9.72
S13 × L1 × 22	2.6	40.93	54.87	4.20
S12 × L1 × 22	2.5	20.57	75.06	4.37
S14 × L1 × 22	2.5	50.88	48.37	0.75
Overall [2]	77.8 [2]	34.59 [2]	60.81 [2]	4.60 [2]

[1] Denotes data that has not been used in the characterization of work intensity. [2] Averages computed by exclusion of data from [1].

Shares of time spent in the three work intensity categories is shown in Table 6. At the sample level, roughly 61% of the time was categorized as moderate intensity work and almost 35% were categorized as light intensity work. The share of light intensity work varied between 18.61 (S12 × L1 × 13) and 54.01% (S5 × L3 × 19) while the share of moderate intensity work varied between 43.76 (S5 × L3 × 19) and 75.06% (S12 × L1 × 22). Nearly 5% of the observed data stood for high intensity work. In this last category, the data was quite heterogeneous, with shares between 0.75 (S14) and 9.72 (S13 working in L1).

3.4. Postural Risk

Figure 3 shows a breakdown per action categories and postural risk indexes estimated at subject, observation day, location and sample level. At sample level, approximately 35% of the analyzed frames were included in the 1st action category, more than half of them were categorized in the 2nd action category and roughly 6% were interpreted as belonging to the 4th action category.

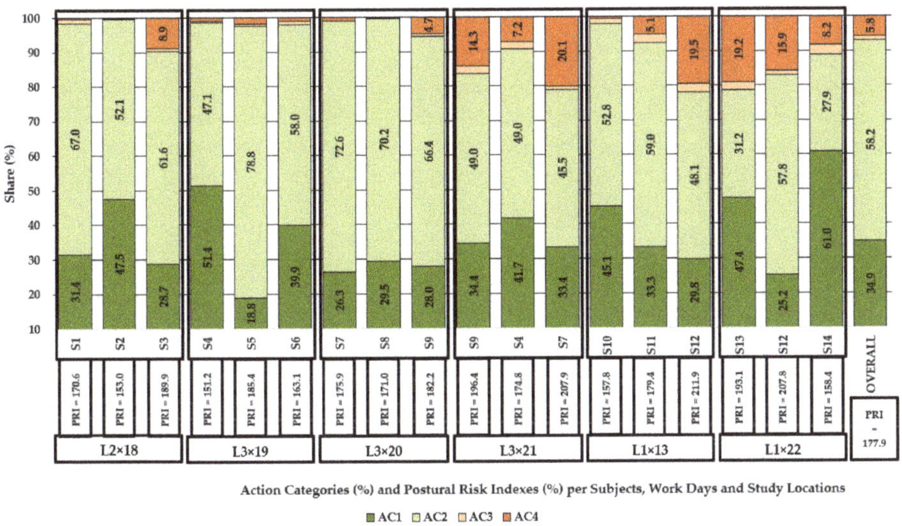

Figure 3. Share of the analyzed frames per action categories and postural risk indexes estimated at subject, location, observation day and sample level.

The postural risk index characterizing the job was found to be of almost 178, indicating rather the categorization of this job in the second action category which requires corrective actions to be taken in the near future. At subject level, on the other hand, distribution on action categories and the computed postural risk indexes were quite variable. Frames attributed to the 1st action category accounted for shares of 18.8 to 61%, with the latter one characterizing the postural behavior of S14; frames attributed to the 2nd action category accounted for shares in the range of 27.9–78.8%, those specific to the 3rd action category accounted for minor shares and those belonging to the 4th category accounted for shares of up to 20.1%. The postural risk indexes varied in between 151.2 (S2 × L2 × 18) and 211.9 (S12 × L1 × 13).

At the sample level (Table 7), back postures were found to be particularly uncomfortable, as in more than 55% of the cases, the subjects were found to have the back bent and twisted or bent forward and sideways. Straight postures of the back were found only in 26% of the cases. In general, the arm postures were found to be comfortable and this situation is related to the characteristics and tool use in this kind of job. Combined with poor postures of the back, legs postures codded by 4, 5 and 6 lead always to the worst postural situation which is characteristic to the fourth action category. It was not the case of the analyzed sample since these legs' postures accounted for only 7%. Therefore, from the postural analysis point of view, the main problems related to potential risks of health impairment were those specific to the back.

Table 7. Share of back, arms and legs postures per codes described by OWAS.

Code	Share of Back Postures (%)	Share of Arms Postures (%)	Share of Legs Postures (%)
1	26.04	99.68	4.59
2	7.77	0.31	56.60
3	9.65	0.01	29.82
4	56.54	NA [1]	3.71
5	NA [1]	NA [1]	3.48
6	NA [1]	NA [1]	0.17
7	NA [1]	NA [1]	1.63

[1] Not applicable according to OWAS method.

4. Discussion

The main aim of this work was to characterize the difficulty and risks associated to manual cultivation operations in hybrid poplar forests. Acknowledging the limitation of the results to male subjects, as well as the fact that indirect observation may still have affected the work behavior of the observed subjects, the first thing which needs to be addressed, even in the conditions of a good utilization of available time for effective work (approximately 70%), is that relating to a particular low efficiency of such operations which was in the range of 8.6–9.0 h per double-pass operated hectare. From this point of view, the first hypothesis of this study was confirmed only from the productivity point of view. Indeed, there is limited information of operational performance metrics for this kind of jobs. Nevertheless, for something similar, de Oliveira et al. [11] found an efficiency rate of approximately 3.3 h per hectare which took 52% of the heart rate reserve during the effective work. The Romanian forestry-related rating system [31], on the other hand, indicates for the same job operational efficiencies in the range of 1.42–4.90 man-hours per 100 m^2, which will probably ensure rest breaks-taking in a sustainable way. One way to improve the efficiency and to balance the effort given by workers would be that of deploying inter-row mechanized cultivation operations on two perpendicular directions since the plantation layouts would enable such an approach. In particular, this could contribute to a reduction of manually operated area to approximately one fourth compared to the current operational layouts.

In terms of physiological workload, worth mentioning that heart rate is a good estimator of the VO_2 indicator [32] that is commonly used to predict the work difficulty in general ergonomic studies [21,22]. Cardiovascular workload, as found in this study indicates that this type of operation tends to overload the workers, therefore confirming the second hypothesis of the study. How the subjects experienced the workload was found to be related to their age. In average, the %HRR metric for the effective work was found to be very close to the threshold of 40% which, according to some authors [10], defines the limit between acceptable and unacceptable workloads. However, this outcome should be interpreted as indicative at least from two points of view. The first one refers to the impossibility to extend the findings to cohorts characterized by anthropometrics that are particularly contrasting to those which built the data from this study. The second one refers to the caution which should be used in the interpretation of data since the %HRR metric was based on the commonly accepted formula for estimating the maximum heart rate, which has its own limitations [33]. Also, an ambulatory trial found heart rates at rest lower when self-measured at home compared to those measured under expert observation [34]. Obviously, such an effect will probably lead to an underestimation of job's difficulty, the same way the exposure to high thermal stress will. As such, and knowing the fact that the climate change affects the health of the workers [14], the thermal stress should be considered in the improvement of work in manual cultivation operations since the climate in the studied area is generally described by hot summers.

Most probably, an increased cardiovascular activity, as found in this study, is related to the type of work, work intensity and the body parts engaged in such work since the job tasks took a great deal of using handwork which is known to affect the heart rate response and characterizes the severity of muscular work [21]. Recovery time of heart rate is dependent on the exercise intensity and may reach more than 30 min [35,36], even if most of the recovery changes may occur in the first 1–2 min [36], while the heart rate response may be sensitive to postural changes [37]. For instance, switching from lying to sitting positions was found to increase the heart rate in some subjects by approximately 10 beats per minute [38]. Therefore, it was not surprising to find that for most of the subjects observed in this study the heart rate reserve was particularly increased also during the rest pauses and during the meal taking. It is difficult to place the manual cultivation operations, in terms of difficulty and risks, amongst other forestry jobs, given the fact that heart response is dependent on many factors such as the age of subjects, gender and their operational environment. Nevertheless, in motor-manual felling, estimates from the same flat-land area and for a worker having an age close to the average of this study [17] were close to those found in this study. In steep terrain forests of Turkey, for instance, harvesting and forest nursery work was found to be difficult to moderate jobs with heart rate reserves of approximately 41 and 32%, respectively [39], while jobs such as cable work in steep terrain [40,41] and cable rigging [42] may take more effort.

Work intensity was found to be light and moderate in most of the surveyed time (more than 95%), therefore partially confirming the third hypothesis of this study. Since ENMO values of up to 0.25 g are characterizing sedentary behaviors and light work such as standing still, dusting, sweeping the floor and self-paced walking [24], this intensity threshold was used to separate light intensity work in this study. In general, vigorous activity is considered to account for more than 21 $mL \times kg^{-1} \times min^{-1}$ VO_2 which roughly corresponds to accelerations corrected by the mean amplitude deviation of 0.45–0.5 g [25]. However, in this study, the intensity of work was considered to be moderate when ENMO had values from 0.25 to 1.0 g, by taking into account also the cardiovascular activity and the behavior or acceleration data in effective working events versus rest pauses. It should be mentioned that even in events such as the meal pauses, the subjects were not found to sit still all the time.

Also, given the position in which the accelerometers were placed, the collected and analyzed data stands, in particular, for the activity of subjects' back. This data may be correlated also with that coming from postural analysis where the back was found to be straight in 26% of the cases and bent, twisted or both in the rest of the cases. This outcome was partially consistent with the last hypothesis of this study. In this regard, the manual cultivation operation seems to be a job that does not require immediate postural redesign since the postural risk indexes were found to be less than 200% in most of the cases. However, the main problem here is that related to the back postures assumed by subjects which were particularly uncomfortable. Working predominantly with the back bent and twisted or bent forward and sideways (56.5% of the cases) may lead to health problems related to the lower back which is a known issue of forest operations jobs [14]. From this point of view, manual cultivation is a job that is even more hazardous compared to manual harvesting operations from Nordic countries [43] and close to that of motor-manual tree felling and processing operations from the area [17]. Compared to other kind of forestry-related partly mechanized jobs such as firewood processing [30] and wood debarking [44], manual cultivation seems to be riskier with the main problems coming from the back postures assumed during the work, since the arms and legs postures were found to be comfortable in most of the cases.

5. Conclusions

The main conclusion of this study is that the manual cultivation operations in poplar forests are rather difficult and hazardous, requiring reengineering tasks from ergonomic and public health points of view. To overcome the effect of small efficiency rates found in this study, mechanization should be extended by approaching the operated plots on two perpendicular directions, limiting this way the manual job to approximately one quarter compared to actual practices. Even if not documented by the available literature, such approaches are seldom used in the Romanian practice. Obviously, this way of extending the mechanized part of operations, will reduce also the continuous physical effort of the upper limbs and back by inter-placing movements from one tree to other, therefore it will lead to an increased use of bigger muscular groups and legs, that could help in attenuating the cardiovascular activity. By such measures, the intensity of manual work will be also decreased and the frequency of poor back postures will improve. Nevertheless, in such cases in which the approach of extending the mechanized operations is not feasible, a correct training of the workers, including a redesign of rest breaks could improve the status quo. These issues may be approached by intervention programs designed to tailor the work tasks, on the one hand, and to properly train the workers, on the other hand. Such approaches are important since the results of this study clearly indicated that the job in manual cultivation operations is characterized by a dynamic work that may overload the heart, upper limbs and the back of the workers. Also, incentives to attract youth in such operations should be developed and implemented at regional and national scale.

Author Contributions: Conceptualization, T.M.-P. and S.A.B.; Data curation, T.M.-P., M.C. and M.V.M.; Formal analysis, M.C. and M.V.M.; Funding acquisition, T.M.-P. and C.I.D.; Investigation, T.M.-P. and M.C.; Methodology, T.M.-P. and S.A.B.; Project administration, M.V.M. and S.A.B.; Resources, C.I.D., F.I. and S.A.B.; Software, S.A.B.; Supervision, S.A.B.; Validation, T.M.-P., M.C., M.V.M., C.I.D. and A.A.B.; Writing—original draft, F.I. and S.A.B.; Writing—review & editing, F.I. and S.A.B.

Funding: This research received no external funding.

Acknowledgments: The authors acknowledge the technical and logistic support of Department of Forest Engineering, Forest Management Planning and Terrestrial Measurements, Faculty of Silviculture and Forest Engineering, Transilvania University of Braşov. The authors would like to thank the local managers of National Forest Administration for agreeing to carry on this study in the forests managed by them and to the subjects who agreed to participate in the study, for their support. This work is part of a PhD thesis developed under the supervision of Doctoral School of the Transilvania University of Braşov. The authors acknowledge the support of the aforementioned organization.

Conflicts of Interest: The authors declare no conflict of interest.

References

1. Dickmann, D.I. Silviculture and biology of short-rotation woody crops in temperate regions: Then and now. *Biomass Bioenerg.* **2006**, *30*, 696–705. [CrossRef]
2. Drew, A.P.; Zsuffa, L.; Mitchell, C.P. Terminology relating to woody plant biomass and its production. *Biomass* **1987**, *12*, 79–82. [CrossRef]
3. Vusić, D.; Šušnjar, M.; Marchi, E.; Spina, R.; Zečić, Ž.; Picchio, R. Skidding operations in thinning and shelterwood cut of mixed stands - Work productivity, energy inputs and emissions. *Ecol. Eng.* **2013**, *61*, 216–223. [CrossRef]
4. Moskalik, T.; Borz, S.A.; Dvořák, J.; Ferencik, M.; Glushkov, S.; Muiste, P.; Lazdiņš, A.; Styranivsky, O. Timber harvesting methods in Eastern European countries: A review. *Croat. J. For. Eng.* **2017**, *38*, 231–241.
5. Boja, N.; Boja, F.; Teusdea, A.; Vidrean, D.; Marcu, M.V.; Iordache, E.; Duţă, C.I.; Borz, S.A. Resource allocation, pit quality, and early survival of seedlings following two motor-manual pit-drilling options. *Forests* **2018**, *9*, 665. [CrossRef]
6. Abrudan, I.V. *Împăduriri*; Transilvania University Press: Braşov, Romania, 2006; p. 200.
7. Corella-Justavino, F.; Jimenez Ramirez, R.; Meza Perez, N.; Borz, S.A. The use of OWAS in forest operations postural assessment: Advantages and limitations. *Bull. Transilv. Univ. Braşov, Series II For. Wood Ind. Agric. Food Eng.* **2015**, *8*, 7–16.
8. Heinimann, H.R. Forest operations engineering and management - the ways behind and ahead of a scientific discipline. *Croat. J. For. Eng.* **2007**, *28*, 107–121.
9. Marchi, E.; Chung, W.; Visser, R.; Abbas, D.; Nordfjell, T.; Mederski, P.S.; McEwan, A.; Brink, M.; Laschi, A. Sustainable forest operations (SFO): A new paradigm in a changing world and climate. *Sci. Total Environ.* **2018**, *634*, 1385–1397. [CrossRef]
10. Potočnik, I.; Poje, A. Forestry ergonomics and occupational safety in high ranking scientific journals from 2005–2016. *Croat. J. For. Eng.* **2017**, *38*, 291–310.
11. de Oliveira, F.M.; Lopes, E.S.; Rodrigues, C.K. Evaluation of the physical work load and biomechanical of workers at manual and semi-mechanized mowing. *Cerne* **2014**, *20*, 419–425. [CrossRef]

12. Deeney, C.; O'Sullivan, L. Work related psychosocial risks and musculoskeletal disorders: potential risk factors, causation and evaluation methods. *Work* **2009**, *34*, 239–248.
13. Enez, K.; Nalbantoglu, S.S. Comparison of risk assessment outputs from OWAS and REBA in forestry timber harvesting. *Int. J. Ind. Ergon.* **2019**, *70*, 51–57. [CrossRef]
14. Gallis, C. Work-related prevalence of musculoskeletal symptoms among Greek forest workers. *Int. J. Ind. Ergon.* **2006**, *36*, 731–736. [CrossRef]
15. Şofletea, N.; Curtu, L. *Dendrologie*, 2nd ed.; Pentru Viaţă Publishing House: Braşov, Romania, 2008; pp. 335–336, ISBN 978-973-85874-4-1.
16. Helander, M. *A Guide to Human Factors and Ergonomics*, 2nd ed.; CRC Press: Boca Raton, FL, USA, 2006; pp. 224–255, ISBN 0-203-68775-2.
17. Cheţa, M.; Marcu, M.V.; Borz, S.A. Workload, exposure to noise, and risk of musculoskeletal disorders: A case study of motor-manual tree felling and processing in poplar clear cuts. *Forests* **2018**, *9*, 300. [CrossRef]
18. Borz, S.A.; Talagai, N.; Cheţa, M.; Gavilanes Montoya, A.V.; Castillo Vizuete, D.D. Automating data collection in motor-manual time and motion studies implemented in a willow short rotation coppice. *Bioresources* **2018**, *13*, 3236–3249. [CrossRef]
19. Björheden, R.; Apel, K.; Shiba, M.; Thompson, M. *IUFRO Forest Work Study Nomenclature*; Swedish University of Agricultural Science: Grapenberg, Sweden, 1995; p. 16.
20. Acuna, M.; Bigot, M.; Guerra, S.; Hartsough, B.; Kanzian, C.; Kärhä, K.; Lindroos, O.; Magagnotti, N.; Roux, S.; Spinelli, R.; et al. Good Practice Guidelines for Biomass Production Studies. Available online: http://www.forestenergy.org/pages/cost-action-fp0902/good-practice-guidelines/ (accessed on 1 April 2019).
21. Rodahl, K. *The Physiology of Work*, 1st ed.; Taylor and Francis: London, UK, 1989; pp. 335–336, ISBN 0-85066-478-0.
22. Åstrand, P.O.; Rodahl, K. *Textbook of Work Physiology-Physiological Bases of Exercise*, 3rd ed.; Human Kinetics: Champaign, IL, USA, 1986; ISBN 978-007-00241-8-6.
23. van Hees, V.T.; Fang, Z.; Langford, J.; Assah, F.; Mohammad, A.; da Silva, I.C.M.; Trenell, M.I.; White, T.; Wareham, N.J.; Barge, S. Autocalibration of accelerometer data for free-living physical activity assessment using local gravity and temperature: an evaluation on four continents. *J Appl. Physiol.* **2014**, *117*, 738–744. [CrossRef]
24. Bakrania, K.; Yates, T.; Rowlands, A.V.; Esliger, D.W.; Bunnewell, S.; Sanders, J.; Davies, M.; Khunti, K.; Edeardson, C.L. Thresholds on raw acceleration data: Euclidian Norm Minus One (ENMO) and Mean Amplitude Deviation (MAD) approaches. *PLoS ONE* **2016**, *11*, e0164045. [CrossRef] [PubMed]
25. Vähä-Ypyä, H.; Vasankari, T.; Husu, P.; Mänttäri, A.; Vuorimaa, T.; Suni, J.; Sievänen, H. Validation of cut-points for evaluating the intensity of physical activity with accelerometry-based Mean Amplitude Deviation (MAD). *PLoS ONE* **2015**, *10*, e0134813. [CrossRef]
26. Karhu, O.; Kansi, P.; Kuorinka, I. Correcting working postures in industry: a practical method for analysis. *Appl. Ergon.* **1977**, *8*, 199–201. [CrossRef]
27. Calvo, A. Musculoskeletal disorders (MSD) risks in forestry: a case study to propose an analysis method. *Agric. Eng. Int.* **2009**, *11*, 1–9.
28. Zanuttini, R.; Cielo, P.; Poncino, D. The OWAS method. Preliminary results for the evaluation of the risk of work-related musculo-skeletal disorders (WMSD) in the forestry sector in Italy. *For. Riv. Selvic. Ecol. For.* **2005**, *2*, 242–255.
29. David, G.C. Ergonomic methods for assessing exposure to risk of factors for work-related musculoskeletal disorders. *Occup. Med.-C* **2005**, *55*, 190–199. [CrossRef] [PubMed]
30. Spinelli, R.; Aminti, G.; de Francesco, F. Postural risk assessment of firewood processing. *Ergonomics* **2016**, *60*, 1–9. [CrossRef] [PubMed]
31. Ministry of Waters, Forests and Environment Protection. *National Forest Administration. Unified Work Time and Production Rates for Forestry, Ministry of Waters*; Forests and Environment Protection: Bucharest, Romania, 1997; p. 146.
32. Dubé, P.A.; Imbeau, D.; Dubeau, D.; Lebel, L.; Kolus, A. Removing the thermal component from heart rate provides an accurate VO_2 estimation in forest work. *Appl. Ergon.* **2016**, *54*, 148–157. [CrossRef] [PubMed]
33. Tanaka, H.; Monahan, K.D.; Seals, D.R. Age-predicted maximal heart rate revisited. *J. Am. Coll. Cardiol.* **2001**, *37*, 153–156. [CrossRef]

34. Lequeuz, B.; Uzan, C.; Rehman, M.B. Does resting heart rate measured by the physician reflect the patient's true resting heart rate? White-coat heart rate. *Indian Heart J.* **2018**, *70*, 93–98. [CrossRef]
35. Javorka, M.; Žila, I.; Balhárek, T.; Javorka, K. Heart rate recovery after exercise: relations to heart rate variability and complexity. *Braz. J. Med. Biol. Res.* **2002**, *35*, 991–1000. [CrossRef] [PubMed]
36. Du, N.; Bai, S.; Oguri, K.; Kato, Y.; Matsumoto, I.; Kawase, H.; Matsuoka, T. Heart rate recovery after exercise and neural regulation of the heart rate variability in 30–40 year old female marathon runners. *J. Sport. Sci. Med.* **2005**, *4*, 9–17.
37. Jones, A.Y.M.; Kam, C.; Lai, K.W.; Lee, H.Y.; Chow, H.T.; Lau, S.F.; Wong, L.M.; He, J. Changes in heart rate and R-wave amplitude with posture. *Chin. J. Physiol.* **2003**, *46*, 63–69.
38. Šipinková, I.; Hahn, G.; Meyer, M.; Tadlánek, M.; Hájek, J. Effect of respiration and posture on heart rate variability. *Physiol. Res.* **1997**, *46*, 173–179.
39. Eroglu, H.; Yilmaz, R.; Kayacan, Y. A study on determining the physical workload of the forest harvesting and nursery-afforestation workers. *Anthropologist* **2015**, *21*, 168–181. [CrossRef]
40. Magagnotti, N.; Spinelli, R. Replacing steel cable with synthetic rope to reduce operator workload during log winching operations. *Small-Scale For.* **2012**, *11*, 223–236. [CrossRef]
41. Spinelli, R.; Ottaviani Aalmo, G.; Magagnotti, N. The effect of a slack-pulling device in reducing operator physiological workload during log winching operations. *Ergonomics* **2014**, *58*, 781–790. [CrossRef]
42. Ottaviani, G.; Talbot, B.; Nitteberg, M.; Stampfer, K. Workload benefits of using synthetic rope strawline in cable yarder rigging in Norway. *Croat. J. For. Eng.* **2010**, *32*, 561–569.
43. Harstela, P. Work postures and strain of workers in Nordic forest work: a selective review. *Int. J. Ind. Ergon.* **1990**, *5*, 219–226. [CrossRef]
44. Spinelli, R.; Aminti, G.; Magagnotti, N.; De Francesco, F. Postural risk assessment of small-scale debarkers for wooden post production. *Forests* **2018**, *9*, 111. [CrossRef]

International Journal of
Environmental Research and Public Health

MDPI

Article

Organisational Climate, Role Stress, and Public Employees' Job Satisfaction

Vicente Pecino [1,2], Miguel A. Mañas [2], Pedro A. Díaz-Fúnez [2], José M. Aguilar-Parra [3,*], David Padilla-Góngora [3] and Remedios López-Liria [4,*]

1. Head Manager of HRM Office & IPTORA Research Team, University of Almería, 04120 Almería, Spain; vpecino@ual.es
2. Department of Psychology & IPTORA Research Team, University of Almería, 04120 Almería, Spain; marodrig@ual.es (M.A.M.); pfunez@ual.es (P.A.D.-F.)
3. Department of Psychology, University of Almería, 04120 Almería, Spain; dpadilla@ual.es
4. Department of Nursing Science, Physiotherapy and Medicine, Hum-498 Research Team, Health Research Centre, University of Almería, 04120 Almería, Spain

* Correspondence: jmaguilar@ual.es (J.M.A.-P.); rll040@ual.es (R.L.-L.)

Received: 19 April 2019; Accepted: 19 May 2019; Published: 21 May 2019

Abstract: The Job Demands-Resources (JD-R) model is an integrative theoretical framework for monitoring workplaces with the aim to increase job engagement and prevent burnout. This framework is of great interest since the management of job resources and demands can negatively affect employees, especially in organisational contexts characterised by high job demands. This study uses the job demands-resources model to investigate the relationships between organisational climate, role stress, and employee well-being (burnout and job satisfaction) in public organisations. This is a descriptive, cross-sectional study. The research participants are 442 public employees. A structural equation model was developed (organisational climate, job satisfaction, burnout, role stress). These confirm that organisational climate is correlated with role stress (−0.594), job satisfaction (0.746), and burnout (−0.408), while role stress is correlated with burnout (0.953) and job satisfaction (−0.685). Finally, there is a correlation between burnout and job satisfaction that is negative and significant (−0.664). The study confirms that a positive organisational climate could lead to less stressed and burned-out workers and, at the same time, to more satisfied employees with improved well-being.

Keywords: organisational climate; role stress; employee' well-being; public administration

1. Introduction

Reforms in the public sector have been a constant of the last 20 years, and there has been a particular focus on developing human factors [1]. These changes have become more necessary with the recent financial crisis, which positioned human resources management as a key internal element towards which many of the administration's new policies should be directed [2,3].

Human factors are the key to improving public services. Bakker [4] states that people who want to change the world for the better often pursue a professional career in public service and are sometimes characterised by a 'general altruistic motivation to serve the interests of a community of people, a state, a nation or humankind' [5]. However, these employees face environments characterised by changes in performance expectations, high work demands, a hierarchical structure and bureaucratisation of work processes [6]; these factors tend to lead to the significant deterioration of employee well-being [7].

The emergence in the late twentieth century of the so-called 'Positive Psychology', which focuses on the positive side of people [8], was crucial to organisational and occupational psychology. This new paradigm has encouraged human resource departments to focus on increasing opportunities, satisfaction, motivation, resources and flexibility to develop people and enhance their well-being [9].

In this sense, we want to analyse how the stressful and motivational characteristics of work environments influence the well-being of employees, and how to create healthy environments [10].

1.1. The Job Demands-Resources Model

The Job Demands-Resources (JD-R) [11] model is an integrative theoretical framework for monitoring workplaces with the aim to increase job engagement and prevent burnout [12]. This framework is of great interest to Positive Organisational Psychology (POP) since the management of job resources and demands can negatively affect employees, especially in organisational contexts characterised by high job demands [13]. Demerouti et al. [11] defined job demands as 'those physical, social, or organisational aspects of the job that require sustained physical or mental effort and are therefore associated with certain physiological and psychological costs' ([11], p. 501). During the past three decades, many studies have shown that job characteristics can have a profound impact on employee well-being (i.e., job satisfaction, burnout, job engagement) and that job demands such as high work pressure, emotional demands, and role stress may lead to satisfaction problems and impaired health [14].

The job resources were defined as 'those physical, psychological, social, or organisational aspects of the job that are either/or functional in achieving work goals; reduce job demands and the associated physiological and psychological costs; stimulate personal growth and development' ([11], p. 501). The job resources are means to the achievement or protection of other valued resources and may be located at the level of the organisation at large, the interpersonal and social relations (i.e., supervisor and co-worker support, team climate), the organisation of work, and at the level of the task [14].

The JD-R model assumes that factors associated with organisations affect employees in two ways: A process of health deterioration, and a motivational process. In the first process, job demands predict the occurrence of burnout, which is associated with negative effects for the organisation and its employees. The motivational process links the existence of labour resources with the emergence of employee engagement, which leads to positive results for both employees and organisations [15].

1.2. Organisational Climate and Role Stress

One of the main job resources is the organisational climate [15]. Organisational climate research is interested in understanding the ways in which workers in an organisation experience and feel the climate, and how it is related to well-being. Schneider, Ehrhart and Macey [16] defined climate as 'the shared meaning organisational members attach to the events, policies, practices, and procedures they experience and the behaviours they see being rewarded, supported and expected'. Thus, organisational climate shows how employees' shared perceptions are connected to their work environment.

Role stress is the most studied job demand involving a natural phenomenon in organisations. It can be defined as a set of expectations, duties and obligations, applied to employees, coming from those who can influence the employees and help to define their roles [17]. It negatively affects employee efficiency [18], becoming an element that decreases employees' well-being [19], and has equally pernicious effects on organisational performance [20]. The theory of role stress examines how characteristics of roles (e.g., conflict, ambiguity, and overload) are perceived and experienced as stressors by role incumbents, leading to affective and physiological symptoms as well as coping responses [21].

In the study of the relationship between organisational climate and role stress (job resources and job demands, respectively), the buffering hypothesis prevails. It suggests that the impact of job demands on employee well-being is weaker when they have a high level of resources [10]. The relationship between organisational climate and role stress is not a new one and has been shown to play a role in employee behaviour. Bakker and Demerouti [22] showed that the direction of this relationship can be positive or negative, and that the difference lies in the level of job resources (social support, job control and feedback) [12]. In this line, Hemingway and Smith [23] explored how organisational climate is associated with increased stress levels and the occurrence of negative behaviours for organisations;

also, Pecino [24], using a sample of public employees, showed how organisational climate is strongly and negatively related to role stress.

1.3. The Motivational Process: Organisational Climate and Job Satisfaction

Job satisfaction is certainly the most researched topic in the history of industrial and organisational psychology [25]. The most relevant definition of job satisfaction is that offered by Locke [26], who defined it as a 'positive or pleasant emotional state resulting from the subjective perception of the person's work experiences'. This topic is of great importance in many models that seek to improve employee well-being [27] and organisational efficiency [28]. Many studies have shown that this variable has positive effects on organisations and their employees [29].

The influence of job resources (organisational climate) on job satisfaction, as an indicator of employee well-being, occurs through a motivational process [30]. Job resources seem to play a motivating role, fostering the learning, growth, and development of employees. Numerous studies have confirmed that the more positively employees perceive the organisational climate, the more satisfied they are [31].

1.4. The Health Deterioration Process: Role Stress and Burnout

Burnout is defined as 'a syndrome of emotional exhaustion, depersonalization, and reduced personal accomplishment that can occur among individuals who work with other people' [32]. There is growing evidence of the negative effects of burnout on employees and their performance [33]. Among the consequences for employees are low job satisfaction and deterioration of their health [34].

The relationship between job demands and burnout, as an indicator of employee well-being, occurs through the health deterioration process [30] and follows the line of the compensatory control model [35]. A study carried out by Buunk et al. [36] showed that intense or prolonged exposure to role stress causes psychological problems (i.e., burnout), as well as physical problems. Recent studies have deepened our understanding of the relationship between role stress and burnout in public employees, finding significant and positive results [37].

1.5. Cross-Links between Processes and Consequences

The organisational climate can affect employees' well-being, directly influencing burnout. Under this hypothesis, Winnubst [38] carried out a pioneering study and concluded that organisational climate is an important antecedent of burnout. Recent studies have shown that formal support groups create organisational climates that decrease stressors such as burnout [39].

Also, the study of the relationship between role stress and job satisfaction is of major importance. Recently, several studies have presented evidence of this relationship in different country, industry, and labour contexts [40,41].

The JD-R model also provides a relationship between the consequences of job demands and those of job resources. A recent longitudinal study by Figueiredo-Ferraz et al. [42], who focused on analysing the relationship between burnout and job satisfaction, found a significant two-way relationship between these variables.

Other findings explained that—relative to private sector employees—public servants became the most engaged by intrinsic factors including work-related resources [43]. Work engagement significantly mediated the relationship between job resources and personal resources of public employees. Public sector workers were more strongly motivated by the desire to work in a supportive working environment. Most observed differences were explained by differences in job content such as skill variety, feedback, or task identity, not by the sector itself [43].

The aim of this study is to analyse the relationship between organisational climate, role stress, burnout, and job satisfaction in public employees. For this purpose, our hypotheses are consistent with previous studies:

Organisational climate will show a significant and negative reciprocal relationship with role stress (hypothesis 1) and a positive reciprocal relationship with job satisfaction (hypothesis 2). Also, role stress will show a significant and positive reciprocal relationship with burnout (hypothesis 3). Furthermore, organisational climate will show a significant and negative reciprocal relationship with burnout (hypothesis 4) and role stress will show a significant and negative reciprocal relationship with job satisfaction (hypothesis 5). Finally, job satisfaction will have a reciprocal relationship, both significant and negative, with burnout (hypothesis 6).

2. Materials and Methods

2.1. Participants and Procedure

Data were collected through online questionnaires in this cross-sectional study. Most participants in the chosen institution completed the questionnaire, for a total of 442 out of 475 public employees. All participants gave written informed consent in accordance with the Declaration of Helsinki. The Ethical Review Committee at the University of Almería (Spain) approved the study (UALBIO2018/027).

In terms of gender, 50.7% of participants were women and 49.3% men. For age, 5.7% of participants were under 36 years old 57.7% were between 36 and 45; 31.2% of them were between 46 and 55; and 5.4% were more than 55 years of age. As for educational level, 11.5% had no formal schooling, primary or secondary education; 25.8% had studied at high school; 61.1% were graduates; and 1.6% held a doctoral degree. In terms of labour status, 96.6% were civil servants and 3.4% were ordinary employees. Their positions at work were as follows: 86.4% were middle managers and workers and 13.6% were head managers. As for work hours, 392 of the participants (88.7 %) worked a morning shift and 50 (11.3%) worked an afternoon shift.

2.2. Instruments

2.2.1. Organisational Climate

A shortened version of the First Organisational Climate/Culture Unified Search 93 (FOCUS-93) questionnaire by Van Muijen et al. [44] was used in this study. It consisted of 12 items using a 7-point Likert scale (ranging from 1 = 'strongly disagree' to 7 = 'strongly agree'). The dimensions contained in the instrument were support, goals, innovation, and rules.

2.2.2. Job Satisfaction

This variable was measured using CSLPS-EAP/33 [45], which consists of 33 items that are answered using a Likert scale with seven responses ranging from 1 = 'strongly dissatisfied' to '7 = strongly satisfied'. The dimensions contained in this instrument are team, retribution, means and conditions, intrinsic, business, workload, autonomy, and objects.

2.2.3. Burnout

This was measured using an adapted version of the Maslasch Burnout Inventory [46], translated by Peiró et al. [47], which consists of nine items answered on a Likert scale with seven responses ranging from 0 = 'never' to 6 = 'every day'. The dimensions contained in this instrument are exhaustion, cynicism, and professional efficacy.

2.2.4. Role Stress

This was measured using a questionnaire composed by Rizzo et al. [48] that was translated by Peiró et al. [49]. It consists of 17 items with a response scale featuring 5 alternatives, ranging from 1 = 'strongly disagree' to 5 = 'strongly agree'. The dimensions evaluated by this instrument are role ambiguity, role conflict and role overload.

2.3. Statistical Analysis

In order to verify the reliability of the dimensions, the internal consistency was assessed using Cronbach's alpha coefficient [50] for each variable and dimension. For each of the four variables under study, a structural equation model was fitted to confirm the dimensions. Finally, to check the relations between the different variables, a structural equation model was developed.

Structural equation models were fitted using the diagonalised weighted least squares (DWLS) [51] or robust maximum likelihood (RML) method [52], depending on the construct to be analysed, since the multivariate normality of the data was not met for any of the dimensions or variables. The univariate normality was checked for each item and skewness and kurtosis measures were obtained. To test the multivariate normality, the Henze-Zirkler test [53] was used.

The DWLS method requires large data sets; specifically, the sample size should be larger than $p > (p + 1)/2$, where p is the number of parameters to be estimated by the structural equation. Therefore, dimensions where the number of items considered in the model was too low could not be fitted using this method. Thus, the method used for those dimensions was RML. Those dimensions were from two variables: Climate and job satisfaction [54].

The goodness of fit for the proposed models was measured using the Tucker-Lewis Index (TLI) and the Comparative Fit Index (CFI). For both, values greater than 0.9 indicate a good fit. Another measure used was the Root Mean Square Error of Approximation, (RMSEA) where values lower than 0.08 indicate a good model fit and the upper limit of the 90% confidence interval should be below the 0.1 cut-off value for a good model fit [55]. The Standardized Root Mean Square Residual (SRMR) is an absolute measure of fit defined as the normalisation of the difference between the observed and predicted correlations. An SRMR value of less than 0.08 is considered as an adequate cut-off point for the goodness of fit [56]. The models were implemented using R software (R Foundation for Statistical Computing, Vienna, Austria) and the Lavaan package [57].

3. Results

First, we performed a confirmatory analysis of the dimensions for each of the variables used in the study, and later we presented a structural equation model for testing the relations between variables.

3.1. Confirmatory Analysis of Climate

Cronbach's alpha for climate was 0.95. The RMSEA and SRMR obtained in the confirmatory analysis for climate were 0.079 (90% CI [0.076, 0.081]) and 0.076, respectively, indicating an acceptable data fit.

The estimated correlation for the dimension ranged from 0.824 between rules and innovation to 0.916 between goal orientation and innovation, indicating strong relationships between them. For rule dimension, item 7 had the lowest impact. Regarding the innovation dimension, items 8 and 28 had the lowest effects in the construct of the dimension. For the support and goal orientation dimension, all items had similar impacts on the constructs.

For the job satisfaction variable, the value of Cronbach's alpha was 0.91. The goodness of fit values of the model were as follows: RMSEA = 0.057 (90% CI [0.053, 0.06]) and SRMR = 0.048. In addition, the values for CFI and TLI were 0.913 and 0.913, respectively, showing a good fit.

The estimated correlations between dimensions ranged from 0.319, between objects and means and conditions, to 0.826 between equipment and workload. The associations between intrinsic, firm, workload, autonomy, and objects were stronger than those between team retribution and conditions. Regarding the salary, autonomy and object dimensions, all items had similar impacts on their constructs. Within the environment/conditions and workload dimensions, the lower parameter estimated was associated with items 15 and 27.

3.2. Confirmatory Analysis of Role Stress

For role stress, the value of Cronbach's alpha was 0.79. The RMSEA value was 0.034 (90% CI [0.023, 0.044]) and the SRMR value was 0.055. The values of CFI and TLI were 0.99 and 0.988, respectively, showing a good fit for the model. The correlations between the dimensions of the construct were positive, with a value of 0.167 for the dimensions of ambiguity and overload, and 0.508 for overload and conflict. Within the ambiguity dimension, the lower parameter estimate was associated with item 1; this item had a weaker impact on the dimension than the rest of them. Regarding the conflict dimension, item 7 had the weakest effect in the construct of the dimension. For the overload dimension, all items had a similar impact.

3.3. Confirmatory Analysis of Burnout

For the burnout variable, Cronbach's alpha was 0.80. The RMSEA was almost 0 (90% CI [0.000, 0.031]), and the SRMR value was 0.038. The CFI and TLI values were both 1, indicating a perfect fit. The correlations between dimensions were positive, with a value of 0.16 for exhaustion and lack of personal accomplishment, and 0.459 for depersonalisation and exhaustion. Within the depersonalisation and lack of personal accomplishment dimensions, the lowest parameter estimated was associated with items 3 and 9; those items had a weaker impact on their respective dimensions than the rest of the items. For the exhaustion dimension, all items had a similar impact.

3.4. Structural Model of Climate as a Determinant of Job Demands

The standardised estimates of the structural equation model testing the relations between all variables are presented in Figure 1. Cronbach's alpha for the construct was 0.76. The measures of goodness of fit for the model were RMSEA = 0.064, (90% CI [0.056, 0.072]), SRMR = 0.082, CFI = 0.967 and TLI = 0.961. (Table 1). The climate variable had a significant direct negative effect on burnout and role stress, and a positive impact on satisfaction; it had a stronger impact on job satisfaction than on burnout and role stress. The correlation between burnout and role stress was positive, while the correlations between job satisfaction and burnout and role stress were negative.

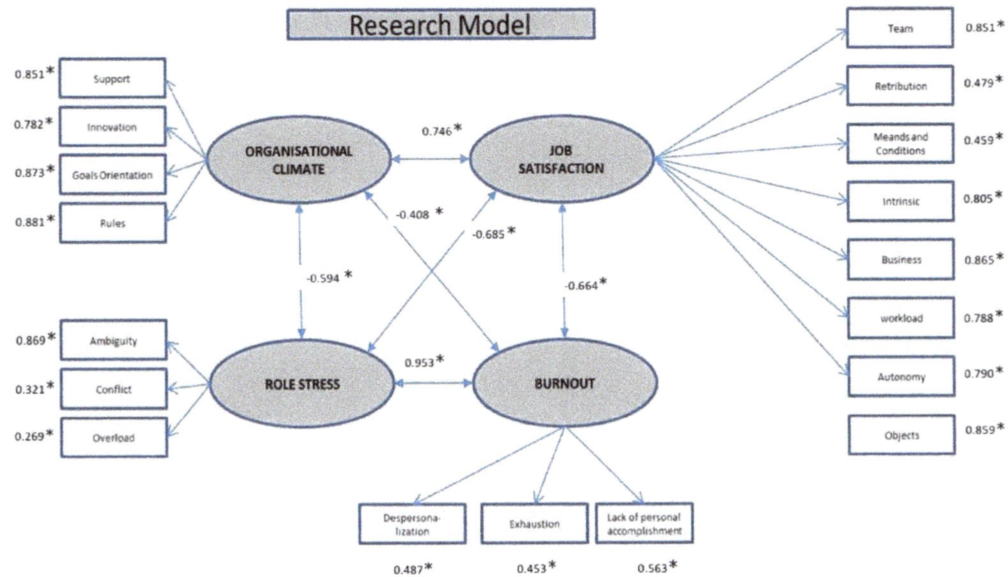

Figure 1. Standardised estimates and goodness of fit parameters for the Research Model. * p-value > 0.01. Crombach's alpha = 0.766. Adjustment made with diagonalised weighted least squares (DWLS). Comparative fit index (CFI) = 0.967; Tucker-Lewis index (TLI) = 0.961; Root mean square error of approximation (RMSEA) = 0.064; Low 90 = 0.056, High = 0.072 and SRMR = 0.082.

Table 1. Estimate parameters for the Job Demands-Resources Model.

Instruments	Variables	Estimated Loads	Std. Error	Z-Value	*p* (>|z|)	Standardised Estimates
Organisational Climate	Support	0.772	0.027	28.787	0.000	0.851
	Innovation	0.553	0.022	25.587	0.000	0.782
	Goal Orientations	0.733	0.026	28.741	0.000	0.873
	Rules	0.685	0.024	28.589	0.000	0.881
Job Satisfaction	Team	0.641	0.034	18.971	0.000	0.851
	Retribution	0.499	0.029	16.955	0.000	0.479
	Means and Conditions	0.450	0.028	16.152	0.000	0.459
	Intrinsic	0.611	0.033	18.468	0.000	0.805
	Business	0.688	0.036	19.247	0.000	0.865
	Workload	0.607	0.031	19.340	0.000	0.778
	Autonomy	0.609	0.033	18.680	0.000	0.790
	Objects	0.717	0.037	19.234	0.000	0.859
Role Stress	Ambiguity	0.511	0.063	8.081	0.000	0.869
	Conflict	0.238	0.030	7.934	0.000	0.321
	Overload	0.249	0.033	7.566	0.000	0.269
Burnout	Depersonalisation	0.413	0.039	10.574	0.000	0.487
	Exhaustion	0.436	0.041	10.535	0.000	0.453
	Lack of personal accomplishment	0.402	0.037	10.810	0.000	0.563
Burnout	Climate	−0.447	0.066	−6.782	0.000	−0.408
Job Satisfaction	Climate	1.121	0.079	14.227	0.000	0.746
Role Stress	Climate	−0.739	0.113	−6.568	0.000	−0.594

4. Discussion

The aim of this work was to study the reciprocal relationships between a job resource (organisational climate), a job demand (role stress) and indicators of employee well-being (burnout and job satisfaction). The results confirmed that organisational climate is significantly and negatively linked to role stress (−0.594), which suggests that the existence of a positive climate would buffer role stress in workers.

In the JD-R model, the direct relationships between demands (role stress) and labour resources (organisational climate) are not specified as positive or negative correlations. Bakker and Demerouti [22] considered this as an empirical question related to the occupational context of the sample under study. Thus, in some organisational contexts, the relationship may be positive and in others negative, depending on variables such as the hierarchy, status, educational level and occupational sector. In the context of public employees, the results obtained confirmed the significant and negative relationships found by previous studies [58].

In this study, climate showed a significant and positive reciprocal influence on job satisfaction (0.746), confirming the motivational process of the JD-R model. Furthermore, previous studies showed that when employees perceive their organisational climate in a more positive way, they are more satisfied [31]. Also, we found that role stress and burnout are significantly and positively related (0.953). Thus, the higher the degree of role stress, the higher the incidence of burnout, which impairs employees' health, as observed in the JD-R model and in previous studies [19,33].

The results confirmed that job demands and resources could interact to positively or negatively affect well-being in two cross-linked relationships [12]. On the one hand, organisational climate showed a significant and negative influence on burnout, which shows that a good climate is related to less burnout. Recent studies have shown that formal support groups create organisational climates that cushion employee stressors related to socio-emotional work such as burnout [59]. On the other hand, the results confirmed that role stress is significantly and negatively related to job satisfaction, which could indicate that higher role stress can lead to lower job satisfaction and, therefore, to worse employee well-being. This result is in line with the findings of recent studies [40,41] and clearly shows how reducing stress levels improves employee satisfaction.

Finally, the results confirmed that job satisfaction has a significant and negative relationship with burnout. In a recent longitudinal study, Figueiredo-Ferraz et al. [42] analysed the relationship between burnout and job satisfaction. They found a significant two-way relationship between the two variables, with more intense effects when job satisfaction was an antecedent of burnout rather than vice versa.

This study represents a step towards understanding the relationships between variables that affect the well-being of employees in public service. These results will be of great interest in the POP field as they will help to promote this viewpoint in the field of human resource management in public administration. The effects of job resources could enhance employees' well-being, increasing satisfaction and preventing burnout [12].

4.1. Practical Implications

The results obtained in this study have important practical implications for managing the employees of public universities. A positive climate is key to enhancing and fostering the well-being of public employees, as the perception of a positive organisational climate leads to more satisfied employees. Such employees are less stressed and suffer from less burnout in their work, which should encourage those responsible for managing people to invest in creating comfortable and positive organisational climates. Such policies would not only help produce more positive results at work, but they would also enhance the development of work in a healthy environment. Furthermore, as was already mentioned when discussing the JD-R model, when a professional job is developed in a job environment characterised by the existence of role stressors, it will have negative effects on the health of employees. Therefore, it is important to establish policies in public administration that help employees have control over their demand level and increase their resources.

4.2. Limitations and Future Directions

However, the results of our study should be considered with the following limitations in mind. First, the results were obtained from self-reports and might be affected by common method variance. Second, the sample was very specific and limited to public employees in a Spanish context; thus, the results cannot be generalised to other types of organisation or public administration. Third, the design of the study had a cross-sectional nature, which prevented us from drawing conclusions about the temporal order of effects and causality relationships. To avoid such limitations, future research should utilise a longitudinal methodology within a multi-method approach [34].

In our changing world, priority should be given to the study of how the well-being of employees in the public sector affects the execution of their duties. Also, the study of different mediating and moderating links in the relation between job demands, resources and well-being in the public context is important. Thus, a more inclusive approach should be taken to examining how work variables affect performance [60]. It will be interesting for future work to consider the multi-level relationships between attitudes, behaviours, and performance aggregated on the team level [61].

5. Conclusions

The study confirms that a positive organisational climate could lead to less stressed and burned-out workers and, at the same time, a higher role stress can lead to lower job satisfaction and, therefore, to worse employee well-being. Organisational climate showed a significant and positive influence on job satisfaction, confirming the motivational process of the JD-R model.

Author Contributions: Conceptualisation, V.P., M.A.M., P.A.D.-F., J.M.A.-P., D.P.-G. and R.L.-L.; Data curation, P.A.D.-F.; Formal analysis, V.P., P.A.D.-F. and J.M.A.-P.; Investigation, M.A.M., D.P.-G. and R.L.-L.; Methodology, V.P., M.A.M., P.A.D.-F. and R.L.-L.; Supervision, V.P. and M.A.M.; Writing—original draft, V.P., P.A.D.-F., J.M.A.-P., D.P.-G. and R.L.-L.; Writing—review & editing, M.A.M., P.A.D.-F., J.M.A.-P., D.P.-G. and R.L.-L.

Funding: This research received no external funding.

Conflicts of Interest: The authors declare no conflict of interest.

References

1. Truss, C. Continuity and change: The role of the HR function in the modern public sector. *Public Adm.* **2008**, *86*, 1071–1088. [CrossRef]
2. Kickert, W. State Responses to the Fiscal Crisis in Britain, Germany and the Netherlands. *Public Manag. Rev.* **2012**, *14*, 299–309. [CrossRef]
3. Lodge, M.; Hood, C. Into an age of multiple austerities? Public management and public service bargains across OECD countries. *Governance* **2012**, *25*, 79–101. [CrossRef]
4. Bakker, A.B. A Job Demands-Resources Approach to Public Service Motivation. *Public Adm. Rev.* **2015**, *75*, 723–732. [CrossRef]
5. Rainey, H.G.; Steinbauer, P. Galloping elephants: Developing elements of a theory of effective government organisations. *J. Public Adm. Res. Theory* **1999**, *9*, 1–32. [CrossRef]
6. Caverley, N. Civil service resiliency and coping. *Int. J. Public Sect. Manag.* **2005**, *18*, 401–413. [CrossRef]
7. Carlotto, M.S.; Gil-Monte, P.R.; Figueiredo-Ferraz, H. Factor analysis of the Spanish Burnout Inventory among public administration employees. *Jpn. Psychol. Res.* **2015**, *57*, 155–165. [CrossRef]
8. Seligman, M.; Csikszentmihalyi, M. Positive psychology: An introduction. *Am. Psychol.* **2000**, *55*, 5–14. [CrossRef]
9. Luthans, F.; Youssef, C.M.; Avolio, B.J. *Psychological Capital: Developing the Human Competitive Edge*; Oxford University Press: Oxford, UK, 2007.
10. Bakker, A.B.; Rodríguez-Muñoz, A.; Derks, D. La emergencia de la psicología de la salud ocupacional positiva. *Psicothema* **2012**, *24*, 66–72. [PubMed]
11. Demerouti, E.; Bakker, A.B.; Nachreiner, F.; Schaufeli, W.B. The Job Demands-Resources Model of Burnout. *J. Appl. Psychol.* **2001**, *86*, 499–512. [CrossRef]

12. Schaufeli, W.B. Applying the Job Demands-Resources model: A 'how to' guide to measuring and tackling work engagement and burnout. *Organ. Dyn.* **2017**, *46*, 120–132. [CrossRef]
13. Bakker, A.B.; Hakanen, J.J.; Demerouti, E.; Xanthopoulou, D. Job resources boost work engagement, particularly when job demands are high. *J. Educ. Psychol.* **2007**, *99*, 274–284. [CrossRef]
14. Bakker, A.B.; Demerouti, E. The job demands-resources model: State of the art. *J. Manag. Psychol.* **2007**, *22*, 309–328. [CrossRef]
15. Bakker, A.B.; Demerouti, E. Job Demands-Resources Theory. In *Wellbeing: A Complete Reference Guide*; Cooper, C., Chen, P., Eds.; Wiley-Blackwell: Chichester, UK, 2014; pp. 37–64.
16. Schneider, B.; Ehrhart, M.G.; Macey, W.H. Perspectives on Organizational Climate and Culture. In *Handbook of Industrial and Organizational Psychology*; Zedek, S., Ed.; American Psychological Association: Washington, DC, USA, 2010; pp. 373–414.
17. Katz, D.; Kahn, R.L. *The Social Psychology of Organizations*; John Wiley: New York, NY, USA, 1978.
18. Kahn, R.; Wolfe, D.; Quinn, R.; Snoek, J.; Rosenthal, R. *Organizational Stress: Studies on Role Conflict and Ambiguity*; Wiley: New York, NY, USA, 1964.
19. Díaz-Fúnez, P.A.; Pecino, V.; Mañas, M.A. Ambigüedad de rol, satisfacción laboral y ciudadanía organizacional en el sector público: Un estudio de mediación multinivel. *Rev. Psicología* **2016**, *34*, 387–412. [CrossRef]
20. Örtqvist, D.; Wincent, J. Prominent consequences of role stress: A meta-analytic review. *Int. J. Stress Manag.* **2006**, *13*, 399–422. [CrossRef]
21. Bliese, P.D.; Edwards, J.R.; Sonnentag, S. Stress and well-being at work: A century of empirical trends reflecting theoretical and societal influences. *J. Appl. Psychol.* **2017**, *102*, 389–402. [CrossRef]
22. Bakker, A.B.; Demerouti, E. Job demands-Resources Theory: Taking Stock and Looking Forward. *J. Occup. Health Psychol.* **2017**, *22*, 273–285. [CrossRef]
23. Hemingway, M.A.; Smith, C.S. Organizational climate and occupational stressors as predictors of withdrawal behaviours and injuries in nurses. *J. Occup. Organ. Psychol.* **1999**, *72*, 285–299. [CrossRef]
24. Pecino, V. Clima Organizacional y sus Consecuencias: Estudios Multinivel en el Sector Público. Unpublished. Ph.D. Thesis, University of Almería, Almería, Spain, June 2016.
25. Judge, T.A.; Klinger, R. Job satisfaction: Subjective well-being at work. In *The Science of Subjective Well-Being*; Eid, M., Larsen, R.J., Eds.; Guilford Press: New York, NY, USA, 2008; pp. 393–413.
26. Locke, E.A. The Nature and Causes of Job Satisfaction. In *Handbook of Industrial and Organizational Psychology*; Dunnette, M.D., Ed.; Rand McNally: Chicago, IL, USA, 1976; pp. 1297–1349.
27. Wright, T.A. The role of "happiness" in organizational research: Past, present and future directions. *Res. Occup. Stress Well-Being* **2005**, *4*, 221–264.
28. Bowen, D.E.; Ostroff, C. Understanding HRM-firm performance linkages: The role of the "strength" of the HRM system. *Acad. Manag. Rev.* **2004**, *29*, 203–221.
29. Bowling, N.A.; Eschleman, K.J.; Wang, Q. A meta-analytic examination of the relationship between job satisfaction and subjective well-being. *J. Occup. Organ. Psychol.* **2010**, *83*, 915–934. [CrossRef]
30. Schaufeli, W.B.; Bakker, A.B. Job demands, job resources, and their relationship with burnout and engagement: A multi-sample study. *J. Organ. Behav.* **2004**, *25*, 293–315. [CrossRef]
31. Pecino, V.; Mañas, M.A.; Díaz-Fúnez, P.A.; López-Puga, J.; Llopis, J.M. Clima y satisfacción laboral en el contexto universitario. *An. Psicología* **2015**, *31*, 658–666. [CrossRef]
32. Maslach, C.; Leiter, M.P. Early predictors of job burnout and engagement. *J. Appl. Psychol.* **2008**, *93*, 498–512. [CrossRef]
33. Gabris, G.T.; Ihrke, D.M. Does performance appraisal contribute to heightened levels of employee burnout? The results of one study. *Public Pers. Manag.* **2001**, *30*, 157–172. [CrossRef]
34. Ganster, D.C.; Rosen, C.C. Work stress and employee health: A multidisciplinary review. *J. Manag.* **2013**, *39*, 1085–1122. [CrossRef]
35. Hockey, G.R.J. Compensatory control in the regulation of human performance under stress and high workload: A cognitive-energetical framework. *Biol. Psychol.* **1997**, *45*, 73–93. [CrossRef]
36. Buunk, B.P.; Jonge, J.; Ybema, J.F.; Wolf, J. Psychosocial Aspects of Occupational Stress. In *Handbook of Organization and Work Psychology*, 2nd ed.; Drenth, P.J.D., Thierry, H., Eds.; Psychology Press: Hove, UK, 1998; pp. 145–182.
37. Guthrie, C.P.; Jones, A. Job Burnout in Public Accounting: Understanding Gender Differences. *J. Manag. Issues* **2012**, *24*, 390–411.

38. Winnubst, J.A. Organizational structure, social support, and burnout. In *Professional Burnout: Recent Developments in Theory and Research*; Schaufeli, W.B., Maslach, C., Marek, T., Eds.; Taylor & Francis: London, UK, 1993; pp. 151–162.
39. Drach-Zahavy, A. How does service workers behavior affect their health? Service climate as a moderator in the service behavior-health relationships. *J. Occup. Health Psychol.* **2010**, *15*, 105–119. [CrossRef] [PubMed]
40. Orgambídez-Ramos, A.; Borrego-Alés, Y.; Mendoza-Sierra, I. Role stress and work engagement as antecedents of job satisfaction in Spanish workers. *J. Ind. Eng. Manag.* **2014**, *7*, 360–372. [CrossRef]
41. Singh, A.P.; Singhi, N. Organizational role stress and social support as predictors of job satisfaction among managerial personnel. *J. Psychosoc. Res.* **2015**, *10*, 1–10.
42. Figueiredo-Ferraz, H.; Grau-Alberola, E.; Gil-Monte, P.R.; García-Juesas, J.A. Burnout and job satisfaction among nursing professionals. *Psicothema* **2012**, *24*, 271–276.
43. Buelens, M.; Broeck, H.V. An analysis of differences in work motivation between public and private sector organizations. *Public Adm. Rev.* **2007**, *27*, 65–74. [CrossRef]
44. Van Muijen, J.; Koopman, P.; De Witte, K.; De Cock, G.; Susanj, Z.; Lemoine, C.; Turnipseed, D. Organizational culture: The Focus Questionnaire. *Eur. J. Work Organ. Psychol.* **1999**, *8*, 551–568. [CrossRef]
45. Lloret, S.; González-Romá, V.; Peiró, J.M. El cuestionario CSLPS-EAP/33: Un Estudio acerca de su validez. *Psicológica* **1993**, *14*, 21–30.
46. Maslach, C.; Jackson, S.E. *MBI: Maslach Burnout Inventory*; University of California: Palo Alto, CA, USA, 1986.
47. Peiró, J.M.; González-Romá, V.; Tordera, N.; Mañas, M.A. Does role stress predict burnout over time among health care professionals? *Psychol. Health* **2001**, *16*, 511–525. [CrossRef]
48. Rizzo, J.R.; House, R.J.; Lirtzman, S.I. Role conflict and ambiguity in complex organizations. *Adm. Sci. Q.* **1970**, *15*, 150–163. [CrossRef]
49. Peiró, J.M.; Meliá, L.; Torres, M.A.; Zurriaga, R. La medida de la experiencia de la ambigüedad en el desempeño: El cuestionario general de ambigüedad de rol en ambientes organizacionales. *Evaluación Psicológica* **1986**, *3*, 27–53.
50. Cronbach, L.J. Coefficient alpha and the internal structure of the tests. *Psychometrika* **1951**, *16*, 297–334. [CrossRef]
51. Jöreskog, K.G.; Sörbom, D. *LISREL 8 User's Reference Guide*; Scientific Software International: Uppsala, Sweden, 1996.
52. Maas, C.J.M.; Hox, J.J. Robustness issues in multilevel regression analysis. *Stat. Neerl.* **2004**, *58*, 127–137. [CrossRef]
53. Henze, N.; Zirkler, B. A class of invariant and consistent tests for multivariate normality. *Commun. Stat. Theory Methods* **1990**, *19*, 3595–3617. [CrossRef]
54. Hox, J.J.; Maas, C.J.M.; Brinkhuis, M.J.S. The effect of estimation method and sample size in multilevel structural equation modeling. *Stat. Neerl.* **2010**, *64*, 157–170. [CrossRef]
55. Hu, L.T.; Bentler, P.M. Cutoff Criteria for Fit Indexes in Covariance Structure Analysis: Conventional Criteria Versus New Alternatives. *Struct. Equ. Model.* **1999**, *6*, 1–55. [CrossRef]
56. Hooper, D.; Coughlan, J.; Mullen, M. Structural Equation Modelling: Guidelines for Determining Model Fit. *Electron. J. Bus. Res. Methods* **2008**, *6*, 53–60.
57. Rosseel, Y. Lavaan: An R package for structural equation modeling. *J. Stat. Softw.* **2012**, *48*, 1–36. [CrossRef]
58. Pecino, V.; Díaz, P.A.; Mañas, M.A. Clima, Estrés y Satisfacción Laboral: Un Estudio Multinivel en el Sector Público. *Rev. Psicol. Soc.* **2017**, *32*, 52–79. [CrossRef]
59. Drach-Zahavy, A. Workplace health friendliness: A cross level model for predicting workers' health. *J. Occup. Health Psychol.* **2008**, *13*, 197–213. [CrossRef]
60. Rosen, C.C.; Chang, C.-H.; Djurdjevic, E.; Eatough, E. Occupational stressors and job performance: An updated review and recommendations. *Res. Occup. Stress Well Being* **2010**, *8*, 1–60.
61. Whitman, D.; Van Rooy, D.L.; Viswesvaran, C. Satisfaction, Cirizenship Behaviors, and Performance in Work Units: A Meta-Analysis of Collective Construct Relations. *J. Pers. Psychol.* **2010**, *63*, 41–81. [CrossRef]

International Journal of
Environmental Research and Public Health

MDPI

Article

Determinants of Parental Satisfaction with Nursing Care in Paediatric Wards—A Preliminary Report

Agnieszka Kruszecka-Krówka [1], Ewa Smoleń [2], Grażyna Cepuch [1], Krystyna Piskorz-Ogórek [3], Mieczysława Perek [1] and Agnieszka Gniadek [4,*]

1 Department of Clinical Nursing, Institute of Nursing and Midwifery, Faculty of Health Sciences, Jagiellonian University Medical College, 31-501 Kraków, Poland; agnieszka.kruszecka-krowka@uj.edu.pl (A.K.-K.); grazyna.cepuch@uj.edu.pl (G.C.); mieczyslawa.perek@uj.edu.pl (M.P.)
2 Chair and Department of Management in Nursing, Faculty of Health Sciences, Medical University of Lublin, 20-059 Lublin, Poland; ewasmolen@op.pl
3 Nursing Department Faculty of Health Sciences, University of Warmia and Mazury, 10-719 Olsztyn, Poland; piskorz@wssd.olsztyn.pl
4 Department of Nursing Management and Epidemiological Nursing, Faculty of Health Sciences, Jagiellonian University Medical College, 30-501 Kraków, Poland
* Correspondence: agnieszka.gniadek@uj.edu.pl; Tel.: +48-124-214-010; Fax: +48-124-294-872

Received: 17 March 2019; Accepted: 17 May 2019; Published: 20 May 2019

Abstract: *Background*: The quality of medical services for a child and their parents are tantamount to a sense of satisfaction with care. Purpose: The assessment of determinants of parental satisfaction with nursing care in paediatric wards. *Methods*: The study covered 336 parents of children hospitalised in paediatric departments and was based on the "EMPHATIC" questionnaire, standardized and adapted to Polish conditions. *Results*: The mean score of the overall parental satisfaction was high, amounting to 4.19 points. The lower level of satisfaction with nursing care was reported in parents of children under the age of 6 years, admitted in an emergency mode with a diagnosed post-trauma condition and those with higher education. The duration of hospitalisation, sex and age of parents did not have an influence on the satisfaction with care. *Conclusions*: The age of the child, admission mode and education of respondents are determinants of parental satisfaction with nursing care.

Keywords: satisfaction with care; nursing care; child; parents

---

1. Introduction

One of the most important goals of modern healthcare management systems is to provide high quality medical services [1]. The functioning of a modern paediatric hospital requires a comprehensive approach to the child's health problems, developmental issues and family situation [2,3]. For the patient, the quality of medical services is tantamount to a subjective sense of satisfaction with care [1,4]. Satisfaction with medical care, including nursing care, is a multidimensional concept which is defined in various ways and depends on the degree of correspondence between meeting expectations of the patient and his/her family and the perception of care they are provided with [5]. It is also an important indicator of satisfaction with the comprehensive hospital care [6,7]. In case of a child, the satisfaction with care is also assessed by parents or guardians [8], who have the right to be present, participate and co-decide medical care issues [9]. A sense of parental satisfaction with care is determined by their individual needs, experiences of previous hospitalisations and changing external factors, including systemic factors [5–8,10,11]. Parents' satisfaction with care may also be influenced by other factors such as child's health condition and its impact on family functioning, child's emotional condition, clinical stage of the disease and maintaining continuity of care from hospital admission to discharge including preparing parents for continuing nursing care in home environment [12–16]. The assessment of parental satisfaction is an important part of the holistic nursing care for a paediatric patient which allows finding parents' attitude towards the services they are provided with [5,7,10], and towards respecting patients' rights during hospitalisation. In such a context the assessment of satisfaction with nursing care has also an important control function and allows for protecting patients and their families from latrogeny [17,18]. The opinions of beneficiaries are also an invaluable source of information allowing for analysing the situation and introducing changes in order to optimise the activities of medical providers according to documented presumptions [12,17,19]. Abilities of the nursing staff to meet patients' expectations contribute to an increase in the competitiveness of a health care unit and patients' positive opinions help to advertise it [20,21]. It can be assumed that a satisfied patient is more likely to follow medical and nursing recommendations and regularly take part in a medical check-up [22–24]. Moreover, patient's high satisfaction from nursing care may determine the satisfaction of the whole nursing team and their work and play an important motivating role [25].

In Poland, the evaluation of satisfaction of parents/guardians with childcare in paediatric departments is a relatively new research area; at the same time, it is one of the priority recommendations for healthcare providers. National research in this area has been so far conducted mainly using non-standardized original questionnaires which makes it impossible to draw objective conclusions and to compare results [8,10]. In Poland, the first study, which was based on the standardized "EMPHATIC" questionnaire developed by Latour et al. [26–30], was carried out in the years 2012–2014 [10,31].

Given the above, there is a need for further research using standardized tools for the assessment of parental satisfaction with nursing care in paediatric departments. The analysis of scientific reports suggests that the implementation of the evaluation of satisfaction with medical care, including nursing care in health facilities should be a priority, because this would allow for finding determinants and optimizing the activities focused on the needs of the child and its family.

Study objective: The assessment of determinants of parental satisfaction with nursing care in paediatric wards.

2. Materials and Methods

2.1. Trial Design and Participants

The study was carried out in the years 2016–2017 in general-paediatric and specialist (non-surgical) departments at the University Children's Hospital and the Provincial Specialist Children's Hospital in Krakow. The study was approved by the directors of the facilities and parents. The study was conducted in a group of 336 parents of children hospitalised in general-paediatric and specialist departments (non-surgical) on the day of discharge from the hospital. After receiving the medical information letter, the parent (being the main caregiver during hospitalisation) completed the questionnaire.

The inclusion criteria were as follows: Permanent or periodic, not shorter than 12 h a day presence of a parent with a child during hospitalisation, hospital stays lasting more than three days, and voluntary consent to participate in the study.

The exclusion criteria included: Unwillingness to participate in the study, hospitalisation lasting less than three days, the absence of parents during hospitalisation or their occasional presence (shorter than 12 h a day), or a terminal period of the child's life.

Parental participation in the study was voluntary and anonymous. Each parent was provided with the full information about the purpose of the study and the possibility of resigning from the participation at any stage without giving a reason.

2.2. Outcome Measures

The study was based on the method of diagnostic survey using a questionnaire technique including:

1. A standardized questionnaire for the evaluation of the level of satisfaction of parents/guardians with nursing care—"EMPHATIC" questionnaire developed by Latour et al. [30], adapted to the Polish conditions by Smoleń and Ksykiewicz-Dorota [31].

The tool uses five major criteria evaluating satisfaction with nursing care for a child and specific criteria: criterion I "Information"—contains eight specific criteria, criterion II "Care and treatment"—contains nine specific criteria, criterion III "Availability"—contains two specific criteria, criterion IV "Parental participation"—contains six specific criteria, criterion V "Professionalism/Professional approach"—contains 14 specific criteria.

Each specific criterion was assessed by parents in a five-point Likert scale from 1 to 5 points, where "1" means "I am very dissatisfied", and "5"—"I am very satisfied". The evaluation of satisfaction was presented using point values, with the accuracy of two decimal places. The assessment score in the range from 4 to 5 is considered as satisfaction with care.

Due to the preliminary character of the study, only the material referring to the main criteria, which was an average value of the scores obtained in detailed criteria, were taken into account in a statistical analysis. No statistical analysis for particular detailed criteria was carried out. What was presented were only the results showing which detailed criteria received from respondents that had the highest and lowest scores.

2. The summary of socio-demographic data: Age of the child, reason for hospitalisation, duration of the child's stay in the ward, the mode of admitting to the hospital, parental age, sex and education.

A division of children into age groups was created in accordance with the paediatric classification corresponding to the developmental stages [32], while the age of parents was assigned to one of three categories: below 30 years of age, 30–40 years of age, above 40 years of age. The questionnaire included an emergency or elective mode of admission to the hospital.

2.3. Statistical Analysis

The statistical analyses were performed using IBM SPSS Software for Windows, Version 23.0 (IBM Corp, Armonk, NY, USA). The elements of descriptive statistics and the following tests were used: V-Cramér, Phi, Tb—Kendall, Tc—Kendall, U Mann-Whitney and Kruskal-Wallis. Threshold of statistical significance for all tests was set at $p < 0.05$.

2.4. Ethics

The study was carried out according to the ethical principles of the Helsinki Declaration. The protocol of the study was approved by the Bioethical Committee of the Jagiellonian University (No. 122.6120.254.2016). Participation in the study was voluntary and written informed consent to participate in the study was sought from all the study subjects.

3. Results

3.1. Participants

The study group consisted of 336 parents. Women accounted for 84.5% ($n = 284$) of the respondents. The mean age of parents was 33.57 (Min 19, Max 59). In specialist departments, 63.1% of children ($n = 212$) were hospitalised and 36.9% ($n = 124$) stayed in general-paediatric wards. The mean duration of hospitalisation was 10.64 days (Min 3, Max 119). The emergency mode of admission to the hospital concerned 66.7% of children ($n = 224$). The details are presented in Table 1.

Table 1. Characteristics of the study group.

Sociodemographic Variables of the Subjects		[%]	[n]
Gender	woman	84.5	284
	man	15.5	52
Age of parents	up to 30 years of age	30.7	103
	30-40 years	46.4	156
	above 40 years of age	15.5	52
	no data available	7.4	25
Education	higher	86.9	292
	secondary	11.6	39
	vocational	1.5	5
Age of child	neonate	1.5	5
	infant	30.4	102
	toddlers and kindergarten period	42.6	143
	early school period	17.3	58
	puberty	8.3	28
Duration of hospitalisation	3–7 days	59.8	201
	8–14 days	24.4	82
	over 14 days	15.8	53

%—response rate; *n*—number of valid answers.

3.2. The Assessment of Parental Satisfaction with Nursing Care

The mean score of overall parental satisfaction with nursing care was 4.19 points. The results of parental evaluation of satisfaction with nursing care were high for the major criteria I–V.

The highest mean score (4.38 points) was obtained for major criterion III "Availability", while the lowest score (4.11 points) was achieved for major criterion II "Care and treatment" and IV "Parental participation".

The assessment of parental satisfaction with nursing care, taking into account specific criteria, showed that for the major criterion V "Professionalism/Professional approach" the highest mean score—4.57 points—was reported for the specific criterion "The nurse provided high-quality care regardless of race, religion, sex and education".

High scores of the parental assessment were also given for the specific criteria: "The immediate environment of the child was clean" (4.56 points), "The hours of visits at the ward were flexible" (4.52 points) and "The child's health was the highest priority for the nurse" (4.47 points). The lowest mean score was obtained for the specific criterion "The nurse introduced herself by name and surname"—2.67 points.

A lower mean score in the assessment of parental satisfaction with care was also achieved for major criterion IV "Parental participation" for the specific criterion "The nurse asked about the expectations of parents/guardians regarding childcare" (3.48 points). The low level of parental satisfaction with care also involved major criterion II "Care and treatment" with respect to providing mental support by a nurse (3.77 points), preparation for care after discharge from the hospital (3.77 points) or emotional support (3.92 points); and the major criterion I "Information" with respect to informing about the course of nursing care on a daily basis (3.78 points), too.

3.3. Parental Satisfaction from Nursing Care and the Reference Level of Polish Hospitals and Their Wards

All main criteria as well as general satisfaction from nursing care were evaluated higher by parents of patients hospitalised in Provincial Hospital than of those hospitalised in University Hospital, however only for the first main criterion "I Information" the differences were statistically significant ($p = 0.005$).

No statistically significant differences between the assessment of particular criteria of satisfaction with nursing were found depending on the ward type—general-paediatric vs. specialist departments ($p > 0.05$).

3.4. Parental Satisfaction with Care vs. the Age of Hospitalised Children

Taking into account the division of children into age groups used in paediatrics, it was shown that compared to parents of children from other age groups, parents of children aged 6 to 12 years better evaluated both the overall satisfaction with nursing care ($p = 0.04$) and the level of satisfaction within the major criterion "I. Information" ($p = 0.02$), "II. Care and treatment" ($p = 0.04$) and "V. Professionalism/Professional approach" ($p = 0.03$).

However, the division of children into only two age groups - up to the age of 6 years (younger children) and above the age of 6 years (older children) statistically significant differences were demonstrated both in terms of the overall satisfaction assessment and the evaluation of all major criteria, with the exception of criterion "III. Availability" (Table 2).

Table 2. Parental satisfaction with nursing team care and the age of hospitalised children.

Child's Age		Criterion Information	Criterion Care and Treatment	Criterion Availability	Criterion Parental Participation	Criterion Professionalism/ Professional Approach	General Satisfaction
Up to 6 years	M	4.04	4.05	4.35	4.05	4.17	4.13
	Me	4.19	4.11	5.00	4.17	4.32	4.26
	n	250.00	250.00	250.00	250.00	250.00	250.00
	SD	0.85	0.81	0.80	0.78	0.68	0.69
Over 6 years	M	4.39	4.31	4.45	4.28	4.39	4.36
	Me	4.50	4.56	5.00	4.33	4.53	4.47
	n	86.00	86.00	86.00	86.00	86.00	86.00
	SD	0.56	0.71	0.79	0.68	0.56	0.57
Total	M	4.13	4.11	4.38	4.11	4.23	4.19
	Me	4.25	4.28	5.00	4.17	4.37	4.32
	n	336.00	336.00	336.00	336.00	336.00	336.00
	SD	0.80	0.79	0.79	0.76	0.66	0.67
p U Mann-Whitney		0.002	0.01	0.30	0.01	0.01	0.01

M—arithmetic mean; Me—median; *n*—number of valid answers; SD—standard deviation; Min—minimum value; Max—maximum value; *p*—significance level.

3.5. Parental Satisfaction with Care vs. Admission Mode to the Hospital, Type of Clinical Diagnosis and Duration of Hospitalisation

Admission to the hospital in an emergency mode was statistically significant, and more often involved children up to the age of 6 years ($p < 0.001$), while older children, i.e., over 6 years of age, were more frequently admitted in an elective mode ($p < 0.001$).

Emergency admission of children to hospital was statistically more common in University Hospital than in Provincial Hospital ($p = 0.001$, Phi = 0.19, $Chi^2 = 11.74$, df = 1).

Emergency hospital admission was significantly more common for children suffering from an acute disease, after an injury or poisoning ($Chi^2 = 107.63$, df = 5, $p < 0.001$, V Kramer = 0.57).

Parents of children admitted to the hospital in an emergency mode was statistically significant, with lower evaluated nursing care within the major criteria: I "Information", II "Care and Treatment", IV "Parental participation" and general satisfaction with care (Table 3).

Table 3. Parental satisfaction with nursing team care and the mode of admitting a child to the hospital.

Mode of Admitting a Child to the Hospital		Criterion Information	Criterion Care and Treatment	Criterion Availability	Criterion Parental Participation	Criterion Professionalism/ Professional approach	General Satisfaction
Elective	M	4.03	4.06	4.35	4.06	4.20	4.14
	Me	4.13	4.22	5.00	4.17	4.37	4.26
	n	224.00	224.00	224.00	224.00	224.00	224.00
	SD	0.85	0.81	0.78	0.77	0.68	0.68
Emergency	M	4.33	4.23	4.42	4.22	4.28	4.30
	Me	4.50	4.33	5.00	4.33	4.37	4.40
	n	112.00	112.00	112.00	112.00	112.00	112.00
	SD	0.66	0.74	0.82	0.73	0.61	0.63
Total	M	4.13	4.11	4.38	4.11	4.23	4.19
	Me	4.25	4.28	5.00	4.17	4.37	4.32
	n	336.00	336.00	336.00	336.00	336.00	336.00
	SD	0.80	0.79	0.79	0.76	0.66	0.67
p U Mann-Whitney		0.003	0.05	0.30	0.04	0.34	0.03

M—arithmetic mean; Me—median; *n*—number of valid answers; SD—standard deviation; Min—minimum value; Max—maximum value; *p*—significance level.

Parents of children diagnosed with post-trauma conditions reported a lower satisfaction level within the main criterion I "Information" than parents of children with another type of clinical diagnosis ($p = 0.011$).

The duration of the child's stay in the hospital did not have an influence on the overall assessment of parental satisfaction with nursing care ($p = 0.48$) and the evaluation within the major criteria: I "Information", II "Care and Treatment", III "Availability", IV "Parental participation" and V "Professionalism/Professional approach" ($p > 0.05$). The lowest satisfaction from nursing care in all main categories was observed in the case of parents of children whose hospitalisation lasted between 8 and 14 days, however, this difference was not statistically significant.

3.6. Satisfaction with Care vs. Parental Sex, Age and the Level of Education

There was no relationship between parental gender ($p = 0.59$), age ($p = 0.19$) and general satisfaction with nursing care and the assessment within all major criteria ($p > 0.05$). It was shown that the satisfaction with nursing care within major criterion II "Care and treatment" ($p = 0.04$) and IV "Parental participation" ($p = 0.03$) were evaluated higher by parents with a lower level of education.

No statistical significance was found for the major criteria I "Information" ($p = 0.11$), III "Availability" ($p = 0.61$), V "Professionalism/Professional approach" ($p = 0.16$) and overall satisfaction assessment ($p = 0.7$).

4. Discussion

Outstanding quality of medical services, which is expressed by the satisfaction of patients and their families, is a challenge for modern health care systems [1]. The assessment of satisfaction with medical care, including nursing care is recognized as a part of the integrated quality management system, setting the direction of changes in modern healthcare facilities [1,2].

The results of studies conducted in the last decade in various scientific centres using standardized research tools [8,10,15,33,34] or original survey questionnaires [16] confirm the high level of parental satisfaction with nursing care or its specific aspects. The results of our research are in line with the trend of the high level of overall parental satisfaction with nursing care.

For the individual major criteria: I "Information", II "Care and Treatment", III "Availability", IV "Parental participation" and V "Professionalism/Professional approach" the score of assessment ranged from 4.11 to 4.38 points. Similarly, like in the study conducted by Smoleń & Ksykiewicz-Dorota [10], the criterion III "Availability" was the highest evaluated by parents. However, the outcomes of the analysis of individual specific criteria turned out to be lower than expected. The lowest score was given for the specific criterion "The nurse introduced herself by name and surname" within the major criterion V "Professionalism/Professional approach".

Finding the reasons for these results would require further research in this area. Perhaps the optimization of activities aimed at making the staff aware of the importance to introduce themselves by name and surname will be a factor improving the perception of the quality of nursing care. It is also relevant that the nursing team provide informational and emotional support [16,34] in which they have full competence [35,36]. It is also necessary to cooperate with parents based on their expectations and prepare them to take care of the child after discharge from the hospital, and this was confirmed by other scientific reports [15,37].

In our study, parents of children over 6 years of age gave higher scores for all the criteria evaluating satisfaction with care. Similar results were obtained by Uysal & Cirlak [33] who proved that parents of seven-year-olds and older children showed higher level of satisfaction with nursing care than parents of children under the age of 7 years. Despite different cultural considerations in the examined groups and various standardized research tools applied in the studies the findings were similar in this aspect, which may confirm that children's age is a universal factor which affects satisfaction from nursing. Therefore, these results can be explained by the specificity of the early developmental periods, which has an impact on the nature of symptoms, adaptation of children to hospital conditions and their reactions to separation from the family environment. These factors may generate higher expectations of parents towards nursing teams [38]. A disparity between expectations of parents and the care they actually receive results in a lower score in the assessment of satisfaction with services. Also, the development of parental caring competence as a child grows up and the process of gaining experience, also related to illness, imply a higher evaluation of services [36]. However, other scientific reports did not confirm the relationship between the age of hospitalised children and parental satisfaction with care [8,34]. This can be caused by an influence of dependent and independent variables, other than those applied in our study, including a significantly smaller number of parents who took part in the study.

Our research proves that parents of children admitted to the hospital in an emergency mode gave lower score for the individual criteria of satisfaction with care (I "Information", II "Care and Treatment", IV "Parental participation") and general satisfaction with care. An emergency admission to the hospital, which is usually associated with a sudden onset of illness or deterioration of the child's health, does not allow for the physical and mental preparation of parents and children for hospitalisation, hindering the process of adaptation and causing fear, which may have an impact on the satisfaction with nursing services. However, Smoleń & Ksykiewicz-Dorota [10] obtain different outcomes. According to the reports provided by them, parents of children admitted to the hospital in an emergency mode higher assessed the possibility of participating and making decisions regarding care than parents of children admitted in an elective mode.

The study found no correlation between the satisfaction with nursing care and the duration of the child's stay in the hospital. According to other scientific reports, the evaluation of the relationship between the satisfaction with care and the duration of hospitalisation was different [8,10,26], which may have been the result of other inclusion criteria to the study group, the use of different research tools or the small size of the study group. It should be pointed out that the longer the children stay in hospital, the better they are adapted to hospitalisation conditions, which is also true about their parents/legal guardians who participate in hospital nursing and treatment. However, when the hospitalisation period is prolonged due to complications, hospital infections or other latrogeny factors, both parents' and patients' reactions can become negative and determine a lower level of satisfaction with nursing. This aspect should definitely be taken into account in further studies.

Like in the studies conducted by other authors, the age and sex of parents were not determinants of the satisfaction with nursing care [16,33,34,39]. However, there are no unambiguous reports in this area [10,12,40]. The diversity of outcomes in research reports and our study results may be influenced by the choice of a research tool, as well as the family model (patriarchal/matriarchal/partnership) or cultural/national influences.

On the other hand, parental education was an important determinant of the level of satisfaction with nursing care. Parents with lower education were more satisfied with services. These results are consistent with the reports provided by other authors [10,41,42]. Perhaps lower parental education is associated with lower awareness of the child's and parental rights in the hospital, the lack of knowledge about the developmental specificity, and consequently less expectations about the nursing team. However, according to the scientific reports provided by Uysal & Cirlak [33] and Aslanabadi & Shahbazi [34], parental education was not related to the level of satisfaction with care.

The analysis of scientific reports and our results indicate that parents of hospitalised children have similar expectations regarding nursing care [8,10,15,16], although their scope may be different and dependent not only on the specificity of the disease, but also on its course, the child's health [26,43], emotional condition of parents [12,44] and previous experiences of hospitalisation [8,36,45]. Moreover, the level of organization of health care in Poland is comparable in all hospitals, which is also true about the health insurance system. Also, there is little diversity in cultural and religious background of the society. While comparing the results of the study with the studies conducted by other authors it should be pointed out that the observed differences may result not only from the choice of research tools used for assessing satisfaction but also from patients' and their parents' expectations, which is determined by a general level of medical care provided, organization of the health care system and also cultural factors. However, scientific research proves that hospitals with good work environments and better professional nurse staffing have more satisfied patients and nurses, and evidence of better quality and safety of care, despite differences in how healthcare is organised, financed and resourced, and in despite of cultural differences [46]. In light of the aforementioned findings, further research in this area is recommended.

4.1. Clinical Implications

The standardized research tool used in the study is available to nursing teams, it does not require psychologists' interpretation, is understandable and easy to use for parents. The awareness of determinants of parental satisfaction will allow for objectivization of results and introduction of measures to optimize both patient and family-oriented services.

4.2. Limitations

The study results should be treated as preliminary and cannot be used to draw general conclusions on parental satisfaction with nursing due to the following: Limited group of subjects, the lack of respondents from small or provincial paediatric hospitals, no assessment of the subjects' emotional state, which may have an impact on their expectations towards nursing care and to determine aforementioned satisfaction, the omission of the parents' earlier experiences of hospitalisations and their influence on the current perception of nursing care.

5. Conclusions

The result of the overall assessment of parental satisfaction with nursing care was high. The highest scores were given for the major criterion III "Availability", while the lowest score was for the major criterion II "Care and Treatment" and IV "Parental participation". The age of the child, the mode of admission and education of the respondents are significant predictors of parental satisfaction with nursing care.

Author Contributions: Conceptualization, A.K.-K. and E.S.; Methodology, A.K.-K. and A.G.; Software, A.K.-K. and E.S.; Validation, E.S.; Formal analysis, A.K.-K., G.C. and A.G.; Investigation, A.K.-K., E.S., M.P. and K.P.-O.; resources, A.K.-K., E.S., M.P. and K.P.-O.; Data curation, A.K.-K. and E.S.; writing—original draft preparation,

A.K.-K, G.C. and E.S.; writing—review and editing, A.K.-K., G.C. and A.G.; visualization, A.K.-K. and A.G.; supervision, A.G.; project administration, A.K.-K.; funding acquisition, A.K.-K.

Funding: This work was supported in part by Grant No. K/ZDS/007057.

Acknowledgments: The authors would like to express their gratitude to nurse Irena Kwarcińska, MSc and Krystyna Twarduś, PhD.

Conflicts of Interest: The authors state that there are no conflicts of interest regarding the publication of this article.

References

1. Al-Abri, R.; Al-Balushi, A. Patient satisfaction survey as a tool towards quality improvement. *Oman Med. J.* **2014**, *29*, 3–7. [CrossRef]
2. Shields, L. What is "family-centered care"? *EJPCH.* **2015**, *3*, 139–144. [CrossRef]
3. Arabiat, D.; Whitehead, L.; Foster, M.; Shields, L.; Harris, L. Parents' experiences of Family Centred Care practices. *J. Pediatr. Nurs.* **2018**, *42*, 39–44. [CrossRef]
4. Georgoudi, E.; Kyriazis, S.; Mihalache, A.; Kourkouta, L. Measurement of patient satisfaction as a quality indicator of hospital health services: The case of outpatient clinics in general hospital. *SJPH.* **2017**, *5*, 128–135. [CrossRef]
5. Risser, N. Development of an instrument to measure patient satisfaction with nurses and nursing care in primary care settings. *Nurs. Res.* **1975**, *24*, 45–52. [CrossRef]
6. Prakash, B. Patient satisfaction. *J. Cutan. Aesthet. Surg.* **2010**, *3*, 151–155. [CrossRef] [PubMed]
7. Otani, K.; Kurz, R.S. The impact of nursing care and other healthcare attributes on hospitalised patient satisfaction and behavioural intentions. *J. Healthc. Manag.* **2004**, *49*, 181–197. [CrossRef]
8. Smoleń, E.; Ksykiewicz-Dorota, A. Nurses' professionalism as a component of evaluation of parents/caregivers satisfaction with nursing care. *Med. Pr.* **2015**, *66*, 549–556. (In Polish) [CrossRef]
9. European Association for Children in Hospital. The 10 articles of a EACH Charter. Available online: https://www.each-for-sick-children.org/ (accessed on 12 December 2018).
10. Smoleń, E.; Ksykiewicz-Dorota, A. Satisfaction with chosen elements of nursing care at the department of paediatrics. *Przeds Zarz.* **2014**, *15*, 215–228. (In Polish)
11. Foster, M.; Whitehead, L.; Arabiat, D.; Frost, L. Parents' and staff perceptions of parental needs during a child's hospital admission: An Australian study. *J. Pediatr. Nurs.* **2018**, *43*, e2–e9. [CrossRef] [PubMed]
12. Matziou, V.; Boutopoulou, B.; Chrysostomou, A.; Vlachioti, E.; Mantziou, T.; Petsios, K. Parent's satisfaction concerning their child's hospital care. *Jpn. J. Nurs. Sci.* **2011**, *8*, 163–173. [CrossRef]
13. Abuqamar, M.; Arabiat, D.H.; Holmes, S. Parents' Perceived Satisfaction of Care, Communication and Environment of the Pediatric Intensive Care Units at a Tertiary Children's Hospital. *J. Pediatr. Nurs.* **2016**, *31*, e177–e184. [CrossRef]
14. Lew, V.K.; Lalwani, K.; Palermo, T.M. Factors affecting parental satisfaction following pediatric procedural sedation. *J. Clin. Anesth.* **2010**, *22*, 29–34. [CrossRef]
15. Fidanci, B.E.; Arslan, F.; Fidanci, K. Parent's Expectations and satisfaction on Paediatrics Clinic. *Transl. Med.* **2014**, *4*, 137. [CrossRef]
16. Fernando, R.R.C.; Senanayake, M.P. Parental satisfaction with communication provided by different health care personnel at Lady Ridgeway Hospital for Children, Colombo. *Sri Lanka J. Child Health* **2012**, *41*, 180–185. [CrossRef]
17. Alsaqri, S. Patient satisfaction with quality of nursing care at governmental hospitals, Ha'il City, Saudi Arabia. *Ann. Agric. Crop. Sci.* **2016**, *6*, 128–142.
18. Tang, W.M.; Soong, C.Y.; Lim, W.C. Patient satisfaction with nursing care: A descriptive study using interaction model of client health behavior. *Int. J. Nurs. Sci.* **2013**, *3*, 51–56. [CrossRef]
19. Abdel Maqsood, A.S.; Oweis, A.I.; Hasna, F.S. Differences between patients' expectations and satisfaction with nursing care in a private hospital in Jordan. *Int. J. Nurs. Pract.* **2012**, *18*, 140–146. [CrossRef]
20. Ksykiewicz-Dorota, A.; Sierpińska, L.; Gorczyca, R.; Rogala-Pawelczyk, G. Polish version of patient satisfaction with nursing care quality questionnaire (PSNCQQ). *Prog. Health Sci.* **2011**, *1*, 51–56.
21. Karaca, A.; Durna, Z. Patient satisfaction with the quality of nursing care. *Nurs. Open* **2019**, *6*, 535–545. [CrossRef]

22. Buchanan, J.; Dawkins, P.; Lindo, J.L.M. Satisfaction with nursing care in the emergency department of an urban hospital in the developing world: A pilot study. *Int. Emerg. Nurs.* **2015**, *23*, 218–224. [CrossRef]
23. Dzomeku, V.M.; Atinga, B.E.; Tulukuu, P.; Mantey, R.E. In-patient satisfaction with nursing care: A case study at Kwame Nkrumah University of Science and Technology hospital. *IJRMHS* **2013**, *2*, 19–24.
24. Fröjd, C.; Swenne, C.L.; Rubertsson, C.; Gunningberg, L.; Wadensten, B. Patient information and participation still in need of improvement: Evaluation of patients' perceptions of quality of care. *J. Nurs. Manag.* **2011**, *19*, 226–236. [CrossRef]
25. Ibrahim, M.M.; El-Khedr, S.M. The relationship between nurses' burnout and mothers' satisfaction with pediatric nursing care. *Int. J. Curr. Res.* **2013**, *5*, 1902–1907.
26. Latour, J.M.; van Goudoever, J.B.; Duivenvoorden, H.J.; van Dam, N.A.; Dullaart, E.; Albers, M.J.; Verlaat, C.W.; van Vught, E.M.; van Heerde, M.; Hazelzet, J.A. Perceptions of parents on satisfaction with care in the paediatric intensive care unit: The EMPHATIC study. *Intensive Care Med.* **2009**, *35*, 1082–1090. [CrossRef]
27. Latour, J.M.; van Goudoever, J.B.; Duivenvoorden, H.J.; Albers, M.J.; van Dam, N.A.; Dullaart, E.; van Heerde, M.; de Neef, M.; Verlaat, C.W.; van Vught, E.M.; et al. Differences in the perceptions of parents and healthcare professionals on paediatric intensive care practices. *Pediatr. Crit. Care Med.* **2011**, *12*, 211–215. [CrossRef] [PubMed]
28. Latour, J.M.; Duivenvoorden, H.J.; Hazelzet, J.A.; van Goudoever, J.B. Development and validation of a neonatal intensive care parent satisfaction instrument. *Pediatr. Crit. Care Med.* **2012**, *13*, 554–559. [CrossRef]
29. Latour, J.M.; Hazelzet, J.A.; Duivenvoorden, H.J.; van Goudoever, J.B. Construction of a parent satisfaction instrument: Perceptions of paediatric intensive care nurses and physicians. *J. Crit. Care.* **2009**, *24*, 255–266. [CrossRef] [PubMed]
30. Latour, J.M.; van Goudoever, J.B.; Duivenvoorden, H.J.; Albers, M.J.; van Dam, N.A.; Dullaart, E.; van Heerde, M.; de Neef, M.; Verlaat, C.W.; van Vught, E.M.; et al. Construction and psychometric testing of the EMPHATHIC questionnaire measuring parent satisfaction in the paediatric intensive care unit. *Intensive Care Med.* **2011**, *37*, 310–318. [CrossRef] [PubMed]
31. Smoleń, E.; Ksykiewicz-Dorota, A. Validation of polish version of the questionnaire for evaluation of parents/caregivers satisfaction with nursing care in a paediatric ward. *Med. Biol. Sci.* **2015**, *29*, 41–46. [CrossRef]
32. Guerra, N.G.; Williamson, A.A.; Lucas-Molina, B. Normal development: Infancy, childhood, and adolescence. In *IACAPAP e-Textbook of Child and Adolescent Mental Health*; Rey, J.M., Ed.; International Association for Child and Adolescent Psychiatry and Allied Professions: Geneva, Switzerland, 2012; pp. 1–39.
33. Uysal, G.; Cirlak, A. The expectations related to nursing and the satisfaction levels of the parents of the children who have acute health problems. *Procedia Soc. Behav. Sci.* **2014**, *152*, 435–439. [CrossRef]
34. Aslanabadi, S.; Shahbazi, S.H. Mothers' satisfaction with nursing care in a Children's Hospital. *Iran J. Nurs.* **2014**, *26*, 61–70.
35. Seliner, B.; Latal, B.; Spirig, R. When children with profound multiple disabilities are hospitalised: A cross-sectional survey of parental burden of care, quality of life of parents and their hospitalised children, and satisfaction with family-centered care. *J. Spec. Pediatr. Nurs.* **2016**, *21*, 147–157. [CrossRef]
36. Ghadery-Sefat, A.; Abdeyazdan, Z.; Badiee, Z.; Zargham-Boroujeni, A. Relationship between parent–infant attachment and parental satisfaction with supportive nursing care. *Iran J. Nurs. Midwifery Res.* **2016**, *21*, 71–76. [CrossRef]
37. Brenner, M.; Larkin, P.J.; Hilliard, C.; Cawley, D.; Howlin, F.; Connolly, M. Parents' perspectives of the transition to home when a child has complex technological health care needs. *Int. J. Integr. Care* **2015**, *15*, e035. [CrossRef]
38. Bsiri-Moghaddam, K.; Basiri-Moghaddam, M.; Sadeghmoghaddam, L.; Ahmadi, F. The concept of hospitalisation of children from the view point of parents and children. *Iran J. Paediatr.* **2011**, *21*, 201–208.
39. Israel-Aina, Y.T.; Odunvbun, M.E.; Aina-Israel, O. Parental satisfaction with quality of health care of children with sickle cell disease at the University of Benin Teaching Hospital, Benin City. *J. Community Med. Primary Health Care* **2017**, *29*, 33–45.
40. Boutopoulou, B.; Petsios, K.; Chrysostomou, A.; Vlachioti, E.; Mantziou, T.; Matziou, V. Parental satisfaction concerning their child's hospital care: A questionnaire survey. *Pediatr. Res.* **2010**, *68*, 39–40. [CrossRef]

41. Solheim, E.; Garratt, A.M. Parent experiences of inpatient paediatric care in relation to health care delivery and sociodemographic characteristics: Results of a Norwegian national survey. *BMC Health Serv. Res.* **2013**, *13*, 512–523. [CrossRef]
42. Erden, I.A.; Pamuk, A.G.; Ocal, T.; Aypar, U. Parental satisfaction with paediatric day case surgery. *M E J Anaesth.* **2006**, *18*, 1113–1121.
43. Ebrahim, S.; Singh, S.; Parshuram, C.S. Parental satisfaction, involvement and presence after paediatric intensive care unit admission. *J. Crit. Care* **2013**, *28*, 40–45. [CrossRef]
44. Tsironi, S.; Koulierakis, G. Factors associated with parents' levels of stress in paediatric wards. *J. Child Health Care* **2018**, *22*, 175–185. [CrossRef]
45. Hakio, N.; Rantanen, A.; Åstedt-Kurki, P.; Suominen, T. Parents' experiences of family functioning, health and social support provided by nurses—A pilot study in paediatric intensive care. *Intensive Crit. Care Nurs.* **2015**, *31*, 29–37. [CrossRef]
46. Aiken, L.H.; Sermeus, W.; Van den Heede, K.; Sloane, D.M.; Busse, R.; McKee, M.; Bruyneel, L.; Rafferty, A.M.; Griffiths, P.; Moreno-Casbas, M.T.; et al. Patient safety, satisfaction, and quality of hospital care: Cross sectional surveys of nurses and patients in 12 countries in Europe and the United States. *BMJ* **2012**, *344*, e1717. [CrossRef]

International Journal of
Environmental Research and Public Health

MDPI

Article

The Effectiveness of a Multidisciplinary Exercise Program in Managing Work-Related Musculoskeletal Symptoms for Low-Skilled Workers in the Low-Income Community: A Pre-Post-Follow-Up Study

Kin Cheung [1,*], Mimi M. Y. Tse [1], Chi Kan Wong [2], Kwan Wai Mui [2], Siu Kan Lee [2], Ka Yan Ma [1], Keith T. S. Tung [1] and Echo Ping Woi Lau [1]

[1] School of Nursing, The Hong Kong Polytechnic University, Hong Kong, China; mimi.tse@polyu.edu.hk (M.M.Y.T.); eunis.ma@polyu.edu.hk (K.Y.M.); keithtung144@gmail.com (K.T.S.T.); echo.lau@polyu.edu.hk (E.P.W.L.)

[2] Caritas Community Development Service, Hong Kong, China; wongchikan64@gmail.com (C.K.W.); muiterence@caritassws.org.hk (K.W.M.); leesiukan@caritassws.org.hk (S.K.L.)

* Correspondence: kin.cheung@polyu.edu.hk; Tel.: +852-27666773; Fax: +852-23649663

Received: 27 March 2019; Accepted: 28 April 2019; Published: 2 May 2019

Abstract: Studies on work-related musculoskeletal symptoms (WRMSs) have been conducted mainly on different types of workforce but not many on low-skilled workers. The purpose of this study was to evaluate the effectiveness of a multidisciplinary exercise program in decreasing the number of body parts with WRMSs for low-skilled workers. This study used a repeated-measures, single-group design. One hundred and five (105) workers participated in eight weekly 90-min sessions (including 45-min workshops and 45-min exercises) in low-income community settings. The exercise program involved a 21-movement stretching exercise and a 10-movement muscle-strengthening exercise. Questionnaire and health-assessment data were collected at the baseline (N = 105) and immediately after the 8-week program (n = 86). The average age of the 105 participants was 50.5 ± 8.7 years (ranging from 31 to 67). Over 80% (n = 87) of them were female, 68.6% (n = 72) were married, and 68.6% (n = 72) had completed secondary school. They reported an average of three body parts with WRMSs at baseline (T0). By the end of the eight weeks (T1), the participants had reduced the number of WRMS-affected body parts, job stress, and incidences of working through pain, and had improved spine flexibility and handgrip strength. The factors significantly affecting the reduction in the number of body parts with WRMSs were change in the workstyle of working through pain, and self-rated health status. Our study has demonstrated that a community-based multidisciplinary program can reduce the number of body parts affected by WRMSs in low-skilled workers in low-income communities.

Keywords: public health; health promotion; occupational health; social class; health inequalities

1. Introduction

Worldwide, work-related musculoskeletal symptoms (WRMSs) are a major public health issue, with musculoskeletal conditions contributing the greatest proportion of lost work productivity [1]. Workers with WRMSs may experience pain, numbness, stiffness, and aching in various body parts [2]. Of all working adults, grassroots working-class workers are the most vulnerable to WRMSs because the nature of their work mostly exposes them to the identified risk factors [3].

Evidence has shown multidimensional programs, including exercise, can prevent/manage WRMSs in different contexts: office workers in Portugal [4]; bus drivers in South Korea [5]; workers requiring prolonged standing in Portugal [6]; and underprivileged migrant workers in a community setting in Korea [7]. A review of 61 studies of the effectiveness of workplace intervention for WRMSs showed that exercise programs, such as stretching and resistance-training, have demonstrated positive effects with moderate-to-strong levels of evidence [8]. Although nearly 60% of the WRMS intervention studies were conducted in office-based workplaces, the review indicated that it would be possible to implement the interventions in non-office settings.

Although the workplace has been recommended as a place for promoting physical activity, this concept is not yet accepted widely [9], particularly in small or medium-sized enterprises. Low-skilled workers might not be a beneficiary group because their workplaces most likely do not offer WRMSs prevention/management programs. In addition to their low education levels, this group might have limited access to WRMSs prevention/management knowledge. Community-based WRMSs prevention/management programs could be an innovative way to target low-skilled workers. Despite limited relevant studies having been conducted, one community-based study with Korean–Chinese migrant workers has shown promising results [7]. These Korean–Chinese migrant workers (of whom 90% were domestic or restaurant workers) rarely received any interventions, such as stretching exercises, which are commonly provided to native Koreans in their workplaces. The results of this randomized control trial study were encouraging, and suggested that community-based stretching exercise programs are feasible and effective in helping low-skilled working-class workers to prevent/manage WRMSs [7].

The aim of this study was to evaluate the effectiveness of a multidisciplinary exercise program in managing WRMSs for low-skilled workers in low-income community settings. The hypotheses were that the workers would reduce the number of their body parts with WRMSs (primary outcomes) and improve their workstyles, self-rated health status, self-rated job stress, self-efficacy, social support, mental health, handgrip strength, and spine flexibility (secondary outcomes) between baseline (T0) and immediate (T1) follow-up measures after the program.

2. Methods

2.1. Study Design, Setting, and Participants

This was a repeated-measures, single-group design study. The participants were recruited from low-income communities through seven Caritas Community Development Service (CCDS) [10] centers from all three regions of Hong Kong. The inclusion criteria were low-skilled workers aged ≥ 18 working full-time or part-time, with at least one body part that had been affected by WRMSs for at least one month. A "low-skilled" job was defined as work not requiring a high level of skill or without formal qualification requirements [11]. This type of job usually plays a supporting role in an organization [12]. Some of the typical low-skilled jobs are cleaning, laboring, general office work, equipment operation, and helping in restaurants [12–14]. The exclusion criteria were engagement in WRMS prevention programs in the workplace at the time of the study, undergoing medical treatment, or doing stretching exercises more than three times a day, five days per week [7].

2.2. Multidisciplinary Exercise Program

Ethical approval was obtained from The Hong Kong Polytechnic University (HSEARS20170815005). The program involved eight weekly 90-min sessions, with a group size of 13–22 participants. Each session consisted of a 45-min workshop and then a total of 45 min of stretching (10.5–15 min) and muscle strengthening (5–10 min) exercises, followed by a question-and-answer period (about 20 min).

The eight WRMS workshop topics, conducted by nurses, physiotherapists, traditional Chinese medicine (TCM) doctor, and social workers, included: (1) Exercise; (2) Health and work; (3) Manual handling; (4) Non-pharmaceutical pain management; (5) TCM; (6) Mental health; (7) Laws and compensation; and (8) Community resources. The teaching material was validated by a panel of seven experts representing the fields of nursing, occupational health, TCM, physiotherapy, and social workers. The content validity of the teaching material was 1.00.

The exercise regime was based on exercises suggested by occupational safety and health authorities [15,16] and validated by four physiotherapists and three nurses. The 21-movement stretching exercise involved neck (6 movements), shoulders (1), upper extremities (2), wrists (4), back (6), and lower extremities (2). The 10-movement muscle strengthening exercise involved neck (6 movements), upper extremities (2) and lower extremities (2). Each movement took 10 seconds and was repeated three times.

The data were collected from a questionnaire (30 min) and health assessments (30 min) conducted at the baseline (T0) and immediately after the program completion (T1). To ensure the consistency of the data-collection procedure, the personnel responsible for collecting the data in each center were trained for two hours by a member of the research team, and their return demonstrations achieved satisfactory results. The same models of equipment were used for the health assessments in each center, to ensure consistency.

2.3. Measurements

The questionnaire was developed based on previous studies and a literature review [17–25]; it was validated by the same panel as the teaching material. The content validity index was 0.99. Some parts of the questionnaire had been tested previously by the investigators or in other local studies. Below is a description of each section:

1. Personal information included age, gender, education level, and job-related information. Self-rated health status was measured with a 4-point Likert scale (from 0 = very poor to 3 = very good). In addition, self-rated job stress was collected using a 5-point Likert scale (from 0 = none to 4 = very stressful).
2. Self-reported musculoskeletal symptoms were assessed by the general Nordic Musculoskeletal Questionnaire (NMQ) about pain, aches or discomfort in different body parts [2]. The NMQ has been used to evaluate the effect of intervention programs in reducing musculoskeletal symptoms [17,18], and it has also been used by the research team with local nursing personnel [18–20].
3. The WRMS knowledge scale, developed by the research team [20], measured knowledge about ergonomic principles, and manual handling. The scale's validity and reliability had been established prior to the study through trialing with local workers [20]. The knowledge scores were tabulated for data analysis by summing the correct responses. Higher scores represented better knowledge. The Cronbach's alpha was 0.60.
4. Workstyle was assessed by using the 24-item Chinese Workstyle Short Form (C-WSF) for WRMSs with a 5-point Likert scale (from 0 = almost never to 4 = almost always) [20]. Workstyle is generally defined as an interactive pattern of a particular worker's behavioral, physiological and cognitive responses to their work demands with both ergonomic and psychological risk factors in work environments [21]. The sums of the subscales were used, with a high score indicating a high frequency of adverse workstyle practices. The internal consistency coefficients for the four subscales were: 0.83 for working through pain (e.g., I feel aching while at work), 0.91 for social reactivity (e.g., I cannot interrupt my work because my other team members will be unhappy with me), 0.88 for demands at work (e.g., I have too many deadlines and I can never finish my work) and 0.52 for breaks (e.g., while at work I occasionally stop working to take a break) [20]. The Cronbach's alpha for the overall C-WSF was 0.91.
5. Self-efficacy for exercise was assessed by two subscales: (a) the 12-item self-efficacy for exercise behaviors [22], and (b) the 5-item self-efficacy scale [23] measuring an individual's confidence for exercise behavior change. Both used 5-Likert scales ranging from "not at all confident" to "extremely confident". The sums of subscales were yielded, with higher scores representing higher levels of self-efficacy for exercise. The Cronbach's alphas for the two subscales were 0.93 and 0.84, respectively.

6. Social support for exercises was assessed by using the 10-item Chinese Social Support and Exercise (SSE) questionnaire with a 5-point Likert scale (0 = "never" to 4 = "very often") [24]. A score for the items in each scale was summated; the higher the score, the greater the level of support. The Cronbach's alphas for family and friends were 0.91 and 0.95, respectively.
7. Depression and anxiety status were assessed to indicate each participant's mental health. Depression was assessed by using the 20-item Center for Epidemiologic Studies Depression Scale (CES-D) with a 4-point Likert scale (0 = rarely or none of the time, to 3 = applied to me very much or most of the time). This measured the frequency of common depressive symptoms over the preceding week. The Chinese version of CES-D had been tested previously with local Chinese patients and good reliability was established ($\alpha = 0.85$) [25]. The scores of all items were summed for the data analysis. The cut-off point for possible depression was ≥ 16. Anxiety was assessed by the criteria from DSM-V. This measured the common anxiety symptoms over the six months [26]. The Cronbach's alphas for depression and anxiety were 0.90 and 0.78, respectively.
8. Six extra items were added to the T1 questionnaire to evaluate the appropriateness of the program's content level, usefulness, teaching pace and session times, the extent to which the program met their expectations, and their overall satisfaction. The items used a 4-point Likert scale of 1 ("poor or useless") to 4 ("very good or very useful").

Spine flexibility was assessed using the sit-and-reach method. The subjects were instructed to sit on the floor with both legs straight and their soles touching the sit-and-reach box. They were then asked to bend their backs, with both palms facing down and fingertips straight ahead, to push the scale on the top of the box. The distance pushed was measured in centimeters. Other health assessments, such as body mass index (BMI), hip-waist ratio (HWR), blood pressure (BP), blood glucose (BG), cholesterol (using a glucometer), and handgrip strength, were also measured.

2.4. Data Analyses

All the analyses were computed by using the Statistical Package for Social Sciences (SPSS, version 24.0). To examine what factors influenced the number of body parts with WRMSs, which was treated as a continuous variable, at the baseline, non-parametric Spearman correlation analyses were used. A series of linear regression analyses with all variables entered at once into the regression model were employed. Factors found to be correlated significantly in the non-parametric test were entered into the univariate regression analyses, and a multivariate regression model was used to identify the contributing factors. The Wilcoxon Signed Ranks tests were adopted to observe any significant changes in the number of body parts with WRMSs and associated factors over the eight-week period. Non-parametric Spearman correlation analyses were then conducted to test whether there was any association between the measured factors and the changes in the number of body parts with WRMSs. For all significant correlated factors, mutually adjusted multiple linear regression analyses were employed, with age and gender included in the model as covariates, to confirm what factors truly contributed to the reduction in the number of body parts with WRMSs. Statistical significance was determined by two tailed tests, with a p-value of < 0.05.

3. Results

3.1. Characteristics of Participants at Baseline (T0)

The average age of the 105 participants was 50.5 ± 8.7 years (ranging from 31 to 67). Over 80% (n = 87) of them were female, 68.6% (n = 72) were married, and 68.6% (n = 72) had completed secondary school. Regarding their employment status, 30.5% (n = 32) were part-time employees. They reported having experienced WRMSs in an average of three body parts at T0. In addition, female workers with depression or anxiety had more body parts with WRMSs ($p < 0.05$). No significant differences were observed among other demographic characteristics (Table 1).

3.2. Factors Associated with Body Parts with WRMSs at Baseline (T0)

Table 2 shows that the number of body parts with WRMSs was significantly correlated with the workstyle of working through pain, social reactivity, the total score for workstyle, self-rated health status, and depressive symptoms.

Under univariate regression analyses, gender, the workstyle of working through pain, social reactivity, depressive symptoms, anxiety and self-rated health status were all found to be significantly associated with the number of body parts with WRMSs. Multivariate regression analysis indicated that gender and the workstyle of working through pain remained as significant factors. Workstyle seems to have been the most influential factor in affecting the number of body parts with WRMSs (Table 3).

3.3. Factors Associated with the Change before and after Intervention (T1-T0)

Immediately after the intervention (T1), 86 (81.9%) participants took part in the follow-up data collection. However, there were no significant differences found in the reported number of body parts with WRMSs between the participants who joined T1 and those who dropped out. Table 4 shows that the number of body parts with WRMSs, sit-and-reach distance, handgrip strength, workstyle of working through pain, and self-rated job stress had changed significantly over time. The number of body parts with WRMSs was reduced by a mean value of 1.05. The workstyle of working through pain and self-rated job stress was also reduced significantly from T0 to T1 (−1.70 and −0.29, respectively). Also, both the sit-and-reach distance and the right-hand grip strength were enhanced by mean values of 1.95 cm and 0.40 kg, respectively, at T1.

Under the univariate model, it was demonstrated that gender and change in the workstyle of working through pain and right-hand grip strength were significantly associated with the change in the number of body parts with WRMSs. After adjusting for potential confounders, changes in the workstyle of working through pain and self-rated health status were the significant factors influencing the reduction in the number of body parts with WRMSs (Table 5).

3.4. Evaluation of the Program

With a response rate of 93.02% (n = 80), the participants rated all aspects of the program positively, with means ranging from 3.33 to 3.44 out of 4.00.

Table 1. Characteristics of participants, and the association of factors and number of body parts with WRMSs at baseline (T0).

Factors			**Number of Painful Body Parts**	**Comparison #**
	N	**%**	**Median**	***p***
TOTAL	105	100.0	3	-
Gender				0.013 *
Male	18	17.1	2	
Female	87	82.9	4	
Marital status				0.239
Single	12	11.4	3	
Married	72	68.6	3	
Divorced	14	13.3	4.5	
Widowed	7	6.7	4	
Education level				0.627
Primary school	26	24.8	3	
Secondary school	72	68.6	3	
Tertiary institute	5	4.8	4	
University or above	2	1.9	2	

Table 1. *Cont.*

Factors			Number of Painful Body Parts	Comparison #
	N	%	Median	*p*
Smoking				0.189
Yes	8	7.6	2.5	
No	97	92.4	3.0	
Drinking				0.812
Yes	3	2.9	4	
No	102	97.1	3	
Stretching				0.948
Yes (≤3 times/day)	48	45.7	3	
No	57	54.3	3	
Need to work overtime				0.246
Yes	18	17.1	4	
No	83	79.0	3	
Job type				0.117
Full time	73	69.5	3	
Part time	32	30.5	4	
Job nature				0.979
Mild labour-intensive job (craft and related worker, sales and service worker, clerical support worker)	52	49.5	3.5	
Labour-intensive job (machine operator, elementary worker, others)	53	50.5	3	
Depression (dichotomous)				0.006 **
Yes	31	29.5	4	
No	73	69.5	3	
Anxiety (dichotomous)				0.012 *
Yes	17	16.2	5	
No	88	83.8	3	

Mann–Whitney test or Kruskal–Wallis test, whichever appropriate. *: $p < 0.05$, **: $p < 0.01$.

Table 2. Correlation table with the number of body parts with WRMSs at baseline (T0).

Variables	*r*	*p*	
Work-related musculoskeletal health knowledge	0.017	0.867	
Work style—Work through pain	0.457	<0.001	***
Work style—Social reactivity	0.298	0.002	**
Work style—Demands at work	0.177	0.074	
Work style—Break	−0.154	0.117	
Work style—Total score	0.295	0.002	**
Self-efficacy for exercise	−0.134	0.174	
Social support from family	−0.036	0.717	
Social support from friends	0.043	0.665	
T0_Sbp_1_mmHg	−0.105	0.286	
T0_Dbp_1_mmHg	0.004	0.964	
T0_pulse_1_bpm	0.116	0.237	
BMI	0.002	0.985	
Wrist-to-hip ratio	0.083	0.400	
Body fat percentage	−0.008	0.936	
Blood sugar level	−0.009	0.926	
Cholesterol level	0.072	0.489	
Sit and reach	0.003	0.977	
Hand grip strength (right)	−0.076	0.443	
Hand grip strength (left)	−0.025	0.799	
Age	−0.077	0.433	
Self-rated health status	−0.346	<0.001	***
Depressive symptoms (score)	0.254	0.009	**
Self-rated job stress	0.182	0.065	

**: $p < 0.01$, ***: $p < 0.001$.

Table 3. Univariate and multivariate regression model studying factors affecting the number of body parts with WRMSs at baseline (T0).

Factors Affecting the Number of Painful Body Parts	Univariate			Multivariate #		
	B	*p*		B	*p*	
Gender	1.467	0.014	*	1.538	0.005	**
Working style						
Work through pain	0.199	0.000	***	0.146	0.004	**
Social reactivity	0.151	0.003	**	0.015	0.793	
Depressive symptoms (score)	0.061	0.005	**	0.009	0.714	
Anxiety (dichotomous)	1.305	0.039	*	0.628	0.331	
Self-rated health status	−1.531	0.000	***	−0.633	0.145	

Mutually adjusted for each other. *: $p < 0.05$, **: $p < 0.01$, ***: $p < 0.001$.

Table 4. Changes in the number of body parts with WRMSs and associated factors over time (T1−T0).

	Baseline—Mean	T1—Mean	Changes (T1−T0)	*p* #	
Number of body parts with WRMSs	3.82	2.77	−1.05	<0.001	***
Sit and reach	25.60	27.55	1.95	<0.001	***
Hand grip (left) (kg)	21.45	21.33	−0.12	0.005	**
Hand grip (right) (kg)	22.75	23.15	0.40	0.001	**
Depression symptoms	12.60	12.18	−0.42	0.578	
Number of workers with anxiety	17	17	0	-	
Self-efficacy for exercise	1.17	1.25	0.08	0.591	
Social support from family	1.02	1.09	0.07	0.237	
Social support from friends	0.89	1.00	0.11	0.880	
Self-rated job stress	1.62	1.33	−0.29	0.027	*
Workstyle—total score	35.64	33.50	−2.14	0.706	
Work through pain	11.93	10.23	−1.70	0.005	**
Social reactivity	5.15	4.84	−0.31	0.794	
Demands at work	16.02	15.74	−0.28	0.538	
Break	2.59	2.68	0.09	0.187	
Self-rated health status	1.60	1.72	0.12	0.197	

Wilcoxon signed-ranks test. *: $p < 0.05$, **: $p < 0.01$, ***: $p < 0.001$.

Table 5. Univariate and multivariate regression model studying factors affecting the change in the number of body parts with WRMSs over time (T1−T0).

Factors Affecting the Number of Body Parts with WRMSs +	Univariate			Multivariate #		
	B	*p*		B	*p*	
Age	0.460	0.097		0.059	0.031	*
Gender	−1.514	0.038	*	−1.618	0.029	*
Working style						
Work through pain	0.209	<0.001	**	0.265	<0.001	***
Social reactivity	−0.024	0.757		−0.092	0.379	
Sit and reach	−0.029	0.641		−0.091	0.104	
Handgrip strength (left)	−0.051	0.315		−0.116	0.108	
Handgrip strength (right)	−0.118	0.013	*	−0.044	0.428	
Depressive symptoms (score)	0.009	0.814		0.011	0.767	
Anxiety (dichotomous)	0.063	0.919		−0.542	0.387	
Self-rated job stress	0.440	0.083		0.346	0.221	
Self-rated health status	−0.094	0.863		1.161	0.031	*

+ All factors refer to the changes over time (T1−T0) in Table 4, except gender, depressive symptoms, self-rated health status, and anxiety (found significant in T0 in Tables 1–3) and age. # Mutually adjusted for each other. *: $p < 0.05$, **: $p < 0.01$, ***: $p < 0.001$.

4. Discussion

Our study is one of the first to develop a WRMS-prevention multidisciplinary program with stretching and muscle-strengthening exercises for low-skilled workers in a low-income community setting. Our results have provided promising evidence of the 2-month program's effectiveness in reducing the number of body parts with WRMSs, job stress, working through pain, improved spine flexibility, and handgrip strength. The factors significantly affecting the reduction in the number of body parts with WRMSs were the change in the workstyle of working through pain, and self-rated health status. In addition, our analyses demonstrated a medium effect size (0.44) with a good statistical power of 0.98.

Our results have also strengthened the evidence that the community could be the setting for WRMSs prevention programs, apart from workplaces. Consistent with Lee et al.'s study [7] in a Korean community, our program not only improved workers' flexibility but also reduced WRMSs and other outcomes. The success of our program could be due to its partnership design, multidisciplinary and multidimensional approaches, and appropriate length (right dose). Studies have shown the ineffectiveness of single interventions (such as ergonomics training or stress management); rather, multidimensional interventions are recommended to tackle the multifactorial nature of WRMSs [4–6,8]. The element of TCM also addressed the cultural needs of the Chinese participants. Furthermore, our exercise duration (15.5–25 min) was longer than that of the Korean study (6 min) [7]. Thus, the community center could serve as a vehicle to reach low-skilled, disadvantaged workers, to allow them to access the WRMSs prevention programs, and to bring them together synergistically [27].

The Workstyle model [21] and the concept of presenteeism (continuing to work despite not feeling well) [28] could be used to explain our results further. Our program might have been able to improve low-skilled workers' musculoskeletal health literacy. For instance, they became more aware that WRMSs are not a necessary consequence of their work, that they are human beings not instruments or machines in the workplace, and that they should take an active role in improving their musculoskeletal health. They might have changed from passivity to becoming active in improving their own WRMSs. Using the Workstyle model, adverse workstyles have been identified as factors associated with WRMSs in office workers [21,29,30] and nursing assistants in nursing homes [31]. Also, working through pain [20,32], self-rated health [20], and self-rated mental health [32] have been found to be associated with WRMSs. Workers with WRMSs tended to have higher presenteeism (such as working through pain) and vice versa [33]. Furthermore, more WRMSs and higher presenteeism have been found to be related to low-skilled workers, low education, low job resources, and longer working hours, and to be more common in female workers [33]. In addition, high presenteeism has been associated with low self-rated health [28,33], and workers with low self-rated health tended to have more WRMSs [33]. Moreover, a population-based study (N = 1615) found that workers with long working hours, working without contracts, and being highly dependent on their wages to contribute to the total household income were associated with higher presenteeism [34]. Reasons given for presenteeism included not wanting to burden colleagues, not being able to afford to be absent for economic reasons, and worrying about being laid off [34]. The factors associated with presenteeism identified in the literature match with the general characteristics of low-skilled workers. Based on the Workstyle model, working with pain is a behavior resulting from limited job resources, financial need to support families, and fear of losing the job (cognitive reasoning and psychological considerations) [21,29]. Additionally, the East Asian hierarchical work structure weakens employees' power to question their seniors or those at management level [32]. Chinese culture also emphasizes self-discipline and the individual's responsibility to others and to society [35]. Because low-skilled workers are at the bottom of the organizational structure [36], they have low bargaining power and are expected to adhere to their job duties and be loyal to the organization. The promising results of our program reflect that the elements of the workshops might have changed the participants' cognitive and psychological appraisals (part of the Workstyle model), with an understanding that presenteeism (working while suffering from pain) could aggravate their WRMSs further.

This study was limited by its single-group pre-and-post study design, with the majority of our participants being female. This might temper the generalizability of our findings. However, we attempted to enhance the representativeness of the study population by including seven different community centers as recruitment sites. Nevertheless, this study provides preliminary evidence for the effectiveness of the program and gives rise to further investigations. A clustered random controlled trial with a robust design, such as a larger sample size with well-matched interventions and a control group, is needed to build up generalizable and representative evidence for the effectiveness of this multidisciplinary exercise intervention program.

There are implications for practice: The findings of our study can help to inform policymakers, employers, and occupational health and safety stakeholders to pay attention to WRMSs, particularly among low-skilled workers. Indeed, the promising results of our study suggest that more resources from policymakers should be allocated to community centers (e.g., non-governmental organizations) to conduct WRMS prevention and management programs. Further studies can explore the concept of the settings approach to improve low-skilled workers' musculoskeletal health literacy. The four core principles of the settings approach, namely, community participation, partnership, empowerment and equity [37], can be used as a framework to guide community-based interventions. Empowerment refers to "the process by which people gain control over the factors and decisions that shape their lives" [38]. Through community participation and partnership with different occupational health and safety stakeholders and employers, community-based programs can empower workers to take control of their own musculoskeletal health. Self-help groups, or even musculoskeletal health ambassadors, could be established in community centers. Those groups or ambassadors could provide further social support to their peers using social media (such as WhatsApp, Line, or WeChat). Addressing musculoskeletal health successfully in low-skilled workers could give them more equitable access to health promotion and to lobby for more resources allocated to communities. The equity approach would enable every low-skilled worker to have the opportunity to access musculoskeletal health and services.

5. Conclusions

Community could be the alternative setting for WRMS prevention programs for low-skilled workers. Our study has demonstrated that a community-based multidisciplinary program can reduce the number of body parts affected by WRMSs in low-skilled workers in low-income communities. Further studies should be conducted to test the program. Healthcare professions and policymakers should explore the concept of the settings approach to allocate resources to community centers in order to empower low-skilled workers to lobby their right for musculoskeletal health.

Author Contributions: K.C.: Planned the study, coordinated the study, drafted, and revised the manuscript. M.M.Y.T.: Planned the study, revised the discussion section, and proofread the manuscript. C.K.W.: Planned the study, coordinated the study, and proofread the manuscript. K.W.M.: Coordinated the intervention, and proofread the manuscript. S.K.L.: Planned the study, coordinated the data collection training, and proofread the manuscript. K.Y.M.: Coordinated the data collection training, drafted the methods section, and proofread the manuscript. K.T.S.T.: Performed data analysis, drafted results section, and proofread the manuscript. E.P.W.L.: Planned the study, and proofread the manuscript. All authors read and approved the final manuscript.

Funding: The study was funded by the Community Chest of Hong Kong and Social Welfare Development Fund.

Acknowledgments: The authors are grateful to all the low-skilled workers for their participation in the study and the funding provided by the Community Chest of Hong Kong and Social Welfare Development Fund.

Conflicts of Interest: The authors declare no conflict of interest.

References

1. World Health Organization. Musculoskeletal Conditions 2018. Available online: http://www.who.int/news-room/fact-sheets/detail/musculoskeletal-conditions (accessed on 8 November 2018).
2. Kuorinka, I.; Jonsson, B.; Kilbom, A.; Vinterberg, H.; Biering-Sørensen, F.; Andersson, G.; Jørgensen, K. Standardised Nordic questionnaires for the analysis of musculoskeletal symptoms. *Appl. Ergon.* **1987**, *18*, 233–237. [CrossRef]
3. Summers, K.; Jinnett, K.; Bevan, S.; The Center for Workforced Health and Performance. *Musculoskeletal Disorders, Workforce Health and Productivity in the United States*; Lancaster University: Lancashire, UK, 2015.
4. Machado-Matos, M.; Arezes, P.M. Impact of a workplace exercise program on neck and shoulder segments in office workers. *Dyna* **2016**, *83*, 63–68. [CrossRef]
5. Lee, J.H.; Gak, H.B. Effects of self stretching on pain and musculoskeletal symptom of bus drivers. *J. Phys. Ther. Sci.* **2014**, *26*, 1911–1914. [CrossRef] [PubMed]
6. Moreira-Silva, I.; Santos, R.; Abreu, S.; Mota, J. The effect of a physical activity program on decreasing physical disability indicated by musculoskeletal pain and related symptoms among workers: A pilot study. *Int. J. Occup. Saf. Ergon.* **2014**, *20*, 55–64. [CrossRef]
7. Lee, H.; Chae, D.; Wilbur, J.; Miller, A.; Lee, K.; Jin, H. Effects of a 12 week self-managed stretching program among Korean–Chinese female migrant workers in Korea: A randomized trial. *Jpn. J. Nurs. Sci.* **2014**, *11*, 121–134. [CrossRef]
8. Van Eerd, D.; Munhall, C.; Irvin, E.; Rempel, D.; Brewer, S.; Van Der Beek, A.J.; Dennerlein, J.T.; Tullar, J.; Skivington, K.; Pinion, C.; et al. Effectiveness of workplace interventions in the prevention of upper extremity musculoskeletal disorders and symptoms: An update of the evidence. *Occup. Environ. Med.* **2016**, *73*, 62–70. [CrossRef]
9. World Health Organization. The Workplace: A priority Setting for Health Promotion. 2018. Available online: http://www.who.int/occupational_health/topics/workplace/en/ (accessed on 4 December 2018).
10. Caritas Community Development Service. Caritas Community Development Service. 2018. Available online: http://cd.caritas.org.hk/02aboutus.htm (accessed on 3 December 2018).
11. Ruhle, S.A.; Suess, S. Presentieeism and Low-Skilled Work—A Conceptual Analysis. Academy of Management Proceedings. *Acad. Manag. Proc.* **2018**. [CrossRef]
12. Human Resources and Skills Development Canada. National Occupational Classification Matrix 2011. 2011. Available online: http://www.immigrationcanadaservices.com/wp-content/uploads/2016/11/Matrix-1.pdf (accessed on 14 December 2018).
13. Immigration Canada Services. Job Opportunities for Low Skilled Workers in Canada. 2017. Available online: http://www.immigrationcanadaservices.com/job-opportunity-for-low-skilled-workers-in-canada/ (accessed on 14 December 2018).
14. Migration Advisory Committee. Migrants in Low-Skilled Work: The Growth of EU and Non-EU Labour in Low-Skilled Jobs and its Impact on the UK. 2014. Available online: https://www.gov.uk/government/organisations/migration-advisory-committee (accessed on 14 December 2018).
15. Occupational Safety and Health Branch Labour Department. More Exercise Smart Work II. 2007. Available online: https://www.labour.gov.hk/eng/public/oh/MESW.pdf (accessed on 14 December 2018).
16. Occupational Safety & Health Council. Stretching Exercise to Prevent Occupational Musculoskeletal Disorders. 2010. Available online: http://www.oshc.org.hk/oshc_data/files/leaflets/2016/CL1319C.pdf (accessed on 14 December 2018).
17. Svensson, A.L.; Strøyer, J.; Ebbehøj, N.E.; Schultz-Larsen, K.; Marott, J.L.; Mortensen, O.S.; Suadicani, P. Multidimensional intervention and sickness absence in assistant nursing students. *Occup. Med.* **2009**, *59*, 563–569. [CrossRef]
18. Szeto, G.P.; Law, K.Y.; Lee, E.; Lau, T.; Chan, S.Y.; Law, S.W. Multifaceted ergonomic intervention programme for community nurses: Pilot study. *J. Adv. Nurs.* **2010**, *66*, 1022–1034. [CrossRef] [PubMed]
19. Cheung, K. The incidence of low back problems among nursing students in Hong Kong. *J. Clin. Nurs.* **2010**, *19*, 2355–2362. [CrossRef]
20. Cheung, K.; Szeto, G.; Lai, G.K.; Ching, S.S. Prevalence of and factors associated with work-related musculoskeletal symptoms in nursing assistants working in nursing homes. *Int. J. Environ. Res. Public Health* **2018**, *15*, 265. [CrossRef] [PubMed]

21. Feuerstein, M. Workstyle: Definition, Empirical Support, and Implications for Prevention, Evaluation, and Rehabilitation of Occupational Upper-Extremity Disorders (Chapter 11). In *Beyond Biomechanics: Psychosocial Aspects of Musculoskeletal Disorders in Office Work*; Taylor Francis: London, UK, 1996.
22. Sallis, J.F.; Pinski, R.B.; Grossman, R.M.; Patterson, T.L.; Nader, P.R. The development of self-efficacy scales for health-related diet and exercise behaviors. *Health Educ. Res.* **1988**, *3*, 283–292. [CrossRef]
23. Marcus, B.H.; Selby, V.C.; Niaura, R.S.; Rossi, J.S. Self-efficacy and the stages of exercise behavior change. *Res. Q. Exerc. Sport* **1992**, *63*, 60–66. [CrossRef]
24. Liang, Y.; Lau, P.W.; Huang, W.Y.; Maddison, R.; Baranowski, T. Validity and reliability of questionnaires measuring physical activity self-efficacy, enjoyment, social support among Hong Kong Chinese children. *Prev. Med. Rep.* **2014**, *1*, 48–52. [CrossRef]
25. Zhang, Y.; Ting, R.Z.; Lam, M.H.; Lam, S.P.; Yeung, R.O.; Nan, H.; Ozaki, R.; Luk, A.O.; Kong, A.P.; Wing, Y.K.; et al. Measuring depression with CES-D in Chinese patients with type 2 diabetes: The validity and its comparison to PHQ-9. *BMC Psychiatry* **2015**, *15*, 198. [CrossRef]
26. American Psychiatric Association. *Desk reference to the diagnostic criteria from DSM-5 (DSM-5). (Taiwanese Society of Psychiatry, Trans)*; American Psychiatric Publishing: Arlington, TX, USA, 2013; ISBN 978-0-89042-556-5.
27. World Health Organization. Introduction to Healthy Settings. 2018. Available online: https://www.who.int/healthy_settings/about/en/ (accessed on 4 December 2018).
28. Skagen, K.; Collins, A.M. The consequences of sickness presenteeism on health and wellbeing over time: A systematic review. *Soc. Sci. Med.* **2016**, *161*, 169–177. [CrossRef]
29. Feuerstein, M.; Huang, G.D.; Pransky, G. *Workstyle and Work—Related Upper Extremity Disorders. Psychosocial Factors in Pain*; Guilford: New York, NY, USA, 1999.
30. Sharan, D.; Parijat, P.; Sasidharan, A.P.; Ranganathan, R.; Mohandoss, M.; Jose, J. Workstyle risk factors for work related musculoskeletal symptoms among computer professionals in India. *J. Occup. Rehabil.* **2011**, *21*, 520–525. [CrossRef]
31. Cheung, K.; Ching, S.S.; Ma, K.Y.; Szeto, G. Psychometric Evaluation of the Workstyle Short Form among Nursing Assistants with Work-Related Musculoskeletal Symptoms. *Int. J. Environ. Res. Public Health* **2018**, *15*, 823. [CrossRef]
32. Maakip, I.; Keegel, T.; Oakman, J. Workstyle and musculoskeletal discomfort (MSD): Exploring the influence of work culture in Malaysia. *J. Occup. Rehabil.* **2015**, *25*, 696–706. [CrossRef]
33. Choi, S.; Yi, Y.; Kim, J. Exposure to adverse social behavior in the workplace and sickness presenteeism among Korean workers: The mediating effects of musculoskeletal disorders. *Int. J. Environ. Res. Public Health* **2018**, *15*, 2198. [CrossRef]
34. Navarro, A.; Salas-Nicás, S.; Moncada, S.; Llorens, C.; Molinero-Ruiz, E. Prevalence, associated factors and reasons for sickness presenteeism: A cross-sectional nationally representative study of salaried workers in Spain, 2016. *BMJ Open* **2018**, *8*, e021212. [CrossRef]
35. Wu, K. Research on Sense of Social Responsibility in China: Looking Back and Looking Forward. *Cross-Cult. Commun.* **2014**, *10*, 140–147.
36. Maxwell, N.L. *Low-Skilled Jobs: The Reality Behind the Popular Perceptions*; California State University, East Bay: Hayward, CA, USA, 2006.
37. World Health Organization. Healthy Settings. 2018. Available online: https://www.who.int/healthy_settings/en/ (accessed on 4 December 2018).
38. World Health Organization. Track 1. Community Empowerment. 2018. Available online: https://www.who.int/healthpromotion/conferences/7gchp/track1/en/ (accessed on 4 December 2018).

International Journal of
Environmental Research and Public Health

MDPI

Article

The Nature and Cost of Readmissions after Work-Related Traumatic Spinal Injuries in New South Wales, Australia

Lisa N. Sharwood [1,2,*], Holger Möller [3], Jesse T. Young [4,5,6,7], Bharat Vaikuntam [1,2], Rebecca Q. Ivers [3,8], Tim Driscoll [9] and James W. Middleton [1,2,10]

1 Faculty of Medicine and Health, University of Sydney, Sydney 2006, Australia; bvai6198@sydney.edu.au (B.V.); james.middleton@sydney.edu.au (J.W.M.)
2 Kolling Institute, John Walsh Centre for Rehabilitation Studies, Sydney 2065, Australia
3 The George Institute for Global Health, University of New South Wales, Sydney 2042, Australia; hmoeller@georgeinstitute.org.au (H.M.); rebecca.ivers@unsw.edu.au (R.Q.I.)
4 Justice Health Unit, Centre for Health Equity, Melbourne School of Population and Global Health, The University of Melbourne, Victoria 3010, Australia; jesse.young@unimelb.edu.au
5 Centre for Adolescent Health, Murdoch Children's Research Institute, Victoria 3052, Australia
6 School of Population and Global Health, The University of Western Australia, Perth 6009, Western Australia, Australia
7 National Drug Research Institute, Curtin University, Perth 6102, Western Australia, Australia
8 School of Public Health and Community Medicine, University of New South Wales, Sydney 2052, Australia
9 School of Public Health, University of Sydney, Sydney 2006, Australia; tim.driscoll@sydney.edu.au
10 Agency for Clinical Innovation, Sydney 2067, Australia
* Correspondence: lisa.sharwood@sydney.edu.au

Received: 11 March 2019; Accepted: 23 April 2019; Published: 29 April 2019

Abstract: This study aimed to measure the subsequent health and health service cost burden of a cohort of workers hospitalised after sustaining work-related traumatic spinal injuries (TSI) across New South Wales, Australia. A record-linkage study (June 2013–June 2016) of hospitalised cases of work-related spinal injury (ICD10-AM code U73.0 or workers compensation) was conducted. Of the 824 individuals injured during this time, 740 had sufficient follow-up data to analyse readmissions ≤90 days post-acute hospital discharge. Individuals with TSI were predominantly male (86.2%), mean age 46.6 years. Around 8% (n = 61) experienced 119 unplanned readmission episodes within 28 days from discharge, over half with the primary diagnosis being for care involving rehabilitation. Other readmissions involved device complications/infections (7.5%), genitourinary or respiratory infections (10%) or mental health needs (4.3%). The mean ± SD readmission cost was $6946 ± $14,532 per patient. Unplanned readmissions shortly post-discharge for TSI indicate unresolved issues within acute-care, or poor support services organisation in discharge planning. This study offers evidence of unmet needs after acute TSI and can assist trauma care-coordinators' comprehensive assessments of these patients prior to discharge. Improved quantification of the ongoing personal and health service after work-related injury is a vital part of the information needed to improve recovery after major work-related trauma.

Keywords: work-related injuries; spinal trauma; record linkage data; cost; rehabilitation; complications; unmet needs; unplanned readmissions

1. Introduction

The immediate period following hospital discharge after acute traumatic injury holds substantial risk for ongoing health, recovery and welfare concerns [1]. Ongoing challenges can include physical limitations, continuing pain and the experience of secondary conditions. These factors can impair participation in previous activities, complicate or hamper the return to work [2] and contribute to financial stress, relationship strain and social exclusion. These factors predispose individuals to deterioration in mental health [3,4]; further impeding recovery from injury. Direct and measurable costs to an injured worker incorporate the loss or change in employment earnings, in addition to legal and medical costs. Indirect and less easily measured costs include pain, impaired function, reduced quality of life, potential for chronic injury and stress on interpersonal relationships [5,6]. Harmful substance use has previously been reported as high in injured populations, and likely compounds this multitude of issues [7,8]. Context-specific costs to the healthcare service for readmissions after acute injury are less well described, yet important to measure.

The incidence and cost of traumatic spinal injuries (TSI) sustained in workplaces in New South Wales (NSW) was recently estimated for the first time. Over a 3-year period, 824 persons sustained TSI in work-related incidents, occupying 13,302 acute care bed days and costing a total of $19,500,000 (95%CI $16 M–$23 M) [9]. The total cost of work-related injury and disease in Australia was estimated at $61.8 billion in 2012–2013, of which NSW bore 28% ($17.3 billion) of the total cost from 31% of cases nationwide [10]. Injuries sustained in this cohort comprised column fractures, spinal cord injury or both; 21% of persons also sustained concomitant head, chest or abdominal traumatic injury. High numbers of these injuries occurred in the construction industry, particularly due to falling from height. This study did not report on any incidence, nature and cost of readmissions to hospital following the acute care period.

Gabbe and Nunn recently reported 40% of patients after traumatic spinal cord injury to experience readmissions within the first 2 years in Victoria [11]. Similar proportions were described by Ruseckaite et al. [12] studying a cohort of patients injured in compensable transport incidents. Over one third of these patients experienced acute care facility readmission within 28 days of injury. Investigating unplanned readmissions in certain injury populations should be routinely undertaken to benchmark discharge planning efforts and therefore assist trauma care coordination.

Unplanned hospital readmissions occurrences within 28 days post the acute-care episode are progressively being used in various jurisdictions internationally as a measure of the quality of hospital care or treatment. In some systems, rates of unplanned readmissions are being used as an indicator of hospital performance that is then linked with funding reimbursements. Previous analysis in NSW has indicated that at least one quarter of unplanned readmissions are linked to "deficiencies in care" [13]. In 2013–2014, the NSW average for unplanned readmissions across all conditions and acute care facilities was 6.8 per cent; higher than the NSW 2021 target of 5.5 per cent [13].

The burden of TSI occurring in workplace settings is of particular interest for national injury prevention bodies, such as Safe Work Australia, who have prioritised a national target of a 30% reduction in serious work-related injury compensation claims by 2022 [14]. Quantification of the extended burden of TSI within the acute care setting complements the evidence informing injury prevention efforts in occupational health and safety, describing more specifically the extent of enduring disability associated with work-related injury.

Therefore, the aim of this population-based study was to measure the post-acute care burden in a cohort of hospitalised traumatic spinal column and cord injuries that occurred while "working for an income" in NSW, Australia. Specifically, following those patients previously identified as sustaining a work-related TSI [9], we describe the incidence of 28- and 90-day readmissions, subsequent to their discharge from acute hospitalisation, investigating readmission etiology and healthcare system costs.

2. Methods

The epidemiology and occupational context of persons who sustained a TSI while "working for an income" in NSW has been previously and fully reported [9]. The Centre for Health Record Linkage (CHeReL) linked NSW Admitted Patient Data Collection (APDC), Registry of Births, Deaths and Marriage and Activity Based Funding (ABF) costing records for all people aged ≥16 years who were hospitalised between 1 June 2013 and 30 June 2016 with a TSI recorded in their index admission due to a work-related incident defined as ICD10-AM [15] code U73.0 or funding by workers compensation in the index admissions. Spinal injuries included all spinal cord and/or column injuries, defined using specific ICD-10-AM codes (Appendix A). NSW is the most populous Australian state with approximately 7.5 million inhabitants residing across 800,000 km^2 in suburban, rural and very remote areas [16].

For the current study, readmissions were identified from APDC records linked with these index admissions. We defined hospital readmissions as being within 28 and 90 days after discharge with a primary diagnosis code related to the index admission. This benchmark was chosen in accordance with definitions from the NSW Bureau of Health Information [17], and the Independent Price Health Authority [18], who determine that readmissions to hospital within 28 days of discharge should be reviewed and considered as "potentially avoidable". These were identified by manual review of the primary diagnosis codes of all admissions within 28 and 90 days, respectively. Readmissions within the first 28 days were consequently nested within those identified within 90 days.

Estimation of the costs of readmission was based on the formula used to calculate the National Weighted Activity Units (NWAUs) assigned to each ABF activity [19]. Weighted Activity Units (WAU) are the weights assigned per hospital separation; we used the 2013/2014 National Pricing Model technical specifications published by the Independent Hospital Pricing Authority [19] (for compatibility with AR-DRG version 6.0x). The WAUs in this study were adjusted for private patient service and private patient accommodation adjustments; a slight difference to NWAUs to avoid distortion by differential funding of public and compensable patients. All patients were assumed to be funded by Medicare for the WAU estimation. The "per separation" cost was defined as the WAU multiplied by the National Efficient Price 2013/2014 ($4993); with higher WAUs thus being more resource intensive.

Descriptive statistics were used to report the prevalence of various factors. Values were reported as mean and standard deviation (SD) for normally distributed continuous variables, proportions for categorical variables and median and interquartile range (IQR) for non-normally distributed continuous variables. All statistical analyses were performed using Stata version 15.0 (Stata Corporation, College Station, TX, USA). Standardised reporting of demographic and other variables, as recommended by De Vivo et al. [20], was followed where possible.

This study was approved by the Cancer Institute NSW, Population & Health Services Research Ethics Committee: AU RED Reference: HREC/16/CIPHS/19, Cancer Institute NSW reference number: 2016/07/647.

3. Results

Between 1 June 2013 and 30 June 2016, 824 individuals sustained a traumatic spinal injury in NSW while working for an income, of which 740 (89.8%) had sufficient follow-up data to analyse readmissions <90 days post-acute hospital discharge (up to 1 April 2016) and were included in the analyses. Of these 740 individuals, 61 (8.2%) experienced a total of 119 (16.1%) readmissions in the first 28 days after their acute care discharge. By 90 days after discharge from acute care, 102 (13.8%) individuals had experienced 250 readmissions.

Characteristics of the primary injury cohort compared with individuals requiring readmissions within 28 and 90 days are described in Table 1. The cohort were predominantly male (86.2%); those aged 45–59 years were the largest age group (34.7%), this was also true for the readmitted proportions (37.7% and 36.3% for 28- and 90-day readmissions, respectively). Almost half of original work-related injuries had occurred as a result of a fall in their workplace (49.2%); over half of these (55.1%) were falls from building structures, scaffolding or ladders.

Table 1. Characteristics of the injured cohort compared with readmitted individuals.

Characteristics	Cohort (n = 740) N (%)	Readmitted <28 days (n = 61) N (%)	Readmitted <90 days (n = 102) N (%)
Sex (male)	638 (86.2)	50 (81.9)	87 (85.3)
Age category years			
16–29	125 (16.9)	7 (11.5)	10 (9.8)
30–44	206 (27.8)	15 (24.6)	28 (27.4)
45–59	257 (34.7)	23 (37.7)	37 (36.3)
60+	152 (20.5)	16 (26.2)	27 (26.4)
Mechanism of injury			
Falls	364 (49.2)	29 (47.5)	48 (47.1)
Transport	223 (30.1)	16 (26.2)	29 (28.4)
Mechanical forces	124 (16.7)	11 (18.0)	18 (17.6)
Other/unspecified	27 (3.6)	5 (8.2)	7 (6.9)
Index Injury #			
Spinal cord injury	44 (5.9)	7 (11.5)	13 (12.7)
Spinal fracture/dislocation	725 (97.9)	60 (98)	101 (99)
Cervical	161 (21.7)	11 (18.0)	20 (19.6)
Thoracic	258 (34.8)	25 (40.9)	36 (35.3)
Lumbosacral	424 (57.3)	35 (57.4)	65 (63.7)
Co-morbid traumatic brain injury	51 (6.9)	8 (13.1)	9 (8.8)
Co-morbid severe chest injury	86 (11.6)	11 (18.0)	19 (18.6)
Co-morbid abdominal injury	27 (3.6)	5 (8.2)	9 (8.8)
Operative procedure index admission	293 (39.5)	19 (31.1)	42 (41.1)
Persons to readmissions ratio	NA	61:119	102:250

Counts injuries, not persons, i.e., some patients have more than one injury. NA: Not applicable

Table 2 displays the principal diagnosis (i.e., primary reason) for the readmission after the index TSI hospitalisation within 28 and 90 days; hence the denominator is the number of admission episodes, not the number of persons. Allied Health Services collectively apportion the majority of primary reasons for admission (56.3% and 59.6%). While this is a broad-reaching category, most individuals requiring readmission in this category were coded as "Care involving use of rehabilitation procedure, unspecified" (88%). All of these individuals had previously been discharged from an acute-care admission. Greater than 10% of the cohort of persons with TSI required readmission for complications of internal fixation devices (including infection), open wound infections and other complaints; 16 persons (13.4%) were readmitted within 28 days and 35 (14%) within 90 days.

The measure of resources required to accommodate these readmissions was counted as bed days and costs. The mean ± SD length of stay for readmissions within 28 days was 3.1 ± 7.0 days, compared with the length of stay for readmissions within 90 days at 4.8 ± 20.3 days. The total number of acute care bed days used by the 102 persons readmitted in 250 episodes was 1232 days at a total cost of $708,464 (95%CI: $417,325–$999,603). The mean ± SD per patient readmission cost was $6946 ± $14,532. The mean costs for 90-day readmissions were highest for patients with spinal cord injuries ($24,558), persons aged 16–29 years ($21,947) and transport incidents occurring on a street/highway ($15,492).

Table 2. Readmissions within 28 and 90 days.

Reason for Readmission *	28 days *N* (%) #	90 days *N* (%) #
Allied Health Service (Z00–Z99)	67 (56.3)	149 (59.6)
Care involving use of rehabilitation procedure, unspecified (Z50.9)	59 (88.0)	99 (66.4)
Other	8 (11.9)	50 (33.5)
Injury and related (S00–T98)	16 (13.4)	35 (14.0)
Mechanical complication/infection of internal device	9 (56.2)	12 (34.3)
Open wound/infection	5 (31.2)	8 (22.8)
Other (suppressed)	2 (12.5)	15 (42.8)
Musculoskeletal & nervous systems, skin, sensory organs (G00–G99, M00–M99, L00–L99, H00–H95)	9 (7.6)	19 (7.6)
Circulatory system (I00–I99)	6 (5.0)	9 (3.6)
Mental & behavioural (F00–F99)	5 (4.2)	9 (3.6)
Digestive & genitourinary systems (K00–K93, N00–N99)	5 (4.2)	12 (4.8)
Respiratory system & infections (J00–J99, A00–B99)	5 (4.2)	5 (2.0)
Not elsewhere classified (R00–R99)	6 (5.0)	12 (4.8)
Total Readmissions	**119**	**250**

* Principal ICD10-AM diagnosis group in brackets (15). # Of total readmission numbers.

4. Discussion

In a cohort of 740 patients who had sustained work-related incident related traumatic spinal injuries during a three-year period, we found that around 8% (n = 61) of these patients experienced 119 inpatient readmissions within 28 days post-acute care discharge. Reasons for unplanned readmissions included requiring allied health interventions (56.3%), injury repair and operative complications (13.4%), circulatory problems including embolus (5%) and mental health problems (4.2%). The mean (SD) per patient cost for acute readmission was $6,946 ($14,532). Total costs of unplanned readmissions in the 90 days post-acute discharge were $708,464 (95%CI: $417,325–$999,602).

Although the recently reported NSW average of unplanned readmissions was 6.8% [13], we found a (disease-specific) readmission rate of 16.1% by 28 days post the index discharge among people who sustained work-related TSI, resulting predominantly from spinal fractures. Hospital performance monitoring in Australia measures a range of indicators including the incidence of hospital-acquired complications and rates of unplanned readmissions. These indices are now linked to government funding; for example, admissions where a hospital acquired complication incurs a payment reduction to hospital reimbursement [18]. Unplanned hospital readmissions can be a signal of issues with the effectiveness, continuity and integration of care provided to patients. As such, the use of patient clinical data in this way can help to drive safety and quality improvement. In this study, it may be that patients discharged to home may have rather benefited from a subsequent rehabilitation admission, avoiding the need to return to an acute care hospital. While rehabilitation admissions still impose a system cost, it is unlikely to be to the same extent. This information is therefore helpful in the discharge planning stage for patients with a traumatic spinal injury.

Our study had some limitations. We did not have access to various important variables about the injured worker, such as ethnicity, level of education and experience, the employment situation (e.g., whether permanent/part-time/casual) and specific occupation. Indigenous status was available but not identified from the APDC collection for this study. We have assumed all the patients to be of non-indigenous status for the estimation of costs using the NWAU-based approach; while we have not provided estimate of the cost impact this may have had, it is not anticipated to vary the current estimates significantly. Furthermore, the APDC District Network Return (DNR) does not include hospitalisation cost data for patients who were admitted to private hospitals across NSW. The degree of under-representation that this presents is uncertain, however such severe injuries are much more likely to be treated within the public hospital system [21]. We used NWAU-based costing approach to estimate the costs over the DNR data-based estimation to include all the public hospital separations in the costing analysis. The cost estimates presented are an under-estimation of the true costs as the separations at private hospitals were excluded from the analysis.

Braaf et al. [22] described the experiences of seriously injured patients within the Victorian state trauma service regarding communication from the health professionals caring for them after their injury. Many patients reported insufficient information, confusion and lack of clear communication to have hampered their discharge from acute care. While we did not interview patients involved in the current study, the high rate of readmissions for care involving rehabilitation suggests an area for improvement in the discharge planning process. Readmission can reflect the underuse of recommended care, adverse events and complications of hospital care, inadequate discharge planning or problems with coordination and integration of care across hospital, primary care and community settings. Patients discharged without sufficient information for continuity of care [23] can deteriorate once out of the acute care setting. Readmissions with infections, open wounds and device complications could likely be avoided with education, support and a general practitioner liaison.

5. Conclusions

Work-related traumatic spinal injuries create a significant burden of cost and disability for the Australian workforce but are preventable and also fall under a current focus of the Safe Work Australia policy to reduce serious injury compensation claims by 30% by 2022. This study demonstrates that the ongoing burden of work-related spinal trauma is not insignificant in the acute period post primary discharge. This study offers evidence of unmet needs after acute TSI and can assist trauma care coordinators' comprehensive assessments of these patients prior to discharge. Improved quantification of the ongoing personal and health service after work-related injury is a vital part of the information needed to improve recovery after major work-related trauma.

Author Contributions: Conceptualisation, L.N.S. and T.D.; Methodology, L.N.S., H.M. and B.V.; Software, H.M. and L.N.S.; Formal Analysis, L.N.S., H.M. and B.V.; Data Curation, L.N.S., H.M. and B.V., Writing—Original Draft Preparation, L.N.S.; Writing—Review and Editing, J.T.Y., J.W.M., R.Q.I., H.M. and T.D.; Supervision, J.W.M.; Project Administration, L.N.S.; Funding Acquisition, L.N.S.

Funding: L.N.S. acknowledges and is supported by funding from icare™.

Acknowledgments: The authors would like to thank the Meteor coding assistant team at the Australian Institute of Health and Welfare for their strategic advice in the clarification of search and usage of activity codes.

Conflicts of Interest: The authors declare no conflict of interest. The founding sponsors had no role in the design of the study; in the collection, analyses, or interpretation of data; in the writing of the manuscript, or in the decision to publish the results.

Appendix A

A. TSI Identification

The dataset combined all patients for whom one of the following ICD-10-AM (International Classification of Diseases—Tenth Revision, Australian Modification) codes have been identified in any separation, and in any position of the diagnostic code list within the NSW Admitted Patient Data Collection (APDC):

S12, S12.0, S12.1, S12.2, S12.21, S12.22, S12.23, S12.24, S12.25, S12.7, S12.8, S12.9, S13.1, S13.10, S13.11, S13.12, S13.13, S13.14, S13.15, S13.16, S13.17, S13.18, S13.2, S13.3, S14.0, S14.10, S14.11, S14.12, S14.13, S14.70, S14.71, S14.72, S14.73, S14.74, S14.75, S14.76, S14.77, S14.78, S22.0, S22.00, S22.01, S22.02, S22.03, S22.04, S22.05, S22.06, S22.1, S24.0, S24.1, S24.10, S24.11, S24.12, S24.7, S24.70, S24.71, S24.72, S24.73, S24.74, S24.75, S24.76, S24.77, S32, S32.0, S32.00, S32.01, S32.02, S32.03, S32.04, S32.05, S34.0, S34.1, S34.3, S34.70, S34.71, S34.72, S34.73, S34.74, S34.75, S34.76, T06.0, T06.1, T09.3.

B. Mechanism of Injury and Activity

Injury mechanism and activity at the time of injury were identified using the following ICD-10 AM codes:

1. Activity of injured person at time of injury
    a. Sports and leisure: U50–U72
    b. Other activity: U73
2. Accidents
    a. Transport accidents: V00–V99
    b. Other external causes of accidental injury: W00–X59
    c. Intentional self-harm: X60–X84
    d. Assault: X85–Y09
    e. Event of undetermined intention: Y20–Y36
    f. Legal intervention and operations of war: Y35–Y36

C. Multiple Trauma

Other injury categories in addition to TSCI were identified using the following ICD-10 AM codes. The other injury categories are:

a. Arm or shoulder injury: S57, S58, S61, S62, S67, S68
b. Hip or leg injury: S71, S72, S73, S77, S78, S79, S81, S82, S83, S87, S88, S91, S92, S93, S97, S98
c. Chest or abdomen injury: S21, S22, S26, S27, S28, S28.0, S28.1, S31, S36, S38
d. Skull or face injury: S01, S02, S05, S08
e. Traumatic brain injury: S06, S07

References

1. Gabbe, B.; Sutherland, A.; Hart, M.; Cameron, P. Population-based capture of long-term functional and quality of life outcomes following major trauma—The experiences of the Victorian State trauma registry. *J. Trauma Inj. Infec. Critic. Care* **2010**, *69*, 532–536. [CrossRef] [PubMed]
2. Dembe, A.; Delbos, R.; Erickson, J.; Banks, S. Associations between employees' work schedules and the vocational consequences of workplace injuries. *J. Occup. Rehabilit.* **2007**, *17*, 641–651. [CrossRef] [PubMed]
3. Degen, R.; MacDermid, J.; Grewal, R.; Drosdowech, D.; Faber, K.; Athwal, G. Prevalence of symptoms of depression, anxiety, and posttraumatic stress disorder in workers with upper extremity complaints. *J. Orthop. Sports Phys. Ther.* **2016**, *46*, 590–595. [CrossRef] [PubMed]
4. O'Hagan, T.; Ballantyne, P.; Vienneau, P. Mental health status of ontario injured workers with permanent impairments. *Can. J. Public Health/Revue Canadienne de Santé Publique* **2012**, *103*, e303–e308. [PubMed]
5. Asfaw, A.; Souza, K. Incidence and cost of depression after occupational injury. *J. Occup. Environ. Med.* **2012**, *54*, 1086–1091. [CrossRef] [PubMed]
6. Asfaw, A.; Pana-Cryan, R.; Bushnell, P.T. Incidence and costs of family member hospitalization following injuries of workers' compensation claimants. *Am. J. Ind. Med.* **2012**, *55*, 1028–1036. [CrossRef] [PubMed]
7. Craig, A.; Guest, R.; Tran, Y.; Middleton, J. Depressive mood in adults with spinal cord injury as they transition from an inpatient to a community setting: Secondary analyses from a clinical trial. *Spinal Cord* **2017**, *55*, 926–934. [CrossRef] [PubMed]
8. Craig, A.; Nicholson, P.K.; Guest, R.; Tran, Y.; Dezarnaulds, A.; Hales, A.; Ephraums, C.; Middleton, J. The occurrence of psychological disorders and co-morbidities following spinal cord injury. *Arch. Phys. Med. Rehab.* **2015**, *96*, 1426–1434. [CrossRef] [PubMed]
9. Sharwood, L.; Mueller, H.; Ivers, R.; Vaikuntam, B.; Driscoll, T.; Middleton, J. The epidemiology, cost, and occupational context of spinal injuries sustained while 'working for income' in NSW: A record-linkage study. *Int. J. Environ. Res. Public Health* **2018**, *15*, 2121. [CrossRef] [PubMed]

10. Safe Work Australia. Cost of Injury and Illness by State 2012–2013. Available online: https://www.safeworkaustralia.gov.au/statistics-and-research/statistics/cost-injury-and-illness/cost-injury-and-illness-state-and (accessed on 22 December 2018).
11. Gabbe, B.J.; Nunn, A. Profile and costs of secondary conditions resulting in emergency department presentations and readmission to hospital following traumatic spinal cord injury. *Injury* **2016**, *47*, 1847–1855. [CrossRef] [PubMed]
12. Ruseckaite, R.; Gabbe, B.; Vogel, A.P.; Collie, A. Health care utilisation following hospitalisation for transport-related injury. *Injury* **2012**, *43*, 1600–1605. [CrossRef] [PubMed]
13. New South Wales Audit Office. *Managing Length of Stay and Unplanned Readmissions in NSW Public Hospitals: New South Wales Auditor-General's Report Performance Audit*; Audit Office of NSW: Sydney, NSW, Australia, 2015.
14. Safe Work Australia. *Australian Work Health and Safety Strategy 2012–2022*; Safe Work Australia: Canberra, Australia, 2012.
15. National Centre for Classification in Health. *ICD-10-AM/ACHI/ACS*, 10th ed.; IHPA; Australian Consortium for Classification Development: Sydney, NSW, Australia, 2017.
16. Australian Bureau of Statistics. *Australian Demographic Statistics*; Australian Bureau of Statistics: Canberra, Australia, 2017.
17. Bureau of Health Information. *Exploring Clinical Variation in Readmission. Return to Acute Care Following Discharge from Hospital, Eight Clinical Conditions, NSW, July 2012–June 2015*; Bureau of Health Information: Sydney, NSW, Australia, 2017.
18. Independent Hospital Pricing Authority. *Consultation Paper on the Pricing Framework for Australian Public Hospital Services 2017–2018*; Independent Hospital Pricing Authority: Sydney, NSW, Australia, 2016.
19. Independent Hospital Pricing Authority. *National Pricing Model Technical Specifications 2013–2014*; Independent Hospital Pricing Authority: Sydney, NSW, Australia, 2013.
20. DeVivo, M.; Biering-Sorensen, F.; New, P.; Chen, Y. Standardization of data analysis and reporting of results from the international spinal cord injury core data set. *Spinal Cord* **2011**, *49*, 596–599. [CrossRef] [PubMed]
21. Badhiwala, J.H.; Lai, C.K.; Alhazzani, W.; Farrokhyar, F.; Nassiri, F.; Meade, M.; Mansouri, A.; Sne, N.; Aref, M.; Murty, N.; et al. Cervical spine clearance in obtunded patients after blunt traumatic injury: A systematic review. *Ann. Intern. Med.* **2015**, *162*, 429–437. [CrossRef] [PubMed]
22. Braaf, S.; Ameratunga, S.; Nunn, A.; Christie, N.; Teague, W.; Judson, R.; Gabbe, B.J. Patient-identified information and communication needs in the context of major trauma. *BMC Health Serv. Res.* **2018**, *18*, 163. [CrossRef] [PubMed]
23. Uitvlugt, E.B.; Siegert, C.E.; Janssen, M.J.; Nijpels, G.; Karapinar-Carkit, F. Completeness of medication-related information in discharge letters and post-discharge general practitioner overviews. *Int. J. Clin. Pharm.* **2015**, *37*, 1206–1212. [CrossRef] [PubMed]

International Journal of
Environmental Research and Public Health

MDPI

Article

Burnout Syndrome in Middle and Senior Management in the Industrial Manufacturing Sector of Mexico

Sharon Macias-Velasquez [1], Yolanda Baez-Lopez [1,*], Aidé Aracely Maldonado-Macías [2], Jorge Limon-Romero [1] and Diego Tlapa [1]

1. Facultad de Ingeniería, Arquitectura y Diseño, Universidad Autónoma de Baja California; Carretera Transpeninsular Ensenada-Tijuana 3917, Colonia Playitas, Ensenada 22860, Baja California, Mexico; idali.macias@uabc.edu.mx (S.M.-V.); jorge.limon@uabc.edu.mx (J.L.-R.); diegotlapa@uabc.edu.mx (D.T.)
2. Department of Industrial Engineering and Manufacturing, Autonomous University of Ciudad Juarez, Ave. del Charro 450 Norte, Cd Juarez 32310, Chihuahua, Mexico; amaldona@uacj.mx

* Correspondence: yolanda@uabc.edu.mx; Tel.: +52-646-175-0744

Received: 26 March 2019; Accepted: 23 April 2019; Published: 25 April 2019

Abstract: Due to globalization and the accelerated growth of technology, ever more employees of companies are affected by burnout syndrome, the psychological nature of which requires a prolonged response to chronic interpersonal stressors in work environments. The present research aims to validate the operability of the Maslach Burnout Inventory-General Survey (MBI-GS) using a sample of 378 professionals belonging to middle and senior management working in companies within the IMMEX sector (comprising the industrial-manufacturing, maquiladora and export services) located in the state of Baja California, Mexico. Firstly, an exploratory factor analysis using the principal components method and Varimax rotation was performed and the results revealed the existence of three factors representing more than 67 percent of the total variance. Secondly, a confirmatory factorial analysis was carried out performing appropriate results for the indices Chi-square goodness-of-fit model, Root Mean Square Error of Approximation (RMSEA), Normed Fit Index (NFI), Comparative Fit Index (CFI), Relative Fit Index (RFI), Parsimony Ratio (PRATIO) and Parsimony Normed Fit Index (PNFI), which are highly recommended by literature in these types of studies. Additionally, construct validity was satisfactorily verified. The factorial solution coincided with the Maslach Burnout Inventory original proposal so that this instrument can be considered a valid and reliable option to analyze the burnout levels in people pertaining to middle and senior management in these types of industries.

Keywords: burnout; construct validity; MBI; industry

1. Introduction

Job stress is a collection of psychological, emotional, cognitive and behavioral reactions to certain overwhelming or demanding aspects of the organization and environment of the workplace. People presenting stress experience tension, anxiety and feelings of impotence at not being able to confront certain situations and, in some cases, repercussions for their physical health [1]. The seriousness of these symptoms will depend on the magnitude of the demands which the employee must fulfill in a certain period of time, their application of self-control and the decision-making freedom they enjoy [2]. Employees with demanding jobs characterized by work-based tension and low levels of decision-making autonomy and social support tend to take more sick-leave [3].

Job stress is among the main work-related problems according to the World Health Organization (WHO), and is a category in which Mexico is ranked first in the world, with 75% of its workers suffering from stress, followed by China and the United States, the two largest economies in the world, with 73% and 59%, respectively [4]. In economic terms, both workers and governments are noting ever higher costs of stress, which infringes on individual companies and the economy in general, affecting productivity [5] through the increased incidence of phenomena such as: working days lost due to absenteeism; internal employee transfers; rate of workplace accidents; client complaints; and, demand for the training of replacement workers [6]. This situation could represent losses of between 0.5% and 3.5% of a country's gross domestic product [7].

In the particular case of Mexico, employee job stress causes losses of between 5 and 40 billion dollars per year [7]. Together with the existing difficulties in controlling other more well-known workplace risks, there is neither sufficient awareness of job stress nor sufficient resources for combatting it, with the concept being introduced into Mexican legislation little by little.

Job stress has been a growing subject of research, with the results obtained clearly showing the relationships among stress, health conditions [8–10], support from work colleagues [11] and behavior showing feelings of insecurity about work [10], to mention but a few areas. An extreme variant known as burnout appears in those individuals who are not able to successfully deal with extended periods of job stress [12,13]. From an existential perspective, the root cause of burnout resides in people's need to believe that their lives are meaningful—that what they do is useful and important [14]. Those people hoping to obtain a meaning from their work develop their profession with highly-motivated and idealistic goals. When such people feel that they have failed, that their work is meaningless, and that they are not making a difference to the world, they begin to experience exhaustion and hopelessness, feelings which will, ultimately, consume them [15].

The concept of burnout was introduced by Maslach and Jackson and is the most widely used concept for this phenomenon in the literature [16]. Burnout began to appear with some regularity in the 1970s in the United States, especially among people working in the human services [17]. The conceptualization of job burnout is understood as a psychological syndrome in response to chronic interpersonal stressors on the job. The three key dimensions of this response are an overwhelming exhaustion, feelings of cynicism and detachment from the job, and a sense of ineffectiveness and lack of accomplishment [17].

The three dimensions of burnout are related to workplace variables in different ways. In general, exhaustion and cynicism tend to emerge from the presence of work overload and social conflict, whereas a sense of inefficacy arises more clearly from a lack of resources to get the job done (e.g., lack of critical information, lack of necessary tools, or insufficient time) [18]. In jobs with high job demands and limited job resources, we expect that employees develop exhaustion, cynicism, and a reduced sense of competence [19].

The main instrument used to measure burnout in a certain population is the Maslach Burnout Inventory-General Survey (MBI-GS), which was developed in response to two demands. The first comprised the study of the phenomenon in areas distinct to the healthcare sector for which it was originally created (MBI-HSS), finding, in some cases, different factorial structures with more than three dimensions, as in Densten [20]. Secondly, more studies have been born of an interest in the burnout caused by professional roles that do not necessarily involve the social demands of interacting with other individuals [21].

The validity of the instrument has been confirmed by various authors. Langballe [22] examined the factorial validity of the MBI-GS across eight different occupational groups in Norway: lawyers, physicians, nurses, teachers, church ministers, bus drivers, and people working in the advertising and information technology industries ($N = 5024$). Separate confirmatory factor analyses showed that the hypothesized three-factor model had sufficient fit in all occupational groups except for the group of people working in advertising. The results support that MBI-GS provides a suitable measurement to assess burnout across a diversity of professions [22]. Huibers et al. [23] carried out a cross-sectional study that compared the MBI-GS with other concepts such as chronic fatigue, finding that fatigued employees shared important characteristics with those suffering from chronic fatigue, independent of their state of burnout.

In the industrial sector, the validity of the Japanese translation of the MBI-GS was studied in a sample of middle management in a manufacturing company, with the results replicating the tri-dimensional structure of the original instrument and supporting the validity of the construct in the sample studied [24]. These studies confirmed factorial validity in the majority of the professions analyzed, maintaining the three-factor structure with which the concept was originally proposed.

Interest in this concept has increased in the last decade, both nationally and internationally [25], with the research panorama related to burnout in Latin America showing a tendency to follow the paradigmatic and methodological guidelines for studies carried out in the United States, Spain and other countries. This is reflected in the fact that the majority of the studies apply the Maslach and Jackson model. With regard to the professions of interest, a tendency to focus on the fields of healthcare and care provision was found, as well as those fields in which a supplier-client interaction can be clearly observed [26].

In Mexico, after nearly 20 years since the first publication on burnout, an increasing amount of research into this area [25] has focused on different professional populations, with teaching [27–30] healthcare [31,32] and high performance athletics [33] among those professions that stand out. The cities in which the highest number of studies on this subject have been conducted are Guadalajara and Mexico City [25].

This study was carried out in the main cities of the state of Baja California due to the great importance it represents to the industrial sector, occupying the first place in the northwest of the country in terms of the total number of people with employment, with a 56.4% participation rate [34].

In Baja California the activity of the maquiladoras began with the establishment of the free trade area in the 1960s, which allowed the duty-free importation of machinery, equipment, raw materials and supplies, after which the maquiladoras were extended to the rest of the region from the northern border, later, to the coasts, other border regions and, finally, to the whole country [35]. According to the data reported about the export manufacturing industry, in 2018, the industrial-manufacturing, maquiladora and export services (IMMEX) experienced a period of growth, with an increase of 0.51% in the number of companies [36]. The state of Baja California occupies the first place in the number of IMMEX companies, with 18.18%, and the second national place of personnel employed in the sector, with 14.64% [37]. In addition, 15,353 million dollars were generated in Baja California as export value, highlighting the importance of this activity in regional economy [35]. Due to the importance of this sector, the personnel of the IMMEX sector were selected to carry out the study, which noted the complexity of the functions they perform and the few studies that have been done on the burnout occurring in the sector, despite the growing industrial activity in the state.

Specifically, those positions at the middle and senior management were analyzed. Related research can be found among other studies conducted on this classification of personnel, such as the analysis of burnout and obesity [38] or burnout and the body weight index, which describe how important it is to take into account additional factors such as genetics or dietary habits [39]. In contrast to previous research, the present study proposes the validity of the instrument MBI-GS for a specific sector, geographic area and professional activity.

The Present Research

Is necessary to broaden the occupational field and regions in which studies on burnout are carried out, improve the research design and information analysis, and ensure the validity of the scales used [25]. The present research aims to validate the operability of the MBI-GS for measuring the burnout construct in a sample of 378 professionals pertaining to middle and senior management in the industrial sector of the state of Baja California, Mexico, whose particular characteristics qualify them for evaluation in the selected sample.

Further to the evaluation of functionality being a fundamental requirement for every instrument used, the present study took into account the fact that the instrument has been translated into Spanish and that its design did not consider aspects of Latin American culture. The study was undertaken in order to validate the burnout construct with the objective of confirming that the instrument is being used correctly, independent of the subject's position in the company, and their gender, age and/or profession [21,40], as other authors have confirmed in their studies.

The study begins by developing an exploratory factorial analysis (EFA) in order to determine the coincidence, in the sample selected, of the tridimensionality of the instrument.

Subsequently, confirmatory factorial analysis (CFA) is conducted with the objective of corroborating that the factorial structure is appropriate for use with the population of middle and senior management in the border region of the country.

Considering that the instrument can be used in any employment context, it is hoped that the application of the instrument in this sector obtains reliable measure of burnout's levels. Specifically, the following hypotheses are tested:

Hypothesis 1: *The tridimensional character of the MBI-GS is maintained for the population of middle and senior management in the industrial sector of the state of Baja California, Mexico.*

Hypothesis 2: *The MBI-GS is a valid and reliable instrument for the measurement of burnout in middle and senior management in the state of Baja California, Mexico.*

2. Materials and Methods

2.1. Instrument Overview

The instrument used to measure burnout in the sample was the Spanish version of the MBI-GS, translated by Moreno et al. [41]. It is the generic version of the MBI Human Services Survey (HSS) used for professions outside the area of health, and comprises 16 items with 7 Likert-scale answer options for each question, where: 0 = on no occasion over the course of the year; 1 = very rarely over the course of the year; 2 = on some occasions over the course of the year; 3 = on many occasions over the course of the year; 4 = frequently over the course of the year; 5 = almost every day; and, 6 = every day. Maslach and Leiter describe the instrument's 3 dimensions: Exhaustion (Exha) is the central quality of burnout and the most obvious manifestation of this complex syndrome and refers to feelings of being overextended and depleted of one's emotional and physical resources [17]. Which could, for example, be exemplified by the questionnaire question "I feel exhausted by the end of my working day".

Cynicism (Cyn) is an attempt to put distance between oneself and service recipients by actively ignoring the qualities that make them unique and engaging people. Their demands are more manageable when they are considered impersonal objects of one's work. It refers to a negative, callous, or excessively detached response to various aspects of the job [17] and could be exemplified by the sentence "I only want to do my job and not be bothered".

The component of reduced efficacy (ProEf) or accomplishment represents the self-evaluation dimension of burnout. It refers to feelings of incompetence and a lack of achievement and productivity at work [17]. Could be represented by the question "In my opinion, I am very good at my job".

Of the 16 items, 10 were characterized negatively and 6 positively, with Table 1 showing the feelings to which each item refers and each identification code used in the research.

Table 1. Codes of the MBI-GS (Maslach Burnout Inventory-General Survey) instrument.

Item Code	Feeling That Represents
1 Totally exhausted	Exhausted emotionally
2 Exhausted	Finishing at the end of day
3 Fatigued	Fatigued at dawn
4 Stressed	Work is stressful
5 Resolve	Able to solve problems
6 Exhausted1	Exhausted by my work
7 Contribution	Make a contribution to work
8 Interest	Loss of interest
9 Enthusiasm	Loss of enthusiasm
10 Good	I'm good at doing my job
11 Carried out	I feel fulfilled
12 Value	Realized worthwhile things
13 Bothered	Do not bother me
14 Indifferent	I have become indifferent
15 Doubt	I doubt the value of my work
16 Efficacy	Effective in doing my job

Based on Moreno [41].

The questionnaire is structured with an introduction, followed by the employee's informed consent and the section of MBI-GS questions, and finishes with the person's demographic data, which include the following: type of management position; size of the company; time in the current position; the respondent's department; type of contract; hours worked per week; academic qualifications; marital status; and, gender.

The research conforms to the provisions of the Declaration of Helsinki in 1995 (as revised in Edinburgh 2000) [42], and all ethical guidelines were followed as required for conducting human research, including adherence to the legal requirements of Mexico.

The database was analyzed using the software IBM® SPSS® Statistics version 23 (IBM company, Chicago, IL, USA), 64 bits edition, with the Amos™ (analysis of moment structures) complementary package [43].

2.2. Methodology

The stages which comprise the methodology developed in the present study are described below.

2.2.1. Sample Selection

The professionals who belong to the middle and senior management of the 930 IMMEX manufacturing companies in the state of Baja California are the subjects of study for this investigation. Not knowing exactly the number of people in these positions, the study population is considered as being unknown. To extract the sample from the population, we used the non-probabilistic method of sampling by quota [44] with two strata, the first case of middle management, including department supervisors, group leaders, engineers and professionals, while the second stratum includes Senior management, including area managers and plant managers.

Contact with the companies to publicize the project was made by telephone and by email with the human resources department. The criterion used to determine the number of individuals to survey for each quota was for the convenience of participation; for the stratum of middle managers, 338 surveys were considered, while for the stratum of top managers there were 40 surveys, integrating a total sample of 378 employees from the state of Baja California, Mexico.

Regarding the sample size required to obtain reliable conclusions from the factorial analysis, we surpass by far what is recommended as a general rule, that indicates that the minimum is to have at least five times as many observations as the number of variables to be analyzed, and the more acceptable sample size would have a 10:1 ratio [45]. Therefore, considering a total of 16 items in the questionnaire, a sample size of 160 responses should be gathered.

2.2.2. Data Analysis

Due to the nature of the participants and settings where they were contacted, we decided to review all collected data during and after collection, similarly to reference [46]. Accordingly, we didn't have missing data in the responses to the MBI-GS questionnaire owing to the fact, that in the event of a missing response, the interviewer asked if it was possible to complete the question with the person concerned. The detection of outliers in the sample was carried out by means of the Mahalanobis d-squared distance, a statistical measurement that represents the distance, in units of standard deviation, of a point relative to the centroid [47].

EFA was used to identify the number and composition of the factors set out in Hypothesis 1. In addition, CFA was used to verify the number of underlying dimensions of the instrument and the pattern of item relationships (factor loadings). CFA also assists in the determination of how a test should be scored [48].

With the objective of determining the pertinence of developing a factorial analysis from a statistical perspective, the adequacy of implementing factorial analysis in the sample was evaluated using the determinant of the correlation matrix; the Bartlett sphericity test; the Kaiser-Meyer-Olkin (KMO) index; and, the measure of sample adequacy (MSA) for each item.

The extraction of factors was achieved via the use of principal component. In order to facilitate interpretation, the initial matrix is rotated by means of the Varimax orthogonal method, which despite not being the simplest analytical solution of the existing methods, does show the clearest separation of the factors [45] and, being independent of the distributional assumptions, is less likely to produce inadequate solutions [49]. Those factors with an eigenvalue greater than 1 were selected for extraction. Subsequently, a CFA was developed with the objective of maintaining the groupings and ensuring that the model shows an adequate fit. The estimation used for the model was undertaken by means of maximum likelihood.

The model fit for the sample was evaluated by means of 7 fit indices: Chi-square (χ^2); Root Mean Square Error of Approximation (RMSEA); Normed Fit Index (NFI); Comparative Fit Index (CFI); Relative Fit Index (RFI); Parsimony Ratio (PRATIO); and, Parsimony Normed Fit Index (PNFI).

3. Results

3.1. *Assessment of Normality*

The normality of each of the variables that comprise the instrument was evaluated by means of the standardized kurtosis index and, taking into account the absolute values obtained, shows that all are below the value of 3 recommended by DeCarlos [50]. The positive kurtosis values are found to be within the range of (0.194, 2.740), while the negative values are found to be within the range of (−0.843, −0.216); therefore, it is possible that the condition of univariate normality is fulfilled for the sample.

Evidence of extreme kurtosis with absolute values higher than 8 [51] is always a cause for concern, given that it is known to be exceptionally prejudicial in analysis used for structural equation modeling.

A prerequisite to verifying that multivariable normality has been fulfilled is to have fulfilled the condition of univariate normality in each observable variable [50]. The evaluation of this type of normality considers the normalized value of multivariate Mardia kurtosis, with the procedure carried out by comparing the Mardia coefficient for the data under study with a calculated value based on the formula $p(p+2)$, where p is the number of variables observed in the model [52]. In this case, the assumption is verified by contrasting the multivariable kurtosis value obtained via the AMOS program with the calculations made using the formula proposed [51]. Considering 16 variables for the instrument, the calculation undertaken with the formula proposed gives a value of 288, while the multivariable kurtosis index was 74.921, which is lower than the value calculated with the formula of reference, enabling the assumption, in this case, of the multivariable normality hypothesis in the data set.

The presence of multicollinearity in the data, the occurrence of which would indicate that distinct variables measure the same or are closely related, was then reviewed. In this sense, the variance inflation factor (VIF) verifies that, if this index is greater than 10, the variable could be redundant [51], while the results for the indices indicate a maximum value of 5.793; therefore, it is possible to conclude that the multicollinearity problem is not present in this data set.

From the database, 25 responses were identified as outliers and eliminated, leaving a total of 378 valid responses from further analysis. This test considered a conservative level of statistical significance with a value of $p < 0.001$ [50].

3.2. Characteristics of the Sample

The representative sample comprised 378 employees, aged from 25 to 60 (Mean ± SD: 34.01 ± 9.41), of whom 36.7% were women, 63.3% were male and 92.2% had an indefinite contract, 5.7% of which were temporary workers and 2% were not specified. With regard to working hours per week, 55.5% of subjects reported spending approximately 48 h in the office, while 22.4% reported a total of 45 h, 11.4% reported 56 or more hours, 6.5% reported 42 h, and, finally, 4.1% reported spending a minimum of 32 h working. Of those interviewed, 91.8% of employees pertain to middle management and 5.7% to senior management. 6.5% of this population has been educated up to secondary level and 20.4% up to high school level, while more than half of the sample (67.3%) has an undergraduate degree and only 5.3% has a postgraduate degree.

3.3. Factor Analysis

3.3.1. Exploratory Factor Analysis

The data were analyzed using an EFA to prove whether the structure of the instrument was similar to that established in Maslach's initial proposal, as well as to identify the existence of items with non significant factorial loadings, which, in some studies, have been eliminated.

Previously to run the EFA, the aforementioned tests were conducted with the sample data, obtaining satisfactory results in all cases. Firstly, the determinant = 3.325×10^{-5} for the correlation matrix was statistically different to zero this result, indicating that there are variables with very high intercorrelations, for which reason the analysis is feasible. Later Bartlett's test of sphericity which is based on testing the null hypothesis that the correlation matrix of measure variables, provided an identity matrix and resulted in an approximate value of $\chi^2 = 3823.886$, with 120 degrees of freedom and the $p = 0.000$. In this case, the null hypothesis is rejected, indicating that the correlation matrix is statistically different to the identity matrix. Finally, the Kaiser-Mayer-Olkin (KMO) test is used to measure the sampling adequacy, and a value of 0.885 was obtained which considered an adequate relationship among the variables [53]. In terms of the measurement of the sampling adequacy (MSA), in which the results for each variable in the anti-image correlation matrix are examined, all exceeded the threshold value of 0.5 [45], which indicates that the reduction of the variables in the present research is adequate. The satisfactory results obtained in this stage allow us to continue with the analysis by indicating that this database is suitable to perform the factor analysis.

The next stage involved the group of the 16 variables into distinct factors that will now represent the original data, with these combinations of the original variables denominated here as dimensions. The extraction of factors obtained values of 6.293 for the first dimension, 3.228 for the second and 1.219 for the last, which, together, represent 67.128% of the total explained variance. Due to the coincidences found with the grouping of the items in the present sample, the resulting dimensions are named according to the original scale [17] as emotional exhaustion (Exha), professional efficiency (ProEf) and cynicism (Cyn). Thus, we found support for Hypothesis 1.

Table 2 presents the results for the significant loadings for each factor on the instrument (16 items), with 0.4 the minimum value considered for determining the influence of the item on the factor relative to the sample size [45]. The grouping of the variables in the factors was clear in terms of the loading values, for which reason no ambiguity was found in determining the factor to which they would pertain.

Table 2. Matrix of rotated component y communalities.

Item Code	Factors			Communalities
	Exha	ProEf	Cyn	
1 Totally Exhausted	0.844			0.734
2 Exhausted	0.871			0.795
3 Fatigued	0.769			0.690
4 Stressed	0.786			0.717
6 Exhausted1	0.753			0.765
5 Resolve		0.658		0.441
7 Contribution		0.688		0.545
10 Good		0.814		0.678
11 Carried out		0.791		0.659
12 Value		0.830		0.694
16 Efficacy		0.763		0.606
8 Interest			0.768	0.786
9 Enthusiasm			0.740	0.761
13 Bother			0.652	0.442
14 Indifferent			0.774	0.748
15 Doubt			0.737	0.679
% Variance	39.334	20.173	7.621	
% Accumulated variance	39.334	59.507	67.128	

Note: Exha: emotional exhaustion; ProEf: professional efficiency; Cyn: cynicism.

According to the results, the Exha factor is characterized by the following items: 1—totally exhausted; 2—exhausted; 3—fatigued; 4—stressed; and, 6—exhausted1. The ProEf factor has high factorial loads for the items: 5—resolve; 7—contribution; 10—good; 11—carried out; 12—value; and, 16—efficacy. Finally, the following items comprise the Cyn factor: 8—interest; 9—enthusiasm; 13—bother; 14—indifferent; and, 15—doubt.

Once the significant loading had been identified, the analysis of the communalities presented in Table 2, which is the extent to which an item correlates with all other items; represents the quantity of explained variance for the factorial model in terms of each variable.

In this case, it was considered that at least half of the explained variance in each variable was obtained, as suggested by Joseph Hair [45]. The portions of the explained variance with the greatest representativeness on the instrument were items 1, 2, 4, 6, 8, 9 and 14, with values above 0.7. It was observed that the acceptable levels of explanation were fulfilled for items 3, 7, 10, 11, 12, 15 and 16, while, finally, two items (5 and 13) were identified with values below established levels, indicating the lack of sufficient explanation for the factorial model analyzed. This stage was finalized, taking into account all the items comprising the instrument for subsequent analysis.

3.3.2. Confirmatory Factorial Analysis

The most direct method for validating the results is to use a confirmatory perspective and evaluate the replicability of the results [45] in the sample of middle and senior management in the maquiladora industry of the state of Baja California. The importance of evaluating the quality of the results lies in ensuring the validity of the conclusions obtained [45]. For this, an objective evaluation was developed by means of a CFA complemented by a literature review that confirmed the grouping of the variables in the dimensions proposed, as well as a prior CFA. In particular, this section is developed with the aim of testing the degree to which the theoretical pattern of factor loading in specific dimensions represents the real data taken from the sample.

Figure 1 presents a measurement model that represents the same factorial structure on which the theoretical relationship proposed by Maslach [17] is based, as constituted by 3 latent correlational dimensions: Exha, with 5 variables and 5 associated errors (*e*); ProEf, with 6 variables and 6 associated errors (*e*); and, finally, Cyn, with 5 variables and 5 associated errors (*e*). These errors refer to inaccuracies in measuring the true variable values associated to every item in the questionnaire.

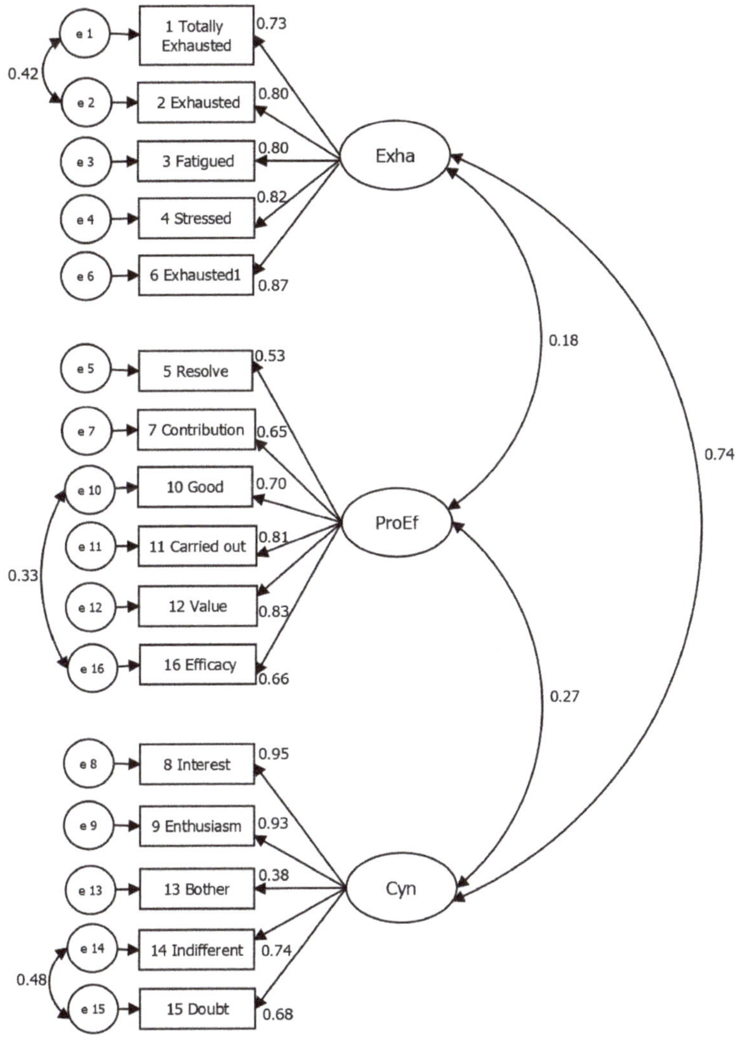

Figure 1. Model of factorial structure for MBI-GS in of middle and senior management in the maquiladora industry of the state of Baja California.

The comparison of the results of the testing of the theoretical measurement model with the reality represented in the sample is examined below, along with an analysis of both the global fit of the model and the validity criteria of the construct.

The global fit of the model is then analyzed, with Table 3 showing the final statistics produced by the CFA. χ^2 represents a traditional value for evaluating the fit of the model. A good fit should show non-significant results with a threshold of 0.05 [54]. The results show an χ^2 of 262.915 with a significant p-value; however, despite its popularity, there are various considerations that limit its use, known by some authors as the "lack of fit" [55] of a measurement, for which reason, it is recommended that it is accompanied by other fit statistics.

Table 3. Summary of the adjustment indices of the measurement model.

Goodness of Fit Statistics
Chi-square (χ^2) = 262.915 (p = 0.000)
Degrees of freedom (df) = 98
Absolute fit indices
Root mean square error of approximation (RMSEA) = 0.067
90 percent confidence interval for RMSEA = (0.057; 0.077)
Incremental fit indices
Normed fit index (NFI) = 0.932
Comparative fit index (CFI) = 0.956
Relative fit index (RFI) = 0.917
Parsimony fit indices
Parsimony Ratio (PRATIO) = 0.817
Parsimony normed fit index (PNFI) = 0.761

The value of the RMSEA index was 0.067, which is lower than 0.08 [56] for the model, with 16 variables measured in a sample of 378 data points. Using 90% of the highly significant confidence interval and a p-value for test of close fit (PCLOSE) of 0.003 for RMSEA gives the conclusion that the true value is found to be between 0.057 and 0.077, which provides additional support for the model fit. The second index considered is the minimum discrepancy (CMIN) in the χ^2 value divided by its degrees of freedom (df), giving a value of 2.683, which is notably lower than 3 [57]. In terms of the incremental fit, the CFI is the most widely used index, which, for this study, has a value of 0.956, which exceeds the threshold value of 0.95 [58].

The NFI index has a value greater than 0.9, with a good fit considered in accordance with Bentler and Bonnet [59], as does the RFI index. The parsimony indices consider the complexity of the model, which results in values considerably lower than other goodness of fit indices [60]. Mulaik et al. [55] state that it is possible to obtain parsimony of fit indices within the region 0.50–1.

The CFA results, with three relationships among the covariances of the error terms, suggest that the MBI measurement model gives a reasonably good fit, which supports continuing with the subsequent evaluations. Considering that one of the primary objectives of the CFA is to evaluate the validity of the construct of a theoretical measurement [45] this paper continues with the subsequent components that include said validity.

3.4. Convergent Validity

3.4.1. Average Variance Extracted (AVE)

The items pertaining to a specific dimension must either converge in or share a high proportion of the common variance, which is known as convergent validity.

The convergent validity was obtained by means of the AVE, calculated as the average of the variance extracted from the standardized loading [45] of the items for each dimension expressed in the following manner (1):

$$AVE = \frac{\sum_{i=1}^{n} L_i^2}{n} \quad (1)$$

where L_i^2 represents the loadings for the factor and i is the item number. For n items, the AVE is calculated as the total of the squared loadings divided by the number of items that comprise each factor. Values greater than 0.5 indicate an adequate convergence, with Table 4 showing values greater than the threshold for the Exha and Cyn dimensions, adequately fulfilling this principle, with the value for the ProEf dimension found to be very close to the established value.

Table 4. Average Variance Extracted and α Cronbach by dimension.

Factors	Items	AVE	α Cronbach
Exha	1 Totally Exhausted 2 Exhausted 3 Fatigued 4 Stressed 6 Exhausted1	0.646	0.908
ProEf	5 Resolve 7 Contribution 10 Good 11 Carried out 12 Value 16 Efficacy	0.494	0.855
Cyn	8 Interest 9 Enthusiasm 13 Bother 14 Indifferent 15 Doubt	0.585	0.841

3.4.2. Reliability

It was necessary to determine whether the questions from the scale are related to each other. The Cronbach alpha index was used to measure the reliability of the internal consistency of the instrument [61]. This index oscillates between 0 and 1, where the closer the index is to 1, the greater the internal consistency of the items analyzed. For reference, values greater than 0.7 are considered acceptable, with results lower than this value considered questionable [62]. A value of 0.882 is obtained for the total instrument, while eliminating Item 13 gives the highest total value for the MBI-GS, 0.891, which coincides with the results of the confirmatory analysis.

The scores obtained for the dimensions for emotional exhaustion give a value of 0.908, the highest value obtained without deleting any of the items, while a value of 0.855 is obtained for professional efficiency without eliminating any item. Finally, it is suggested that, for cynicism, Item 13 is again eliminated, leading to the alpha value rising from 0.841 to 0.907. As shown in Table 4, despite the suggested elimination of an item from the Cyn dimension, the α values surpass 0.8, giving good internal consistency in the items comprising each dimension.

3.5. Discriminant Validity

This type of validity shows whether the dimensions forming the general concept of MBI are truly different to each other or whether it would be possible to group all the items in one single construct for the measurement model. This value is established by means of the AVE test and should be greater when compared with the estimated correlations for the other dimensions. Table 5 shows that the AVE values found on the diagonal are higher than the estimated correlations; therefore, for this example, the discriminant validity shows evidence that each construct is unique and can be used to analyze part of the phenomenon.

Table 5. Correlations among the dimensions, average variance extracted and squared correlations.

	Exha	ProEf	Cyn
Exha	0.804 [a]		
ProEf	0.184	0.703 [a]	
Cyn	0.742	0.268	0.765 [a]

Note: [a] Root square of AVE.

The results shown in the confirmatory factor analysis, as well as the tests of convergent and discriminant validity, confirm that the MBI-GS is a valid and reliable instrument for measuring burnout in middle and senior management in the state of Baja California, Mexico, as predicted by hypothesis 2.

4. Discussion

Taking into account the various studies that have been developed around the subject of chronic job stress, the main objective of the present research is to evaluate the operability of the MBI instrument by means of factorial validation analysis.

Further to being the most commonly used instrument [26] in the literature for detecting the degrees of burnout, one of the main advantages of the MBI is its validity, with high significant correlations found for the distinct sectors where it has been applied, in the analysis of professions providing social assistance, such as nurses [63], police officers [64], and teachers [65], or even in the comparison of employees by gender [66].

The results of the present study reveal this to be the most adequate instrument for evaluating burnout syndrome in middle and senior management [67]. Taking a maximum of approximately 5 min to complete, it is, therefore, viable for application in companies where there is limited time for activities of this nature (the application of questionnaires, guided tours, etc.); moreover, it is designed for upper and senior management, who are responsible for formulating, articulating and executing strategy and policy within their organizations and who often work more than 48 h per week.

As a limitation to this type of study, we have the fact that the participation of workers is voluntary, so the study can discard the opinion of people who do not agree to participate and there is a risk of bias in the information. However, for this particular study, the strategy was to present the project to senior management, through the Human Resources department, explaining the benefits of the same for the workers and convincing them of their participation, so there was no resistance to providing answers.

From the initial statistical analysis stage, the data in the model showed the existence of three correlated dimensions (Exha, ProEf and Cyn) on which the construct can be formulated. The factorial loading for the items obtained higher values than those previously established and enabled the easy identification as to which dimension they pertain. The tests undertaken to verify the adequacy of model were completed satisfactorily. For verifying the amount of explained variance via commonality analysis, 2 items were detected, items 5 and 13, with low values compared to the established threshold. The strategy for these two largely unrepresentative items was to conserve them in the model, firstly because all the conditions were correctly fulfilled in prior analysis, and secondly because the values are slightly lower than 0.5 and, in accordance with Hair [44] are not considered low commonalities. However, the possibility of eliminating them at some point was not discounted.

A CFA was developed to provide a confirmatory focus for the established theoretical measure and, in contrast with the EFA, the number of factors were specified *a priori*, as well as the number of variables loaded on these factors. From a confirmatory perspective, the fit for the model suggests the inclusion in the evaluation of at least one absolute index of fit and an incremental index of fit, in addition to Hair's [45] χ^2 results; however, the present study evaluated 7 indices, obtaining satisfactory results for each. The Chi-square (χ^2) test, the RMSEA and its respective confidence interval were considered for the absolute fit, while, for the incremental fit, the NFI, CFI and RFI were considered, and, finally, PRATIO and PNFI were evaluated for the parsimony fit.

The modification index (MI) analysis suggested the following correlations for residual errors, with values above 27.59 for items 14–15, 1–2 and 10–16 for cynicism, emotional exhaustion and professional efficiency, respectively. This correlation represented improvements in model fit with direct evidence in the indices described above, whose final values are those presented. Studies have been found which confirm the three-factor original model that enables correlation among residual errors, showing a better fit for healthcare professionals [21], lawyers, priests, teachers and drivers [22].

The extracted variance test was carried out to complement the analysis of the validity of the construct. While analyzing the estimations of the standardized weight applied to the AVE calculation, values ranging from 0.535 to 0.949 were observed. However, a value lower than 0.384 was obtained in the factor for Item 13 on the scale for cynicism, a result which coincided with the findings of Bria et al. [21], who reported a value of 0.21 for the same items, the lowest obtained in their research, which was, however, conducted with healthcare professionals and, thus, is distinct to the profession featured in the present study.

The Cronbach alpha method was used to evaluate internal consistency for each dimension of the instrument, whose values suggest that it is robust, obtaining $\alpha_{Exha} = 0.90$, $\alpha_{ProEf} = 0.85$ and $\alpha_{Cyn} = 0.84$. These results were compared with averaged values from 7 studies [25], obtaining $\alpha_{Exha} = 0.86$, $\alpha_{ProEf} = 0.75$ and $\alpha_{Cyn} = 0.60$, from which it can be clearly observed that, in all dimensions, the values are lower than the results, showing a better level of consistency for the sample data.

5. Conclusions

The importance of a having a valid instrument in place at the beginning of any project lies in the reliability of the results obtained in the final stages. For this reason, this study centered on investigating the grouping of the factors that have an impact on the burnout measured with the MBI-GS, which is considered the predominant instrument on an international level, used in up to 90% of studies [68]. It comprises 16 items mainly related to the individual-work interaction, leaving the feelings generated by workplace relations in second place, for example whether the people with whom the subject interacts could be the cause of burnout [69].

The results of the theoretically-founded factorial statistical analysis conducted in the study confirm the original three-factor structure proposed, with 6 items obtained for professional efficiency, 5 for emotional exhaustion, and 5 for cynicism.

The Hypothesis 1 was accepted because the exploratory analysis confirmed the factorial structure of the instrument, with this result confirmed in the subsequent stage.

The Hypothesis 2 was accepted based on the fulfillment of not only the indices of fit for the model, but also the convergent and discriminant validity and reliability on which the construct's validity is based. The instrument has been shown to be adequate for detecting burnout syndrome in middle and senior management in the state of Baja California, Mexico.

The timely detection of burnout syndrome by companies will have repercussions in terms of the work climate and productivity, and also for the personal fulfillment of the employee.

In the international context, on World Day for Safety and Health at Work in 2013, the International Labor Organization (ILO) stated that, despite the fact that some workplace risks have decreased, an increase in new work-related health conditions has been registered without the application of adequate prevention, protection and control measures. Ergonomic risk factors are included among these emerging workplace risks.

It is for the above reason that ergonomic risk factors demand a governmental commitment to strengthen occupational health and safety to ensure dignified or decent work, through policies, strategic lines of action and projects with a preventive focus, in order to guarantee healthy and safe working conditions. With the health effects of these factors on employees being well-known, it is of the utmost importance to attend to them.

Author Contributions: Formal analysis, S.M.-V. and Y.B.-L.; Investigation, S.M.-V., Y.B.-L. and A.A.M.-M.; Methodology, D.T.; Validation, J.L.-R.

Funding: This research received external funding granted through the CONACYT-INS project (FRONTERAS CIENCIA) 2016-01-2433.

Conflicts of Interest: The authors declare no conflict of interest.

References

1. Houtman, I.; Jettinghoff, K.; Cedillo, L. Sensibilizando Sobre el Estrés Laboral en los PaÍses en Desarrollo, un Riesgo Moderno en un Ambiente Tradicional de Trabajo. Available online: http://www.who.int/iris/handle/10665/43770 (accessed on 29 January 2018).
2. American Institute of Stress, AIS. Workplace Stress. Available online: https://www.stress.org/workplace-stress/ (accessed on 18 January 2018).
3. Sundquist, J.; Östergren, P.-O.; Sundquist, K.; Johansson, S.-E. Psychosocial Working Conditions and Self-Reported Long-Term Illness: A Population-Based Study of Swedish-Born and Foreign-Born Employed Persons. *Ethn. Health* **2003**, *8*, 307–317. [CrossRef] [PubMed]
4. Forbes. Mexicanos, Los Más Estresados del Mundo Por su Trabajo. Available online: https://www.forbes.com.mx/mexicanos-los-mas-estresados-del-mundo-por-su-trabajo/ (accessed on 29 May 2018).
5. La torre, G.; Sestili, C.; Mannocci, A.; Sinopoli, A.; De Paolis, M.; De Francesco, S.; Rapaccini, L.; Barone, M.; Iodice, V.; Lojodice, B.; et al. Association between Work Related Stress and Health Related Quality of Life: The Impact of Socio-Demographic Variables. A Cross Sectional Study in a Region of Central Italy. *Int. J. Environ. Res. Public Health* **2018**, *15*, 159. [CrossRef] [PubMed]
6. Gamero, C. Evaluación del coste por pérdida de jornadas laborales asociado al estrés laboral: Propuesta para España. *Estud. Econ. Apl.* **2010**, *28*, 1–20.
7. Senado de la República. Gaseta del Senado Gobierno de México. Available online: http://www.senado.gob.mx/64/gaceta_del_senado/documento/77826# (accessed on 27 June 2018).
8. Kang, M.; Koh, S.; Cha, B.; Park, J.; Woo, J.; Chang, S. Association Between Job Stress on Heart Rate Variability and Metabolic Syndrome in Shipyard Male Workers. *Yonsei Med. J.* **2004**, *45*, 838–846. [CrossRef]
9. González, M.; Landero, R. Confirmación de un modelo explicativo del estrés y de los síntomas psicosomáticos mediante ecuaciones estructurales. *Rev. Panam. Salud Publica* **2008**, *23*, 7–18. [CrossRef]
10. Wu, X.; Li, Y.; Yao, Y.; Luo, X.; He, X.; Yin, W. Development of Construction Workers Job Stress Scale to Study and the Relationship between Job Stress and Safety Behavior: An Empirical Study in Beijing. *Int. J. Environ. Res. Public Health* **2018**, *15*, 2409. [CrossRef]
11. Yang, T.; Shen, Y.-M.; Zhu, M.; Liu, Y.; Deng, J.; Chen, Q.; See, L.-C. Effects of Co-Worker and Supervisor Support on Job Stress and Presenteeism in an Aging Workforce: A Structural Equation Modelling Approach. *Int. J. Environ. Res. Public Health* **2016**, *13*, 72. [CrossRef] [PubMed]
12. Yu, X.; Wang, P.; Zhai, X.; Dai, H.; Yang, Q. The Effect of Job Stress on Job Burnout Among Teachers: The Mediating Role of Self-efficacy. *Soc. Indic. Res.* **2015**, *122*, 701–708. [CrossRef]
13. Aranda, C.; Pando, M.; Salazar, J.G. Síndrome de Burnout en trabajadores de diversas actividades económicas en México. *Rev. Iberoam. Psicol. Cienc. Tec.* **2015**, *8*, 23–28.
14. Yiu-kee, C.; Tang, C.S. Existential Correlates of Burnout Among Mental Health Professionals in Hong-Kong. *J. Ment. Health Couns.* **1995**, *17*, 220–229.
15. Malach-Pines, A.; Keinan, G. Stress and Burnout: The Significant Difference. *Pers. Individ. Dif.* **2005**, *39*, 625–635. [CrossRef]
16. Książek, I.; Stefaniak, T.J.; Stadnyk, M.; Książek, J. Burnout syndrome in surgical oncology and general surgery nurses: A crosssectional study. *Eur. J. Oncol. Nurs.* **2011**, *15*, 347–350. [CrossRef]
17. Maslach, C.; Schaufeli, W.B.; Leiter, M.P. Job Burnout. *Ann. Rev. Psychol.* **2001**, *52*, 397–422. [CrossRef] [PubMed]
18. Maslach, C. Job Burnout: New Directions in Research and Intervention. *Curr. Dir. Psychol. Sci.* **2003**, *12*, 189–192. [CrossRef]
19. Bakker, A.B.; Demerouti, E.; Taris, A.W.T.; Schaufeli, W.B.; Schreurs, P.J.G. A Multigroup Analysis of the Job Demands-Resources Model in Four Home Care Organizations. *Int. J. Stress Manag.* **2003**, *10*, 16–38. [CrossRef]
20. Densten, I.L. Re-thinking burnout. *J. Organ. Behav.* **2001**, *22*, 833–847. [CrossRef]

21. Bria, M.; Spânu, F.; Bâban, A.; Dumitrascu, D.L. Maslach Burnout Inventory—General Survey: Factorial Validity and Invariance Among Romanian Healthcare Professionals. *Burn. Res.* **2014**, *1*, 103–111. [CrossRef]
22. Langballe, E.M.; Falkum, E.; Innstrand, S.T.; Aasland, O.G. The Factorial Validity of the Maslach Burnout Inventory–General Survey in Representative Samples of Eight Different Occupational Groups. *J. Career Assess.* **2006**, *14*, 370–384. [CrossRef]
23. Huibers, M.J.H.; Beurskens, A.J.H.M.; Prins, J.B.; Kant, I.J.; Bazelmans, E.; van Schayck, C.P.; Knottnerus, J.A.; Bleijenberg, G. Fatigue, Burnout, and Chronic Fatigue Syndrome Among Employees on Sick Leave: Do Attributions Make the Difference? *Occup. Environ. Med.* **2003**, *60*, i26–i31. [CrossRef]
24. Kitaoka-Higashiguchi, K.; Nakagawa, H.; Morikawa, Y.; Ishizaki, M.; Miura, K.; Naruse, Y.; Kido, T.; Higashiyama, M. Construct Validity of the Maslach Burnout Inventory-General Survey. *Stress Health* **2004**, *20*, 255–260. [CrossRef]
25. Juárez-García, A.; Idrovo, Á.J.; Camacho-Ávila, A.; Placencia-Reyes, O. Burnout Syndrome in Mexican Population: A Systematic Review. *Salud Ment.* **2014**, *37*, 157–174. [CrossRef]
26. Bambula, F.D.; Gómez, I.C. La investigación sobre el síndrome de burnout en latinoamérica entre 2000 y el 2010. *Psicol. Desde Caribe* **2016**, *33*, 113–131.
27. Arias, F.A.; González, M.E.G. Estrés, agotamiento profesional (burnout) y salud en profesores de acuerdo a su tipo de contrato. *Cienc. Trab.* **2009**, *11*, 172–176.
28. Aldrete Rodriguez, M.G.; Preciado Serrano, M.L.; Franco, S.; Pérez, J.A.; Aranda, C. Factores psicosociales laborales y síndrome de burnout, diferencias entre hombres y mujeres docentes de secundaria, zona metropolitana de Guadalajara, México. *Cienc. Trab.* **2008**, *10*, 138–142.
29. Gil-Monte, P.R.; Noyola Cortes, V.S. Estructura factorial del Cuestionario para la Evaluación del Síndrome de Quemarse por el Trabajo en maestros mexicanos de educación primaria. *Rev. Mex. Psicol.* **2011**, *28*, 7–84.
30. Roga, S.U.; Sandoval Ocana, J.I.; Gil-Monte, P.R. Prevalencia del síndrome de quemarse por el trabajo (SQT) (burnout) en maestros mexicanos. *Inf. Psicol.* **2007**, 53–63.
31. García, R.C.; Oviedo, A.M.; Santillán, M.L.V.; Velázquez, V.H.; Fiesco, M.d.S.P. Prevalencia del Síndrome de Burnout en personal de enfermería de dos hospitales del Estado de México. *Fundam. Human.* **2009**, *19*, 179–193.
32. Gholami, T.; Pahlavian, A.H.; Akbarzadeh, M.; Motamedzade, M.; Moghaddam, R.H. The role of burnout syndrome as a mediator for the effect of psychosocial risk factors on the intensity of musculoskeletal disorders: A structural equation modeling approach. *Int. J. Occup. Saf. Ergon.* **2016**, *2*, 283–290. [CrossRef] [PubMed]
33. Reynaga Estrada, P.; Pando Moreno, M. Relación del Síndrome de Agotamiento Crónico (Burnout) con el Trastorno Potencial en Jóvenes deportistas. *Invest Salud* **2005**, *7*, 153–160.
34. Instituto Nacional de Estadística y Geografía, INEGI. Censos económicos 2014. Available online: http://internet.contenidos.inegi.org.mx/contenidos/productos/prod_serv/contenidos/espanol/bvinegi/productos/nueva_estruc/702825077952.pdf (accessed on 20 June 2018).
35. Secretaria de Economía, SE. Invest in Baja. IMMEX (La Industria Manufacturera Maquiladora y de Servicios de Exportación). Available online: http://www.investinbaja.gob.mx/en/business-environment/manufacture-options (accessed on 19 August 2018).
36. Banco de Información económica. Available online: https://www.inegi.org.mx/sistemas/bie/ (accessed on 5 August 2018).
37. Programa de la industria manufacturera, maquiladora y de servicios de exportación (IMMEX)—2007 en adelante. Available online: https://www.inegi.org.mx/programas/immex/default.html#Tabulados (accessed on 8 October 2018).
38. Macias, S.; Baez, Y.; Maldonado-Macias, A.; Limon, J.; Tlapa, D. Burnout and obesity in Middle and Upper Management in the Manufacturing Industry of Baja California. In *Advanced Macroergonomics and Sociotechnical Approaches for Optimal Organizational Performance*; IGI Global: Hershey, PA, USA, 2018; p. 335.
39. Armenta-Hernández, O.D.; Maldonado-Macías, A.; García-Alcaraz, J.; Avelar-Sosa, L.; Realyvasquez-Vargas, A.; Serrano-Rosa, M.A. Relationship between Burnout and Body Mass Index in Senior and Middle Managers from the Mexican Manufacturing Industry. *Int. J. Environ. Res. Public Health* **2018**, *15*, 541. [CrossRef] [PubMed]
40. Maslach, C.; Leiter, M. Early predictors of job burnout and engagement. *J. Appl. Psychol.* **2008**, *93*, 498–512. [CrossRef]
41. Moreno-Jimenez, B.; Rodríguez-Carvajal, R.; Escobar Redonda, E. La evaluación del burnout profesional. Factorialización del MBI-GS. Un análisis preliminar. *Ansiedad y Estrés* **2001**, *7*, 69–78.
42. World Medical Association. Declaration of Helsinki. World Medical Association 2000. Available online: https://www.wma.net/wp-content/uploads/2018/07/DoH-Oct2000.pdf (accessed on 26 March 2019).
43. Arbuckle, J.L. *IBM SPSS Statistics 20 Core System. User's Guide, 2013*; IBM Corporation: Armonk, NY, USA. (in press)

44. Tashakkoru, A.; Teddlie, C. *Handbook of Mixed Methods in Social & Behavioral Research*, 2nd ed.; SAGE Publications: New York, NY, USA, 2003; pp. 278–283. ISBN 9781412972666.
45. Hair, J.F.; Black, W.C.; Babin, B.J.; Anderson, R.E. *Multivariate Data Analysis*, 7th ed.; Pearson Education Limited: Harlow, UK, 2014; pp. 60–579. ISBN 1-292-02190-X.
46. Muyanja, C.; Nayiga, L.; Brenda, N.; Nasinyama, G. Practices, knowledge and risk factors of street food vendors in Uganda. *Food Control* **2011**, *22*, 1551–1558. [CrossRef]
47. Byrne, B.M. *Structural Equation Modeling with AMOS: Basic Concepts, Applications, and Programming*, 2nd ed.; Routledge Taylor & Francis Group: New York, NY, USA, 2010; pp. 101–360. ISBN 978-0-8058-6372-7.
48. Brown, T. *Confirmatory Factor Analysis for Applied Research*, 2nd ed.; Guilford Press: New York, NY, USA, 2015; ISBN 9781462515363.
49. Fabrigar, L.; Wegener, D.; MacCallum, R.; Strahan, E. Evaluating the Use of Exploratory Factor Analysis in Psychological Research. *Psychol. Methods* **1999**, *4*, 272–299. [CrossRef]
50. DeCarlo, L. On the Meaning and Use of Kurtosis. *Psychol. Methods* **1997**, *2*, 292–307. [CrossRef]
51. Kline, R.B. *Principles and Practice of Structural Equation Modeling*, 2nd ed.; Kenny, D.A., Ed.; The Guilford Press: New York, NY, USA, 2005; pp. 49–101. ISBN 1-57230-690-4.
52. Raykov, T.; Marcoulides, G.A. *An Introduction to Applied Multivariate Analysis*; Routledge Taylor & Francis Group: New York, NY, USA, 2008; pp. 20–389. ISBN 978-0-8058-6375-8.
53. Kaiser, H.F.; Rice, J. Little Jiffy, Mark IV. *Educ. Psychol. Meas.* **1974**, *34*, 111–117. [CrossRef]
54. Barrett, P. Structural Equation Modelling: Adjudging Model Fit. *Pers. Indiv. Differ. J.* **2007**, *42*, 24–815. [CrossRef]
55. Mulaik, S.A.; James, L.R.; Van Altine, J.; Bennett, N.; Lind, S.; Stilwell, C.D. Evaluation of Goodness-of-fit Indices for Structual Equation Models. *Psych. Bull.* **1989**, *105*, 430–445. [CrossRef]
56. MacCallum, R.; Browne, M.; Sugawara, H. Power Analysis and Determination of Sample Size for Covariance Structure Modeling. *Psychol. Methods* **1996**, *1*, 130–149. [CrossRef]
57. Bollen, K.A. *Structural Equations with Latent Variables*; Wiley: New York, NY, USA, 1989; pp. 248–489. ISBN 978-0-471-01171-2.
58. Hu, L.; Bentler, P. Cutoff Criteria for Fit Indexes in Covariance Structure Analysis: Conventional Criteria Versus New Alternatives. *Struct. Equ. Modeling* **1999**, *6*, 1–55. [CrossRef]
59. Bentler, P.; Bonnet, D. Significance Tests and Goodness of Fit in the Analysis of Covariance Structures. *Psych. Bull.* **1980**, *88*, 588–606. [CrossRef]
60. Hooper, D.; Coughlan, J.; Mullen, M. Structural Equation Modelling: Guidelines for Determining Model Fit. *Electron. J. Bus. Res. Method* **2008**, *6*, 53–60. [CrossRef]
61. Cronbach, L.J. Coefficient alpha and the internal structure of tests. *Psychometrika* **1951**, *16*, 297–334. [CrossRef]
62. George, D.; Mallery, P. *IBM SPSS Statistics 23 Step by Step: A Simple Guide and Reference*, 14th ed.; Routledge: New York, NY, USA, 2016; ISBN 0134320255.
63. Hayter, M. Utilizing the Maslach Burnout Inventory to measure burnout in HIV/AIDS specialist community nurses: The implications for clinical supervision and support. *Prim. Health Care Res.* **2000**, *1*, 243–253. [CrossRef]
64. Gil, P.R. Validez factorial de la adaptación al español del Maslach Burnout Inventory-General Survey. *Salud Públi. México* **2002**, *44*, 33–40.
65. Hakanen, J.J.; Bakker, A.B.; Schaufeli, W.B. Burnout and work engagement among teachers. *J. School Psychol.* **2006**, *43*, 495–513. [CrossRef]
66. Purvanova, R.K.; Muros, J.P. Gender differences in burnout: A meta-analysis. *J. Vocat. Behav.* **2010**, *77*, 168–185. [CrossRef]
67. Macias, S.I.; Baez, Y.; Maldonado, A.; Tlapa, D.; Limon, J. *Comparison of the Techniques to Measure the Burnout in the Medium and Higher Controls of the Manufacturing Industry*; Congreso Internacional de Ergonomía: Mexicali, Baja California, Mexico, 20 April 2018; Available online: http://www.semac.org.mx/images/stories/libros/Libro%20SEMAC%202018.pdf (accessed on 26 March 2019).

68. Scheufeli, W.; Enzmann, D. *The Burnout Companion to Study and Practice: A Critical Analysis*, 1st ed.; Taylor & Francis Group: New York, NY, USA, 1998; p. 224. ISBN 9780748406982.
69. Martínez, P.A. El síndrome de Burnout. Evolución conceptual y estado actual de la cuestión. *VivatAcademia* **2010**, 112. [CrossRef]

International Journal of
Environmental Research and Public Health

MDPI

Article

The Mediating Role of Job Strain in the Transformational Leadership–Safety Behavior Link: The Buffering Effect of Self-Efficacy on Safety

Byung-Jik Kim [1,2] and Se-Youn Jung [3,*]

1 Sogang Business School, Sogang University, Seoul 04107, Korea; kimbj82@business.kaist.edu
2 College of Business, Korea Advanced Institute of Science and Technology, Seoul 02455, Korea
3 Prime College, Korea National Open University, Seoul 03087, Korea
* Correspondence: jseyoun@knou.ac.kr

Received: 15 March 2019; Accepted: 18 April 2019; Published: 21 April 2019

Abstract: Although some previous studies have examined the impact of transformational leadership on safety behavior, those works have paid relatively less attention to the intermediating role of employees' job strain in the link as well as contingent variables that moderate the relationship. Considering that not only job strain substantially affects employees' perceptions, attitudes, and behaviors in an organization, but also there are some contextual factors that moderate the relationships, we investigated intermediating mechanisms (i.e., mediator and moderator) in the relationship between transformational leadership and safety behavior. Relying on the context-attitude-behavior framework, we conducted a structural equation modeling analysis with a moderated mediation model. Specifically, we hypothesized that the level of an employee's job strain would mediate the transformational leadership–safety behavior link. We also hypothesized that an employee's self-efficacy regarding safety would moderate the association between job strain and safety behavior. Using survey data from 997 South Korean employees, we found that all of our hypotheses were supported. The findings suggest that the level of an employee's job strain mediates and elaborately explains the transformational leadership–safety behavior link. Moreover, an employee's self-efficacy regarding safety is a buffering factor which decreases the harmful effects of job strain on safety behavior.

Keywords: transformational leadership; safety behavior; job strain; self-efficacy regarding safety; moderated mediation model

1. Introduction

Accidents at work have been considered as an important topic due to their profound impact on human life at the physical, mental, and economic levels. Accidents at work function as a fatal blow not only to the victims, but also to their firms and the national economy. The mental and physical damages caused by accidents at work usually make the daily life of the victims devastating for a lifetime. Furthermore, companies with accidents at work are more likely to suffer serious economic losses and long recovery periods. Therefore, efforts to reduce accidents at work are highly required to protect employees' well-being as well as firms' sustainability.

According to Bird and his colleague's domino theory [1], before the occurrence of an accident, a "precursor" appears which functions as the direct cause of the accident. Among various precursors, employees' unsafe behavior (e.g., impulsive or careless behavior) has been regarded as one of the most direct antecedents of an accident. To enhance the quality of employees' safety behavior, previous studies have suggested various factors influencing safety behavior. For example, the job demand–resources (JD-R) model [2,3] suggests a useful conceptual model which describes the impact of various physical, psychological, and organizational factors on safety outcomes. The model points out that two types of working conditions including job demands and job resources significantly affect safety outcomes such as safety behavior, accidents, and injuries. The job demands dimension consists of various components that are negatively associated with safety behavior, including a bad physical environment, a high level of work pressure, complexities, and risks. In addition, the job resources dimension consists of various factors that are positively related to safety behavior, including knowledge, autonomy, and a supportive environment (e.g., social support, leadership, a safety climate).

Among the various antecedents, in this paper, we focus on leadership styles, especially transformational leadership, due to its critical role in explaining various organizational outcomes by affecting employees' cognitions, emotions, and behavior [4–6]. Transformational leadership is defined as a leadership style "broadening and elevating followers' goals and providing them with confidence to perform beyond the expectations specified in the implicit or explicit exchange agreement" [6]. Although some scholars have investigated the relationship between transformational leadership and employees' safe behavior [7–9], we believe that there are some research gaps to be additionally addressed.

First, the previous studies which delved into the association between transformational leadership and safety behavior have underexplored the importance of job strain in explaining the intermediating mechanism of the relationship. Job strain can be defined as an employee's negative perceptions, emotions, and physiological states which emerge when an employee recognizes that he or she cannot adequately deal with various external stimuli such as interpersonal relationships, job characteristics, and the work environment [10–13]. The concept has been known to critically influence employees' perceptions, attitudes, and behaviors by diminishing cognitive/emotional/physical abilities to implement his or her tasks and duties. Then, eventually, it deteriorates the quality of his or her performance in an organization [11–13]. In other words, job strain of employees functions as a critical construct which not only explains the influence of transformational leadership on employees in an organization, but also predicts their important attitudes or behaviors. Despite its significant theoretical and practical impact on employees in an organization, to the best of our knowledge, there has not been any research to have considered job strain as a critical mediator in explaining the influence of transformational leadership on employees' safe behavior. Although some previous studies have suggested a bivariate relationship between transformational leadership and job strain [7] as well as between job strain and safety behavior [12], those did not examine the entire relationship among the three variables in an integrated manner based on an overarching theoretical ground. By investigating the intermediating role of job strain with a theoretically overarching basis, we can provide an elaborate explanation on how transformational leadership positively affects safety behavior at work. Thus, examining the role of job strain in describing the association is highly required.

Second, previous studies on the transformational leadership–safety behavior link have paid less attention to the contingent or contextual factors that moderate the relationship. These studies have focused on various intermediators in the link. For example, Shen and his colleagues [9] reported that transformational leadership influences employees' safety behavior through the sequential mediating roles of safety-specific leader-member exchange (LMX), safety climate, safety knowledge, and safety motivation. Although finding various mediating factors in the relationship between transformational leadership and safety behavior is very important, it is not enough to elaborately describe the influence of transformational leadership on safety behavior because the mediating variables cannot fully explain the association in all situations or contexts. In other words, the explanation of the mediators is limited to a certain situation or context. Thus, we suggest that examining contingent variables (i.e., moderators) in the link would contribute to elaborating the transformational leadership–safety behavior literature.

To deal with these issues, in the present study, we have investigated the intermediating effect of job strain between transformational leadership and safety behavior, as well as the moderating effect of self-efficacy regarding safety on the job strain–safety behavior link. The theoretical logic is based on the context-attitude-behavior model [14,15], which explains the mediation structure. Grounded on it, we expect that transformational leadership, as one of the important contexts, may build employees' behavior (i.e., safety behavior) by affecting their attitude (i.e., job strain). Based on previous works, we suggest that transformational leadership would decrease the level of employees' job strain [7,16,17] and that employees' job strain would increase safety behavior [12,18–21]. In the present study, considering that stress indicates changes in well-being because of various stressors while strain means lowered levels of well-being or functioning (e.g., exhaustion, tension, anxiety, and rumination) [11,12,17], we focus on strain of employees at work.

In addition, we propose that there may be contingent factors that moderate the relationship between job strain and safety behavior. Although job strain may diminish the quality of employees' safety behavior, some buffering factors can weaken the negative influence of job strain on safety behavior. Among those factors, we have focused on employees' self-efficacy regarding safety since the concept of self-efficacy has been regarded as one of the most fundamental factors which explain an individual's perceptions, attitudes, and behavior [22,23]. Based on Eden and Zuk's definition [24], we have defined self-efficacy regarding safety as an individual's overall estimate or expectation of his or her ability to effectively deal with safety-related situations.

When an employee has a high level of self-efficacy regarding safety, he or she can protect himself/herself from the harmful influences of job strain. Furthermore, the employee may feel that he or she has enough abilities to effectively deal with the harmful effects of job strain at work. Through this, the negative psychological and physical states from job strain would not substantially diminish the quality of safety behavior. On the contrary, if the level of an employee's self-efficacy regarding safety is low, he or she may feel that he or she cannot adequately deal with many issues from unsafe situations at work. Then, the negative influences of job strain may be facilitated and amplified, being considerably damaging to his or her safe behavior.

To empirically test the above hypotheses, by utilizing data from 997 employees in South Korea, we conducted a structural equation modeling (SEM) analysis with a moderated mediation model.

2. Theories and Hypotheses

2.1. Transformational Leadership and Job Strain

Some previous works on leadership have shown that transformational leadership decreases the degree of an employee's job strain [7,16,17]. According to Cummings and Cooper [25], stress can be defined as "the force that causes a strain in the physical and psychological states by escaping from the state of stability". As the concept of stress develops, there have been a lot of discussions about the concept as well as attempts to describe it in terms of industrial/organizational psychology and organizational behavior theories [11,12]. In the present study, considering that stress indicates changes in well-being because of various stressors while strain means lowered levels of well-being or functioning (e.g., exhaustion, tension, anxiety, and rumination) [11,12,17], we have focused on strain of employees at work. An employee's job strain has been considered as an important factor which diminishes cognitive/emotional/physical abilities to implement his or her tasks and duties, eventually deteriorating the quality of his or her performance [10–13]. Based on many previous works on job strain, we have defined job strain as an employee's negative perceptions, emotions, and physiological states which emerge from recognizing that he or she cannot adequately deal with various external stimuli such as interpersonal relationships, job characteristics, or the work environment [11–13,26,27].

Through providing employees with a higher level of inspirational motivation, idealized influence, supportive caring, and intellectual challenges, transformational leadership can reduce various uncomfortable perceptions and emotions in an organization [7,16,17]. Specifically, we suggest that each of the sub-dimensions of transformational leadership may decrease the level of employees' job strain as follows.

First, a leader with transformational leadership is likely to provide inspirational motivation to his or her followers. Through this, the followers of the leader may pursue noble values and goals beyond their own ego-centric interests [28,29]. Then, the followers may try to proactively cooperate with their colleagues to achieve novel objectives, which tend to be collective-level. Through this collaborative atmosphere, the followers may feel that they are safe and trusted by colleagues in the organization. Those positive perceptions would decrease their level of job strain.

Second, through idealized influence, a leader with transformational leadership can provide psychological safety to his or her followers, directly contributing to reducing their job strain [28]. The followers of transformational leadership are likely to regard the leaders as their role model, identifying with their leader [30]. Through this identification, the followers would feel that they are competent enough to achieve collective and noble goals like their transformational leader. Their positive perceptions and feelings would alleviate their job strain.

Third, a transformational leader tends to stimulate employees to think differently with traditional practices. Through this intellectual stimulation, the followers may try to solve various work problems with novel approaches [30]. The new approaches would help the followers to reframe their stressful experiences in positive and effective ways [31]. Furthermore, in the process of stimulation, followers may effectively solve difficult problems in an organization. Their positive experiences would enhance a follower's sense of self-efficacy, facilitating the more efficient problem-solving ability of followers. By virtue of it, the level of employees' job strain would be decreased.

Lastly, by providing individual consideration, a transformational leader is likely to reduce employees' job strain. It is self-explanatory that the leadership style can decrease the level of employees' strain since the leader's supportive caring for followers in an individual manner would function as a psychological base for them. The followers may feel that their negative emotions such as anxiety, fatigue, and anger in the process of working are healed and restored, by relying on the psychological base [5,28]. Based on the reasons described above, we suggest that transformational leadership is negatively associated with employees' job strain in an organization.

Hypothesis 1. *Transformational leadership is negatively related to employees' job strain.*

2.2. Employee's Job Strain and Safety Behavior

Safety behavior has been considered as one of the most important safe performances in an organization, being defined as employees' behaviors which seek to prevent mental and physical hazards [12,32–34]. Many previous works have reported that safety behavior is closely associated with occupational injuries and accidents in various industries [33,35–37].

Based on previous studies [12,18–21], we suggest that job strain would decrease the level of an employee's safety behavior. As job strain increases, employees may experience functional diminishment in their cognitive/emotional/physical areas [18–20]. The loss of such functions has a serious adverse effect on an employee's abilities pertinent to both attention and prevention for safety [12,18–20]. According to the explanation of the stress–thought model, stress not only increases psychological anxiety and physical fatigue, which cause deterioration of cognitive functions, but also makes normal thinking impossible [19,20]. Considering that adequate situational judgments and decision-making processes are essential for conducting proper safety behavior, stress can have a critical and harmful effect on safety behavior. In addition, according to extant works which have explored the relationship between emotions and decision-making processes [38,39], individuals are likely to experience negative emotions when they are under stress. Then, these negative experiences would lower the level of their logical thinking and judgment ability, eventually resulting in impulsive decision-making and unsafe behavior [38,39]. Based on the above studies, we can hypothesize that job strain will reduce the level of employees' safety behavior.

Hypothesis 2. *An employee's strain is negatively related to his or her safety behavior.*

2.3. Mediating Role of Job Strain between Transformational Leadership and Safety Behavior

As described above, we suggest that an employee's job strain would mediate the relationship between transformational leadership and safety behavior. Based on the above arguments, we believe that transformational leadership may enhance the level of an employee's safety behavior by diminishing his or her job strain at work.

To integrate our hypotheses, which are described above, based on a theoretical ground, we have relied on the context–attitude-behavior framework [14,15] that bolsters the mediation structure. This perspective suggests that a variety of contexts at work (e.g., organizational systems, rules, leadership, and environments) are important preceding factors which significantly affect the attitudes and behavior of employees. Grounded on it, we expect that transformational leadership, as one of the critical contexts, would create employees' behavior (i.e., safety behavior) by affecting their attitude (i.e., job strain). Previous works theoretically and empirically bolster our hypotheses by demonstrating the negative association between transformational leadership and job strain [7,16,17] and job strain and safety behavior [12,18–21]. Thus, we hypothesize as follows.

Hypothesis 3. *Employees' job strain mediates the relationship between transformational leadership and safety behavior.*

2.4. Moderating Effect of Employees' Self-Efficacy regarding Safety between Job Strain and Safety Behavior

We suggest that there may be contingent factors which moderate the relationship between job strain and safety behavior. Although job strain would decrease the quality of an employee's safety behavior, there may be some buffering factors which can diminish the negative impact of job strain on safety behavior. Among various buffering factors, in this paper, we have focused on employees' self-efficacy regarding safety because the concept of self-efficacy has been known as one of the most fundamental variables which explain individuals' perceptions, attitudes, and behavior [22,23].

According to Bandura, self-efficacy is defined as the "beliefs in one's capabilities to organize and execute courses of action required in managing prospective situations. Efficacy beliefs influence how people think, feel, motivate themselves, and act" [22]. Previous works have reported the significant role of self-efficacy in various organizational outcomes [22–24]. This concept is considered as a both task-specific and general variable, and it has been known as a dispositional trait that significantly explains individual behaviors across various situations [40]. In this research, we have applied the concept into safety-related contexts. Thus, based on Eden and Zuk's definition [24], we have defined self-efficacy regarding safety as an individual's overall estimate or expectation of his or her ability to effectively deal with safety-related situations.

We believe that an employee's self-efficacy regarding safety can function as a buffering factor that diminishes the negative effects of job strain on the employee's safety behavior. As described above, job strain would deteriorate the quality of an employee's safety behavior. The employee's anxiety and physical fatigue at work which originate in job strain would diminish his or her cognitive functions, directly destroying adequate safe-related decision making. However, if the employee has a high level of self-efficacy regarding safety, he or she can protect himself/herself from the harmful influence of job strain. By virtue of the high-level of self-efficacy, he or she may feel considerable competence in effectively dealing with the harmful effects of job strain. Then, the negative psychological and physical states from job strain may no longer significantly decrease the quality of his or her safety behavior.

In contrast, when an employee has a low level of self-efficacy regarding safety, he or she may feel that he or she cannot deal with various problems from unsafe situations at work (e.g., how to implement safe-related rules and procedures or how to decrease the possibility of safe accidents). In that situation, the negative impact of job strain would be facilitated and amplified, significantly damaging the employee's cognitive abilities. Then, the quality of safe-related decision-making would be substantially decreased, critically destroying his or her safe behavior. Thus, we propose that an employee's self-efficacy regarding safety may moderate the relationship between job strain and the employee's safety behavior (Please see Figure 1).

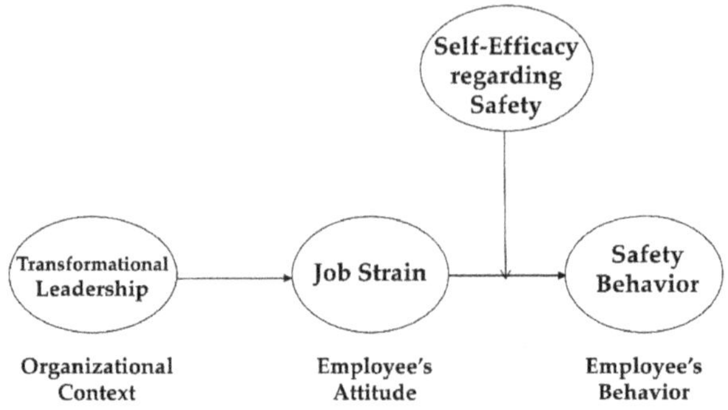

Figure 1. Framework of research model.

Hypothesis 4: *An employee's self-efficacy regarding safety may moderate the relationship between his or her job strain and safety behavior.*

3. Method

3.1. Data Collection

Considering the residence and industry of the respondents, we chose and contacted companies which had more than 15 employees. Then, considering the size of the company, roughly 3–8 employees were randomly selected. Survey-trained researchers conducted the survey using structured questionnaires. When the quality of the response was bad, the survey was conducted again. Through these processes, data from 997 employees from 103 firms who adequately responded to all the items were utilized in the analysis. The characteristics of the sample are described below (Please see Table 1).

Table 1. Descriptive characteristics of our sample.

Characteristic	Percent
Gender	
Male	74.8%
Female	25.2%
Age	
20s	38.8%
30s	42.5%
40s	15.8%
Above 50s	2.9%
Education	
Below high school diploma	35.1%
Community college	16.4%
Bachelor	43.6%
Master's degree or more	3.4%
Tenure (in year)	
Below 5	45.1%
5 to 10	36.2%
10 to 15	10.6%
15 to 20	4.8%
20 to 25	2.6%
Above 25	1.7%

Table 1. *Cont.*

Characteristic	Percent
Firm size	
Above 1000	8.7%
500–1000 members	14.8%
300–499 members	13.1%
100–299 members	32.6%
50–99 members	25.5%
Below 50 members	5.3%
Industry Type	
Manufacturing	53.5%
Transportation	11.0%
Construction	8.9%
Information service and telecommunications	3.2%
Sales	6.9%
Health and welfare	8.6%
Financial/insurance	6.2%
Research and development (R & D)	1.7%

3.2. Measures

We measured the research variables with a five-point Likert scale (1 = strongly disagree, 5 = strongly agree). Then, we computed internal consistency of the variables by using Cronbach alpha values.

3.2.1. Transformational Leadership

We utilized 13 items that were adapted from the Multifactor Leadership Questionnaire (MLQ) to measure transformational leadership. The scale was developed by Bass and Avolio [30], consisting of four sub-dimensions: Idealized influence, inspirational motivation, intellectual stimulation, and individual consideration. The 13 items were selected by the suggestions of previous studies on transformational leadership [5–7]. Sample items were "the leader in my organization is a role model I want to be" and "my leader articulates a compelling vision of the future". The Cronbach alpha value was 0.92.

3.2.2. Job Strain

To measure the level of job strain, we utilized 10 items of the job strain scale by adapting the scale of DeJoy and his colleagues [41]. The 10 items of job strain were selected by the authors because those adequately reflected the core components of the measure [41]. Sample items were "I feel nervous and strain because of work" and "I feel nervous when I work". The Cronbach alpha value was 0.85.

3.2.3. Safety Behavior

We utilized 8 items of the Neal and Griffin's [36] scale to measure safety behavior. The scale consisted of two sub-dimensions: Safety participation (SP) and safety compliance (SC). Sample items included "I use all necessary safety equipment to do my job" (SC) and "I put in extra effort to improve the safety of workplace" (SP). The value of Cronbach alpha was 0.94.

3.2.4. Self-Efficacy regarding Safety

To measure the level of employees' self-efficacy regarding safety, we utilized four items by adapting the self-efficacy scale of Bandura [42]. Sample items were "I am confident in reducing the risk of accidents" and "I am capable of maintaining and improving the safety of my workplace". The value of Cronbach alpha was 0.89.

3.2.5. Control Variables

Considering that various factors can influence employees' safety behavior [33], we included employees' gender, tenure, position, and education level in our analysis to control for employees' safety behavior.

3.3. Statistical Analysis

Frequency analysis and correlation analysis were performed using the SPSS 21.0 program. Furthermore, we conducted a structural equation modeling (SEM) analysis by using the Amos 21.0 program. SEM, unlike the existing multiple regression analysis methodology, is capable of "simultaneously" analyzing the direct or indirect path between variables in an integrated model.

Considering the suggestion of Anderson and Gerbing [43], we took a two-step approach which includes the measurement model and the structural model. To evaluate the model fit of our hypothesized model, various fit indices such as the comparative fit index (CFI), the turker–lewis index (TLI), and the root mean square error of approximation (RMSEA) were utilized. According to previous studies [44,45], when the values of CFI and TLI of a certain model are greater than 0.90 and the value of RMSEA is less than 0.06, then the model can be considered as a good model. Based on this, bootstrapping analysis was conducted to confirm whether the indirect effect of our research model was significant.

4. Results

4.1. Descriptive Statistics

The descriptive statistics of this research are shown in Table 2. The main research variables including the independent variable, mediator, moderator, and dependent variable were highly correlated.

Table 2. Means, standard deviations, and correlations between variables.

Variable	Mean	SD	1	2	3	4	5	6	7
1. Gender	1.25	0.44	-						
2. Tenure (year)	6.254	5.66	−0.19 **	-					
3. Position	2.57	0.53	0.29 **	−0.43 **	-				
4. Education level	3.12	0.99	−0.13 **	−0.22 **	−0.14 **	-			
5. Transformational Leadership	3.25	0.64	−0.10 **	0.02	−0.10 **	−0.01	-		
6. Job Strain	2.84	0.66	0.13 **	−0.03	−0.00	0.03	−0.17 **	-	
7. Safety Behavior	3.44	0.78	−0.18 **	0.16 **	−0.10 **	−0.11 **	0.28 **	−0.15 **	-
8. Self-Efficacy regarding Safety	3.37	0.80	−0.24 **	0.19 **	−0.15 **	−0.13 **	0.28 **	−0.12 **	0.74 **

Note: * $p < 0.01$. With regard to gender, male is coded as 1, and female is coded as 2. With regard to position, general manager or higher are coded as 5, deputy general manager and department manager as 4, assistant manager as 3, clerk as 2, and others below clerk as 1. With regard to education, "below high school diploma" level is coded as 4, "community college" level as 3, "bachelor's" level as 2, and "master's degree or more" level is coded as 1.

4.2. Measurement Model

To check whether the level of discriminant validity was appropriate, we conducted a confirmatory factor analysis (CFA) for the research variables which were evaluated by the same employee (i.e., transformational leadership, job strain, safety behavior, and self-efficacy regarding safety). The four-factor model had a good fit to the observations ($\chi2$ (df = 140) = 594.71; CFI = 0.965; TLI = 0.958; RMSEA= 0.057). Then, we conducted sequential chi-square ($\chi2$) difference tests to compare the four-factor model with the three-factor, two-factor, and single-factor model, respectively. Specifically, considering that safety behavior and self-efficacy were very highly correlated, we made the two-factor model which loaded the two variables on the same factor The results of the test showed that the four-factor model had the best fit among all alternative models. Therefore, we believe that the research variables are distinctive (Please see Table 3).

Table 3. Chi-square difference tests among alternative measurement models.

Model	χ^2	*df*	CFI	TLI	RMSEA	Δdf	$\Delta\chi^2$	Preference
1 Single Factor Model	3653.07	146	0.733	0.687	0.155			
2 Factor Model that integrates (1) TL with job strain, (2) safety behavior with self-efficacy regarding safety	2309.20	145	0.835	0.806	0.122	1	1343.87	2 Factor Model
3 Factor Model that integrates self-efficacy with safety behavior	1092.36	143	0.928	0.914	0.082	2	1216.84	3 Factor Model
4 Factor Model	594.71	140	0.965	0.958	0.057	3	497.65	4 Factor Model

Note: CFI means comparative fit index, TLI means turker–lewis index, and RMSEA means root mean square error of approximation. In addition, Tl means transformational leadership.

4.3. Structural Model

4.3.1. Result of Mediation Analysis

We established a moderated mediation model by utilizing the SEM technique. In the analysis, the association between transformational leadership and safety behavior was mediated by employees' job strain.

The fit indices of our hypothetical model (Model 1) was good enough: $\chi 2 = 323.22$ (df = 77), CFI = 0.960, TLI = 0.945, and RMSEA = 0.057. In the model, all the control variables (i.e., gender, position, tenure, and education level) were not statistically significant. The model demonstrated that transformational leadership was significantly and negatively associated with job strain ($\beta = -0.20$, $p < 0.001$), and job strain was significantly and negatively related to safety behavior ($\beta = -0.06$, $p < 0.05$). The results suggest that Hypothesis 1 and 2 were supported.

4.3.2. Result of Moderation Analysis

To test the moderating effect of employees' self-efficacy regarding safety, we built a moderated mediation model which simultaneously included both the mediation structure and moderation structure. The moderation effect of employees' self-efficacy regarding safety on the association between job strain and safety behavior was tested by the model (see Figure 2). As described above, job strain and safety behavior were transformed into mean-centered variables and the interaction term was calculated by multiplying the two transformed variables [46]. Please consider that centered variables are useful in (i) estimating the interaction terms without loss of correlations and (ii) decreasing and testing multicollinearities among research variables. In addition, we tested whether there was a multicollinearity bias between job strain and self-efficacy regarding safety by using the SPSS program. To test this, we calculated the variance inflation factors (VIF) and tolerances [47]. The VIF for job strain and self-efficacy regarding safety was 1.02 and 1.02, respectively, and the tolerance statistics were 0.99 and 0.99, respectively. Because the obtained VIF values were smaller than 10, as well as the tolerance statistics above 0.2, we can conclude that the two variables (job strain and self-efficacy regarding safety) were relatively free from the issue of multicollinearity.

The coefficient of the interaction term ($\beta = 0.07$, $p < 0.01$) was significant, implying that employees' self-efficacy regarding safety functions as a moderator in the association between job strain and safety behavior. In other words, when the level of an employee's self-efficacy regarding safety is high, the negative effect of job strain on safety behavior is decreased. Thus, the results support Hypothesis 4.

4.4. Bootstrapping Analysis

We conducted bootstrapping analysis with a sample of 5000 to test Hypothesis 3, which suggested that there is a mediating effect of job strain between transformational leadership and safety behavior. Note that the mediation effect is significant at a 5% level when the 95% bias-corrected confidence interval (CI) for the mediation effect does not include zero [48]. In the analysis, the bias-corrected CI for the effect on the pathway from transformational leadership to safety behavior via job strain excluded zero (95% CI = (0.01, 0.04)). Thus, the result indicates that the mediation effect of job strain on the path was significant at the level of 5%, supporting Hypothesis 3.

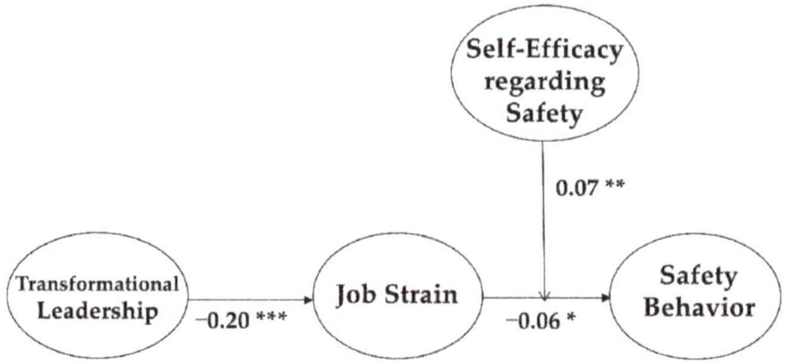

Figure 2. The standardized estimate values of the final model. Notes: * $p < 0.05$, ** $p < 0.01$, *** $p < 0.001$.

5. Discussion

In the present paper, we examined the underlying mechanisms of the relationship between transformational leadership and safety behavior. To empirically test our hypotheses, data from employees in South Korea were utilized. By conducting a moderated mediation model analysis with the SEM technique, we found that employees' job strain mediated the association between transformational leadership and safety behavior. In addition, employees' self-efficacy regarding safety functioned as a moderator in the relationship between job strain and safety behavior. In this section, some theoretical and practical implications can be drawn from our results.

5.1. Theoretical Implication

We believe that this research may contribute to extending transformational leadership and safety behavior literature by providing these theoretical implications.

First, we delved into the mediating role of job strain to explain the influence of transformational leadership on employees' safe behavior. Previous works which examined the association between these variables had paid less attention to the significance of job strain in describing intermediating processes in the link. Considering that employees' job strain substantially influences employees' perceptions, attitudes, and behaviors, eventually decreasing the quality of various organizational outcomes [10–13], our attempt to reveal the important role of job strain as a mediator in the transformational leadership–safety behavior link would be meaningful. Through it, we expect that this research may contribute to elaborating transformational leadership and safety behavior literature.

Second, we found a contingent factor which moderated the relationship between transformational leadership and employees' safety behavior. Although some previous studies have reported mediators in the link, those have paid less attention to the contingent or contextual factors which moderate the relationship. Of course we acknowledge that investigating mediators in the link would be highly required. However, to elaborately explain the intermediating mechanisms in the transformational leadership–safety behavior link, it is highly required to find certain conditions or contexts under which the mediators work well, since the mediating variables cannot always intermediate the link in all situations. Therefore, we expect that our finding that employees' self-efficacy regarding safety functions as a buffering factor to decrease harmful effects of job strain on safety behavior would enrich previous works on transformational leadership and safety behavior.

5.2. Practical Implications

We expect that our findings may provide business leaders with practical implications. First, leaders or top management teams who want to enhance employees' safety behavior through implementing transformational leadership would get some insights from this paper. Our results demonstrated that transformational leadership can increase the quality of an employee's safety behavior through decreasing his or her job strain. Thus, to check whether their attempt to enhance employees' safety behavior through facilitating transformational leadership is successful, the top management teams or leaders should monitor the changes in the level of employees' job strain as an indicator. If the level of job strain has not changed or has even increased, this would indicate that their transformational leadership does not function effectively enough to boost employees' safety behavior. In addition, the leaders using transformational leadership should focus their leadership behavior on employees' job strain by implementing "job strain-specific" leadership.

Second, the findings demonstrated that employees' self-efficacy regarding safety functions as a buffering factor in the association between employees' job strain and safety behavior. We expect that the results may emphasize the importance of employees' individual characteristics in preventing the harmful effects of job strain on safety behavior. As the finding suggests, an employee's job strain is not always harmful to his or her safety behavior. Its negative impact would be minimized when the employee has a high-level of self-efficacy regarding how to implement safe-related procedures and how to decrease the possibility of safe accidents. Therefore, we suggest that top management teams or leaders should attempt to foster employees' self-efficacy regarding safety by providing them with safe education programs, safety guidance, and safety systems in an organization.

5.3. Limitations and Suggestions for Future Studies

Although we believe that this research has valuable implications from the theoretical and empirical point of view, it has some limitations which need to be addressed. First, in this study, we found that transformational leadership affects safety behavior through "psychological factors" such as job strain. However, prior to such psychological factors, "physical environments" or "physical states of employees" may affect safety behavior. Further studies are needed to verify this. Second, although we conducted a SEM analysis to test our mediation hypothesis, we could not adequately reveal the causal relationships that our research hypotheses claim since this study only utilized cross-sectional data. This should be complemented and alleviated by not only utilizing a longitudinal research design but also by considering the influence of third variables or alternative explanations [49]. In addition, future studies should deal with the fundamental concern that cross-sectional data cannot adequately describe and explain the interaction effects between variables. Third, the data of this study were collected through participants' self-reports. Since the employee's behavior which is reflected in the self-report survey may be different from his or her actual behavior, there needs to be adequate supplementation. For example, a third party's observation or behavioral assessment can be good alternative ways to collect data. Fourth, because the same respondents responded to our survey at the same time, they cannot be free from the common method bias problem. The problem is likely to lead to an overestimation of the correlation between the variables. This limitation needs to be dealt with. Lastly, this paper could not fully utilize the entire items of each measure for our research variables (i.e., transformational leadership and job strain). Although we chose core and essential items from the original version of the measures, future studies should use the full items of the original measures. Fifth, in this study, we only focused on employees' positive behavior, such as safety behavior, when we investigated the impact of transformational leadership in an organization. However, considering that negative behavior of employees also critically influences organizational outcomes, future studies are needed to deal with negative behavior such as unsafe behavior or counterproductive work behavior. Lastly, this paper did not adequately deal with the issue of nesting of data. Considering that some respondents may be nested into the same organization, the respondents are likely to share the same culture, climate, and leadership style. Thus, the perceptions of the respondents on their transformational leadership tend to be more similar within the organization than between organizations. This research could not deal with this issue. To complement it, additional multi-level approaches are recommended.

6. Conclusions

Although this study has various limitations, we believe that it contributes to deepening the transformational leadership and safety behavior literature by investigating a mediating factor between transformational leadership and safety behavior, as well as a contingent factor through which job strain influences safety behavior. Specifically, through this study, we have shown two important findings. First, transformational leadership reduces the level of employees' job strain, and then the reduced strain ultimately increases their level of safety behavior. Second, although job strain decreases the quality of employees' safety behavior, their self-efficacy regarding safety functions as a buffering factor by moderating the relationship. The findings show that an employee's job strain plays an intermediating role in connecting transformational leadership with safety behavior. We also demonstrated the importance of self-efficacy regarding safety in minimizing the negative effects of job strain on safety behavior.

Author Contributions: B.-J.K. and S.-Y.J. contributed to all the processes including writing of the original draft, conceptualization, data collection, formal analysis, and methodology of this paper.

Funding: This research received no external funding.

Conflicts of Interest: The authors declare no conflict of interest.

References

1. Bird, F.E.; Cecchi, F.; Tilche, A.; Mata-Alvarez, J. *Management Guide to Loss Control*; Institute Press: Atlanta, GA, USA, 1974.
2. Bakker, A.B.; Demerouti, E. The job demands–resources model: State of the art. *J. Manag. Psychol.* **2007**, *22*, 309–328. [CrossRef]
3. Demerouti, E.; Bakker, A.B.; Nachreiner, F.; Schaufeli, W.B. The job demands–resources model of burnout. *J. Appl. Psychol.* **2001**, *86*, 499–512. [CrossRef] [PubMed]
4. Bass, B.M. Leadership: Good, better, best. *Organ. Dyn.* **1985**, *13*, 26–40. [CrossRef]
5. Carmeli, A.; Sheaffer, Z.; Binyamin, G.; Reiter-Palmon, R.; Shimoni, T. Transformational leadership and creative problem-solving: The mediating role of psychological safety and reflexivity. *J. Crea. Behav.* **2014**, *48*, 115–135. [CrossRef]
6. Dvir, T.; Eden, D.; Avolio, B.J.; Shamir, B. Impact of transformational leadership on follower development and performance: A field experiment. *Acad. Manag. J.* **2002**, *45*, 735–744.
7. Hoffmeister, K.; Gibbons, A.M.; Johnson, S.K.; Cigularov, K.P.; Chen, P.Y.; Rosecrance, J.C. The differential effects of transformational leadership facets on employee safety. *Saf. Sci.* **2014**, *62*, 68–78. [CrossRef]
8. Mullen, J.; Kelloway, E.K.; Teed, M. Employer safety obligations, transformational leadership and their interactive effects on employee safety performance. *Saf. Sci.* **2017**, *91*, 405–412. [CrossRef]
9. Shen, Y.; Ju, C.; Koh, T.; Rowlinson, S.; Bridge, A. The impact of transformational leadership on safety climate and individual safety behavior on construction sites. *Int. J. Environ. Res. Public Health* **2017**, *14*, 45. [CrossRef]
10. Gill, A.S.; Flaschner, A.B.; Shachar, M. Mitigating stress and burnout by implementing transformational-leadership. *Int. J. Contemp. Hosp. Manag.* **2006**, *18*, 469–481. [CrossRef]
11. Michie, S. Causes and management of stress at work. *Occup. Environ. Med.* **2002**, *59*, 67–72. [CrossRef] [PubMed]
12. Sonnentag, S.; Frese, M. Stress in organizations. In *Comprehensive Handbook of Psychology*; Industrial and Organizational Psychology; Borman, W.C., Ilgen, D.R., Klimoski, R.J., Eds.; Wiley: New York, NY, USA, 2003; Volume 12, pp. 453–491.
13. Spector, P.E.; Dwyer, D.J.; Jex, S.M. Relation of job stressors to affective, health, and performance outcomes: A comparison of multiple data sources. *J. Appl. Psychol.* **1988**, *73*, 11. [CrossRef]
14. Martin, K.D.; Cullen, J.B. Continuities and Extensions of Ethical Climate Theory: A Meta-Analytic Review. *J. Bus. Ethics* **2006**, *69*, 175–194. [CrossRef]
15. Shin, Y.; Sung, S.Y.; Choi, J.N.; Kim, M.S. Top Management Ethical Leadership and Firm Performance: Mediating Role of Ethical and Procedural Justice Climate. *J. Bus. Ethics* **2015**, *129*, 43–57. [CrossRef]

16. Barling, J.; Loughlin, C.; Kelloway, E.K. Development and test of a model linking safety-specific transformational leadership and occupational safety. *J. Appl. Psychol.* **2002**, *87*, 488. [CrossRef] [PubMed]
17. Bundi, S.M.; Lewa, P.; Ndwiga, M. Effects of Transformational Leadership on Work Stress among Top Managers in State Owned Enterprises (SOEs) in Kenya. *Eur. J. Bus. Manag.* **2016**, *7*, 185–194.
18. Gilboa, S.; Shirom, A.; Fried, Y.; Cooper, C. A meta-analysis of work demand stressors and job performance: Examining main and moderating effects. *Pers. Psychol.* **2008**, *61*, 227–271. [CrossRef]
19. Sampson, J.M.; DeArmond, S.; Chen, P.Y. Role of safety stressors and social support on safety performance. *Saf. Sci.* **2014**, *64*, 137–145. [CrossRef]
20. Steffy, B.D.; Jones, J.W.; Murphy, L.R.; Kunz, L. A demonstration of the impact of stress abatement programs on reducing employees' accidents and their costs. *Am. J. Health Promot.* **1986**, *1*, 25–32. [CrossRef] [PubMed]
21. Wallace, J.C.; Edwards, B.D.; Arnold, T.; Frazier, M.L.; Finch, D.M. Work stressors, role-based performance, and the moderating influence of organizational support. *J. Appl. Psychol.* **2009**, *94*, 254. [CrossRef] [PubMed]
22. Bandura, A. Exercise of personal and collective efficacy in changing societies. In *Self-efficacy in Changing Societies*; Bandura, A., Ed.; Cambridge University Press: Cambridge, UK, 1997; pp. 1–45.
23. Gist, M.E.; Mitchell, T.R. Self-efficacy: A theoretical analysis of its determinants and malleability. *Acad. Manag. Rev.* **1992**, *17*, 183–211. [CrossRef]
24. Eden, D.; Zuk, Y. Seasickness as a self-fulfilling prophecy: Raising self-efficacy to boost performance at sea. *J. Appl. Psychol.* **1995**, *80*, 628. [CrossRef] [PubMed]
25. Cummings, T.G.; Cooper, C.L. A cybernetic framework for studying occupational stress. *Hum. Relat.* **1979**, *32*, 395–418. [CrossRef]
26. Havlovic, S.J.; Keenan, J.P. Coping with work stress: The influence of individual differences. *J. Soc. Behav. Personal.* **1995**, *6*, 179–192.
27. Parker, D.F.; DeCotiis, T.A. Organizational determinants of job stress. *Organ. Behave. Hum. Perform.* **1983**, *32*, 160–177. [CrossRef]
28. Kim, B.J.; Park, S.; Kim, T.H. The effect of transformational leadership on team creativity: Sequential mediating effect of employee's psychological safety and creativity. *Asian J. Technol. Innov.* **2019**, 1–18. [CrossRef]
29. Jung, D.; Avolio, B. Opening the black box: An experimental investigation of the mediating effects of trust and value congruence on transformational and transactional leadership. *J. Organ. Behav.* **2000**, *21*, 949–964. [CrossRef]
30. Bass, B.M.; Avolio, B.J. *Improving Organizational Effectiveness through Transformational Leadership*; SAGE: Thousand Oaks, CA, USA, 1994.
31. Rowold, J.; Schlotz, W. Transformational and transactional leadership and followers' chronic stress. *Lead. Rev.* **2009**, *9*, 35–48.
32. Burke, M.J.; Sarpy, S.A.; Tesluk, P.E.; Smith-Crowe, K. General safety performance: A test of a grounded theoretical model. *Pers. Psychol.* **2002**, *55*, 429–457. [CrossRef]
33. Christian, M.S.; Bradley, J.C.; Wallace, J.C.; Burke, M.J. Workplace safety: A meta-analysis of the roles of person and situation factors. *J. Appl. Psychol.* **2009**, *94*, 1103. [CrossRef]
34. Griffin, M.A.; Neal, A. Perceptions of safety at work: A framework for linking safety climate to safety performance, knowledge, and motivation. *J. Occup. Health. Psychol.* **2000**, *5*, 347. [CrossRef]
35. Clarke, S. The relationship between safety climate and safety performance: A meta-analytic review. *J. Occup. Health. Psychol.* **2006**, *11*, 315. [CrossRef] [PubMed]
36. Neal, A.; Griffin, M.A. A study of the lagged relationships among safety climate, safety motivation, safety behavior, and accidents at the individual and group levels. *J. Appl. Psychol.* **2006**, *91*, 946. [CrossRef] [PubMed]
37. Seo, H.C.; Lee, Y.S.; Kim, J.J.; Jee, N.Y. Analyzing safety behaviors of temporary construction workers using structural equation modeling. *Saf. Sci.* **2015**, *77*, 160–168. [CrossRef]
38. Maule, O.S.A.J. *Time Pressure and Stress in Human Judgment and Decision Making*; Svenson, O., Maule, A.J., Eds.; Springer Science and Business Media: New York, NY, USA, 1993.
39. Wickens, C.D.; Lee, J.D.; Liu, Y.; Becker, S.G. *An Introduction to Human Factors Engineering*; Pearson: Upper Saddle River, NJ, USA, 2009.
40. Lennings, C.J. An evaluation of a generalized self-efficacy scale. *Personal. Individ. Differ.* **1994**, *16*, 745–750. [CrossRef]

41. DeJoy, D.M.; Wilson, M.G.; Vandenberg, R.J.; McGrath-Higgins, A.L.; Griffin-Blake, C.S. Assessing the impact of healthy work organization intervention. *J. Organ. Occup. Psychol.* **2010**, *83*, 139–165. [CrossRef]
42. Bandura, A. *Multidimensional Scales of Perceived Self-efficacy*; Stanford University: Stanford, CA, USA, 1990.
43. Anderson, J.C.; Gerbing, D.W. Structural Equation Modeling in Practice: A Review and Recommended Two-Step Approach. *Psychol. Bull.* **1988**, *103*, 411–423. [CrossRef]
44. Browne, M.W.; Cudeck, R. Alternative Ways of Assessing Model Fit. *Sage focus Ed.* **1993**, *154*, 136. [CrossRef]
45. Cheung, G.W.; Lau, R.S. Testing Mediation and Suppression Effects of Latent Variables: Bootstrapping with Structural Equation Models. *Organ. Res. Methods* **2008**, *11*, 296–325. [CrossRef]
46. Hayes, A.F.; Preacher, K.J. *Conditional Process Modeling: Using Structural Equation Modeling to Examine Contingent Causal Processes*; IAP Information Age Publishing: Charlotte, NC, USA, 2013; pp. 219–226.
47. Brace, N.; Kemp, R.; Snelgar, R. *SPSS for Psychologists: A Guide to Data Analysis Using SPSS for Windows*; Palgrave: London, UK, 2003.
48. Shrout, P.E.; Bolger, N. Mediation in Experimental and Nonexperimental Studies: New Procedures and Recommendations. *Psychol. Methods* **2002**, *7*, 422–445. [CrossRef]
49. Conway, J.M.; Lance, C.E. What reviewers should expect from authors regarding common method bias in organizational research. *J. Bus. Psychol.* **2010**, *25*, 325–334. [CrossRef]

International Journal of
Environmental Research and Public Health

MDPI

Article

Prevalence of Noise-Induced Hearing Loss Among Tanzanian Iron and Steel Workers: A Cross-Sectional Study

Israel P. Nyarubeli [1,2,3,*], Alexander M. Tungu [4], Bente E. Moen [1,3] and Magne Bråtveit [3]

1. Centre for International Health, Department of Global Public and Primary Care, University of Bergen, Årstadveien 21, 5020 Bergen, Norway; Bente.Moen@uib.no
2. Department of Environmental and Occupational Health, Muhimbili University of Health and Allied Sciences, P.O. Box 65015, Dar es Salaam, Tanzania
3. Research Group for Occupational and Environmental Medicine, Department of Global Public and Primary Care, University of Bergen, 5020 Bergen, Norway; Magne.Bratveit@uib.no
4. Department of Physiology, Muhimbili University of Health and Allied Sciences, P.O. Box 65001, Dar es Salaam, Tanzania; alextungu@yahoo.co.uk

* Correspondence: israelpau2004@yahoo.co.uk

Received: 8 March 2019; Accepted: 13 April 2019; Published: 16 April 2019

Abstract: Iron and steel factory workers in Tanzania are likely to develop noise-induced hearing loss (NIHL) due to exposure to high sound levels. Studies on hearing status in this population are lacking. The aims of this study were to determine prevalence of NIHL among iron and steel workers and compare hearing thresholds at different frequencies with a control group. We conducted a cross-sectional study among 221 iron and steel workers exposed to average noise level of 92 dB(A), compared with 107 primary school teachers recruited as controls and exposed to average noise level of 79.7 dB(A). We used a questionnaire-based interview to collect information on socio demographic characteristics and other confounding variables. Hearing loss was defined as hearing threshold levels ≥25 dB hearing loss in either ear at 3000, 4000 or 6000 Hz. The prevalence of hearing loss was significantly higher among the exposed group than among the controls, i.e. 48% and 31%, respectively. There were significant differences in hearing thresholds between the exposed and control groups at 3000, 4000, 6000, and 8000 Hz. Hearing loss was more frequent among workers exposed to higher noise levels than among the controls suggesting that iron and steel workers run a higher risk of developing hearing loss.

Keywords: audiometry; occupational; noise-induced hearing loss; hearing threshold; exposed; iron and steel; Tanzania

---

1. Introduction

Noise-induced hearing loss (NIHL) is an underestimated public health concern [1,2]. Globally, the magnitude of disabling hearing loss (above 40 dB) from all causes has increased in the past two decades from 120 to 466 million people from 1995 to 2018 [3,4]. Estimates of the prevalence of hearing loss related to noise exposure above 85 dB(A) vary in the range of 7–21% or higher [5]. Prevalence is estimated to be higher in the low and middle-income countries compared to the findings in other parts of the world [4]. This may be due to ongoing economic investments in industrialization coupled with challenges related to an inadequate public health policy, lack of regulatory frameworks and limited resources spent on preventive measures.

Studies highlight noise exposure as one major risk factor contributing to hearing loss [1,4,5]. Other suggested risk factors for hearing loss include increasing age, [6–8] smoking, [5] exposure to organic solvents, [9] the use of ototoxic medicines, [5,9] gender, vibration, genetics, ear surgery, ear infections and illnesses [5,10]. In addition, exposure to noise has been associated with increased risks of cardiovascular diseases and diabetes [5,11–14].

Studies conducted in Sub-Saharan Africa (SSA) have mainly focused on the mining sector and indicate, for instance, that the prevalence of hearing loss in this industry was 37% in Zimbabwe and 47% in Tanzania [15,16]. Despite the presence of hearing conservation programmes aimed at prevention, the prevalence of hearing loss was above 50% among gold miners in South Africa, while it was 21% among stone crushers in Ghana [8,17]. To our knowledge, there are no published studies on hearing loss in large iron and steel factories in SSA. One study among iron and steel mill workers in Western Africa, specifically Nigeria, found a hearing loss prevalence of 28% and 57% in the better and the worse ears, respectively [18]. This prevalence is almost twice as high as that found in the general adult population in Uganda [10]. One must take into account that the definition and presentation of hearing loss may differ from study to study [1]. Nevertheless, the prevalence of hearing loss is still alarming.

In Tanzania, like in other SSA countries, investments in the manufacturing industries, including iron and steel industries, create jobs for a significant large number of employees. Globally the demand for steel is increasing, and this sector has provided employment for 50 million people [19]. The construction of new infrastructures such as bridges, flyover exchange roads, buildings, towers and railways obviously create numerous workplaces. Although the construction of industrial-level infrastructure represents significant increase in economic assets across SSA, little is known about the prevalence of NIHL in these industries, and documentation is scarce to inform policy-makers and stakeholders working in preventive health services. In a recent study, the eight-hour average noise level among iron and steel workers in Tanzania was 92 dB(A), and 90% of the measurements were above the occupational exposure limit of 85 dB(A). The workers did not use hearing protection devices [20] implying that the workers are at increased risk of developing NIHL. There is a need for assessing NIHL in this working group with a view to developing a plan for implementation of a hearing conservation programme. Therefore, the aims of this study were to determine the prevalence of NIHL among iron and steel workers, and to compare the hearing thresholds at different frequencies between these workers and a control group exposed to a low level of occupational noise.

2. Materials and Methods

2.1. Study Population

This cross-sectional study was conducted from June 2016 until June 2017 and involved permanent male workers from four iron and steel factories in Tanzania exposed to noise. Characteristics and details of noise-exposure assessments in these factories have been presented elsewhere [20]. The results showed a personal, mean equivalent noise exposure ($L_{EX,8h}$) for these workers of 92.0 dB(A) [20].

Controls were male teachers from 34 public primary schools in Tanzania. This control group was chosen because they were expected to be exposed to low levels of occupational noise [5,21–23]. In the control group, 24 full-shift noise measurements from six primary schools were conducted using personal dosimeters (type 4448, Brüel and Kjær, DK-2850 Nærum, Denmark) attached to the teacher's shoulder (ISO standard 9612:2009). The 8-hour equivalent noise exposure among these controls at work was 79.7 dB(A).

The sample size calculation was based on the estimated prevalence of hearing loss among workers exposed to loud noise at work. Since there was no available information about hearing loss among noise exposed workers or among the general population in Tanzania, the sample size was calculated based on a community baseline survey conducted in Uganda that found the prevalence of hearing loss among adults to be 12% [10]. In our study the effect of noise on hearing loss was hypothesized to be doubled i.e., 24%. To achieve 90% power and be able to detect a difference in hearing loss between noise exposed workers and a non-exposed group at a significance level of 0.05 (Using Open-Epi online calculator Version 3.3a, OpenEpi, Atlanta, GA, USA) [24], totally 230 exposed workers was needed. We added 10% to account for non-responders, providing a total sample size of 253 workers.

2.2. Study Participants

A total of 376 permanent workers (253 from four iron and steel factories and 123 teachers from 34 public primary schools) were randomly selected by using a table of random numbers from the provided list of workers and were invited to participate in the study (Figure 1). Workers list was provided by the respective employers. We held meetings with both the management for each factory and the administration at the public primary school where we presented the purpose of the project and asked for a research permit. Each of these partners referred us to a contact person who helped the research team in the planning of the research activities. The study participants were informed of the purpose of the project and those who agreed to participate, provided written consent. This paper presents the audiometry results.

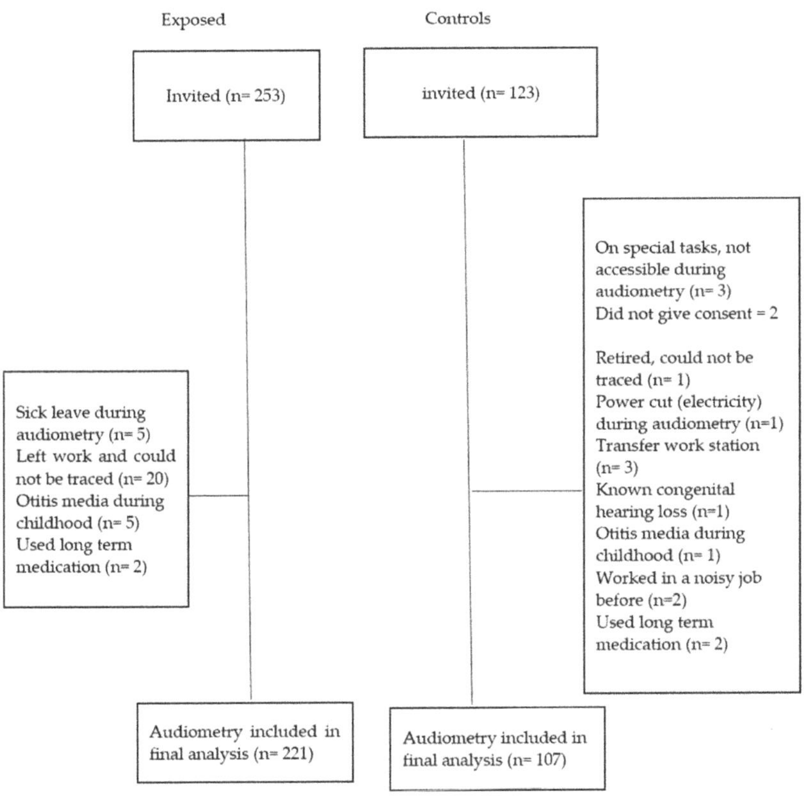

Figure 1. Flow chart describing the participants in the study of hearing loss among exposed iron and steel factory workers (n = 221) and controls—primary school teachers (n = 107) in Tanzania.

We used information collected through a structured interview with both exposed participants and controls to exclude the following categories of workers from the data analysis: those with congenital hearing loss, history of otitis media during childhood and those reported to have worked in noisy job among the controls. In addition, we excluded those who reported using long-term medication because the participants did not have adequate knowledge of the type of medication they used. Thus, we ended with a total of 328 (221 exposed and 107 controls) persons taking audiometric measurements (Figure 1).

The participants were instructed to avoid areas with high level of noise for a minimum of 12 h prior to audiometric examinations to minimize the possibility of temporary threshold shift (TTS).

The duration since last occupational noise exposure (free noise exposure) was recorded before the audiometric test was administered [25,26].

2.3. Interview Questionnaire and Checklist

A structured interview questionnaire was used to collect information on demographic characteristics and factors that may influence hearing loss. These included age (in years), number of years of employment, history of noise exposure at work (yes/no), current smoking (yes/no), present use of long-term medication (yes/no), exposure to chemicals/organic solvents (yes/no), use of hearing protection while working in noisy areas (yes/no), ear infections as a child or adult (yes/no), head injury/trauma (yes/no), tinnitus (yes/no). In addition, information about otitis in childhood (yes/no), known congenital hearing loss (yes/no), any relatives with hearing loss and any history of ear-related medical condition (diabetes and hypertension) was collected. This information was collected before the audiometry day and used to exclude participants before audiometry (Figure 1).

Prior to otoscopy, but on the same day as the audiometry, participants were interviewed using a checklist indicating whether they had symptoms of upper respiratory infections (e.g., running nose) (yes/no), ear discharge (yes/no), time and date they left work (hours) and the most recent time they were exposed to high noise at a level that made it difficult to communicate. Afterwards, otoscopy was performed by an occupational physician; in circumstances when the ear canal was completely obstructed with wax or cerumen, the latter were removed, and a new appointment was scheduled for audiometry. This also applied to participants with upper respiratory infections; the test was postponed until they were asymptomatic.

2.4. Pure Tone Audiometry

Audiometric measurements (pure tone audiometry) were conducted in an ear-screening locally-constructed booth in a quiet room at the headquarters of the Occupational Safety and Health Authority (OSHA) in Tanzania. The same technical personnel conducted all audiometric tests using a standardized protocol. Background noise in the test booth was monitored by a calibrated hand-held Sound Level Meter (Brüel and Kjær, type 2250), and checked for conformity with ISO 8253-1:2010 standard [27]. The highest background noise level (L_{max}) in the booth was 51 dB at 31.5 Hz. For best results, audiometry was conducted in the morning before any work exposure. In addition, the city is less noisy in the morning compared to other times of the day when the participants could potentially be exposed to a higher level of environmental noise. Pure tone audiometry was conducted using an Interacoustics AD226 (Interacoustics, DK-5500, Middelfart, Denmark) with Amplivox Audiocup earphones having lower test limit of −10 dB. The equipment was pre-calibrated. Test frequencies were 250–8000 Hz in the order starting with 1000, 2000, 3000, 4000, 6000, 8000, 500, 250 and finish at 1000 Hz [27]. A manual test procedure was used in compliance with ISO 8253-1:2010 [26–28].

2.5. Data Analysis

Descriptive statistics were presented as mean and standard deviation or percentage. Chi-square and independent samples *t*-tests were used to compare categorical and continuous descriptive variables, respectively. NIHL was defined as hearing threshold level ≥25 dB hearing loss in either ear at 3000, 4000 or 6000 Hz [29].

Potential determinants of hearing loss were identified. Age was categorized into three age groups (tertiles) based on the age distribution among the controls. Duration of work was categorized arbitrarily into three groups (≤2 years, 2–10 years, 11–37 years). History of ear-related medical conditions (diabetes, hypertension, ear infections and head injury) was combined into a dichotomized variable (yes/no), current smoking (yes/no), relatives with hearing impairment (yes/no), tinnitus (yes/no) and previous noisy work (yes/no). A chi-square test was used to explore the relationship between these variables and hearing loss in exposed participants compared with controls.

The intercorrelation between participant's age and duration of work determinants was tested with the Pearson correlation test. In multiple regression analyses, we chose the determinant that contributed most to the hearing loss.

We used log binomial regression models with a 95% confidence interval (CI) to ascertain differences in hearing loss (yes/no) between exposed and controls within each age strata and within the total group of workers while adjusting for the significant determinants selected from Chi-square analyses and the correlation test.

We computed the mean hearing threshold for the different test frequencies for both exposed participants and controls, as well as for the three age groups within the main exposure groups. For each test frequency, multiple linear regression was used to analyze for differences between exposed and controls, while adjusting for age as a continuous variable, previous noisy work and history of ear-related medical condition.

The exposed group had a mean exposure duration of 5 years (range: 0–24 years) and a L_{Aeq8h} of 92 dB(A) [20]. Within the three age groups (≤2 years, 2–10 years, 11–37 years) the mean duration of exposure in these factories were 1, 5, and 17 years, respectively. We calculated the predicted noise-induced permanent threshold shift (NIPTS) corresponding to these three mean exposure durations according to ISO 1999 section 6.3, that provides a formula and method that predicts NIPTS at 1000, 2000, 3000, 4000 and 6000 Hz as a function of the logarithm of exposure duration (d) (in years), and the square of noise exposure level (L_{Aeq8h}), with frequency specific constants u, v, and L_0 (a sound pressure level, defined as a function of a given constant value for each frequency in decibels [30]:

$$\text{NIPTS} = [u + v\log_{10}(d)]\,(L_{Aeq8h} - L_0)^2 \quad (1)$$

We used IBM SPSS Statistics, Version 25 (Allen & Unwin, 83 Alexander Street, Crown Nest, NSW, Australia) for data analysis and set a parameter of $p < 0.05$ as statistical significance. NIPTS was estimated using Microsoft Excel (Office 365, Microsoft Corporation, Redmond, WA, USA).

2.6. Ethical Clearance

We obtained ethical clearance from The Regional Committee of Medical and Health Research Ethics (REK-VEST) in Norway (number 2016/635/REK sør-øst dated 20 May 2016); and later from The Muhimbili University of Health and Allied Sciences (MUHAS) Ethics Committee in Tanzania number 2016-06-24/AEC/Vol. XI/38 dated 24 June 2016. Each iron and steel factory and primary school administration was contacted individually, and all of them granted permission to conduct the study. Individual participants were contacted and informed about the research objectives and activities to be conducted and gave written consent. Information that was collected was treated as confidential and was not accessed by unauthorized parties. We used participants' identification instead of names in data collection, processing and analysis.

3. Results

The participation rate was 87% for both the exposed and controls. The exposed group was significantly younger than the controls (independent sample t-test; $p < 0.001$) (Table 1). There was a significant difference between exposed and controls for the three descriptive variables; age group, duration of work and previous noisy work, (Chi square test; $p < 0.001$) but not for the other variables i.e., current smoking, tinnitus, relative with hearing impairment and history of ear-related medical condition (Table 1). Among the exposed, 67% of the workers fell in the youngest age group (18–35 years) (Table 1). In addition, there were significant differences in hearing loss between exposed and controls for the four determinants—age group, duration of work, previous noisy work and history of ear-related medical condition (Chi-square test; $p < 0.05$). The overall prevalence of hearing loss was significantly higher (Chi square test, $p = 0.003$) among exposed workers (48%) than among the controls (31%) (Table 2).

Table 1. Descriptive characteristics of the participants in the study among noise-exposed (n = 221) and control (n = 107) workers in Tanzania.

Characteristics	Descriptive		p-Value
	Exposed (n (%))	Controls (n (%))	
Age: Mean (SD)	32 (8)	40 (7)	<0.001 [a]
Age group (years) (group mean for Exposed))			
18–35 (27)	149 (67.4)	36 (33.6)	<0.001 [b]
36–43 (39)	58 (26.2)	37 (34.6)	
44–59 (47)	14 (6.3)	34 (31.8)	
Total	221 (100.0)	107 (100.0)	
Duration of work (years) (group mean for Exposed)			
≤2 (1)	86 (38.9)	-	<0.001 [b]
3–10 (5)	108 (48.9)	27 (25.2)	
11–37 (17)	27 (12.2)	80 (74.8)	
Current smoking			
no	183 (82.8)	96 (89.7)	
yes	38 (17.2)	11 (10.3)	0.07
Previous noisy work			
no	178 (80.5)	107 (100.0)	
yes	43 (19.5)	-	<0.001 [b]
Tinnitus			
no	202 (91.4)	104 (97.2)	
yes	19 (8.6)	3 (2.8)	0.06
Relative with hearing impairment			
no	199 (90.0)	96 (89.7)	
yes	22 (10.0)	11 (10.3)	0.9
History of ear-related medical condition			
no	176 (79.6)	93 (86.9)	
yes	45 (20.4)	14 (13.1)	0.01 [b]

[a] independent samples t-test; [b] Chi-square test.

Table 2. Prevalence of hearing loss among exposed (n = 221) and control (n = 107) workers in Tanzania.

Variable	Hearing Loss [a] (n (%))			
	Exposed	Controls	Chi-Square Test (p-Value)	Prevalence Ratio 95% Confidence Interval) †
Age group (years)				
18–35	63 (42.3)	5 (13.9)	0.002 *	2.5 (0.93, 6.76)
36–43	34 (58.6)	12 (32.4)	0.013 *	1.7 (0.79, 3.47)
44–59	10 (71.4)	16 (47.0)	0.124	1.5 (0.58, 3.70)
All	107 (48.4)	33 (30.8)		1.3 (1.10, 1.62)

[a] Hearing loss defined as ≥25 dB in either ear at 3000, 4000 or 6000 Hz; † log-binomial analysis within each age group, adjusted for age as a continuous variable, previous noisy work and history of ear-related medical condition; * $p < 0.05$.

Hearing loss increased with advancing age among both exposed and controls (Table 2). Within the age-groups, there were significant differences in hearing loss between exposed and the controls for the youngest and middle-aged group (Chi square test, p 1 = 0.002; p 2 = 0.013) but not for the older age group (Table 2).

Results from the log binomial regression model, adjusted for age, previous noisy work and history of ear-related medical condition, showed a statistically higher risk of hearing loss among exposed workers compared to controls, with a prevalence ratio of 1.3. When performing the analysis within each age stratum, the youngest age group (18–35 years) had the highest prevalence ratio (2.5), although it was not statistically significant (Table 2).

The mean hearing threshold between exposed and control workers at 3000, 4000 and 6000 Hz differed significantly (independent samples *t*-test, $p < 0.05$) (Table 3). In linear regression analyses within each age stratum, there were significant differences in hearing threshold between exposed and controls for the frequencies 4000 and 6000 Hz within the youngest age group (18–35 years) adjusting for age as a continuous variable, previous noisy work and history of ear-related medical condition (Figure 2). In analogous analyses, the hearing threshold for the frequencies 3000, 4000 and 6000 Hz were significantly different in the 36–43 years age group, and in the age group 44–59 years, only the frequency 6000 Hz was significantly different (Figure 2).

Table 3. Hearing threshold of the worse ear among noise exposed and controls for the tested frequencies.

Workers' Group	Number of Workers	Mean Hearing Thresholds in Decibel (dB) for Each Frequency							
		250	500	1000	2000	3000	4000	6000	8000
Exposed	221	17.0 (6.1)	19.0 (5.2)	19.4 (6.0)	19.6 (7.3)	23.6 (8.9) [a]	25.0 (9.7) [a]	24.3 (10.6) [a]	16.0 (9.7) [a]
Control	107	17.2 (5.5)	18.0 (5.7)	19.7 (5.2)	18.8 (8.1)	20.8 (8.0)	21.7 (8.8)	19.6 (9.2)	13.6 (9.8)

[a] independent samples *t*-test, $p < 0.05$.

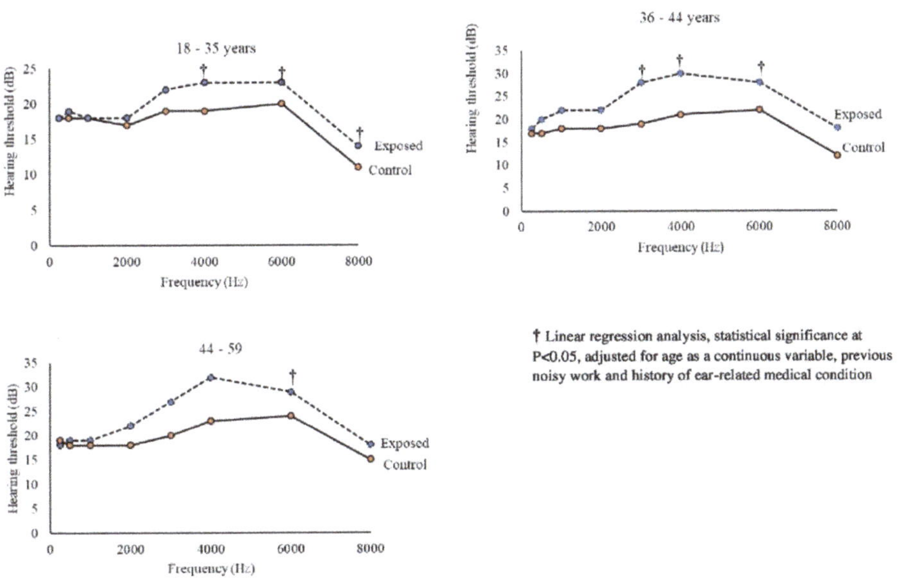

Figure 2. Hearing threshold of noise-exposed male workers (n = 221) (dotted lines) compared with male controls (n = 107) (solid lines) in Tanzania, stratified into age groups (triplets).

Table 4 shows the age-stratified differences in hearing thresholds for the different test frequencies in exposed and controls. The regression coefficients show that for the frequencies with significant findings, the difference between exposed and controls was about 3–6 dB among the youngest age group, 4–6 dB in the middle-aged group and about 10 dB for the oldest age group.

Table 4. Hearing threshold at the tested frequencies stratified by age groups among exposed iron and steel factory workers (n = 221) and controls (n = 107) in Tanzania.

Age Group	Audiometry Frequency (Hz)													
	250		500		1000		3000		4000		6000		8000	
	β	95% CI	β	95% CI	β	95% CI	β	95% CI	β	95% CI	β	95% CI	β	95% CI
18–35	0.16	−2.31, 2.63	−1.54	−3.47, 0.39	−0.53	−2.57, 1.52	−3.05	−6.19, 0.11	−4.94 *	−8.57, −1.31	−5.84 *	−10.16, −1.52	−4.90 *	−8.66, −1.14
36–43	−0.14	−3.06, 2.77	−1.92	−4.63, 0.79	−1.45	−4.54, 1.64	−5.70 *	−10.11, −2.27	−6.37 *	−10.93, −1.81	−4.32 *	−8.73, 0.09	−3.36	−7.51, 0.79
44–59	−0.72	−5.51, 4.07	−2.47	−6.52, 1.59	−1.07	0.67, −6.20	−6.85	−14.66, 0.95	−4.95	−13.23, 3.33	−10.22 *	−18.87, −1.58	−6.00	−15.41, 3.41

Linear regression analysis, adjusted for age as a continuous variable, previous noisy work and history of ear-related medical condition. * Statistical significant at $p < 0.05$.

The mean hearing threshold among the participants in the 18–35 age group was similar to the predicted NIPTS according to ISO 1999 at the lower frequencies (1000, 2000 and 3000 Hz), while it was about 1 dB higher than ISO 1999 for the higher frequencies (4000 and 6000 Hz) (Figure 3a). For the 36–44 and 45–59 age groups, the hearing threshold for the higher frequencies were lower (3, 1 dB and 6, 4dB lower, respectively) for same frequencies than that the NIPTS predicted by ISO 1999 (Figure 3b,c).

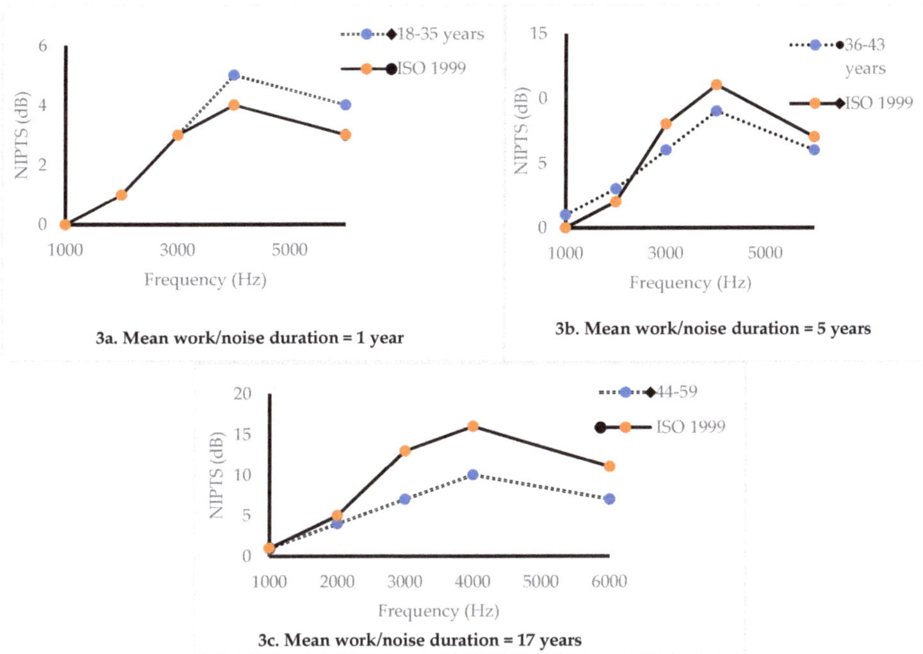

Figure 3. (**a**–**c**) Mean of the measured hearing threshold by audiometry (dotted lines) and median noise-induced permanent threshold shift (NIPTS) predicted by ISO 1999 (solid lines) for the three age-groups of iron and steel workers in Tanzania exposed to an average noise level of L_{Aeq8h} of 92 dB(A) for the mean duration of noise exposure within each age group.

4. Discussion

We found a higher prevalence of hearing loss among Tanzanian iron and steel factory workers compared to controls i.e., 48% vs. 31% respectively. In addition, a comparison of hearing thresholds between the two groups for the frequencies 4000 and 6000Hz revealed significant differences. To our knowledge, this is the first study in SSA to document the prevalence of hearing loss among workers exposed to noise in iron and steel factories.

In the present study, we found a significantly higher prevalence of NIHL among iron and steel workers than the controls. The noise exposed workers were exposed to a mean noise level of 92 dB(A), without using hearing protection devices [20]. At this noise level, it is likely that the workers develop NIHL [31,32]. A study conducted among Indian iron and steel workers exposed to noise levels above 90 dB(A) found an even higher prevalence of NIHL than we found. Over 90% of the workers engaged in casting and forging had hearing loss in the higher frequencies i.e., 4000 and 6000 Hz [33]. This is likely due to differences in the nature of work, including tasks and tools used during the steel production process. For example, the Indian study was done in small and medium factories with the forging and casting tasks frequently characterized by impulse noise that might cause hearing damage at higher frequencies [34]. By contrast, our study was done in larger-scale factories with a relatively higher level of mechanization. Another study done in Nigeria also found higher prevalence in the worse ear

(57%) among steel mill workers exposed to 75–93 dB(A), with pure tone averages of 30 dB, 31 dB and 32 dB for the finishing, mill floor and mechanical departments respectively, as compared to a pure tone average of 21 dB among administrative workers with lower noise exposure (49 dB(A)) [18]. In Nepal, the prevalence among workers in a steel factory was comparable to our study, i.e., 40% and 46% for the right and left ear, respectively. However, the study excluded workers over 45 years and information on factory characteristics were not available [35]. Another study done in Nepal among 115 small-scale metal industry workers and 123 controls found lower prevalence for the exposed (30%) and only 4% for the controls [36]. The difference in prevalence between the Nepal study and our study may be due to the definition used to define hearing loss [1,36]. However, the high prevalence presented based on these studies suggests that noise exposure among iron and steel workers contribute substantially to hearing loss [37].

Age is one of the main factors for the development of hearing loss. To adjust for age can be difficult in statistical analyses. In the present study, we stratified the working population into three age groups and found a borderline increased risk for hearing loss among the younger age group (18–35 years), and significant differences between exposed and controls in hearing thresholds for the frequencies of 4000 and 6000Hz. The significant difference in the dip for the 4000 and 6000 Hz frequencies is a sign indicating hearing loss due to noise exposure in this age stratum [17,18,38,39]. Similar findings have been shown among gold miners in South Africa where the greatest difference in hearing threshold between age strata was found among the younger age group (16–40 years) at the noise dip of 4000 Hz [7]. Therefore, it is essential that noise control measures, including hearing conservation programmes should be established particularly to protect workers from developing NIHL.

In this study we found higher estimates of NIPTS than predicted by ISO 1999 standard for 18–35 years at frequencies of 4000 and 6000 Hz. These frequencies are likely to be affected by noise exposure [40]. The characteristics of noise, size of ear canal and other factors determines the location of notch for the higher frequencies [41]. However, the notch at these frequencies and especially at 4000 Hz is an established clinical sign and may be valuable in confirming the diagnosis of NIHL [40,42]. In addition, Our NIPTS estimates, though generally lower than that of ISO 1999 predictions, show similar patterns especially at higher frequencies. This result differs from a study conducted in United States which reported estimates in agreements to that of ISO 1999 [43]. The lower results and estimates from our study may be explained partly by differences in reference population characteristics. ISO 1999 standard was prepared based on populations from developed and industrialized countries such as United States and with steady state noise [30], which it is difficult to compare results to our study that had mixed noise characteristics. However, although the hearing threshold in the age range 44–59 years was somewhat lower than predicted from the ISO 1999, the overall results suggests that noise exposure among the iron and steel workers leads to an increased risk of NIPTS.

The control group in our study had a significant lower prevalence of hearing loss compared to the exposed workers at higher frequencies. The measured hearing loss in this group was lower than that recorded among the controls in South African miners study for the higher test frequencies i.e., 31% versus 46% respectively [8]. The control group in the South Africa study was the administration group, and this makes it difficult to compare with our study. Moreover, the control group in the South Africa study was not screened for previous noise exposure as we did in our study. The participants in our control group were screened for several factors responsible for hearing loss and were thus expected to have low prevalence. This indicates that there might be factors other than noise that may have contributed to the hearing loss in the South African study. In Tanzania, there are no published data on community hearing profile among adults. Community studies conducted in other African countries such as Nigeria and Egypt found a lower prevalence of hearing loss (defined as hearing threshold >25 dB) than we found i.e., 18% and 16%, respectively [44]. However, in these community studies, there is no information on noise exposure profile among the participants, and this makes it difficult to compare with the control group in our study. Based on the selection of examined workers, including the control group, we think that it is likely that occupational noise exposure has contributed to the difference in hearing loss between our two groups.

Strengths of this study are the high response rate among the participants, the use of a control group from workplaces with low sound levels, and the use of standardized methods for audiometry. In addition, it was possible to control for the effect of age in hearing thresholds by stratification of age groups while adjusting for age as a continuous variable within the age strata. The statistical analyses made it possible to adjust for potential confounding factors related to hearing loss, such as current smoking, previous noise exposure, tinnitus, history of ear-related medical conditions, duration of work and relatives with hearing impairments. The use of calibrated research equipment and devices together with adherence to the novel procedure related to audiometry testing and ISO 8253-1:2010 standard for ambient noise improved the findings.

Our study had some limitations; The design of the study was cross-sectional, and this reduces the possibility to conclude regarding the causal relationship between noise at work and hearing loss. Still, this study indicates that the sound levels are of importance to the registered hearing losses in this working population, as the frequencies involved are in the upper frequency area and the sound levels measured were above 85 dB(A). A longitudinal study would have provided a better exposure-effect association. Information collected through interview questionnaire might introduced recall bias. To minimize this bias, we used the same trained research personnel and method for both the exposed and the controls. In addition, in many societies today, people listen to music at high volume levels, and this may affect their hearing ability. We have limited information about leisure time exposure to noise among our study participants, but we have no reason to believe that the workers in iron and steel factories are more exposed to leisure time sound than are the control workers. In addition, iron and steel workers spent most of their time during the day at work. Lastly, it was impractical to monitor workers at their homes before audiometry.

5. Conclusions

Based on these findings, this study should be a wake-up call for stakeholders in the establishment and should serve to encourage the implementation of noise control measures such as the use of hearing protection devices in these workplaces. The information we found on the high prevalence of hearing loss may be used by policy and decision-makers in awareness creation programmes aimed at noise control such as establishing hearing conservation programmes and preventive services among working populations exposed to noise [33].

Author Contributions: I.P.N., B.E.M., M.B. and A.M.T. were involved in project conceptualization, methodology, validation, formal analysis, data curation, writing (original draft preparation), writing (review and editing) and visualization. I.P.N., J.A.H. and A.M.T. were involved in investigation. In addition, B.E.M. and M.B. were involved in resources, supervision and project administration.

Funding: This work was financially supported by the Norwegian State Educational Loan Fund (Lånekassen). We also wish to thank the Norwegian Programme for Capacity Development in Higher Education and Research for Development (NORHED) for providing equipment for this study.

Acknowledgments: The authors are indebted to administrators in the four factories and 34 primary schools for hosting the project and allowing workers to participate. We thank the workers for their participation. Likewise, our gratitude goes to the field research assistant (Ms. Judith A. Haule), the Muhimbili University of Health and Allied Sciences and the Occupational Safety and Health Authority in Tanzania for their helpful involvement in this work.

Conflicts of Interest: The authors declare no conflict of interest.

References

1. Rabinowitz, P.M. The Public Health Significance of Noise-Induced Hearing Loss. In *Noise-Induced Hearing Loss: Scientific Advances*; Springer Handbook of Auditory Research 40; le Prell, C.G., Henderson, D., Fay, R.R., Popper, A.N., Eds.; Springer Science + Business Media, LLC: New York, NY, USA, 2012; pp. 13–25. ISBN 978-1-4419-9523-0.

2. Daniell, W.E.; Swan, S.S.; McDaniel, M.M.; Camp, J.E.; Cohen, M.A.; Stebbins, J.G. Noise exposure and hearing loss prevention programmes after 20 years of regulations in the United States. *Occup. Environ. Med.* **2006**, *63*, 343–351. [CrossRef]
3. World Health Organization (WHO). Prevention of Blindness and Deafness: Global Estimates on Prevalence of Hearing Loss, Estimates 2018. Available online: http://www.who.int/pbd/deafness/estimates/en/ (accessed on 14 August 2018).
4. Nelson, D.I.; Nelson, R.Y.; Concha-Barrientos, M.; Fingerhut, M. The global burden of occupational noise-induced hearing loss. *Am. J. Ind. Med.* **2005**, *48*, 446–458. [CrossRef]
5. Lie, A.; Skogstad, M.; Johannessen, H.A.; Tynes, T.; Mehlum, I.S.; Nordby, K.C.; Engdahl, B.; Tambs, K. Occupational noise exposure and hearing: A systematic review. *Int. Arch. Occup. Environ. Health* **2015**, *89*, 351–372. [CrossRef]
6. Macca, I.; Scapellato, M.L.; Carrieri, M.; Maso, S.; Trevisan, A.; Bartolucci, G.B. High-frequency hearing thresholds: Effects of age, occupational ultrasound and noise exposure. *Int. Arch. Occup. Environ. Health* **2015**, *88*, 197–211. [CrossRef] [PubMed]
7. Strauss, S.; Swanepoel, D.W.; Becker, P.; Eloff, Z.; Hall, J.W., III. Noise and age-related hearing loss: A study of 40 123 gold miners in South Africa. *Int. J. Audiol.* **2014**, *53*, 66–75. [CrossRef] [PubMed]
8. Strauss, S.; Swanepoel, D.W.; Becker, P.; Eloff, Z.; Hall, J.W., III. Prevalence and degree of noise-induced hearing loss in South African gold miners: Original research. *Occup. Health South. Afr.* **2012**, *18*, 20–25.
9. Campo, P.; Morata, T.C.; Hong, O. Chemical exposure and hearing loss. *Dis. Mon.* **2013**, *59*, 119–138. [CrossRef]
10. Westerberg, B.D.; Lee, P.K.; Lukwago, L.; Zaramba, S.; Bubikere, S.; Stewart, I. Cross-sectional survey of hearing impairment and ear disease in Uganda. *J. Otolaryngol. Head Neck Surg.* **2008**, *37*, 753–758.
11. Chang, T.Y.; Liu, C.S.; Young, L.H.; Wang, V.S.; Jian, S.E.; Bao, B.Y. Noise frequency components and the prevalence of hypertension in workers. *Sci. Total Environ.* **2012**, *416*, 89–96. [CrossRef]
12. Fischer, M.E.; Schubert, C.R.; Nondahl, D.M.; Dalton, D.S.; Huang, G.H.; Keating, B.J.; Klein, B.E.K.; Klein, R.; Tweed, T.S.; Cruickshanks, K.J. Subclinical atherosclerosis and increased risk of hearing impairment. *Atherosclerosis* **2015**, *238*, 344–349. [CrossRef]
13. Ismaila, S.O.; Odusote, A. Noise exposure as a factor in the increase of blood pressure of workers in a sack manufacturing industry. *Beni-Suef Univ. J. Basic Appl. Sci.* **2014**, *3*, 116–121. [CrossRef]
14. Lee, J.H.; Kang, W.; Yaang, S.R.; Choy, N.; Lee, C.R. Cohort study for the effect of chronic noise exposure on blood pressure among male workers in Busan, Korea. *Am. J. Ind. Med.* **2009**, *52*, 509–517. [CrossRef]
15. Musiba, Z. The prevalence of noise-induced hearing loss among Tanzanian miners. *Occup. Med.* **2015**, *65*, 386–390. [CrossRef]
16. Chadambuka, A.; Mususa, F.; Muteti, S. Prevalence of noise induced hearing loss among employees at a mining industry in Zimbabwe. *Afr. Health Sci.* **2013**, *13*, 899–906. [CrossRef]
17. Kitcher, E.D.; Ocansey, G.; Tumpi, D.A. Early occupational hearing loss of workers in a stone crushing industry: Our experience in a developing country. *Noise health* **2012**, *14*, 68–71. [CrossRef]
18. Ologe, F.E.; Akande, T.M.; Olajide, T.G. Occupational noise exposure and sensorineural hearing loss among workers of a steel rolling mill. *Eur. Arch. Otorhinolaryngol.* **2006**, *263*, 618–621. [CrossRef]
19. World Steel Association. Worlds Steel in Figures 2015. Available online: https://www.worldsteel.org/media-centre/press-releases/2015/world-Steel-in-figures-2015-is-available-online.html (accessed on 22 April 2018).
20. Nyarubeli, I.P.; Tungu, A.M.; Bråtveit, M.; Sunde, E.; Kayumba, A.V.; Moen, B.E. Variability and determinants of occupational noise exposure among iron and steel factory workers in Tanzania. *Ann. Work Expo. Health* **2018**, *62*, 1109–1122. [CrossRef]
21. Shield, B.; Dockrell, J.E. External and internal noise surveys of London primary schools. *J. Acoust. Soc. Am.* **2004**, *115*, 730–738. [CrossRef]
22. Sarantopoulos, G.; Lykoudis, S.; Kassomenos, P. Noise levels in primary schools of medium sized city in Greece. *Sci. Total Environ.* **2014**, *482–483*, 493–500. [CrossRef]
23. Silva, L.T.; Oliveira, I.S.; Silva, J.F. The impact of urban noise on primary schools. Perceptive evaluation and objective assessment. *Appl. Acoust.* **2016**, *106*, 2–9. [CrossRef]
24. Dean, A.G.; Soe, M.M. OpenEpi: Open Source Epidemiologic Statistics for Public Health, Version 3.03a. Available online: http://www.openepi.com/ (accessed on 7 March 2019).

25. National Institute for Occupational Safety and Health (NIOSH). Criteria for A Recommended Standard: Occupational Noise Exposure Revised Criteria 1998. NIOSH, Ed.; Cincinnati, Ohio. Available online: https://www.cdc.gov/niosh/docs/98-126/pdfs/98-126.pdf (accessed on 1 August 2018).
26. Franks, J.R. Hearing measurement. In *Occupational Exposure to Noise: Evaluation, Prevention and Control*; World Health Organization, Ed.; WHO Electronic Book; WHO: Dortmund, The Netherlands, 2001; Chapter 8; pp. 183–232.
27. International Organization for Standardization (ISO). *Acoustics-Audiometric Test Methods—Part1: Pure Tone Air and Borne Conduction Audiometry*; ISO standard 8253-1:2010; ISO: Geneva, Switzerland, 2010.
28. British Society of Audiology (BSA). Recommended Procedure: Pure Tone Air Conduction and Borne Conduction Threshold Audiometry with or without Masking. 80 Brighton Road, Reading Berkshire, RG6 1PS, UK: British Society of Audiology; 2011. Available online: http://www.thebsa.org.uk/wp-content/uploads/2014/04/BSA_RP_PTA_FINAL_24Sept11_MinorAmend06Feb12.pdf (accessed on 9 November 2017).
29. The Norwegian Labour Inspection Authority. *Audiometric Testing in Noise Exposed Workers*; The Norwegian Labour Inspection Authority: Trondheim, Norway, 2013. (In Nowegian)
30. International Organization for Standardization (ISO). *Acoustics-Estimation of Noise-Induced Hearing Loss*; ISO standard 1999:2013; ISO: Geneva, Switzerland, 2013.
31. Rabinowitz, P.M.; Galusha, D.; McTague, M.F.; Slade, M.D.; Wesdock, J.C.; Dixon-Ernst, C. Tracking occupational hearing loss across global industries: A comparative analysis of metrics. *Noise Health* **2012**, *14*, 21–27. [CrossRef]
32. Lutman, M.E. What is the risk of noise-induced hearing loss at 80, 85, 90 dB(A) and above? *Occup. Med.* **2000**, *50*, 274–275. [CrossRef]
33. Singh, L.P.; Bhardwaj, A.; Kumar, D.K. Prevalence of permanent hearing threshold shift among workers of Indian iron and steel small and medium enterprises: A study. *Noise health* **2012**, *14*, 119–128.
34. Mantysalo, S.; Vuori, J. Effects of impulse noise and continuous steady state noise on hearing. *Br. J. Ind. Med.* **1984**, *4*, 122–132. [CrossRef]
35. Agarwal, G.; Nagpure, P.S.; Gadge, S.V. Noise Induced Hearing Loss in Steel Factory workers. *Int. J. Occup. Saf. Health* **2015**, *4*, 34–43. [CrossRef]
36. Whittaker, J.D.; Robinson, T.; Acharya, A.; Singh, D.; Smith, M. Noise-induced hearing loss in small-scale metal industry in Nepal. *J. Laryngol. Otol.* **2014**, *128*, 871–880. [CrossRef]
37. Dobie, R.A. The burdens of age-related and occupational noise-induced hearing loss in the United States. *Ear Hear.* **2008**, *29*, 565–577. [CrossRef]
38. Sulkowski, W.J. Hearing impairment caused by impulse noise: Survey in the drop forging industry. *Scand. Audiol. Suppl.* **1980**, *12*, 307–317.
39. Kamal, A.A.; Mikael, R.A.; Faris, R. Follow-up of hearing thresholds among forge hammering workers. *Am. J. Ind. Med.* **1989**, *16*, 645–658. [CrossRef]
40. McBride, D.I.; Williams, S. Audiometric notch as a sign of noise induced hearing loss. *Occup. Environ. Med.* **2001**, *58*, 46–51. [CrossRef]
41. Kirchner, D.B.; Evenson, C.E.; Dobie, R.A.; Rabinowitz, P.M.; Crawford, J.; Kopke, R.; Hudson, T.W. Occupational Noise Induced Hearing Loss. ACOEM task force on Occupational Hearing Loss. ACOEM guidance statement. *J. Occup. Environ. Med.* **2012**, *54*, 106–108. [CrossRef] [PubMed]
42. Rabinowitz, P.M.; Galusha, D.; Slade, M.D.; Dixon-Ernst, C.; Sircar, K.D.; Dobie, R.A. Audiogram Notches in Noise-Exposed Workers. *Ear Hear.* **2006**, *27*, 742–750. [CrossRef] [PubMed]
43. Dobie, R.A. Noise-induced permanent threshold shifts in occupational noise and hearing survey: An explanation for elevated risk estimates. *Ear Hear.* **2007**, *28*, 580–591. [CrossRef] [PubMed]
44. Mulwafu, W.; Kuper, H.; Ensink, R.J. Prevalence and causes of hearing impairment in Africa. *Trop. Med. Int. Health* **2016**, *21*, 158–165. [CrossRef]

International Journal of
Environmental Research and Public Health

MDPI

Article

The Role of Motor Learning on Measures of Physical Requirements and Motor Variability During Repetitive Screwing

Tessy Luger *, Robert Seibt, Monika A. Rieger and Benjamin Steinhilber

Institute of Occupational and Social Medicine and Health Services Research, University Hospital and University of Tübingen, Wilhelmstraße 27, 72074 Tübingen, Germany; robert.seibt@med.uni-tuebingen.de (R.S.); monika.rieger@med.uni-tuebingen.de (M.A.R.); benjamin.steinhilber@med.uni-tuebingen.de (B.S.)

* Correspondence: tessy.luger@med.uni-tuebingen.de; Tel.: +4970712984364

Received: 31 January 2019; Accepted: 2 April 2019; Published: 6 April 2019

Abstract: We investigated whether physical requirements and motor variability decreased over days in novices during a repetitive screwing task. Fifty-seven subjects performed one hour of repetitive screwing and fastening on three days, separated by 2–7 days. The average physical requirement and relative cycle-to-cycle variability (coefficient of variation, i.e., CV) were calculated from continuous recordings of electromyography of four arm muscles (biceps brachii, triceps brachii, flexor carpi radialis, extensor digitorum), forearm acceleration, and electrocardiography. Muscle activity levels, heart rate, and forearm acceleration decreased from day 1 to day 2 (range: ~4% to ~20%) and/or 3 (range: ~4% to ~28%). Not all muscles showed a similar pattern. Activity of the extensor digitorum and biceps brachii decreased already between days 1 and 2 (range: ~6% to ~13%), whereas activity of the flexor carpi radialis and triceps brachii decreased between days 1 and 3 (range: ~13% to ~20%). No changes in physical requirement were detected between days 2 and 3. Relative motor variability did not change across days, except that variability of forearm acceleration increased from day 1 to 3 (~5%). This study found consistent changes in physical requirements and indicated that several arm muscles show earlier decreases of muscular activity, like the extensor digitorum, compared to other body parts, like the flexor carpi radialis. Moreover, movement strategies may develop differently than muscle activation strategies, based on the different developments of physical requirements and motor variability. The development of physical requirements in industrial tasks is part of daily living and starts at task onset, highlighting the importance of task familiarization and the randomization of experimental conditions in scientific studies.

Keywords: manual materials handling; electromyography (EMG); motor control; experience; electrocardiography; kinematics

1. Introduction

During our entire lives we acquire new skills, adapt to new situations, and learn to make decisions, which is known as "motor learning" [1]. Motor learning is an ongoing process and is initiated in movement preparations, during which our motor system explores the environment and the different possibilities to gradually improve motor control ("reinforcement learning") [2]. Performing a movement results from the synchronous interaction of multiple systems with the environment ("dynamic systems model") [3,4]. Within this dynamic systems model, our central nervous system (CNS) has to choose a pathway, from a vast number of movement options, to perform the action. In other words, our CNS has to overcome the "degrees of freedom (DOF) problem" and has to select one strategy to execute the desired movement [3]. This reflects the high redundancy of our motor system, with the plausible consequence that our actions become highly variable as well and that we are unable to repeat the exact same movement in repetitive occupational tasks. This phenomenon is termed motor variability, which has been defined as variance in movement of an individual who performs under similar task conditions [5].

The study of Madeleine et al. [6] illustrates that experienced workers showed more motor variability than novices. Sandlund et al. [7] even proposed that motor variability could be considered an individual or personal factor predicting which workers would be prone to develop work-related musculoskeletal disorders (WRMSD), theoretically implying that there could be an optimal level of motor variability. Several studies showed muscular activity levels and motor learning being negatively associated, meaning that muscular activity decreases along the process of motor learning in gaining experience [6,8]. Furthermore, muscular activity was higher when exposed to new environments compared to familiar environments [9,10].

In an occupational context, researchers and practitioners aim to design workplaces by means of ergonomics tools or work organization (e.g., task rotation) that lead to a decreased workload and reduce the risk of WRMSD. In this respect, the role of motor variability in relation to WRMSD has caught the attention of many researchers. Mainly, laboratory studies have been conducted to assess motor variability in an occupational context, since experienced workers from the field have limited availability and conducting field studies generally requires additional resources. Laboratory studies often include inexperienced subjects or novices to test what the effect of ergonomically improved tools or conditions is in a specific work simulation, judged by measures of physical requirements, work performance, and motor variability (e.g., [11,12]). Measures of physical requirements are the static, median or mean, and peak levels of muscular activity, according to the exposure variation analysis [13], median or mean of kinematic variables like joint angles, movement velocity or acceleration, and median or mean of the heart rate. Measures of motor variability are linear metrics like cycle-to-cycle standard deviation or coefficient of variation [14], or nonlinear metrics like entropy-based metrics and coordination metrics [15]. The difficulty of interpreting laboratory assessments among novices is that motor learning may influence study results and respective effects, expressed in terms of, e.g., muscular effort, could be misinterpreted. For example, early phases of the motor learning process could result in higher levels of muscle activity, as shown in a previous study [16].

The aim of this study is to investigate whether physical requirements and motor variability of novices, as a function of adjusted motor control strategies, change over a three-day repeated fine motor task. For investigating the physical requirements, we calculated the static (10th percentile), median (50th percentile), and peak (90th percentile) levels of muscular activity, the mean forearm acceleration, and the mean heart rate. For investigating motor variability, we calculated the cycle-to-cycle variability (coefficient of variation, CV) of muscular activity and forearm acceleration. We have used an exploratory approach because this study was originally not designed to investigate aspects of motor learning, but to assess the test-retest reliability of different normalization procedures of surface electromyography [17]. We hypothesized that measures of physical requirements and motor variability would decrease over days. With the results of this study, we aim to highlight methodological issues that should be considered when designing studies to minimize misinterpretation of results and increase practical relevance and whether we can rely on performing just one measurement to assess the risk of musculoskeletal disorders.

2. Materials and Methods

2.1. Study Population

Subjects were excluded if they had any acute or cardiovascular diseases, impaired range of motion of the neck and upper extremities, or neurological impairments. A total of 65 subjects were recruited for study participation, of which 8 dropped-out due to methodological or organizational issues. The final study population consisted of 57 healthy subjects, of which 30 were female and 27 were male. Details with regard to the subjects can be found in Table 1. All subjects were inexperienced, meaning that none of them had specific experience in the repetitive task with the two specific screwing and fastening tools. The study (260/201BO2) was approved by the local ethics committee of the University of Tübingen (Germany) and all subjects signed the informed consent prior to participation.

Table 1. Description of the study population, as a whole and broken down by sex. Results are displayed as value or as mean ± standard deviation (SD).

	Whole Population	Females	Males
Study population [N]	57	30	27
Age [years]	34.8 ± 14.0	36.5 ± 14.9	32.9 ± 13.0
Height [cm]	174.3 ± 8.9	167.4 ± 5.2	181.9 ± 5.1
Weight [kg]	73.3 ± 13.5	66.2 ± 9.8	81.1 ± 12.8
Handedness [N left/N right]	4/53	1/29	3/24
Sport [hours/week]	5.2 ± 4.5	3.9 ± 2.3	6.8 ± 5.8

2.2. Experimental Design

Subjects performed a repetitive screwing task with their dominant hand on a wooden plate that was positioned in front of them. The height of this plate was individually adjusted, so that the middle of the vertical screwing rows was aligned with the elbow height of the subjects while they were standing upright, with the hand palms facing anterior and the thumbs pointing lateral. For 60 min, subjects screwed 72 screws (4.5 × 45 mm, T-Start T20, 4 g, SPAX International GmbH & Co. KG, Ennepetal, Germany) into the wooden plate (multiplex, 30 mm thick), which was split into 12 vertical rows of six screws each. With their non-dominant hand the subjects positioned the 6 screws, taken from the container that was positioned close to their non-dominant hand, and screwed them in one after another with their dominant hand using a T-handle screwdriver (e.g., T-handle 336, T15, handle cross size 80 mm, shaft length 200 mm, 162 g incl. 3 g bit, Wiha, Germany; Figure 1), after which they pressed a buzzer (phase 1). Then, the subjects changed tools and fastened the same 6 screws with their dominant hand using a torque screwdriver (7443 pistol, 232 g incl. 3 g bit, Wera, Germany; Figure 1), after which they pressed a buzzer again (phase 2). These actions were repeated 12 times until all 12 vertical rows were filled with 6 screws. Due to using torx head screws, the amount of forward directed force was low. The torque screwdriver used for fastening released a click at a predetermined torque of 5 Nm. The buzzer was sampled along with the muscle activity recordings.

Subjects visited the laboratory on three days, separated by 2 to 7 days. At day 1, subjects performed for a period of ~10 min, during which they familiarized with, i.e., got acquainted with, the task. Subjects were considered familiar with the task when they were able to perform screwing and fastening with the two tools provided and work at the predetermined work pace. Following familiarization and at days 2 and 3, the subjects were prepared for the measurements, performed reference measurements for electromyographic (EMG) normalization, and performed the one-hour task.

The work pace of the subjects was controlled using visual feedback, i.e., a vertical bar representing a timeline showed the time that was left to fulfill screwing (phase 1) and fastening (phase 2) of each of the 12 rows. Work pace was predetermined based on the standardized, predetermined motion-time measurement system MTM [18], a system often used in industrial production planning. For both phases together we chose pace MTM-85 to allow all subjects to fulfill the task in the given time without developing muscular fatigue. This pace corresponded to 242 s for screwing (6 screws; phase 1) and 28 s for fastening (6 screws; phase 2), adding up to 270 s for one vertical row. Since we controlled the amount of work and the work pace and since we observed that all subjects screwed in the screws completely, we can conclude that performance was equal within subjects across days and also across subjects.

2.3. Experimental Design

2.3.1. Muscular Activity

Electrical activities of the following four dominant superficial muscles of the hand-arm system that are involved in grasping and screwing, as verified in pilot measurements and as deduced from previous studies [19,20], were measured: The M. triceps brachii, M. biceps brachii, M. flexor carpi radialis, and M. extensor digitorum. Their electrical activity was recorded using surface EMG. We placed pre-gelled Ag/AgCl surface electrodes (35 × 26 mm, 15 mm active area diameter, Kendall™ H93SG ECG Electrodes, Covidien, Zaltbommel, the Netherlands) in a bipolar configuration with an inter-electrode distance of 26 mm (center-to-center) on the muscle belly, according to Criswell [21]. A ground electrode, used to equalize the electrical ground level of the measurement device to the subject's electrical level and to minimize electromagnetic interferences, was placed on the seventh cervical vertebra. Prior to electrode placement we shaved the skin, in case of body hair, and prepared it with an abrasive paste (Skin Prep Gel, Nuprep®, Aurora, USA).

EMG signals were differential amplified, analogue filtered (2nd order high pass filter, –3 dB at 4 Hz; 11th order low pass filter, –3 dB at 1300 Hz), sampled (4096 Hz), analyzed, and stored using a combined data analyzer and logger (PS11-UD, THUMEDI® GmbH & Co. KG, Thum, Germany; overall CMRR > 96 dB; overall effective noise < 0.8 μV RMS; linearity type ±0.25 dB at 20–1100 Hz). The device real-time transformed the data into the frequency domain (1,024-point Fast Fourier Transformation, Bartlett-window, 50% overlap) and digitally high-pass filtered the signal (11th order; –3 dB at 20 Hz). Power line interferences (50 Hz and its first seven harmonics) were removed by replacing it by the spectral values of a 4-Hz wide bandwidth around its center frequency by means of both spectral neighbors. The root-mean-square (RMS) of the electrical activity (μV) and median power frequency (MPF (Hz)) were real-time calculated from the power spectrum (250-millissecond moving window with 50 % overlap) and stored synchronously to the raw data by the PS11 device. An example recording of the RMS of the triceps brachii is provided in Figure S1 (Supplementary Material).

Normalization

Prior to the experimental task, we collected EMG during four 15-s submaximal reference voluntary contractions (RVC) with fixed force levels (Table 2). Each RVC targeted one of the four muscles, biceps brachii, triceps brachii, extensor digitorum, or flexor carpi radialis. The RVCs were measured using a self-developed measuring device in which the subject took a standardized position. With the upper body in an upright position, the forearm was placed horizontally and the upper arm perpendicular to the forearm. For determining the force of the biceps brachii and triceps brachii muscles, the force cell was positioned underneath the cushion below the distal end of the forearm. For determining the force of the extensor digitorum and flexor carpi radialis in the forearm, the force cell was positioned underneath the metacarpal bones in the hand. A monitor was connected to the force cell to give subjects visual feedback on the force level of the muscle contraction. Every RVC was followed by a recovery period of ~1 min. Electrical activity of the muscles was recorded during the RVCs and the middle 10 s of a steady-state period was used for EMG normalization. All RMS values were expressed as a percent of the electrical activity during the RVC, i.e., reference voluntary electrical activity (%RVE; Table 2), by dividing the experimental electrical activity level (μV) by the reference electrical activity level (μV) and multiplying by 100%.

Table 2. Descriptions of submaximal reference voluntary contractions (RVC) of the four target muscles, with corresponding force levels at which subjects had to sustain the RVC.

Target muscle	RVC Procedure	Force Level [N] [1]
M. triceps brachii	Producing a downward force, elbow extension.	80
M. biceps brachii	Producing an upward force, elbow flexion.	110
M. flexor carpi radialis	Producing an upward force, wrist flexion.	60
M. extensor digitorum	Producing a downward force, wrist extension.	60

[1] The force levels [N] were determined during pilot measurements among five subjects to correspond moderate force levels of ~40% maximal force.

Parameters

From the recordings of muscular activity, we determined the low or static level (10th percentile, RMS_{10}), the median level (50th percentile, RMS_{MEDIAN}), and the high level (90th percentile, RMS_{90}) according to the amplitude probability distribution [22]. These parameters were determined for the overall task, screwing only (phase 1), and fastening only (phase 2). In addition, we calculated the within-day change of the MPF and RMS_{MEDIAN} to assess whether there were signs of electromyographic muscular fatigue, determined as an increased RMS_{MEDIAN} concomitant with a decreased MPF [23].

We calculated the relative cycle-to-cycle variability of RMS during screwing (phase 1) and fastening (phase 2) as a metric reflecting the size of motor variability. We defined one work cycle of screwing as screwing 1 screw (~40 s) and one work cycle of fastening as fastening 6 screws belonging to 1 vertical row (~28 s), resulting in 72 screwing and 12 fastening work cycles per day. The relative variability was assessed by calculating the RMS coefficient of variation (CV) per experimental day (RMS_{CV}), i.e., the square root of the mean variance of RMS across screwing and fastening work cycles, divided by the RMS_{MEAN} of the screwing and fastening work cycles.

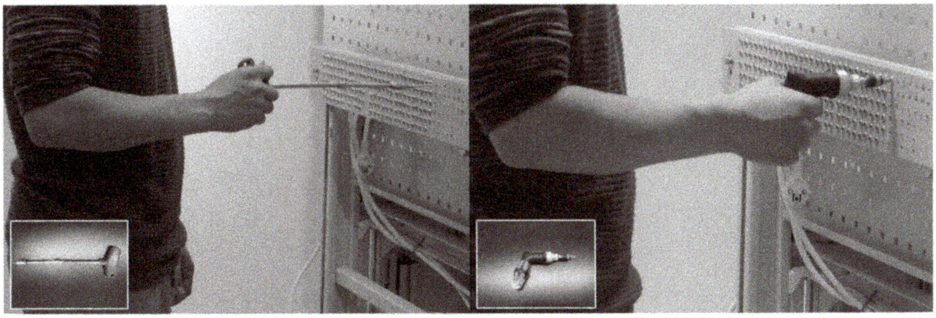

Figure 1. Experimental task setup with an example of screwing using the t-handle screwdriver (left) and an example of fastening using the torque screwdriver (right).

2.3.2. Heart Rate

The electrical activity of the heart was recorded using electrocardiography (ECG) by two pre-gelled Ag/AgCl surface electrodes (35 × 26 mm, Kendall™ H93SG ECG Electrodes, Covidien, Zaltbommel, the Netherlands) placed ~5 cm cranial and ~3 cm left-lateral from the distal end of the sternum and over the anterior to midaxillary line at the fifth left rib. The PS11 sampled (1000 Hz) and recorded the ECG signal (PS11-UD, THUMEDI® GmbH & Co. KG, Thum, Germany), from which we calculated the mean heart rate (HR_{MEAN}) for the overall task, for the screwing part (phase 1), and for the fastening part (phase 2).

2.3.3. Forearm Acceleration

Acceleration of the forearm was sampled (4096 Hz) and recorded (PS11-UD, THUMEDI® GmbH & Co. KG, Thum, Germany) using a single-axis accelerometer (resolution 0.005 m/s^2) placed ventral over the extensor digitorum, 2 to 3 cm ventral of the styloid process ulnaris, using double-sided adhesive tape. Its orientation, i.e., its sensitive axis, was the orthogonal of the forearm bones ulna and radius. The position and orientation were chosen to avoid mechanical interference with the EMG recording electrodes. The accelerometer measured the flexion-extension and rotational acceleration of the forearm. The RMS of the acceleration data was real-time calculated (250-millissecond moving window with 50% overlap), from which we determined the mean (ACC_{MEAN}) for the overall task, screwing only (phase 1), and fastening only (phase 2). Similar as for muscular activity, we calculated the relative cycle-to-cycle variability of the forearm acceleration (ACC_{CV}), for each experimental day, by dividing the square root of the mean variance across all work cycles for screwing and fastening by the ACC_{MEAN}.

2.4. Statistical Analysis

We checked whether the parameters were normally distributed by visually inspecting the histograms and skewness and kurtosis values [24,25]. Based on these explorations, RMS_{10}, RMS_{MEDIAN}, RMS_{90}, and RMS_{CV} were not normally distributed and were therefore log-transformed before the statistical analyses. We performed repeated-measures analysis of variance (RM-ANOVA) on the mean parameters (i.e., RMS_{10}, RMS_{MEDIAN}, RMS_{90}, HR_{MEAN}, and ACC_{MEAN}) of the overall one-hour task, with day as the within-subject factor. We also performed RM-ANOVA (day as within-subject factor) on the mean parameters of phases 1 and 2 separately (i.e., RMS_{10}, RMS_{MEDIAN}, RMS_{90}, RMS_{CV}, HR_{MEAN}, ACC_{MEAN}, and ACC_{CV}). In case of a significant main effect of day, we performed post hoc tests using Student's T-Tests with Bonferroni correction and calculated Cohen's *d* effect sizes using the pooled standard deviation of the two respective days as a standardizer [26]. All statistical analyses were performed with JMP (JMP® 13.1.0) and statistical significance was accepted for the main effects when $p < 0.05$ or, for the Bonferroni-corrected post hoc comparisons, when $p < 0.0167$ (i.e., 0.05 divided by three comparisons). Effect sizes were considered small ($d \geq 0.2$), medium ($d \geq 0.5$), or large ($d \geq 0.8$), as suggested by Cohen [27].

3. Results

All data with statistical outcomes are summarized in Table S1 (Supplementary Material). Data of a different number of subjects was available for each parameter due to failed or unreliable recordings, of which the specific number of subjects is mentioned in Table S1 (Supplementary Material).

3.1. Muscular Fatigue

None of the muscles showed signs of muscular fatigue. Only the flexor carpi radialis showed a significant decrease in RMS_{MEDIAN} concomitant with a significant increase in MPF, which actually points towards the opposite of muscular fatigue, i.e., recovery of muscular strength [23].

3.2. Muscular Activity

3.2.1. M. Triceps Brachii

The factor day had a significant effect on RMS_{MEDIAN} and RMS_{90} during the overall task ($F = 8.88$, $p < 0.001$), the screwing phase ($F = 7.64$, $p < 0.001$), and the fastening phase ($F = 5.81$, $p < 0.01$). For the overall task, RMS_{MEDIAN} decreased from day 1 (11.80 ± 9.56 %RVE) to day 2 (10.31 ± 8.33 %RVE; $p < 0.01$, $d = 0.16$) and from day 1 (11.80 ± 9.56 %RVE) to day 3 (9.32 ± 6.84 %RVE; $p < 0.001$, $d = 0.30$). For screwing, RMS_{MEDIAN} decreased from day 1 (13.74 ± 11.12 %RVE) to day 2 (12.08 ± 10.17 %RVE; $p < 0.01$, $d = 0.16$) and from day 1 (13.74 ± 11.12 %RVE) to day 3 (10.98 ± 9.18 %RVE; $p < 0.001$, $d = 0.29$).

For fastening, RMS_{MEDIAN} decreased from day 1 (10.23 ± 7.97 %RVE) to day 3 (8.23 ± 6.05 %RVE; $p < 0.01$, $d = 0.29$). RMS_{90} decreased in the overall task ($F = 5.27$, $p < 0.01$) from day 1 (38.03 ± 26.13 %RVE) to day 3 (30.82 ± 17.73 %RVE; $p < 0.01$, $d = 0.33$), in the screwing phase also ($F = 4.38$, $p < 0.05$) from day 1 (38.25 ± 26.20 %RVE) to day 3 (31.74 ± 18.83 %RVE; $p < 0.01$, $d = 0.29$), and in the fastening phase ($F = 9.09$, $p < 0.001$) from day 1 (48.47 ± 36.00 %RVE) to day 2 (31.18 ± 31.80 %RVE; $p < 0.01$, $d = 0.16$) and from day 1 (48.47 ± 36.00 %%RVE) to day 3 (39.26 ± 25.81 %RVE; $p < 0.001$, $d = 0.30$; Figure 2). No changes in RMS_{10} or RMS_{CV} were found between days.

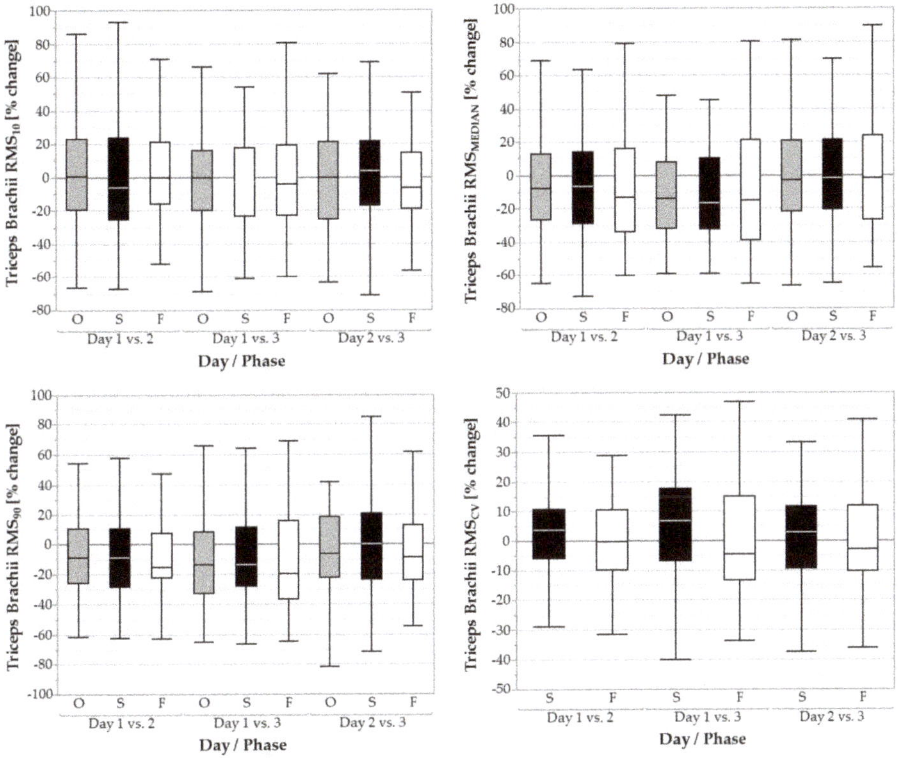

Figure 2. Boxplots of the 10th, 50th, and 90th percentile muscular activity (RMS_{10}, RMS_{MEDIAN}, RMS_{90}) and coefficient of variation (RMS_{CV}) of the triceps brachii over three days for the overall task (O, grey filled boxplots), the screwing phases (S, black filled boxplots), and the fastening phases (F, white filled boxplots).

3.2.2. M. Biceps Brachii

RMS_{MEDIAN} of the overall task was significantly influenced by day ($F = 5{,}89$, $p < 0.01$), with day 1 holding higher values (28.83 ± 15.01 %RVE) than day 2 (25.51 ± 13.82 %RVE; $p < 0.01$, $d = 0.23$) and day 3 (25.50 ± 13.60 %RVE; $p < 0.01$, $d = 0.23$; Figure 3). RMS_{MEDIAN} for the screwing phase also showed a significant effect of day ($F = 3.25$, $p < 0.05$) but post hoc tests revealed no significant pairwise comparisons. RMS_{90} was significantly influenced by day during fastening (F = 14.64, p < 0.001) with a decrease from day 1 (148.33 ± 69.01 %RVE) to 2 (122.52 ± 62.60 %RVE; $p < 0.001$, $d = 0.36$) and also from day 1 (148.33 ± 69.01 %RVE) to 3 (114.85 ± 58.87 %RVE; $p < 0.001$, $d = 0.49$). RMS_{10} and RMS_{CV} did not change between days.

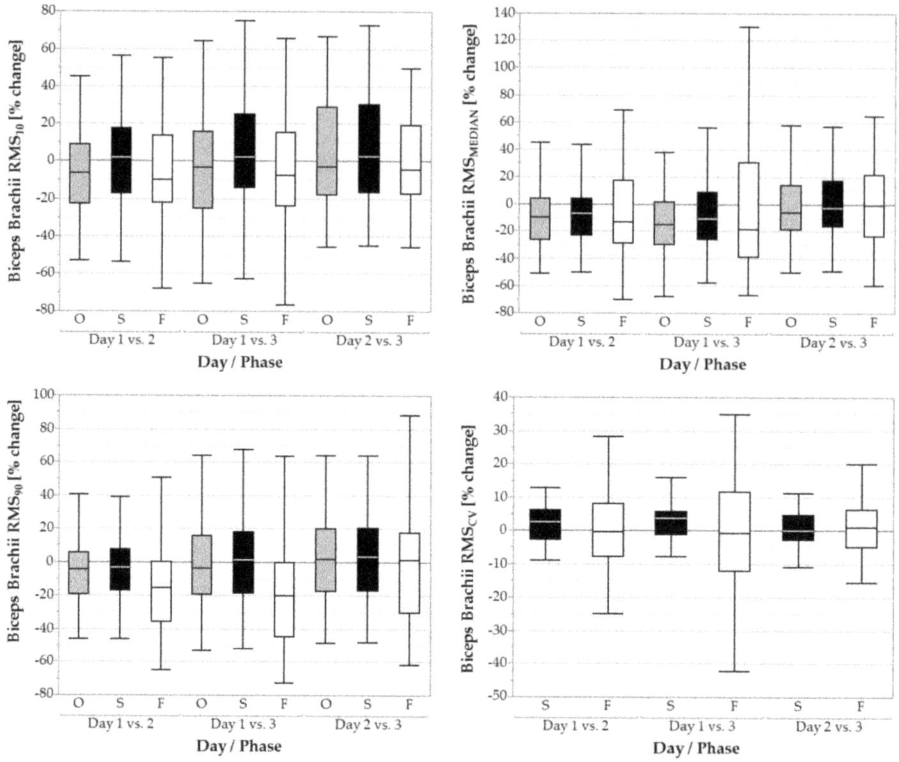

Figure 3. Boxplots of the 10th, 50th, and 90th percentile muscular activity (RMS_{10}, RMS_{MEDIAN}, RMS_{90}) and coefficient of variation (RMS_{CV}) of the biceps brachii over three days for the overall task (O, grey filled boxplots), the screwing phases (S, black filled boxplots), and the fastening phases (F, white filled boxplots).

3.2.3. M. Flexor Carpi Radialis

During the fastening phase, RMS_{90} was significantly influenced by day (F = 4.09, $p < 0.05$; Figure 4). Post hoc tests showed a decreased RMS_{90} from day 1 (65.90 ± 80.80 %RVE) to 3 (52.52 ± 53.75 %RVE; $p < 0.01$, d = 0.20). No significant difference between days was found for RMS_{10}, RMS_{MEDIAN}, or RMS_{CV}.

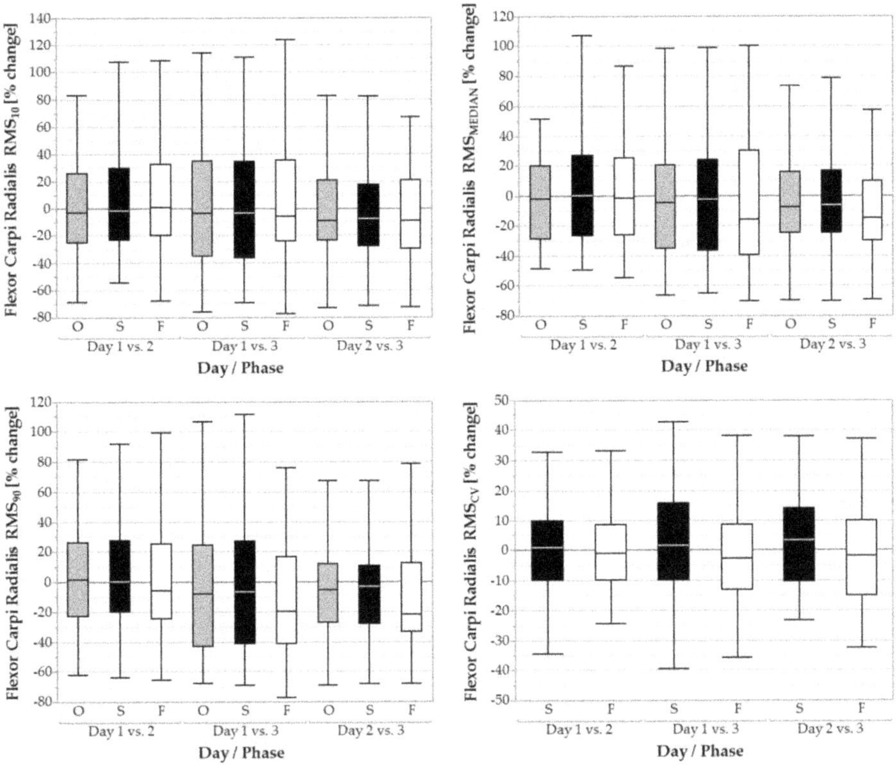

Figure 4. Boxplots of the 10th, 50th, and 90th percentile muscular activity (RMS_{10}, RMS_{MEDIAN}, RMS_{90}) and coefficient of variation (RMS_{CV}) of the flexor carpi radialis over three days for the overall task (O, grey filled boxplots), the screwing phases (S, black filled boxplots), and the fastening phases (F, white filled boxplots).

3.2.4. M. Extensor Digitorum

We found a significant main effect of day for RMS_{MEDIAN} in the overall task ($F = 8.56$, $p < 0.001$), during screwing ($F = 6.32$, $p < 0.01$), and during fastening ($F = 3.31$, $p < 0.05$). During the overall task, RMS_{MEDIAN} decreased from day 1 (45.29 ± 22.23 %RVE) to 2 (42.51 ± 23.57 %RVE; $p < 0.05$, $d = 0.12$) and from day 1 (45.29 ± 22.23 %RVE) to 3 (40.46 ± 22.00 %RVE; $p < 0.001$, $d = 0.22$). RMS_{MEDIAN} decreased from day 1 (50.34 ± 25.56 %RVE) to 3 (46.00 ± 26.25 %RVE) during screwing ($p < 0.001$, $d = 0.17$) and decreased from day 1 (34.76 ± 18.44 %RVE) to 3 (31.76 ± 19.19 %RVE) during fastening ($p < 0.05$, $d = 0.16$). RMS_{10} differed significantly between days for the overall task ($F = 18.35$, $p < 0.001$), screwing ($F = 13.72$, $p < 0.001$), and fastening ($F = 3.50$, $p < 0.05$; Figure 5). In the overall task, RMS_{10} decreased from day 1 (12.70 ± 7.06 %RVE) to 2 (10.13 ± 6.59 %RVE; $p < 0.001$, $d = 0.38$) and from day 1 (12.70 ± 7.06 %RVE) to 3 (9.12 ± 5.84 %RVE; $p < 0.001$, $d = 0.55$). In the screwing phase, RMS_{10} decreased from day 1 (17.45 ± 9.45 %RVE) to 2 (15.03 ± 8.73 %RVE; $p < 0.01$, $d = 0.27$) and from day 1 (17.45 ± 9.45 %RVE) to 3 (14.04 ± 8.07 %RVE; $p < 0.001$, $d = 0.39$). In the fastening phase, RMS_{10} decreased from day 1 (16.43 ± 9.30 %RVE) to 3 (15.18 ± 10.42 %RVE; $p < 0.05$, $d = 0.13$). The factor day also significantly influenced RMS_{90} for the overall task ($F = 5.96$, $p < 0.01$), screwing ($F = 5.24$, $p < 0.01$), and fastening ($F = 4.27$, $p < 0.05$). RMS_{90} decreased from day 1 (83.00 ± 45.24 %RVE) to 3 (75.60 ± 43.64 %RVE) in the overall task ($p < 0.001$, $d = 0.17$), decreased from day 1 (84.22 ± 47.10 %RVE) to 3 (77.29 ± 45.61 %RVE) in the screwing phase ($p < 0.01$, $d = 0.15$) and decreased from day 1 (84.14 ± 38.57 %RVE) to 3

(76.82 ± 38.52 %RVE) in the fastening phase ($p < 0.01$, $d = 0.19$). No significant effect of day on RMS_{CV} was found.

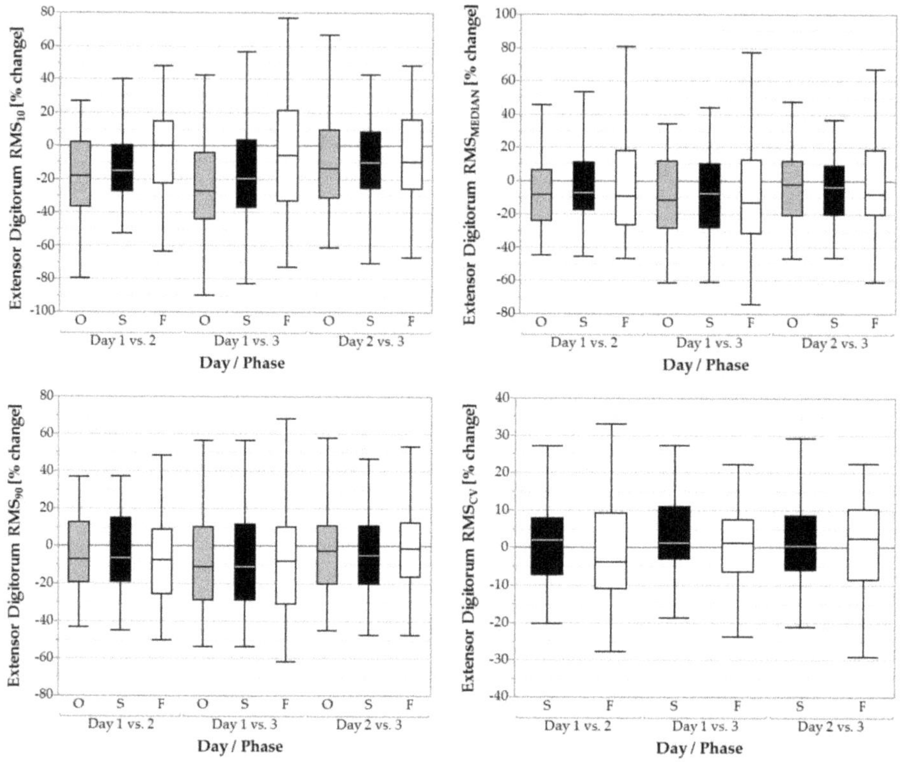

Figure 5. Boxplots of the 10th, 50th,and 90th percentile muscular activity (RMS_{10}, RMS_{MEDIAN}, RMS_{90}) and coefficient of variation (RMSV) of the extensor digitorum over three days for the overall task (O, grey filled boxplots), the screwing phases (S, black filled boxplots), and the fastening phases (F, white filled boxplots).

3.3. Heart Rate

HR_{MEAN} differed significantly between days (Figure 6) for the overall task ($F = 5.91$, $p < 0.01$), screwing ($F = 9.38$, $p < 0.001$), and fastening ($F = 6.35$, $p < 0.01$). For the overall task, HR_{MEAN} decreased from day 1 (91 ± 15 bpm) to 2 (88 ± 12 bpm; $p < 0.01$, $d = 0.27$) and from day 1 (91 ± 15 bpm) to 3 (88 ± 11 bpm; $p < 0.01$, $d = 0.28$). For screwing, HR_{MEAN} decreased also from day 1 (92 ± 15 bpm) to 2 (88 ± 12 bpm; $p < 0.001$, $d = 0.27$) and from day 1 (92 ± 15 bpm) to 3 (88 ± 11 bpm; $p < 0.001$, $d = 0.29$). For fastening it decreased from day 1 (89 ± 15 bpm) to 2 (85 ± 12 bpm; $p < 0.01$, $d = 0.28$) and from day 1 (89 ± 15 bpm) to 3 (85 ± 12 bpm; $p < 0.01$, $d = 0.29$).

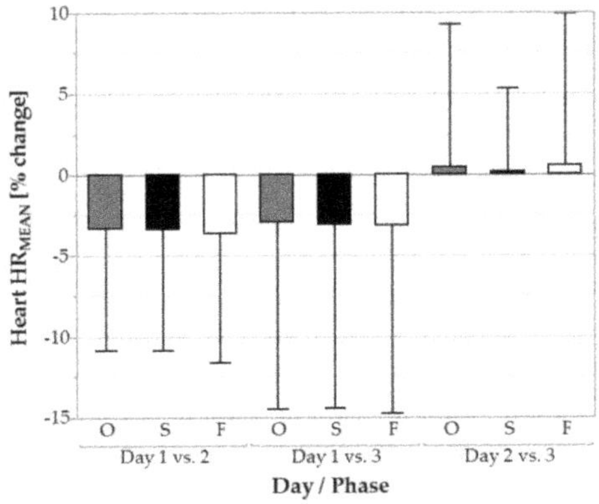

Figure 6. Average heart rate (HR_{MEAN}) over the three days for the overall task (O, grey filled plots), the screwing phases (S, black filled plots), and the fastening phases (F, white filled plots). Error bars represent the SD across subjects.

3.4. Forearm Acceleration

ACC_{MEAN} significantly decreased over days in the overall task ($F = 13.66$, $p < 0.001$) and over the screwing phases ($F = 9.10$, $p < 0.001$; Figure 7). For the overall task, ACC_{MEAN} decreased from day 1 (237.13 ± 56.34 mm/s^2) to 2 (218.65 ± 51.36 mm/s^2; $p < 0.001$, $d = 0.34$) and from day 1 (237.13 ± 56.34 mm/s^2) to 3 (209.45 ± 49.66 mm/s^2; $p < 0.001$, $d = 0.52$). For screwing, ACC_{MEAN} decreased also from day 1 (261.84 ± 65.51 mm/s^2) to 2 (244.35 ± 60.95 mm/s^2; $p < 0.01$, $d = 0.28$) and from day 1 (261.84 ± 65.51 mm/s^2) to 3 (235.34 ± 58.49 mm/s^2; p < 0.001, d = 0.43). We found a main effect of day for ACC_{CV} during fastening ($F = 3.59$, $p < 0.05$). Post hoc tests revealed that ACC_{CV} significantly increased from day 1 (1.52 ± 0.29) to day 3 (1.61 ± 0.36; $p < 0.01$, $d = -0.25$).

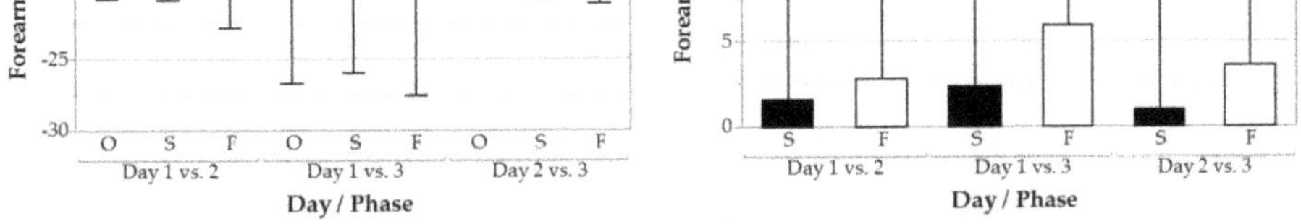

Figure 7. Average acceleration (ACC_{MEAN}) and coefficient of variation (ACC_{CV}) of the forearm over three days for the overall task (O, grey filled plots), the screwing phases (S, black filled plots), and the fastening phases (F, white filled plots). Error bars represent the SD across subjects.

4. Discussion

The objective of this study was to investigate whether physical requirements and motor variability decreased over three days of repetitive screwing among novices. The results largely support our hypothesis, showing a decrease over days in the static, median, and peak EMG activity levels for the extensor digitorum and biceps brachii, but to a lesser extent for the flexor carpi radialis and triceps brachii. No significant differences in physical requirements between days 2 and 3 were detected.

Similarly, acceleration of the forearm and heart rate decreased over days. We found no support for the hypothesis that relative cycle-to-cycle variability of the muscles decreased over days, whereas the relative variability of forearm acceleration significantly increased over days.

4.1. Biomechanical and Cardiovascular Control Strategies

The simulated screwing task activated several upper and lower arm muscles, of which we have measured only a selection. It hereby appeared that the biceps brachii produced the highest activity levels as can be indicated from the normalized EMG values, which relates to its main function of lower arm supination [28] and the T -handle torx screwdriver not requiring much grip force.

The extensor digitorum and triceps brachii clearly decreased their median and peak muscle activity. Similar findings were reported by previous studies that found reductions in muscular activity as a result of motor learning during training (e.g., [29–31]). The overall lowered muscular activity production for the same occupational task may indicate that the early stage of motor learning is a process at the level of the central nervous system, which is supported by the decreased heart rate of ~4 bmp (similar to ~4%) over days, since a decreased heart rate reflects less inhibited parasympathetic activation of the autonomic nervous system [32].

Observing the behaviour of all four muscles separately made us conclude that not all behaved similarly over the three days. The flexor carpi radialis and biceps brachii mainly contributed to the fastening phase of the experimental task, since their peak muscular activity levels decreased between day 1 and days 2 and 3, especially during fastening. On the other hand, the triceps brachii and extensor digitorum showed the most prominent changes during the overall task, as indicated by their decreased median and peak activity levels from day 1 to days 2 and 3. These results indicate that the flexor muscles became more efficient, especially during fastening, and may benefit more from specific training than the extensor muscles that showed less specific changes between the three days.

The strong decreased forearm acceleration after the first day, especially during screwing, could point to a more efficient motor program that has significantly developed already after one day. The resulting movement patterns of screwing being smoother on days 2 and 3 may have resulted in more muscle relaxation, as reflected by the decreased static muscular activity level of the extensor digitorum. Note that all changes in physical requirements were detected at day 2 or 3, compared to day 1. This may indicate that the first day is highly important for developing motor control strategies, whereas no significant changes or improvements happen between days 2 and 3.

4.2. Motor Variability

The amount of motor variability of muscular activity levels remained equal over days in this study, which could imply that the screwing task was not new enough or too simple to provoke developments in motor variability, or that the follow-up was not long enough to be able to find significant developments. The relative variability of forearm acceleration, on the other hand, showed a slight but significant increase regarding the first two days (rate of ~7% increase). This strongly implies that movement strategies and muscular activation strategies develop in a different way. As suggested by previous studies, motor control strategies are optimized with increasing work experience, which could evoke an increased motor variability as a strategy to adapt to performance constraints such as muscular fatigue [33,34] and acute or chronic pain [35].

4.3. Practical Implications

4.3.1. Importance of Familiarization and Randomization

This study with a within-subject design showed decreased muscular activity and acceleration patterns among novices who gain experience in performing a simple screwing task repeated over three days. Decreases were most prevalent between day one and the other two days but were absent between days 2 and 3. This finding indirectly highlights the importance of both sufficient familiarization to experimental tasks and randomization of experimental conditions in studies. Familiarization is especially important when designing a study including repeated measures, to decrease the influence of early stages in the motor learning process. However, it is not clear how much familiarization time is needed, as this probably highly depends on the task complexity. For example, in a study among novice and expert butchers, Madeleine, et al. [36] showed that motor strategies are in development during a six-month follow-up. This does not mean that follow-up times or familiarization periods should be equal to or longer than six months, because this is unrealistic to strive for in studies. However, familiarization should not be too short and include at least some physical practice. Based on the current study results, a two-minute familiarization period, as used by Qin et al. [37], might be too short to reliably measure and interpret physical requirements of occupational tasks. Not reporting task familiarization at all, like Wang et al. [38] did, makes the reader assume that familiarization was not part of the experimental protocol at all and could mean that outcomes were influenced by early stages of the motor learning process. Since the first day of this repetitive task seemed to be most prominent in developing motor control strategies, researchers should provide enough familiarization when investigating occupational tasks.

For comparing different experimental conditions, one can use a between-subject design or a within-subject design. In a between-subject design, classically, subjects are randomly assigned to a group (control vs. intervention). In a within-subject design, subjects will perform all experimental conditions (cross-over design) and are randomly assigned to a sequence of experimental conditions. In most cases, the randomization is performed counterbalanced, meaning that first the number of sequences or the number of subjects per group is determined, after which the assignment to one of the conditions or sequences is based on randomization. The well-known reasons to apply randomization in studies are twofold as follows: (1) Decreasing systematic errors created by a specific experimental manipulation [39] and (2) increasing generalizability or external validity [40]. In addition, we emphasize that randomization may also decrease effects of lack of or insufficient familiarization. This means that an over- or underestimation of the original research question is equally distributed across conditions or across intervention groups. When having a close look at the recent conference proceedings of the International Ergonomics Association 2018 [41], only six of the 223 short papers published, mention randomization in their study. This emphasizes that few studies take randomization into consideration and, as a result, the quality of the study and, therefore, also the relevance of the outcomes may decrease. We therefore recommend applying randomization when possible and, especially when recruiting novices (e.g., students), including a familiarization phase to decrease most of potential motor learning effects.

4.3.2. Motor Variability in An Occupational Context

This study assessed the functional development of motor variability in a manual materials handling task over three days. Although we could not find changes in motor variability over three days, previous studies showed that experienced workers show more variable movement patterns [6], which may indicate that experienced workers are already in the final improvement stage of motor learning where they have developed movement behaviour enabling them to adapt to environmental constraints [42,43]. Furthermore, motor variability has also been suggested to play a beneficial role with respect to internal constraints, such as muscular fatigue [33], pain [44], and external constraints, such as task precision and pace [45]. Confounding factors are also suggested to play a role in the association between motor variability and internal/external constraints, such as sex [46], age [47], and health status. Our current knowledge about the role of motor variability in relation to the aforementioned concepts is still limited. However, when we continue studying motor variability in occupational settings, we might be able to (1) identify workers who are more prone to develop musculoskeletal disorders than others and (2) design (individually adjusted) work tasks and workstations in such a way that motor variability can be promoted [48].

4.4. Methodological Considerations

Our study supports the hypothesis that muscular activity decreased over three days of repetitive screwing and fastening among novices, although it should be noted that our sample size was rather large due to the exploratory design, which is usually not suitable to examine a hypothesis. In general, effect sizes of the reported results were rather small and only few results were accompanied by moderate effect sizes (d = 0.50), including the high muscular activity level of the biceps brachii, the static activity level of the extensor digitorum, and forearm acceleration. Muscular co-contraction has been related to aspects of motor learning in a previous study, [16], by calculating a complex index including the muscular activity and torque levels around a joint, which was beyond the scope of this study.

5. Conclusions

This study showed that physical requirements start developing at task onset, as reflected by the measures of muscular activity, acceleration, and heart rate. However, not all of these measures showed a similar pattern over days, i.e., the extensor digitorum and biceps brachii already showed changes between days 1 and 2, whereas the flexor carpi radialis and triceps brachii showed changes between days 1 and 3. This may indicate the more prominent role of both arm extensor muscles in the screwing and fastening task, regarding the earlier changes. However, changes between days 2 and 3 in physical requirements were absent. Motor variability of the selected muscles did not change between days, but variability of forearm acceleration increased from day 1 to 3, which may reflect that movement strategies develop differently than muscular activation strategies. We emphasize that these developments are part of daily life and should be considered when designing and interpreting studies in terms of task familiarization and randomization of experimental conditions.

Supplementary Materials: The following are available online at http://www.mdpi.com/1660-4601/16/7/1231/s1, Figure S1: Example of a recording of the electrical activity of the triceps brachii of subject 823. The graphs show the raw RMS signal for day 1 (upper), day 2 (middle), and day 3 (lower); Table S1: Results of the one-way repeated measures analysis of variance with the within-subject factor 'day'.

Author Contributions: The specific contributions of each author were as follows: conceptualization, T.L., R.S., M.A.R., and B.S.; methodology, T.L.; software, R.S.; validation, T.L.; formal analysis, T.L.; investigation, R.S. and B.S.; resources, B.S.; data curation, T.L., R.S., and B.S.; writing—original draft preparation, T.L.; writing—review and editing, T.L., R.S., M.A.R., and B.S.; visualization, T.L.; supervision, T.L., M.A.R., and B.S.; project administration, R.S. and B.S.; funding acquisition, M.A.R.

Funding: The work of the Institute of Occupational and Social Medicine and Health Services Research Tübingen is supported by an unrestricted grant of the employers' association of the metal and electric industry Baden-Württemberg (Südwestmetall).

Acknowledgments: We would like to thank Sarah Arnold, Anja Meyer, Felix Epple, and Theresa Kreidler for their assistance in the data analysis.

Conflicts of Interest: The authors declare no conflict of interest.

References

1. Wolpert, D.M.; Diedrichsen, J.; Flanagan, J.R. Principles of sensorimotor learning. *Nat. Rev. Neuros.* **2011**, *12*, 739–751. [CrossRef] [PubMed]
2. Sutton, R.S.; Barto, A.G. *Reinforcement Learning: An Introduction*; MIT Press: Cambridge, MA, USA, 1998.
3. Bernshteĭn, N.A. *The Co-ordination And Regulation of Movements*; Pergamon Press: Oxford, UK, 1967.
4. Scholz, J.P. Dynamic pattern theory–some implications for therapeutics. *Phys. Therap.* **1990**, *70*, 827–843. [CrossRef]
5. Newell, K.M.; Slifkin, A.B. The nature of movement variability. In *Motor Behavior and Human Skill: A Multidisciplinary Approach*; Piek, J.P., Ed.; Human Kinetics: New York, NY, USA, 1998.
6. Madeleine, P.; Lundager, B.; Voigt, M.; Arendt-Nielsen, L. Standardized low-load repetitive work: Evidence of different motor control strategies between experienced workers and a reference group. *Ergonomics* **2003**, *185*, 689–698. [CrossRef]

7. Sandlund, J.; Srinivasan, D.; Heiden, M.; Mathiassen, S.E. Differences in motor variability among individuals performing a standardized short-cycle manual task. *Human Movem. Sci.* **2017**, *51*, 17–26. [CrossRef] [PubMed]
8. Chen, Y.T.; Kwon, M.; Fox, E.J.; Christou, E.A. Altered activation of the antagonist muscle during practice compromises motor learning in older adults. *J. Neurophys.* **2014**, *112*, 1010–1019. [CrossRef] [PubMed]
9. Thoroughman, K.A.; Shadmehr, R. Electromyographic correlates of learning an internal model of reaching movements. *J. Neurosci.* **1999**, *19*, 8573–8588. [CrossRef] [PubMed]
10. Milner, T.E.; Cloutier, C. Compensation for mechanically unstable loading in voluntary wrist movement. *Experim. Brain Res.* **1993**, *94*, 522–532. [CrossRef]
11. Luger, T.; Mathiassen, S.E.; Srinivasan, D.; Bosch, T. Influence of work pace on upper extremity kinematics and muscle activity in a short-cycle repetitive pick-and-place task. *Ann. Work Expos. Health* **2017**, *61*, 356–368. [CrossRef] [PubMed]
12. Samani, A.; Srinivasan, D.; Mathiassen, S.E.; Madeleine, P. Variability in spatio-temporal pattern of trapezius activity and coordination of hand-arm muscles during a sustained repetitive dynamic task. *Experim. Brain Res.* **2017**, *235*, 389–400. [CrossRef]
13. Hägg, G.M.; Luttmann, A.; Jäger, M. Methodologies for evaluating electromyographic field data in ergonomics. *J. Electromyogr. Kinesiol.* **2000**, *10*, 301–312. [CrossRef]
14. Srinivasan, D.; Samani, A.; Mathiassen, S.E.; Madeleine, P. The size and structure of arm movement variability decreased with work pace in a standardised repetitive precision task. *Ergonomics* **2015**, *58*, 128–139. [CrossRef]
15. Samani, A.; Srinivasan, D.; Mathiassen, S.E.; Madeleine, P. Nonlinear metrics assessing motor variability in a standardized pipetting task: Between- and within-subject variance components. *J. Electromyogr. Kinesiol.* **2015**, *25*, 557–564. [CrossRef]
16. Osu, R.; Franklin, D.W.; Kato, H.; Gomi, H.; Domen, K.; Yoshioka, T.; Kawato, M. Short- and long-term changes in joint co-contraction associated with motor learning as revealed from surface emg. *J. Neurophysiol.* **2002**, *88*, 991–1004. [CrossRef]
17. Steinhilber, B.; Seibt, R.; Rieger, M.A. Test-retest-reliability of different normalization procedures of surface electromyography for the use in occupational settings. In *Eight International Conference on Prevention of Work-related Musculoskeletal Disorders (PREMUS 2013)*; Busan, South Korea, 2013; p. 220.
18. Maynard, H.B.; Stegmerten, G.J.; Schwab, J.L. *Methods-Time Measurement*; McGraw-Hill: New York, NY, USA, 1948.
19. Yoo, W.G. Effects of the different screwdriver handle sizes on the forearm muscles activities and wrist motion during screw-driving work. *J. Phys. Thera. Sci.* **2013**, *25*, 885–886. [CrossRef]
20. Cederqvist, T.; Lindberg, M. Screwdrivers and their use from a swedish construction industry perspective. *Appl. Ergon.* **1993**, *24*, 148–157. [CrossRef]
21. Criswell, E. *Cram's Introduction to Surface Electromyography*, 2nd ed.; Jones & Bartlett Learning Publishers: Sudbury, MA, USA, 2010.
22. Jonsson, B. Quantitative electromyographic evaluation of muscular load during work. *Scandinav. J. Rehabil. Med.* **1978**, *10*, 69–74.
23. Luttmann, A.; Jager, M.; Sokeland, J.; Laurig, W. Electromyographical study on surgeons in urology. Ii. Determination of muscular fatigue. *Ergonomics* **1996**, *39*, 298–313. [CrossRef]
24. Kim, H.Y. Statistical notes for clinical researchers: Assessing normal distribution (2) using skewness and kurtosis. *Restorat. Dent. Endodont.* **2013**, *38*, 52–54. [CrossRef] [PubMed]
25. Kim, H.Y. Statistical notes for clinical researchers: Assessing normal distribution (1). *Restorat. Dent. Endodont.* **2012**, *37*, 245–248. [CrossRef] [PubMed]
26. Lakens, D. Calculating and reporting effect sizes to facilitate cumulative science: A practical primer for t-tests and anovas. *Front. Psychol.* **2013**, *4*, 863. [CrossRef] [PubMed]
27. Cohen, J. *Statistical Power Analysis for The Behavioural Sciences*; Routledge Academic: New York, NY, USA, 1988.
28. Gielen, C.C.A.M.; van Zuylen, E.J. Coordination of arm muscles during flexion and supination. *Neuroscience* **1986**, *17*, 527–539. [CrossRef]
29. Seidel, O.; Carius, D.; Kenville, R.; Ragert, P. Motor learning in a complex balance task and associated neuroplasticity: A comparison between endurance athletes and nonathletes. *J. Neurophysiol.* **2017**, *118*, 1849–1860. [CrossRef]

30. Lohse, K.R.; Sherwood, D.E.; Healy, A.F. How changing the focus of attention affects performance, kinematics, and electromyography in dart throwing. *Hum. Movem. Sci.* **2010**, *29*, 542–555. [CrossRef]
31. Zachry, T.; Wulf, G.; Mercer, J.; Bezodis, N. Increased movement accuracy and reduced emg activity as the result of adopting an external focus of attention. *Brain Res. Bull.* **2005**, *67*, 304–309. [CrossRef]
32. Srinivasan, D.; Mathiassen, S.E.; Hallman, D.M.; Samani, A.; Madeleine, P.; Lyskov, E. Effects of concurrent physical and cognitive demands on muscle activity and heart rate variability in a repetitive upper-extremity precision task. *Europ. J. Appl. Physiol.* **2016**, *116*, 227–239. [CrossRef]
33. Falla, D.; Farina, D. Periodic increases in force during sustained contraction reduce fatigue and facilitate spatial redistribution of trapezius muscle activity. *Experim. Brain Res.* **2007**, *182*, 99–107. [CrossRef]
34. Srinivasan, D.; Mathiassen, S.E. Motor variability in occupational health and performance. *Clin Biomech.* **2012**, *27*, 979–993. [CrossRef]
35. Madeleine, P.; Mathiassen, S.E.; Arendt-Nielsen, L. Changes in the degree of motor variability associated with experimental and chronic neck-shoulder pain during a standardised repetitive arm movement. *Experim. Brain Res.* **2008**, *185*, 689–698. [CrossRef]
36. Madeleine, P.; Voigt, M.; Mathiassen, S.E. The size of cycle-to-cycle variability in biomechanical exposure among butchers performing a standardised cutting task. *Ergonomics* **2008**, *51*, 1078–1095. [CrossRef]
37. Qin, J.; Lin, J.H.; Buchholz, B.; Xu, X. Shoulder muscle fatigue development in young and older female adults during a repetitive manual task. *Ergonomics* **2014**, *57*, 1201–1212. [CrossRef]
38. Wang, J.; Bartuzi, P.; Roman-Liu, D. Influence of upper extremity position on emg signal measures calculated in time, frequency and time-frequency domains. *Acta Bioeng. Biomech.* **2013**, *15*, 83–91. [PubMed]
39. Field, A. *Discovering Statistics Using IBM Spss Statistics*; SAGE Publications Ltd.: London, UK, 2013.
40. Fonaraw, G.C. Randomization - there is no substitute. *JAMA Cardiology* **2016**, *1*, 633–635. [CrossRef]
41. IEA. Proceedings of the 20th congress of the international ergonomics association (iea 2018) - volume vii: Ergonomics in design, design for all, activity theories for work analysis and design, affective design, 20th Congress of the International Ergonomics Association, Florence, Italy, 26–30 August 2018; Bagnara, Italy.
42. Davids, K.; Glazier, P.; Araújo, D.; Bartlett, R. Movement systems as dynamical systems. *Sport Med.* **2003**, *33*, 245–260. [CrossRef]
43. Dhawale, A.K.; Smith, M.A.; Olveczky, B.P. The role of variability in motor learning. *Ann. Rev. Neuros.* **2017**, *40*, 479–498. [CrossRef] [PubMed]
44. Madeleine, P.; Madsen, T.M. Changes in the amount and structure of motor variability during a deboning process are associated with work experience and neck-shoulder discomfort. *Appl. Ergonom.* **2009**, *40*, 887–894. [CrossRef]
45. Srinivasan, D.; Mathiassen, S.E.; Samani, A.; Madeleine, P. The combined influence of task accuracy and pace on motor variability in a standardised repetitive precision task. *Ergonomics* **2015**, *58*, 1388–1397. [CrossRef]
46. Côté, J.N. A critical review on physical factors and functional characteristics that may explain a sex/gender difference in work-related neck/shoulder disorders. *Ergonomics* **2012**, *55*, 173–182. [CrossRef]
47. Krüger, M.; Eggert, T.; Straube, A. Age-related differences in the stabilization of important task variables in reaching movements. *Motor Contr.* **2013**, *17*, 313–319. [CrossRef]
48. Gaudez, C.; Gilles, M.A.; Savin, J. Intrinsic movement variability at work. How long is the path from motor control to design engineering? *Appl. Ergonom.* **2016**, *53 Pt A*, 71–78. [CrossRef]

International Journal of
Environmental Research and Public Health

MDPI

Article

Time Spent Working in Custody Influences Work Sample Test Battery Performance of Deputy Sheriffs Compared to Recruits

Robert G. Lockie [1,*], Robin M. Orr [2], Matthew R. Moreno [1], J. Jay Dawes [3] and Joseph M. Dulla [4]

1 Department of Kinesiology, California State University, Fullerton, CA 92831, USA; moreno.matthewr@csu.fullerton.edu
2 Tactical Research Unit, Bond University, Robina, QLD 4229, Australia; rorr@bond.edu.au
3 Department of Health Sciences, University of Colorado-Colorado Springs, Colorado Springs, CO 80918, USA; jdawes@uccs.edu
4 Recruit Training Unit, Training Bureau, Los Angeles County Sheriff's Department, Los Angeles, CA 90022, USA; JMDulla@lasd.org
* Correspondence: rlockie@fullerton.edu; Tel.: +1-657-278-4971

Received: 4 March 2019; Accepted: 24 March 2019; Published: 28 March 2019

Abstract: This study determined the influence of years spent working in custody on fitness measured by a state-specific testing battery (Work Sample Test Battery; WSTB) in deputy sheriffs. Retrospective analysis was conducted on one patrol school class (51 males, 13 females) divided into three groups depending on time spent working in custody: DS24 (<24 months; $n = 20$); DS2547 (25–47 months; $n = 23$); and DS48+ (≥48 months; $n = 21$). These groups were compared to a recruit class (REC; 219 males, 34 females) in the WSTB, which comprised five tasks completed for time: 99-yard (90.53-m) obstacle course (99OC); 165-pound (75-kg) dummy drag; six-foot (1.83-m) chain link fence (CLF) and solid wall (SW) climb; and 500-yard (457.2-m) run (500R). A univariate analysis of covariance (ANCOVA) (controlling for sex and age) with Bonferroni post hoc determined significant between-group differences. DS48+ were slower in the 99OC compared to the REC ($p = 0.007$) and performed the CLF and SW slower than all groups ($p \leq 0.012$). DS24, DS2547, and DS48+ were all slower than REC in the 500R ($p \leq 0.002$). Physical training should be implemented to maintain fitness and job-specific task performance in deputy sheriffs working custody, especially considering the sedentary nature of this work.

Keywords: aerobic fitness; body drag; fence climb; foot pursuit; job-specific; law enforcement officer; obstacle course; police; tactical

1. Introduction

Law enforcement can be a physically demanding profession; during a shift, on-duty officers may be required to drive vehicles [1], pursue suspects [2–4], clear obstacles [5], discharge firearms [6,7], and exert force and apprehend offenders [5,7–9]. Recruits must undergo specific training before they can become law enforcement officers (LEOs). The academy setting is where recruits are trained to tolerate the physical rigors of the profession while also learning the required procedures and skills necessary for policing [5,10–12]. As a result, most agencies have set standards that must be achieved by recruits when they are tested in job-specific tasks and physical fitness [2,12]. Failure to achieve these standards will generally mean a recruit will be separated from their academy and they will not graduate to become an LEO [12].

One example of a job-specific examination of physical skills is the Work Sample Test Battery (WSTB), which must be completed by law enforcement recruits before they graduate from law enforcement academies in California, USA [5,13]. As described by Lockie et al. [5], the WSTB consists of five tests that are completed for time: a run around a 99-yard (90.53-m) obstacle course (99OC); a body drag (BD) with a 165-pound (74.84-kg) dummy; a climb over a six-foot chain link fence (CLF); a climb over a six-foot solid wall (SW); and a 500-yard (457.2-m) run (500R). According to guidelines set by California's Peace Officer Standards and Training (POST), these job-specific tests must be completed within specific time limits, which results in points being allocated to each task [13]. A minimum score of 384 in the WSTB is required. Recruits attain points within each task relative to their time to perform each task [5,13]. A faster task completion results in a greater point allocation [5,13].

Despite the importance of the WSTB being an indication of job task performance for recruits [13], once they graduate, they no longer have to maintain any performance standard. Indeed, few law enforcement agencies (LEAs) mandate that their LEOs meet standards of physical fitness over the course of their career [14,15]. As a result of this, many LEOs experience a decline in physical fitness over time. Although this could be related to age-related declines in physical performance [16,17], there are other factors that can also contribute. Orr et al. [15] compared the physical fitness of police academy cadets (recruits in the context of this study) and incumbent officers. The results indicated that male cadets were superior in muscular endurance (measured by push-ups and sit-ups completed in 60 s) and aerobic fitness (measured by 2.4 km run time) when compared to the aged-matched incumbent LEOs. The female cadets were superior in maximal strength (measured by a one-repetition maximum bench press) and upper-body endurance (push-ups completed in 60 s) compared to the female LEOs. Orr et al. [15] suggested the nature of law enforcement occupations, which feature a low volume of work-related physical activity, significantly impacted the maintenance of fitness in the LEOs. Given that superior strength, endurance, and aerobic capacity have been related to better performance in the WSTB [5], any declines in these qualities could negatively impact job performance, as indicated by tests such as the WSTB.

Decreases in fitness and job-specific task performance could be exacerbated for LEOs who spend extended periods of time in an environment where the job demands are lower than those encountered when on patrol, such as when working in custody. Custody facilities can include jails, detention, or court lockup facilities [18]. Although LEOs working in custody may be required to respond to emergencies and physically confront and restrain inmates, the predominant job tasks are low-intensity. This includes processing and supervising inmates, office work, and cell searches [18–20]. In accordance with these expected lower intensity job conditions, agencies that hire individuals for custody-only positions (e.g., custody assistants) generally do not mandate the testing of physical fitness in these individuals [18,21,22]. As custody assistants are a non-warranted position who work under the directives of sworn personnel [18], LEOs generally need to work in custody facilities as well. For deputy sheriffs from certain agencies in the USA, their first position after graduating academy is working in custody. Deputy sheriffs may spend several months to several years working in custody, depending on whether there are available patrol positions at the station they are assigned to. The length of time they spend in custody could influence their fitness and ability to complete job-specific tasks, which is an issue if they move onto patrol duties after working custody. However, there has been no analysis of the effects that time spent completing custody work could have on the fitness of deputy sheriffs.

Therefore, a cross-sectional analysis of deputy sheriffs from one patrol school class was conducted to analyze the influence of time spent working in custody on WSTB performance and compared to established WSTB standards for recruits from this LEA [5]. As the WSTB is used as an indicator for job preparedness in deputy sheriffs [5,13], it is assumed that if WSTB performance is maintained, the deputy sheriffs would be more physically prepared for the demands of patrol. It was hypothesized that the recruits would be faster in the WSTB tasks when compared to the deputy sheriffs. It was further hypothesized that deputy sheriffs who had spent more time working in custody would also be slower in the WSTB tasks.

2. Materials and Methods

2.1. Subjects

Retrospective analysis on one patrol school class from one LEA comprised of 64 deputy sheriffs (age: 32.28 ± 6.54 years; height: 1.76 ± 0.08 m; body mass: 86.02 ± 16.10 kg), which included 51 males (age: 30.92 ± 5.74 years; height: 1.75 ± 0.07 m; body mass: 90.98 ± 13.76 kg) and 13 females (age: 37.62 ± 6.96 years; height: 1.61 ± 0.03 m; body mass: 66.57 ± 7.56 kg), was conducted. All deputy sheriffs from this patrol school class completed the WSTB, and only data from their time in patrol school were provided by the LEA to the researchers. Additionally, only the WSTB times for the deputy sheriffs were provided to the researchers, and not what would be the derived point allocation. The deputy sheriff data were compared to recruits from four academy classes from the same agency who successfully passed the WSTB. The data from these recruits have been previously published by Lockie et al. [5]. The recruit sample was comprised of 253 recruits (age: 26.69 ± 5.26 years; height: 1.75 ± 0.10 m; body mass: 79.69 ± 12.29 kg); 219 males (age: 26.69 ± 5.35 years; height: 1.77 ± 0.08 m; body mass: 81.94 ± 10.98 kg) and 34 females (age: 26.68 ± 4.68 years; height: 1.62 ± 0.09 m; body mass: 64.43 ± 9.57 kg). All class cohorts started their academy within a calendar year in southern California, USA. Based on the retrospective nature of this analysis, the institutional ethics committee approved the use of pre-existing data (HSR-17-18-370).

2.2. Procedures

The data in this study were collected by staff working for one LEA. The staff were all trained by a certified Tactical Strength and Conditioning Facilitator who verified the proficiency of the staff members. Age, height, body mass, and time spent working in custody were recorded at the start of patrol school. Patrol school was a three-week skills refresher program completed by incumbents who had been working in custody, as they did not complete any patrol duties during this time. Deputy sheriffs self-reported the time they had spent working in custody. For the recruits, age, height, and body mass were recorded at the start of the 22-week academy training period [5]. For the deputy sheriffs and recruits, height was measured barefoot using a portable stadiometer (Seca, Hamburg, Germany), while body mass was recorded by electronic digital scales (Health o Meter, Neosho, Missouri, USA). The deputy sheriffs completed the WSTB within the first week of patrol school, between 0700–1200 (7:00 a.m.–12:00 p.m.). As noted by Lockie et al. [5], the WSTB for the recruits was completed during the final weeks of academy depending on the class schedule, and typically between 0500–1200 (5:00 a.m.–12:00 p.m.). The weather conditions for testing for both patrol school and the academy classes were typical of the climate of southern California during a calendar year. Although conducting testing outdoors is not ideal, there was no indoor testing facility available for this LEA, and these procedures were typical of staff from the LEA [5,12,18,21–24].

2.3. Work Sample Test Battery (WSTB)

As noted, the WSTB is mandatory for LEAs in California, and recruits must attain a certain standard (minimum score of 384) in order to graduate from academy [13]. The focus of this study was the time required to complete each task in the WSTB rather than the point allocation. The procedures for each assessment have been presented by Peace Officer Standards and Training [13] and previously published by Lockie et al. [5] but are documented here as well. All tests were performed outdoors on structures specifically designed for the LEA training facility. Deputy sheriffs and recruits wore physical training attire (i.e., no equipment) during completion of the WSTB. The order of test completion may have varied between deputy sheriffs and recruits depending on time constraints, but the 500R was always completed last. This follows stated guidelines from POST, whereby WSTB events can be completed in any order as long as the 500R is the final event [13]. Deputy sheriffs and recruits were provided the opportunity for two attempts for each test (with a minimum of two minutes rest between attempts). Time was recorded to the nearest 0.1 s by a handheld stopwatch for each attempt, and the fastest time was recorded. Timing via stopwatches is standard practice in LEA testing [5,9,10,12,17,18,25–27]. Furthermore, testers trained in the use of stopwatch timing procedures for running and exercise tests can record reliable data [28].

99-yard obstacle course run (99OC): This test was designed to simulate a foot pursuit and is shown in Figure 1. The 99-yard (90.53-m) course was completed as quickly as possible, and deputy sheriffs and recruits were to remain on the concrete track throughout the course. During the run, individuals also needed to step over three 6-inch × 6-inch (0.15 × 0.15 m) simulated curbs and one 34-inch (0.86-m) high obstacle.

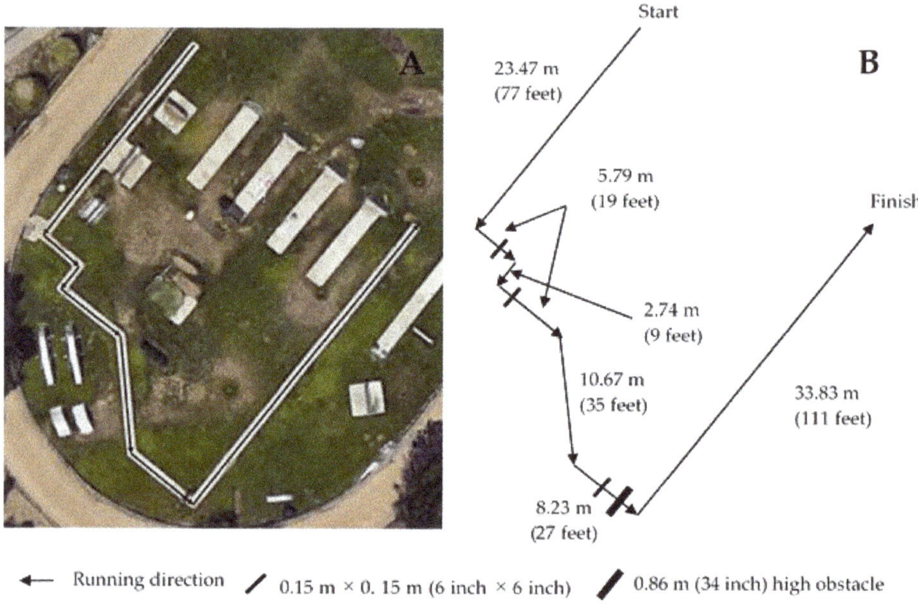

Figure 1. The 99-yard obstacle course. (**A**) Aerial map of the course. (**B**) Dimensions and running direction.

Body drag (BD): Deputy sheriffs and recruits were required to drag a 165-pound (74.84-kg) dummy a distance of 32 feet (9.75 m). Individuals needed to pick up the dummy by wrapping their arms underneath the arms of the dummy and lifting it to a standing position by extending the hips and knees. Once the individual was standing with the dummy and they informed the tester they were ready, timing was initiated, and the individuals had to drag the dummy as quickly as possible by walking backwards over the required distance.

Chain link fence climb (CLF): Deputy sheriffs and recruits started 5 yards (4.57 m) away from the fence, and once the test was initiated, they were required to run up to and scale the fence with whatever technique they deemed most appropriate. However, they could not use any side supports on the fence to assist their climb. If the individual did not initially climb the fence in their first attempt within a trial, they could continue attempting to climb, but the time continued to run within the test. Once the individual cleared the fence, they were to land and run 25 yards (22.86 m) as fast as possible to complete the test.

Solid wall fence climb (SW): The same instructions and procedures for the CLF were provided for the SW, with the only difference being the type of wall that needed to be climbed.

500 yard run (500R): This test simulated a long-distance foot pursuit. The 500-yard (457.2-m) distance was marked on an athletics track, and deputy sheriffs and recruits were instructed to cover this distance as quickly as possible.

2.4. Statistical Analysis

All statistical analyses were computed using the Statistics Package for Social Sciences (Version 25.0; IBM Corporation, New York, NY, USA). Descriptive statistics (mean ± SD) were calculated for each test parameter. The sample was divided into four groups: REC (recruits; n = 253); DS24 (deputy sheriffs who worked in custody for ≤24 months; n = 20); DS2547 (deputy sheriffs who worked in custody for 25–47 months; n = 23); and DS48+ (deputy sheriffs who worked in custody for ≥48 months; n = 21). These time periods were selected to provide a relatively equitable group distribution across the deputy sheriffs. Levene's test for equality of variances was used to ascertain the homogeneity of variance for the data, with significance set as $p < 0.05$. If data were found to be heterogeneous, the alpha level required for between-group significant interactions was adjusted to $p < 0.01$ to reduce the chance of making a Type I error. A univariate analysis of covariance (ANCOVA) was used to ascertain whether there were significant differences between the groups. The ANCOVA analysis was utilized due to the robustness of these procedures when used with a large sample, even with unequal group sizes [29,30]. Sexes were combined within each of the groups, as there are no corrections for sex in the WSTB [13]. Nonetheless, sex was used as a covariate, as numerous studies have documented sex differences in the physical performance of law enforcement populations [16,18,23,24,31]. Body mass and WSTB data were also analyzed with age as an additional covariate, as age can influence body mass and fitness test performance [15–17]. If a significant interaction between the groups was found, a Bonferroni post hoc adjustment for multiple pairwise comparisons was adopted ($p < 0.05$). Similar to previous research [12,23], effect sizes (d) were also calculated for the between-group comparisons, where the difference between the means was divided by the pooled SD [32]. A d less than 0.2 was considered a trivial effect; 0.2 to 0.6 a small effect; 0.6 to 1.2 a moderate effect; 1.2 to 2.0 a large effect; 2.0 to 4.0 a very large effect; and 4.0 and above an extremely large effect [33]. Differences between the mean times for the WSTB tasks through the time points established with the REC and deputy sheriff groups (REC were considered the baseline or 0 months; DS24: up to 24 months working in custody; DS2547: 25–47 months working in custody; DS48+: 48 months or greater working in custody) were also calculated. This was done to ascertain whether there was a certain time point where a clear decline in performance of a WSTB task could be established so as to provide support to findings from the ANCOVA.

3. Results

Descriptive data for the WSTB for all groups are shown in Table 1, while the effect size data are shown in Table 2. Homogenous data were indicated for age (F_3 = 1.297, p = 0.276), height (F_3 = 1.297, p = 0.133), body mass (F_3 = 0.747, p = 0.525), 99OC (F_3 = 0.630, p = 0.596), and the BD (F_3 = 0.472, p = 0.702). The alpha level for significance for these data was set to $p < 0.05$. Heterogeneous data were indicated for the CLF (F_3 = 14.615, $p < 0.001$), SW (F_3 = 9.612, $p < 0.001$), and the 500R (F_3 = 10.668, $p < 0.001$). The alpha level for significance for these data was set to $p < 0.01$.

There was a significant interaction for age (F_3 = 22.535, p = 0.006). REC was younger than all other groups ($p \leq 0.020$; moderate-to-large effects); DS24 and DS2547 were younger than DS48+ ($p \leq 0.007$; moderate effects). There was no significant between-group interactions for height (F_3 = 22.535, p = 0.584). When controlling for sex and age, there was a significant interaction for body mass (F_3 = 4.870, p = 0.003). However, the post hoc analysis indicated that even though there was a moderate effect for the difference between REC and DS48, this comparison did not achieve significance (p = 0.059). There was a significant interaction for the 99OC (F_3 = 3.880, p = 0.010), with DS48+ being significantly slower than REC (p = 0.007), which had a moderate effect. There were also moderate effects for the faster 99OC times for DS24 and DS2547 compared to DS48+, but neither achieved significance (p = 0.410 and 0.437, respectively). There was no significant interaction for the BD (F_3 = 0.464, p = 0.708). There was a significant interaction for the CLF (F_3 = 6.408, $p < 0.001$) and SW (F_3 = 5.547, p = 0.001). DS48+ performed both the CLF ($p \leq 0.004$; all moderate effects) and SW ($p \leq 0.012$; moderate effects for comparisons with REC and DS24) significantly slower than all other groups. There was a significant interaction for the 500R (F_3 = 19.649, $p < 0.001$), with all deputy sheriff groups being significantly slower than REC ($p \leq 0.002$; moderate-to-large effects).

Table 1. Descriptive data (mean ± SD) for age, height, body mass, and the Work Sample Test Battery (WSTB) tasks [99-yard obstacle course (99OC), body drag (BD), chain link fence climb (CLF), solid wall climb (SW), and 500-yard run (500R)] in recruits (REC), and deputy sheriffs who had spent ≤24 months (DS24), 25–47 months (DS2547), and ≥48 months (DS48+) working in custody.

Variables	REC (n = 253)	DS24 (n = 20)	DS2547 (n = 23)	DS48+ (n = 21)
Age (years)	26.69 ± 5.26	30.30 ± 6.36 *	30.30 ± 5.35 *	36.33 ± 6.26 *,§,ϕ
Height (m)	1.75 ± 0.10	1.74 ± 0.07	1.74 ± 0.09	1.71 ± 0.10
Body mass (kg)	79.69 ± 12.29	88.99 ± 13.68	85.46 ± 15.08	83.79 ± 19.35
99OC (sec)	18.49 ± 1.63	18.83 ± 1.60	19.13 ± 1.81	20.64 ± 2.25 *
BD (sec)	5.41 ± 3.19	4.64 ± 0.84	5.08 ± 0.68	6.17 ± 1.77
CLF (sec)	7.83 ± 1.20	7.60 ± 1.62	7.69 ± 1.89	9.78 ± 2.41 *,§,ϕ
SW (sec)	7.75 ± 1.37	7.63 ± 2.09	7.86 ± 1.82	9.83 ± 4.45 *,§,ϕ
500R (sec)	89.20 ± 7.99	100.75 ± 15.08 *	108.09 ± 38.80 *	113.19 ± 18.76 *

* Significantly ($p < 0.05$) different from REC; § Significantly ($p < 0.05$) different from DS24; ϕ Significantly ($p < 0.05$) different from DS2547.

Table 2. Pairwise effect size data between REC and deputy sheriffs who had spent ≤24 months (DS24), 25–47 months (DS2547), and ≥48 months (DS48+) working in custody for age, height, body mass, and the WSTB tasks (99OC, BD, CLF, SW, and 500R).

Variables	REC-DS24	REC-DS2547	REC-DS48+	DS24-DS2547	DS24-DS48+	DS2547-DS48+
Age	0.62 *	0.68 *	1.67 §	<0.01	0.96 *	1.04 *
Height	0.12	0.11	0.40	<0.01	0.35	0.32
Body mass	0.72 *	0.42	0.25	0.25	0.31	0.10
99OC	0.21	0.37	1.09 *	0.18	0.93 *	0.74 *
BD	0.33	0.14	0.29	0.58	1.10 *	0.81 *
CLF	0.16	0.09	1.02 *	0.05	1.06 *	0.97 *
SW	0.07	0.07	0.63 *	0.12	0.63 *	0.58
500R	0.96 *	0.67	1.66 §	0.25	0.73 *	0.17

* Moderate effect for the pairwise comparison; § Large effect for the pairwise comparison.

Figure 2 displays the difference in the mean times for the WSTB tasks through the time points established with the deputy sheriff groups (REC: baseline; DS24: up to 24 months working in custody; DS2547: 25–47 months working in custody; DS48+: 48 months or greater working in custody). For the 99OC, BD, CLF, and SW, there was a notable change in task performance past 48 months of custody work (which, as stated, was significantly different from the baseline for the 99OC, CLF, and SW; Table 1). For the 500R, the most pronounced change in performance time came after 24 months, before this was reduced in subsequent time points. Nonetheless, all of these were significantly different from the baseline established by the REC (Table 1).

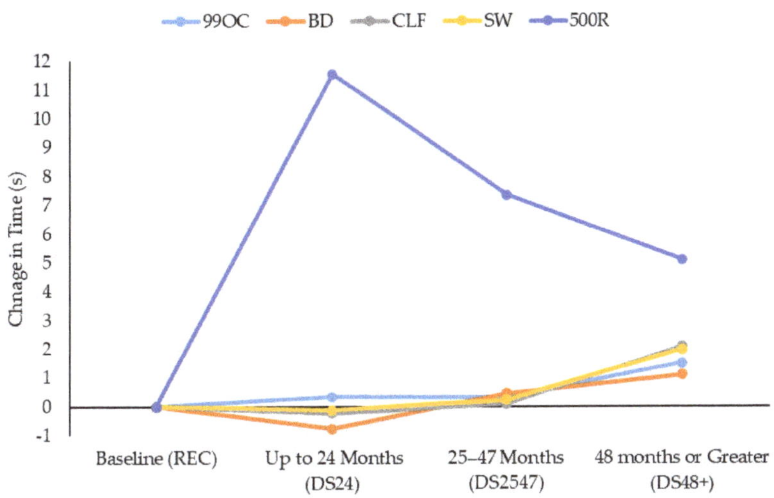

Figure 2. Difference in mean times for each WSTB task (99OC, BD, CLF, SW, and 500R) through the time points established in this study with the deputy sheriff groups (REC: baseline; DS24: up to 24 months working in custody; DS2547: 25–47 months working in custody; DS48+ 48 months or greater working in custody).

4. Discussion

This study analyzed the influence of time spent working in custody on a state-specific job-specific testing battery called the WSTB in deputy sheriffs. It was hypothesized that a longer time spent working in custody would result in poorer WSTB performance in deputy sheriffs when compared to recruits and other deputy sheriffs who had spent less time working in custody facilities. The results provided support to these hypotheses. The DS48+ group performed poorer in the 99OC, CLF, SW, and 500C compared to the REC, and in the CLF and SW compared to the other deputy sheriff groups as well. All deputy sheriff groups were slower in the 500R compared to the REC. In support of previous research [15], these results suggest that LEAs should implement some form of physical training programs for their incumbent deputy sheriffs to maintain their fitness and job-specific skills. This is potentially even more important for deputy sheriffs who have to spend time working in custody before they move onto patrol duties. This is because the general duties of custody can be relatively low-intensity [20], especially compared to those that can be required on patrol (e.g., pursuing and restraining offenders, urgent driving, obstacle clearance) [34,35].

As expected, there were significant differences in age between the REC and deputy sheriff recruits. The mean age for the REC was typical for this agency [5,12,23,24,26,36], and it would be expected that the deputy sheriffs would be older, as they are several months or years into their career. The height and body mass of the REC was also typical for this agency [5,12,23,24,26,36]. Body mass tends to increase in males and females from their 20's to 30's [37]. However, in this study, there were no significant differences between the groups in body mass. Body mass is important to monitor in LEOs and deputy sheriffs, as increased body mass and fat can be indicative of increased cardiovascular disease risk [38–41], which is a major health issue in law enforcement populations [42–44]. Numerous authors have recommended that LEOs (inclusive of deputy sheriffs) should maintain physical activity across their career to ensure better health and fitness [15,25,42]. As is discussed in this paper, this could impact their performance of job-specific tasks as well.

The 99OC is designed to simulate a foot pursuit within an urban area [13]. Lockie et al. [5] detailed that the 99OC had small correlations with fitness tests such as push-ups, sit-ups, mountain climbers, pull-ups, and a 201-m run in recruits. All of these tests place some emphasis on anaerobic energy systems [45], which indicates the importance of these qualities in the performance of the 99OC, and by extension, a foot pursuit. The results from this study showed that DS48+ were slower in the 99OC compared to the REC. It would be expected that the REC would be faster in the 99OC, as they were at the end of their 22-week academy designed to specifically train them for policing duties [5]. For those deputy sheriffs who had spent 48 months or longer working in custody, the combination of the demands of law enforcement shift work (e.g., irregular and long hours) [15,46] with the low-intensity demands of custody work [18–20] likely contributed to the decline in physical characteristics contributing to a slower 99OC. Given that the DS48+ were moving to a patrol position, this would suggest that some form of physical training should be completed during the custody period to minimize any declines in fitness that could influence the performance of a job-specific task, such as a foot pursuit. Rossomanno et al. [25] found that a six-month supervised exercise program for LEOs that incorporated aerobic training and calisthenics could improve time to complete an obstacle course incorporating specific policing skills (e.g., running, jumping, obstacle clearance, dummy drag, and shooting). The LEA from this study should also consider implementing this type of program, especially for deputy sheriffs who need to work a patrol position after custody.

The 500R is also a maximum running task designed to simulate foot pursuit; in this instance, one conducted over a longer distance [13]. Similar to the 99OC, Lockie et al. [5] found that the 500R had small-to-moderate correlations with fitness tests such as push-ups, sit-ups, mountain climbers, pull-ups, and a 201-m run in recruits. In addition, due to the duration of the run placing demands on the aerobic system [45], the 500R also had a large correlation with the 2.4-km run. However, in contrast to the 99OC, all deputy sheriff recruits performed the 500R slower than the REC. This drop in performance was notable from the first time point established in this study (up to 24 months), as opposed to the 99OC, where the significant drop in performance only occurred past 48 months. These data suggest the decline in physiological characteristics important for the 500R (e.g., aerobic capacity) occurs early during a deputy sheriff's custody tenure. As aerobic fitness training tends to be emphasized in LEA academy training [5,12,47,48], it would be expected that REC would be faster in the 500R. Additionally, Orr et al. [15] documented that the incumbent male LEOs were slower in the 2.4-km run compared to cadets, while Lockie et al. [17] found 2.4-km run times tended to get slower with advancing age in incumbent male officers. Given the relationship between the 500R and 2.4-km run [5], if performance in the 2.4-km run declines, it could be surmised that the 500R would decline also. As for the 99OC, if the 500R is viewed as being indicative of a foot pursuit, deputy sheriffs who come from working in custody should attempt to maintain their high-intensity running capacity and aerobic fitness before beginning their patrol tenure. This should occur either at the individual-level or with the provision of structured physical training from the LEA.

Lockie et al. [5] stated that the CLF and SW provide a test of how well a recruit can scale an obstacle such as that they might encounter in urban areas. Upper-body strength measured by pull-ups and muscular endurance measured by push-ups and sit-ups completed in 60 s have been found to relate to faster CLF and SW performance in law enforcement recruits [5]. Declines in upper-body strength and endurance, which have been shown for incumbent officers compared to cadets [15] and across different age groups [16,17], could negatively impact fence climbing tasks. In this study, the DS48+ group performed the CLF and SW slower than all other groups. The physiological characteristics important for obstacle climbing tasks may be maintained to some extent in deputy sheriffs post-academy, with notable changes only occurring after a longer period working in custody (i.e., 48 months or greater). Nevertheless, these results again emphasize the need for structured physical training for deputy sheriffs during their time in custody, as the change in work hours [15,46] and greater volume of low-intensity work [18–20] appear to negatively impact job-specific task performance. The implementation of consistent exercise could maintain performance in climbing tasks. Indeed, a four-foot wall climb was part of the obstacle course detailed by Rossomanno et al. [25].

In contrast to the other WSTB tasks, there were no significant differences between any of the groups in the BD. The BD in the WSTB simulates a victim drag or civilian rescue type scenario [5], which is often assessed in LEOs [3–5]. Lockie et al. [5] suggested that lower-body strength should contribute to this task, given the need for the individual to pick up the dummy from the ground and extend the legs to move to a standing position. However, absolute strength training is not often a focus of law enforcement academy training, with greater preference being given to aerobic training and calisthenics [5,12,47,48]. On the surface, it could be suggested that when compared to the REC, deputy sheriffs maintained the strength required to perform the BD during their tenure in custody. However, if the REC did not complete much absolute strength training during their academy [5,12,47,48], it could be that they are not that strong regardless of their performance in the BD. Taken further, that would mean the deputy sheriffs would not have a higher ceiling of strength to lose during their time in custody. However, these conclusions are speculative, and much further research is needed on the BD. This includes documenting relationships between lower-body strength and the BD, how absolute strength training could influence BD performance, and whether changes in absolute lower-body strength negatively impacts the BD.

There are certain study limitations to this study that should be noted. This study was cross-sectional in nature, and the researchers were unable to compare the current data from the deputy sheriffs to when they were recruits graduating from academy. Future research should track deputy sheriff recruits from their time in academy to their time spent working in custody and in patrol positions to provide a more accurate picture of the effects of the occupation on fitness and job-specific task performance. This study utilized only one patrol school class, which featured 64 deputy sheriffs. This was a much smaller sample when compared to the REC, thus caution should be exercised when applying these results to other law enforcement populations. More research on a greater number of deputy sheriffs who have worked in custody is required, although the results from this study did reflect previous research, which found declines in the physical fitness of LEOs over time [15–17]. Although the REC would likely have completed the WSTB to the best of their ability so as to graduate academy, the motivation for the deputy sheriffs to perform the WSTB maximally may have been lower than the REC. This could have influenced the results from the deputy sheriff groups. Furthermore, the WSTB is only mandatory in the state of California in the USA [5,13]. Other states and countries may use different job-specific testing protocols, and these should be analyzed specifically for each agency, state, or country. Additionally, more general tests of fitness common to law enforcement populations (e.g., push-ups, sit-ups, jump tests, medicine ball throws, maximal running tests) [2,5,10,12,15–18,21–24,26,49–51] could be adopted in future research to track fitness changes relative to time spent working in custody for deputy sheriffs. These tests can be easier to administer while also representing the underlying physical qualities (e.g., strength, power, endurance, running speed) important for job tasks [52].

5. Conclusions

In conclusion, the results from this study indicated that deputy sheriffs who had worked in custody facilities for longer periods of time had poorer performance in WSTB tasks. Specifically, deputy sheriffs who had spent 48 months or greater were slower in the 99OC, CLF, SW, and 500R compared to recruits at the end of academy and deputy sheriffs who had worked for less time in custody. Deputy sheriffs who worked for 48 months or less were slower in the 500R compared to recruits. BD performance was not significantly different between recruits and deputy sheriffs, although that may be a function of a lack of strength training during academy, which would mean there is less absolute strength to decline when a deputy sheriff begins work in custody. These results suggest that structured physical training completed by the individual or provided by the LEA should be implemented to maintain fitness and job-specific task performance in deputy sheriffs. This is especially important for those deputy sheriffs who are leaving custody to begin working in a patrol position, as they will need to be able to perform the tasks that are assessed by the WSTB.

Author Contributions: Conceptualization, R.G.L. and J.M.D.; Methodology, R.G.L., R.M.O., M.R.M., J.J.D., and J.M.D.; Investigation, R.G.L., R.M.O., M.R.M., J.J.D., and J.M.D.; Data Curation, R.G.L., M.R.M., and J.M.D.; Writing-Original Draft Preparation, R.G.L.; Writing-Review & Editing, R.G.L., R.M.O., M.R.M., J.J.D., and J.M.D.

Funding: This research received no external funding.

Acknowledgments: The authors would like to thank the training instructors for facilitating this research, and the California State University, Fullerton tactical research team for collating the data.

Conflicts of Interest: The authors declare no conflict of interest.

References

1. Lockie, R.G.; Dawes, J.J.; Kornhauser, C.L.; Holmes, R.; Orr, R.M. Young officers drive faster, but older officers crash less: Results of a police pursuit driving course. *Police Sci. Aust. N. Z. J. Evid. Based Policy* **2018**, *3*, 37–41.
2. Dawes, J.J.; Lindsay, K.; Bero, J.; Elder, C.; Kornhauser, C.; Holmes, R. Physical fitness characteristics of high vs. low performers on an occupationally specific physical agility test for patrol officers. *J. Strength Cond. Res.* **2017**, *31*, 2808–2815. [CrossRef]
3. Schram, B.; Hinton, B.; Orr, R.; Pope, R.; Norris, G. The perceived effects and comfort of various body armour systems on police officers while performing occupational tasks. *Ann. Occup. Environ. Med.* **2018**, *30*, 15. [CrossRef]
4. Schram, B.; Orr, R.; Pope, R.; Hinton, B.; Norris, G. Comparing the effects of different body armor systems on the occupational performance of police officers. *Int. J. Environ. Res. Public Health* **2018**, *15*, 893. [CrossRef]
5. Lockie, R.G.; Dawes, J.J.; Balfany, K.; Gonzales, C.E.; Beitzel, M.M.; Dulla, J.M.; Orr, R.M. Physical fitness characteristics that relate to Work Sample Test Battery performance in law enforcement recruits. *Int. J. Environ. Res. Public Health* **2018**, *15*, 2477. [CrossRef]
6. Kayihan, G.; Ersöz, G.; Özkan, A.; Koz, M. Relationship between efficiency of pistol shooting and selected physical-physiological parameters of police. *Policing* **2013**, *36*, 819–832. [CrossRef]
7. Orr, R.; Pope, R.; Stierli, M.; Hinton, B. Grip strength and its relationship to police recruit task performance and injury risk: A retrospective cohort study. *Int. J. Environ. Res. Public Health* **2017**, *14*, 941. [CrossRef]
8. Dawes, J.J.; Kornhauser, C.L.; Crespo, D.; Elder, C.L.; Lindsay, K.G.; Holmes, R.J. Does body mass index influence the physiological and perceptual demands associated with defensive tactics training in state patrol officers? *Int. J. Exerc. Sci.* **2018**, *11*, 319–330.
9. Dawes, J.J.; Orr, R.M.; Siekaniec, C.L.; Vanderwoude, A.A.; Pope, R. Associations between anthropometric characteristics and physical performance in male law enforcement officers: A retrospective cohort study. *Ann. Occup. Environ. Med.* **2016**, *28*, 26. [CrossRef]
10. Cocke, C.; Dawes, J.; Orr, R.M. The use of 2 conditioning programs and the fitness characteristics of police academy cadets. *J. Athl. Train.* **2016**, *51*, 887–896. [CrossRef]
11. Orr, R.M.; Ford, K.; Stierli, M. Implementation of an ability-based training program in police force recruits. *J. Strength Cond. Res.* **2016**, *30*, 2781–2787. [CrossRef]
12. Lockie, R.G.; Balfany, K.; Bloodgood, A.M.; Moreno, M.R.; Cesario, K.A.; Dulla, J.M.; Dawes, J.J.; Orr, R.M. The influence of physical fitness on reasons for academy separation in law enforcement recruits. *Int. J. Environ. Res. Public Health* **2019**, *16*, 372. [CrossRef]
13. Peace Officer Standards and Training. Work Sample Test Battery Proctor Manual. 2012. Available online: https://post.ca.gov/post_docs/regulationnotices/2012-05/WrkSmplTestBattryProctrMan.pdf (accessed on 15 August 2018).
14. Bell, M. Implementing Physical Fitness Standards and Training in Law Enforcement. Criminal Justice Institute. 2007. Available online: https://www.cji.edu/site/assets/files/1921/fitnessprogram5.pdf (accessed on 21 March 2019).
15. Orr, R.; Dawes, J.J.; Pope, R.; Terry, J. Assessing differences in anthropometric and fitness characteristics between police academy cadets and incumbent officers. *J. Strength Cond. Res.* **2018**, *32*, 2632–2641. [CrossRef]
16. Dawes, J.J.; Orr, R.M.; Flores, R.R.; Lockie, R.G.; Kornhauser, C.; Holmes, R. A physical fitness profile of state highway patrol officers by gender and age. *Ann. Occup. Environ. Med.* **2017**, *29*, 16. [CrossRef]
17. Lockie, R.G.; Dawes, J.J.; Kornhauser, C.L.; Holmes, R.J. A cross-sectional and retrospective cohort analysis of the effects of age on flexibility, strength endurance, lower-body power, and aerobic fitness in law enforcement officers. *J. Strength Cond. Res.* **2019**, *33*, 451–458. [CrossRef]

18. Lockie, R.G.; Orr, R.M.; Stierli, M.; Cesario, K.A.; Moreno, M.R.; Bloodgood, A.M.; Dulla, J.M.; Dawes, J.J. The physical characteristics by sex and age for custody assistants from a law enforcement agency. *J. Strength Cond. Res.* **2018**. [CrossRef]
19. Jamnik, V.K.; Thomas, S.G.; Burr, J.F.; Gledhill, N. Construction, validation, and derivation of performance standards for a fitness test for correctional officer applicants. *Appl. Physiol. Nutr. Metab.* **2010**, *35*, 59–70. [CrossRef]
20. Jamnik, V.K.; Thomas, S.G.; Shaw, J.A.; Gledhill, N. Identification and characterization of the critical physically demanding tasks encountered by correctional officers. *Appl. Physiol. Nutr. Metab.* **2010**, *35*, 45–58. [CrossRef]
21. Lockie, R.G.; Dulla, J.M.; Stierli, M.; Cesario, K.A.; Moreno, M.R.; Bloodgood, A.M.; Orr, R.M.; Dawes, J.J. Associations between body mass and physical fitness assessments in male custody assistants from a law enforcement agency. *J. Aust. Strength Cond.* **2018**, *26*, 43–49.
22. Lockie, R.G.; Fazilat, B.; Dulla, J.M.; Stierli, M.; Orr, R.M.; Dawes, J.J.; Pakdamanian, K. A retrospective and comparative analysis of the physical fitness of custody assistant classes prior to academy training. *Sport Exerc. Med. Open J.* **2018**, *4*, 44–51. [CrossRef]
23. Lockie, R.G.; Dawes, J.J.; Orr, R.M.; Stierli, M.; Dulla, J.M.; Orjalo, A.J. An analysis of the effects of sex and age on upper- and lower-body power for law enforcement agency recruits prior to academy training. *J. Strength Cond. Res.* **2018**, *32*, 1968–1974. [CrossRef]
24. Cesario, K.A.; Dulla, J.M.; Moreno, M.R.; Bloodgood, A.M.; Dawes, J.J.; Lockie, R.G. Relationships between assessments in a physical ability test for law enforcement: Is there redundancy in certain assessments? *Int. J. Exerc. Sci.* **2018**, *11*, 1063–1073.
25. Rossomanno, C.I.; Herrick, J.E.; Kirk, S.M.; Kirk, E.P. A 6-month supervised employer-based minimal exercise program for police officers improves fitness. *J. Strength Cond. Res.* **2012**, *26*, 2338–2344. [CrossRef]
26. Lockie, R.G.; Stierli, M.; Dawes, J.J.; Cesario, K.A.; Moreno, M.R.; Bloodgood, A.M.; Orr, R.M.; Dulla, J.M. Are there similarities in physical fitness characteristics of successful candidates attending law enforcement training regardless of training cohort? *J. Trainol.* **2018**, *7*, 5–9. [CrossRef]
27. Beck, A.Q.; Clasey, J.L.; Yates, J.W.; Koebke, N.C.; Palmer, T.G.; Abel, M.G. Relationship of physical fitness measures vs. occupational physical ability in campus law enforcement officers. *J. Strength Cond. Res.* **2015**, *29*, 2340–2350. [CrossRef]
28. Hetzler, R.K.; Stickley, C.D.; Lundquist, K.M.; Kimura, I.F. Reliability and accuracy of handheld stopwatches compared with electronic timing in measuring sprint performance. *J. Strength Cond. Res.* **2008**, *22*, 1969–1976. [CrossRef]
29. Rheinheimer, D.C.; Penfield, D.A. The effects of Type I error rate and power of the ANCOVA F Test and selected alternatives under nonnormality and variance heterogeneity. *J. Exp. Educ.* **2001**, *69*, 373–391. [CrossRef]
30. Olejnik, S.F.; Algina, J. Parametric ANCOVA and the rank transform ANCOVA when the data are conditionally non-normal and heteroscedastic. *J. Educ. Behav. Stat.* **1984**, *9*, 129–149. [CrossRef]
31. Birzer, M.L.; Craig, D.E. Gender differences in police physical ability test performance. *Am. J. Police* **1996**, *15*, 93–108. [CrossRef]
32. Cohen, J. *Statistical Power Analysis for the Behavioral Sciences*, 2nd ed.; Lawrence Earlbaum Associates: Hillsdale, NJ, USA, 1988.
33. Hopkins, W.G. How to interpret changes in an athletic performance test. *Sportscience* **2004**, *8*, 1–7.
34. Silk, A.; Savage, R.; Larsen, B.; Aisbett, B. Identifying and characterising the physical demands for an Australian specialist policing unit. *Appl. Ergon.* **2018**, *68*, 197–203. [CrossRef] [PubMed]
35. Decker, A.; Orr, R.M.; Pope, R.; Hinton, B. Physiological demands of law enforcement occupational tasks in Australian police officers. *J. Aust. Strength Cond.* **2016**, *24*, 78–79.
36. Lockie, R.G.; Ruvalcaba, T.R.; Stierli, M.; Dulla, J.M.; Dawes, J.J.; Orr, R.M. Waist circumference and waist-to-hip ratio in law enforcement agency recruits: Relationship to performance in physical fitness tests. *J. Strength Cond. Res.* **2018**. [CrossRef]
37. Fryar, C.D.; Gu, Q.; Ogden, C.L.; Flegal, K.M. Anthropometric reference data for children and adults: United States, 2011–2014. *Vital Health Stat.* **2016**, *3*, 1–46.

38. Seidell, J.C.; Perusse, L.; Despres, J.P.; Bouchard, C. Waist and hip circumferences have independent and opposite effects on cardiovascular disease risk factors: The Quebec Family Study. *Am. J. Clin. Nutr.* **2001**, *74*, 315–321. [CrossRef]
39. Church, T.S.; Cheng, Y.J.; Earnest, C.P.; Barlow, C.E.; Gibbons, L.W.; Priest, E.L.; Blair, S.N. Exercise capacity and body composition as predictors of mortality among men with diabetes. *Diabetes Care* **2004**, *27*, 83–88. [CrossRef]
40. Klein, S.; Allison, D.B.; Heymsfield, S.B.; Kelley, D.E.; Leibel, R.L.; Nonas, C.; Kahn, R. Waist circumference and cardiometabolic risk. *Diabetes Care* **2007**, *30*, 1647–1652. [CrossRef]
41. De Koning, L.; Merchant, A.T.; Pogue, J.; Anand, S.S. Waist circumference and waist-to-hip ratio as predictors of cardiovascular events: Meta-regression analysis of prospective studies. *Eur. Heart J.* **2007**, *28*, 850–856. [CrossRef]
42. Franke, W.D.; Anderson, D.F. Relationship between physical activity and risk factors for cardiovascular disease among law enforcement officers. *J. Occup. Med.* **1994**, *36*, 1127–1132. [CrossRef]
43. Ramey, S.L.; Downing, N.R.; Knoblauch, A. Developing strategic interventions to reduce cardiovascular disease risk among law enforcement officers: The art and science of data triangulation. *Am. Assoc. Occup. Health Nurses J.* **2008**, *56*, 54–62. [CrossRef]
44. Zimmerman, F.H. Cardiovascular disease and risk factors in law enforcement personnel: A comprehensive review. *Cardiol. Rev.* **2012**, *20*, 159–166. [CrossRef] [PubMed]
45. McKardle, W.D.; Katch, F.I.; Katch, V.L. *Exercise Physiology: Nutrition, Energy, and Human Performance*; Wolters Kluwer Health: Baltimore, MD, USA, 2015.
46. Ramey, S.L.; Perkhounkova, Y.; Moon, M.; Tseng, H.C.; Wilson, A.; Hein, M.; Hood, K.; Franke, W.D. Physical activity in police beyond self-report. *J. Occup. Environ. Med.* **2014**, *56*, 338–343. [CrossRef]
47. Cesario, K.A.; Moreno, M.R.; Bloodgood, A.M.; Dulla, J.M.; Lockie, R.G. Heart rate responses of a custody assistant class to a formation run during academy training. In Proceedings of the Southwest American College of Sports Medicine's 37th Annual Meeting, Long Beach, CA, USA, 20–21 October 2017.
48. Moreno, M.R.; Cesario, K.A.; Bloodgood, A.M.; Dulla, J.M.; Lockie, R.G. Heart rate response of a custody assistant class to circuit training during the academy period. In Proceedings of the Southwest American College of Sports Medicine's 37th Annual Meeting, Long Beach, CA, USA, 20–21 October 2017.
49. Moreno, M.R.; Lockie, R.G.; Kornhauser, C.L.; Holmes, R.J.; Dawes, J.J. A preliminary analysis of the relationship between the multistage fitness test and 300-m run in law enforcement officers: Implications for fitness assessment. *Int. J. Exerc. Sci.* **2018**, *11*, 730–738.
50. Lockie, R.G.; Moreno, M.R.; Bloodgood, A.M.; Cesario, K.A. Practical assessments of power for law enforcement populations. *TSAC Rep.* **2018**, *49*, 6–12.
51. Orr, R.M.; Caust, E.; Hinton, B.; Pope, R. Selecting the best of the best: Associations between anthropometric and fitness assessment results and success in police specialist selection. *Int. J. Exerc. Sci.* **2018**, *11*, 785–796. [PubMed]
52. Gumieniak, R.; Jamnik, V.; Gledhill, N. Physical fitness bona fide occupational requirements for safety-related physically demanding occupations; Test development considerations. *Health Fit. J. Can.* **2011**, *4*, 47–52.

International Journal of
Environmental Research and Public Health

MDPI

Article

Significant Impacts of Work-Related Cerebrovascular and Cardiovascular Diseases among Young Workers: A Nationwide Analysis

Ya-Yuan Hsu [1,2], Ray Wang [3] and Chyi-Huey Bai [2,4,5,*]

1 Division of Labor Market, Institute of Labor, Occupational Safety, and Health, Ministry of Labor, Taipei 221, Taiwan; yayuarn@mail.ilosh.gov.tw
2 School of Public Health, College of Public Health, Taipei Medical University, Taipei 110, Taiwan
3 Institute of Epidemiology and Preventive Medicine, College of Public Health, National Taiwan University, Taipei 100, Taiwan; romanray92@gmail.com
4 Department of Public Health, College of Medicine, Taipei Medical University, Taipei 110, Taiwan
5 Research Center of Health Equity, College of Public Health, Taipei Medical University, Taipei 110, Taiwan
* Correspondence: baich@tmu.edu.tw; Tel.: +886-(2)2736-1661 (ext. 6510); Fax: +886-(2)2738-4831

Received: 25 January 2019; Accepted: 12 March 2019; Published: 18 March 2019

Abstract: *Background*: While occupational factors linked to the onset of cerebrovascular and cardiovascular diseases (CVDs) have been reported among workers, much remains unknown about the impacts that occupation has on the onset of CVDs in various age groups. We attempted to describe temporal trends in total and work-related CVDs (WRCVDs) rates stratified by age and year and explore the relative contributions of work to the CVD risk. *Methods*: This study was conducted using two populations from the Labor Insurance Database as the working population and the National Health Insurance Research Database as the general population. We included all people aged 15–75 years from 2006 to 2013. All CVD events and WRCVD events were identified. A Poisson regression was used to estimate the morbidity rate ratio (RR) stratified by age and period, and an RR adjusted for residual confounding was also used. *Results*: Incident CVD rates increased with aging in the general population (from 1113.55 to 1853.32 per 100,000 persons), and WRCVD rates increased in the working population over time (from 2.10 in 2006 to 8.60 in 2013 per 100,000 persons). In the age and period analysis, CVD attacks showed disparities in different populations. The RR of the WRCVD risk was mainly in the working population aged >45 years, and the RR of the CVD risk occurred in the oldest group (aged 55–64 years) of the general population. The population-attributable risk of working exposure was 13.5%. After eliminating residual confounding factors, higher population attributed risk (PAR) work-related excessive CVD risk mainly occurred in workers aged 25–34 and 35–44 years. A decreasing PAR trend was found in the age groups as follows: 15–24, 25–34, 35–44, 45–54, and 55–64 years, with percentages of 17.64%, 16.89%, 16.46%, 10.6%, and 0.65%, respectively. *Conclusions*: There is evidence that period and age trends of CVD rates differed between the working population and general population. Relative effects attributed to work were more severe in younger workers, particularly in workers aged <55 years.

Keywords: work-related cerebrovascular and cardiovascular diseases; occupation; Poisson regression; rate ratio

1. Introduction

In recent years, work overload, inducing cerebrovascular and cardiovascular diseases (CVDs), has become a global epidemic issue [1,2]. Globalization has fostered socioeconomic changes, demographic transitions, and rapid industrialization, leading to various occupational classes suffering from attacks of CVDs [3–6]. The annual number of CVD-related deaths is projected to increase from 17 million in

2008 to 25 million by 2030 [7]. Working populations represent 50% of total CVD deaths, and at least 25% of work disability is related to CVDs [1,5]. The global burden of mortality from work-related diseases may be as high as 5.2 million [8,9].

Risk factors for CVDs in workers include age, occupation type, lifestyle, and behavioral and social determinants. Previously, causal relationships with CVDs were found for work stress [10], long working hours causing work overload [11], job insecurity [12], and physicochemical factors [1]. Numerous studies have suggested that a macro-level of the sociopolitical context influences occupational diseases [13–15].

In Taiwan, the government recognizes CVD attacks caused by overwork as work-related (WR)-CVDs [16]. An occupational disease record and compensation system was established by the Taiwanese government. The Ministry of Labor in Taiwan produced diagnostic guidelines for occupational CVDs that were first promulgated in 1991, and guidelines for work-related CVD (WDCVD) criteria were revised in 2004 and 2010 [17].

There is a growing evidence of a causal relationship between work stress and CVD incidence [16], but there is less evidence of the contribution to the macro dimension of occupational CVDs. While the revised guidelines were able to more correctly guarantee a WRCVD declaration, they were insufficient in providing the relative contribution of work to the risk of CVDs. Therefore, we assessed the annual age-specific WRCVD rates in the working population as well as CVD attack rates in the general population from 2006 to 2013. We also attempted to explore possible impacts of CVD risks and the relative contributions of age and working year.

2. Methods

2.1. Data Sources

This study was conducted using the Labor Insurance Database (LID) for the working population and the National Health Insurance (NHI) Research Database (NHIRD) for the general population. Historical records of occurrences of occupational accidents, diseases, and death events in the working population are compiled by the Bureau of Labor Insurance, Ministry of Labor [17]. All work-related information (such as work-related attacks) for all employees in Taiwan is included in the LID. Approximately 99% of people in Taiwan participate in the NHI program. The Longitudinal Health Insurance Database 2005 (LHID2005), a subset of the NHIRD database, was released by the National Health Research Institute from the Ministry of Health and Welfare [18]. The LHID2005 contains claims data of 1,000,000 beneficiaries randomly selected from the Registry of Beneficiaries of the NHIRD in 2005. This database contains registration files and original claims data for reimbursement.

2.2. Study Populations and Case Ascertainment

We included all populations aged 15–75 years from 2006 to 2013. Only subjects with missing age or year were excluded from the populations (total < 0.3% every year). In the working population, WRCVD events were identified according to records of registered work-related CVD accidents and deaths. The denominator is based on the number of insured working persons of that age and period. There were 8,681,139 participants in 2006, 8,799,404 participants in 2007, 8,795,243 participants in 2008, 9,029,277 participants in 2009, 9,397,603 participants in 2010, 9,725,755 participants in 2011, 9,709,501 participants in 2012, and 9,745,793 participants in 2013. In the general population, participants discharged with a related diagnosis from inpatient visits, outpatient visits, or deaths were defined as CVD event cases. Onset time was set as the first date of having a CVD diagnosis. Patients with newly diagnosed CVDs were identified as patients who had at least two ambulatory visits over 3 months or one inpatient visit. All registrants of that age and period were included as the denominator of the general population. There were 679,831 persons in 2006, 696,554 persons in 2007, 712,656 persons in 2008, 736,068 persons in 2009, 757,013 persons in 2010, 768,543 persons in 2011, 774,429 persons in 2012, and 780,150 persons in 2013.

2.3. Definition of WRCVDs and CVDs

In the working population, the guidelines recognized as WRCVD injury or death events included: (1) cerebrovascular diseases (cerebral hemorrhage, cerebral infarction, subarachnoid hemorrhage, and brain damage caused by severe hypertension), and (2) heart diseases (myocardial infarction, acute heart failure, dissecting aneurysm of the aorta, angina pectoris, serious cardiac arrhythmia, cardiac arrest, and sudden cardiac death). In the general population, CVDs were identified according to claims data. According to the ninth revision of the International Classification of Diseases (ICD-9), WRCVD and CVD codes were identified as follows—acute myocardial infarction: 410; congestive heart failure: 428; dissection of the aorta: 441; cerebral thrombosis with cerebral infarction: 434.01; cerebral embolism with cerebral infarction: 434.11; subarachnoid hemorrhage: 430; intracerebral hemorrhage: 431; and hypertensive encephalopathy: 437.2. Ultimately, 408 observed WRCVD events from the working population and 109,236 observed CVD events from the general population were found.

2.4. Statistical Analysis

The LID and NHIRD are supervised separately by two departments, and they could not be linked at an individual level. Grouped data of CVD or WRCVD and related population size by age and year were extracted from the databases. These participants were separated into six age categories: 15–24, 25–34, 35–44, 45–54, 55–64, and ≥65 years, and these were calculated every calendar year during 2006~2013. Crude annual age-specific CVD morbidity (first-ever-in-a-lifetime event) and/or attack rates (all events, including recurrent events) with 95% confidence intervals (CIs) per 100,000 persons were calculated. A generalized estimation equation (GEE) with a log link and Poisson assumption (as a log-linear model) were used. The model with CVD or WRCVD events as the dependent variable and population size as the offset was conducted using pooled technology.

Insurance payment and occupational disease registration rules varied with age and year during the study period. Two sets of models for each age group and each period were separately used: models adjusted for age and period, and age–period models additionally adjusted for residual confounding.

The residual adjustments were made for two reasons. First, the LHID2005 is a subset database of the whole population, and the sampling fractions in each age and period are unknown. Second, the background exposure of the general population could not be separated from the working population. This method is common in the analysis of vaccine population vs. total population [19,20], such as in the example presented by Vamos et al. [21]. Therefore, individuals who were and those who were not in the working population should have similar CVD risks after background adjustment, with an expected morbidity rate ratio (RR) of 1.0 for the general population. The effect estimates of risk in the general population were used to adjust for the residual confounding that occurred in the working population as the adjusted RR ($RR_{adjusted}$).

$$RR_{adjusted} = \text{Exp}(\beta_{\text{working pop}} - \beta_{\text{general pop}})$$

To calculate 95% CIs for the $RR_{adjusted}$, we resampled 500 times and 10,000 persons each time from the distribution of the observed populations in each age and period group. After taking the difference of each of the 500 sampled estimates, the 2.5th and 97.5th percentiles of the distribution were used to obtain 95% CIs for the adjusted RRs. The population-attributable risk (PAR) percentage for working was also calculated using the standardized rates as a supporting analysis. All statistical analyses were performed with SAS®v.9.3 software (SAS, Cary, NC, USA).

2.5. Ethics

Ethical approval was obtained from the Taipei Medical University-Joint Institutional Review Board (approval no.: TMU-JIRB N201510071).

3. Results

Figure 1 and Table S1 show the percentages stratified by age among persons who suffered from CVDs in the working and general populations. WRCVDs had greater percentage contributions, than in the general population, among persons aged 45–54 (42.16%) and 35–44 years (25.49%) in the working population. In contrast, higher CVD attack rates were found in the older age group ≥65 years (61.69%) in the general population than in the working population.

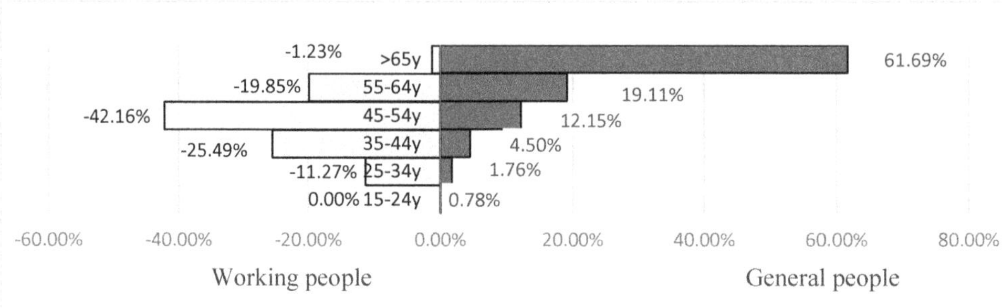

Figure 1. Comparisons of percentage of persons suffering from WRCVDs and CVDs in the working and general populations in Taiwan, 2006–2013, stratified by age. WRCVDs: work related cerebrovascular and cardiovascular diseases. CVDs: cerebrovascular and cardiovascular diseases. y: year.

Table 1 reports the number of event and annual age-specific CVD attack rates (per 100,000) in the working and general populations. In the working population, WRCVD attack rates increased approximately four-fold from 2006 to 2013 (2.10 to 8.60 per 100,000 persons). In the same interval, CVD rates in the general population slowly increased (1113.55 to 1853.32 per 100,000 persons) approximately two-fold. A significant age trend was shown in the general population, but such a trend was not seen in observations of WRCVDs.

Table 1. Annual event number and age-specific attack rates (per 100,000) of WRCVDs and CVDs in working and general populations.

Age Group (Year)	2006	2007	2008	2009	2010	2011	2012	2013
Working population								
15–24	0 0.00	0 0.00	0 0.00	0 0.00	0 0.00	0 0.00	0 0.00	0 0.00
25–34	1 0.04	7 0.27	4 0.15	2 0.07	3 0.11	8 0.28	13 0.47	8 0.29
35–44	6 0.26	11 0.48	7 0.30	9 0.38	14 0.58	19 0.76	15 0.58	23 0.88
45–54	5 0.23	16 0.73	15 0.68	8 0.35	24 1.03	43 1.81	41 1.74	20 0.85
55–64	6 0.77	10 1.17	5 0.59	3 0.32	11 1.04	7 0.60	23 2.02	16 1.40
≥65	0 0.00	0 0.00	1 1.41	2 3.57	0 0.00	1 1.74	0 0.00	1 1.71
Total	18 2.10	44 5.18	32 5.15	24 5.89	52 5.71	78 8.65	92 9.48	68 8.60

Table 1. *Cont.*

Age Group (Year)	2006	2007	2008	2009	2010	2011	2012	2013
General population								
15–24	103 82.07	111 90.21	98 81.24	107 87.59	114 93.22	96 77.67	106 85.06	119 94.91
25–34	225 158.32	223 153.08	215 143.93	222 144.45	241 153.43	282 180.66	254 170.34	262 181.92
35–44	524 376.66	554 396.79	560 403.33	566 404.20	651 462.34	692 488.88	668 466.95	697 483.13
45–54	1377 1086.85	1426 1099.32	1535 1154.03	1623 1185.95	1737 1241.42	1818 1283	1842 1290.35	1919 1338.76
55–64	1853 2632.21	2036 2660.95	2180 2646.14	2418 2725	2812 2926.51	3010 2906.89	3243 2924.97	3326 2866.08
≥65	5422 7133.84	6193 7554.28	7009 7928.19	8223 8691.93	9729 9647.96	10,176 9970.51	10,239 9844.15	10,400 9710.91
Total	9504 1113.55	10,543 1216.38	11,597 1318.42	13,159 1462.64	15,282 1670.51	16,074 1753.15	16,352 1798.21	16,723 1853.32

Event/attack rates (per 100,000) are shown. WRCVDs: work related cerebrovascular and cardiovascular diseases. CVDs: cerebrovascular and cardiovascular diseases.

The trends of annual age-specific WRCVD attack rates and CVD attack rates are displayed in Figure 2a,b. WRCVD attack rates generally increased with age (shown in Figure 2a). Moreover, in the general population, a marked increase occurred in the age group ≥65 years, which had the highest CVD rates (as shown in Figure 2b).

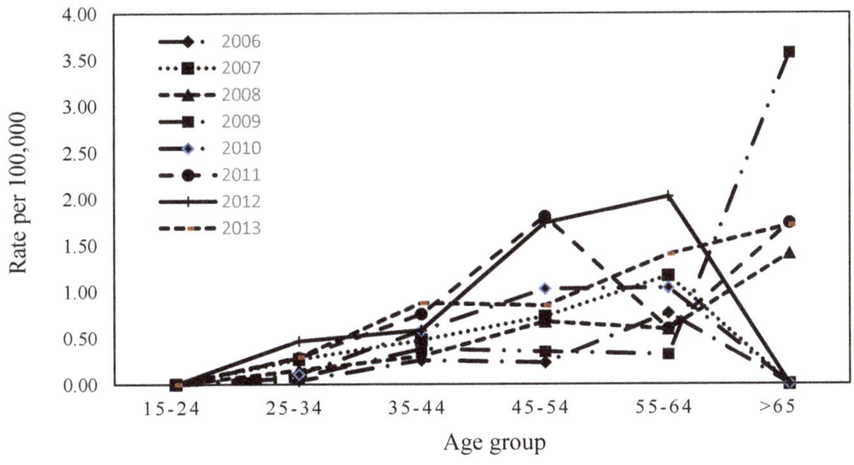

(a)

Figure 2. *Cont.*

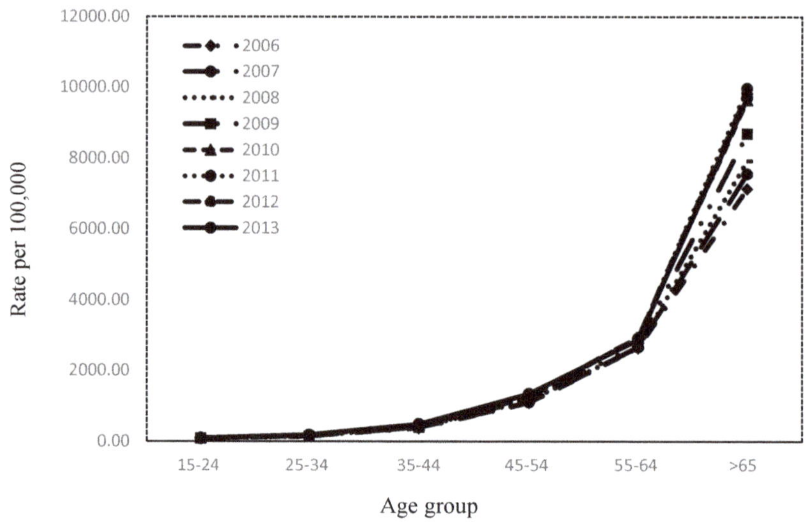

(b)

Figure 2. Trends of annual age-specific WRCVD rates and CVD rates (**a**) in the working population and (**b**) in the general population. WRCVDs: work related cerebrovascular and cardiovascular diseases. CVDs: cerebrovascular and cardiovascular diseases.

An age–period model was used to estimate the RR and 95% CI for WRCVDs and CVDs, and results are shown in Table 2. The population aged ≥65 years was a very different population in the working population than in the general population. Therefore, persons aged ≥65 years old were excluded from the final analysis.

In the working population, period RRs were strongly significant in 2007 and 2010~2013 as compared to 2006 as the reference. An approximate four-fold increase in the WRCVD risk was indicated from 2006 to 2010–2013. Such significant effects of WRCVDs were also found in workers aged 25–64 years. The RRs for WRCVDs increased with age, but we found that the risk rose only two-fold. The highest risk (RR = 1.84; 95% CI = 1.37–2.46) in the 55–64-year age group was shown in comparison to that aged 35–44 years. In the general population, all RRs for CVD onset in each period and age group were significant.

In order to examine the evolution of workers suffering CVD risk disparities across periods and ages, we presented the RRs of CVDs in Table 2. For each concentration of work effect, adjusted RRs were calculated using RRs from the working and general populations. The adjusted RR slightly increased over time, with a considerable increase in 2012 (adjusted RR = 3.84; 95% CI: 2.38–5.61). Of note, there was an observed increase in the adjusted RR in the age group 25–34 years (adjusted RR = 1.08; 95% CI: 0.66–1.94), which significantly decreased in workers aged ≥45 years. At 55–64 years of age, contributions of the effect of work on the CVD risk were slight (adjusted RR = 0.29) but still strongly significant (95% CI: 0.20–0.37).

PARs contributed by working were also calculated using standardized rates. After age and year standardization, the PAR of working exposure was 13.45% (95% CI = 13.2–13.7%). There was a decreasing PAR trend in the age categories 15–24, 25–34, 35–44, 45–54, and 55–64 years, and the percentages were 17.64% (95% CI = 17.4–17.9%), 16.89% (95% CI = 16.7–17.1%), 16.46% (95% CI = 16.2–16.7%), 10.6% (95% CI = 10.4–10.8%) and 0.65% (95% CI = 0.58–0.69%) when standardized by year.

Table 2. Morbidity rate ratios (RRs) and 95% confidence intervals (CIs) for WRCVDs and CVDs by age and period in the working and general populations.

	Working Population				General Population				RR adj †	95% CI of RR adj ‡
	Slope	RR	95% CI	*p* Value	Slope	RR	95% CI	*p* Value		
Period										
2006	Reference	1			Reference	1			1	
2007	0.87	2.39	(1.38–4.13)	0.0019	0.02	1.02	(0.97–1.06)	0.4407	2.35	(1.51–3.40)
2008	0.51	1.67	(0.93–2.98)	0.0839	0.03	1.03	(0.99–1.07)	0.2063	1.62	(1.06–2.50)
2009	0.13	1.14	(0.61–2.12)	0.6842	0.05	1.05	(1.01–1.10)	0.0127	1.08	(0.69–1.58)
2010	0.95	2.58	(1.51–4.40)	0.0005	0.12	1.13	(1.09–1.18)	<0.0001	2.28	(1.45–3.28)
2011	1.3	3.67	(2.20–6.13)	<0.0001	0.14	1.15	(1.11–1.20)	<0.0001	3.19	(2.18–4.66)
2012	1.48	4.41	(2.66–7.31)	<0.0001	0.14	1.15	(1.10–1.20)	<0.0001	3.84	(2.38–5.61)
2013	1.16	3.2	(1.90–5.38)	<0.0001	0.15	1.16	(1.11–1.20)	<0.0001	2.76	(1.85–3.93)
Age										
15–24	−23.98	0	(-)	0.9993	−1.62	0.2	(0.18–0.21)	<0.0001	0	
25–34	−0.92	0.4	(0.28–0.57)	<0.0001	−1.00	0.37	(0.35–0.39)	<0.0001	1.08	(0.66–1.94)
35–44	Reference	1			Reference	1			1	
45–54	0.57	1.76	(1.38–2.25)	<0.0001	1.02	2.78	(2.69–2.87)	<0.0001	0.63	(0.45–0.83)
55–64	0.61	1.84	(1.37–2.46)	<0.0001	1.85	6.35	(6.18–6.58)	<0.0001	0.29	(0.20–0.37)

RR adj †: exp (β labor insurance–β health insurance), 95% CI of RR. ‡: resampling by bootstrapping 500 times. The 2.5th and 97.5th percentiles of the distribution were used to obtain 95% CIs for the adjusted RR. -: unable to estimate. WRCVDs: work related cerebrovascular and cardiovascular diseases. CVDs: cerebrovascular and cardiovascular diseases.

4. Discussion

As far as we know, this is the first longitudinal study to present the attributes of WRCVDs considered as occupational diseases by workers' compensation systems for comparison to all CVDs in the general population. By comparing two population-based databases from national labor and health insurance, we found disparities between the working and general populations in CVD attack rates. A PAR of 13.45% was contributed from working exposure in populations aged 15–64. The contribution from occupations to CVD risk significantly decreased with age, from an $RR_{adjusted}$ of 0.63 at 45–54 years to an $RR_{adjusted}$ of 0.29 at 55–64 years, when compared to the reference group (persons aged 35–44 years) The PARs of working exposure also decreased with increasing age. This demonstrates that work and work-related factors are very significant risk factors in younger populations.

Three major findings were shown when we looked at temporal and age differences from the age–period analysis. First, WRCVDs and CVDs attacks increased with aging and period in populations aged 15–75 years from 2006 to 2013. However, their performances were different. Second, the magnitude of the differences in CVDs between the working and general populations substantially varied by age, with the largest disparities observed particularly among young and middle-aged adults in the main labor force. A pattern of adjusted RRs and PAR was shown, with significantly higher impacts focused on WRCVDs in young workers. In contrast, aging prominently led to increased CVD onset in the general population. Finally, disparities in period-specific adjusted RRs from CVDs for 2009 and 2013 were modest. However, they were all >1, indicating a substantial improvement in the reporting and registration of job-related CVDs after the revised guidelines were promulgated.

In our study, the age–period model was used to adjust for age and period influences [22], and RRs denoted the ratios of morbidity rates as a relative indicator for the reference group after adjustment. Taking account of background age and period trends, $RR_{adjusted}$ was used to adjust residual confounding in the general population. In our observations, the annual CVD attack rates from 2006 to 2013 ranged from 1114 to ~1853 per 100,000. These findings are similar to those in developed countries including the United States, Australia, and Britain [23,24]. As far as we know, age is the strongest risk factor for CVDs in the population, and the aging of the population is projected to continue. We adjusted for the age effect in our age–period model analysis. In addition, the NHIRD population is a representative sample of the general population in Taiwan, which was good for excluding residual confounding.

In our analysis, the working population WRCVD attack rate increased with age. However, the age distribution of CVD events differed between the two populations. Among 109,236 CVD events in the general population, 61.69% were among people aged $\geq$65 years. However, among 408 WRCVDs, 42.16% were among workers 45–54 years old and 25.49% were among workers 35–44 years old. After eliminating background residual confounding, attributable work-related excessive CVD risk mainly occurred in workers aged 45–54 and 35–44 years. The effect was huge, i.e., fourfold ($RR_{adjusted}$ from 0.29 at 55–64 years to 0.6–1.0 at 35–54 years). A Scottish study indicated that premature death from coronary heart disease remains a major contributor to the most affluent groups aged 35–44 and 45–54 years [25,26]. Since middle-aged workers in Japan have been reported to experience prolonged working hours and occupational stress related to CVD risk [27], much evidence has focused on associations between CVDs and occupational factors such as working hours and stress [28].

In a worldwide diagnosis of guidelines for occupational CVDs made in different periods, the governments of Taiwan, Japan, and Korea only recognize CVDs caused by overwork as WRCVDs. The Taiwan Labor Department published "Guidelines for the Diagnosis of Work-Related Cardiovascular Diseases" in 2004 and revised it to be more sensitive in December 2010. Our study showed the higher adjusted RRs of CVDs in 2007 and 2012. The WRCVD attack rate increased from 5.71 in 2010 to 8.60 in 2013 per 100,000 people in the post-2010 revised guideline period. Similarly, the Japanese government recognized WRCVD diagnostic criteria in late 2001, and a gradual increase was found in total compensated CVD occupational diseases [15]. Nevertheless, the Korean government produced occupational health standards in 2003 and found that compensated CVDs accounted for 26%

of the total compensated diseases in 2003, which was a dramatic increase, but the proportion dropped to 7% by 2009 [1]. Reducing compensatory CVDs may be attributable to many preventive activities carried out by governments and employers, but occupational health policy advocacy may increase the annual recognition of WRCVDs. The possible directions need further study.

We provided an exploratory descriptive tool to examine the occupation-attributed relative risk by age and period by taking account of the residual confounding of unknown background factors. Most notably, the present study is the first to examine combined national labor and health insurance databases, which was ideal and strengthened the results. The CVD diagnosis was performed according to ICD-9 codes. WRCVD events were identified through the application and review of guidelines from the government, which identified occupational causes of acute circulatory diseases. The population size was representative and was based on national insurance databases of the workforce and general population. Therefore, the findings in this study are reasonable to present as epidemiological evidence.

Three limitations should be considered in this study. First, the application accuracy of occupational diseases is related to a willingness to recognize occupational causes of injuries or health problems. These assessments included personal exposures to environmental risk factors, for example, from evidence of job insecurity, working hours, job intensification, and management [29,30]. This might vary by age, period, social culture, and country. Problems are also related to the historical background of workers' demands for protection and prevention or compensation and their employers seeking to deny or reduce their liability for work-related diseases and injuries. Second, CVD identification in the general population is based on ICD-9 codes. Due to data extraction limitations, all attack cases included recurring events. However, the stratum-specific rate ratio may have a lower impact in estimation because the extraction criteria for each group are the same. Finally, most WRCVD registered events are recorded for males. The estimations are unstable in some strata in separating by gender. This issue should be considered in the future.

5. Conclusions

CVDs occurred in different periods and age groups in the two insurance system databases. The relative effects attributed to work were more severe in the younger population. Persistent intensive assessment and management of overwork and preventing WRCVDs among young workers are important [31,32]. It should be noted that monitoring regimens across subgroups, as well as the most effective timing and efficacy of primary, secondary, and tertiary preventive interventions for public health policies should be determined in future studies.

Supplementary Materials: The following are available online at http://www.mdpi.com/1660-4601/16/6/961/s1, Table S1: Percentage stratified by age and year among persons who suffered CVDs in the working and general populations.

Author Contributions: Data curation, Y.-Y.H. and R.W.; funding acquisition, C.-H.B.; investigation, C.-H.B.; methodology, C.-H.B.; project administration, C.-H.B.; supervision, C.-H.B.; writing—original draft, Y.-Y.H.

Funding: This study was supported by the Institute of Labor, Occupational Safety, and Health (awarded to ILOSH) and Ministry of Labor, and Ministry of Science and Technology (MOST 107-2314-B-038-072-MY3) in Taiwan.

Acknowledgments: This work was supported by the Council of Labor Affairs, Institute of Labor Occupational Safety and Health in Taiwan.

Conflicts of Interest: The authors declare no conflict of interest.

References

1. Park, J.; Kim, Y.; Hisanaga, N. Work-related cerebrovascular and cardiovascular diseases (WR-CVDs) in Korea. *Ind. Health* **2011**, *49*, 3–7. [CrossRef] [PubMed]
2. Kang, M.Y.; Hong, Y.C. Crossover effect of spouse weekly working hours on estimated 10-years risk of cardiovascular disease. *PLoS ONE* **2017**, *12*, e0182010. [CrossRef] [PubMed]
3. Schnall, P.L.; Dobson, M.; Landsbergis, P. Work, Stress, and Cardiovascular. In *The Handbook of Stress and Health: A Guide to Research and Practice*; Wiley-Blackwell: Hoboken, NJ, USA, 2017; p. 99.

4. Schnall, P.L.; Dobson, M.; Landsbergis, P. Globalization, Work, and Cardiovascular Disease. *Int. J. Health Serv.* **2016**, *46*, 656–692. [CrossRef] [PubMed]
5. Tsutsumi, A. Prevention and management of work-related cardiovascular disorders. *Int. J. Occup. Med. Environ. Health* **2015**, *28*, 4–7. [CrossRef] [PubMed]
6. Moutsatsos, C. Economic globalization and its effects on labor. In *Unhealthy Work: Causes, Consequences, Cures*; Schnall, P., Dobson, M., Roskam, E., Eds.; Baywood: Amityville, NY, USA, 2009.
7. World Health Organization. Cardiovascular Diseases (CVDs): Key Facts. 2017. Available online: www.who.int/mediacentre/factsheets/fs317/en/ (accessed on 20 July 2018).
8. Takala, J. Global estimates of fatal occupational accidents. *Epidemiology* **1999**, *10*, 640–646. [CrossRef] [PubMed]
9. World Health Organization. *Global Status Report on Noncommunicable Diseases 2010*; WHO Press: Geneva, Switzerland, 2011.
10. Pereira, D.; Elfering, A. Social Stressors at Work, Sleep Quality and Psychosomatic Health Complaints—A Longitudinal Ambulatory Field Study. *Stress Health* **2014**, *30*, 43–52. [CrossRef]
11. Bannai, A.; Tamakoshi, A. The association between long working hours and health: A systematic review of epidemiological evidence. *Scand. J. Work Environ. Health* **2014**, *40*, 5–18. [CrossRef]
12. Bosman, J.; Rothmann, S.; Buitendach, J. Job insecurity, burnout and work engagement: The impact of positive and negative affectivity. *SA J. Ind. Psychol.* **2005**, *31*, 48–56. [CrossRef]
13. Kortum, E.; Leka, S.; Cox, T. Psychosocial risks and work-related stress in developing countries: Health impact, priorities, barriers and solutions. *Int. J. Occup. Med. Environ. Health* **2010**, *23*, 225–238. [CrossRef]
14. Cheng, Y. Policy responses to work-related stress: Examining Taiwan's experiences from a welfare state regime perspective. *Saf. Sci.* **2015**, *78*, 111–116. [CrossRef]
15. Park, J.; Kim, Y.; Cheng, Y.; Horie, S. A comparison of the recognition of overwork-related cardiovascular disease in Japan, Korea, and Taiwan. *Ind. Health* **2012**, *50*, 17–23. [CrossRef]
16. Park, J. Impact of Acute Coronary Syndrome (ACS) on Work-relatedness evaluation in cerebrovascular and cardiovascular diseases among workers. *J. Occup. Health* **2006**, *48*, 141–144. [CrossRef]
17. Bureau of Labor Insurance, Ministry of Labor. Available online: http://www.bli.gov.tw/sub.aspx?a=SWZ8zZiGOW4%3d (accessed on 1 December 2017).
18. National Health Insurance Administration, Ministry of Health and Welfare, Taiwan. 2014. Available online: http:/nhird.nhri.org.tw/date_01.html (accessed on 1 December 2017).
19. Lin, D.Y.; Psaty, B.M.; Kronmal, R.A. Assessing the sensitivity of regression results to unmeasured confounders in observational studies. *Biometrics* **1998**, *54*, 948–963. [CrossRef]
20. Weiner, M.G.; Xie, D.; Tannen, R.L. Replication of the Scandinavian simvastatin survival study using a primary care medical record database prompted exploration of a new method to address unmeasured confounding. *Pharmacoepidemiol. Drug Saf.* **2008**, *17*, 661–670. [CrossRef]
21. Vamos, E.P.; Pape, U.J.; Curcin, V.; Harris, M.J.; Valabhji, J.; Majeed, A.; Millett, C. Effectiveness of the influenza vaccine in preventing admission to hospital and death in people with type 2 diabetes. *CMAJ* **2016**, *188*, E342–E351. [CrossRef]
22. Yang, Y.; Land, K.C. *Age-Period-Cohort Analysis: New Models, Methods, and Empirical Applications*; CRC Press: Boca Raton, FL, USA, 2013.
23. Korda, R.J.; Soga, K.; Joshy, G.; Calabria, B.; Attia, J.; Wong, D.; Banks, E. Socioeconomic variation in incidence of primary and secondary major cardiovascular disease events: An Australian population-based prospective cohort study. *Int. J. Equity Health* **2016**, *15*, 189. [CrossRef]
24. Scarborough, P.; Wickramasinghe, K.; Bhatnagar, P.; Rayner, M. *Trends in Coronary Heart Disease 1961–2011*; British Heart Foundation: London, UK, 2011.
25. O'Flaherty, M.; Bishop, J.; Redpath, A.; McLaughlin, T.; Murphy, D.; Chalmers, J.; Capewell, S. Coronary heart disease mortality among young adults in Scotland in relation to social inequalities: Time trend study. *BMJ* **2009**, *339*, b2613. [CrossRef]
26. O'Flaherty, M.; Ford, E.; Allender, S.; Scarborough, P.; Capewell, S. Coronary heart disease trends in England and Wales from 1984 to 2004: Concealed leveling of mortality rates among young adults. *Heart* **2008**, *94*, 178–181. [CrossRef]
27. Uehata, T. Long working hours and occupational stress-related cardiovascular attacks among middle-aged workers in Japan. *J. Hum. Ergol.* **1991**, *20*, 147–153.

28. Kivimäki, M.; Jokela, M.; Nyberg, S.T.; Singh-Manoux, A.; Fransson, E.I.; Alfredsson, L.; Bjorner, J.B.; Borritz, M.; Burr, H.; Casini, A.; et al. Long working hours and risk of coronary heart disease and stroke: A systematic review and meta-analysis of published and unpublished data for 603,838 individuals. *Lancet* **2015**, *386*, 1739–1746. [CrossRef]
29. Fujino, Y.; Iso, H.; Tamakoshi, A.; Inaba, Y.; Koizumi, A.; Kubo, T.; Yoshimura, T.; Japanese Collaborative Cohort Study Group. A prospective cohort study of shift work and risk of ischemic heart disease. *Am. J. Epidemiol.* **2006**, *164*, 128–135. [CrossRef]
30. Kawachi, I.; Colditz, G.A.; Stampfer, M.J.; Willett, W.C.; Manson, J.E.; Speizer, F.E.; Hennekens, C.H. A prospective study of shift work and risk of coronary heart disease in women. *Circulation* **1995**, *92*, 3178–3182. [CrossRef]
31. Assmann, G.; Carmena, R.; Culle, P.; Fruchart, J.C.; Jossa, F.; Lewis, B.; Mancini, M.; Paoletti, R. Coronary heart disease: Reducing the risk—A worldwide view. *Circulation* **1999**, *100*, 1930–1938. [CrossRef]
32. Grundy, S.M.; Balady, G.J.; Criqui, M.H.; Fletcher, G.; Greenland, P.; Hiratzka, L.F.; Miller, N.H.; Etherton, K.P.; Krumholz, H.M.; LaRosa, J.; et al. Primary prevention of coronary heart disease: Guidance from Framingham. A statement for healthcare professionals from the AHA task force on risk reduction. *Circulation* **1998**, *97*, 1876–1887. [CrossRef]

International Journal of
Environmental Research and Public Health

MDPI

Article

Behaviors and Attitudes of Polish Health Care Workers with Respect to the Hazards from Blood-Borne Pathogens: A Questionnaire-Based Study

Anna Garus-Pakowska [1,*] and Mariusz Górajski [2]

[1] Department of Hygiene and Health Promotion; Medical University of Lodz, 90-752 Lodz, Poland
[2] Department of Econometrics, University of Lodz, 90-214 Lodz, Poland; mariusz.gorajski@uni.lodz.pl
* Correspondence: anna.garus-pakowska@umed.lodz.pl; Tel.: +48-4-2272-5288

Received: 30 January 2019; Accepted: 8 March 2019; Published: 12 March 2019

Abstract: Blood-borne infections represent an important occupational health issue in health care settings. The aim of this study was to analyze behaviors of health care workers (HCWs) in the field of needlestick injuries (NSIs) as well as to learn about their attitudes to patients infected with blood-borne viruses. A total of 487 HCWs based at 26 hospitals in Poland completed an anonymous self-administered questionnaire in the period of October–December 2015. Data was analyzed using descriptive statistics and multiple logistic regression. Of the HCWs, 44.8% suffered superficial wounds, and 17.9% HCWs were cut deeply at least once. The most frequent causes of injuries were: rush (31.4%), unpredictable patient behavior (29%), and lack of attention (27%). The rate of underreporting NSIs was 45.2%. Males showed more than three times higher chance of not reporting injuries (odds ratio (OR) 3.495, 95% Confidence Interval (CI): 1.65–7.49). The nurses more often took off their protective gloves to make the procedure easier ($p = 0.036$). Taking off protective clothes was positively associated with long work experience (OR 1.16, 95% CI: 0.995–1.36). Recapping concerned 15.5% of doctors, 8.2% of nurses, and 11.2% of paramedics. 25.9% HCWs feared infection in the workplace, and every tenth HCW refused to help the infected patient. The longer the work experience, the greater the concern about the possibility of infection (OR 1.33, 95% CI: 0.99–1.78). Most HCWs were more cautious when dealing with an infected patient and in their opinion infected patients should be required to inform HCWs of their serological status and such information should be compulsorily transferred between different health institutions. The emphasis in the training of HCWs in the future should be on classes perfecting practical skills like paying more attention to reporting NSIs, improving occupational behaviors like avoiding needle recapping, and on the development of appropriate attitudes towards patients infected with HIV, HBV, or HCV.

Keywords: needlestick injuries; sharp injury; health care workers; occupational exposure; risk factors; knowledge; behaviors; underreporting; hospitals; Poland

---

1. Introduction

Among the more than 60 different pathogens transmitted through the bloodstream, and thus threatening workers in health care settings hepatitis B virus (HBV), hepatitis C virus (HCV), and human immunodeficiency virus (HIV) are the most common and carry a serious risk of complications. They also cause social consequences, such as stigma and discrimination, and economic consequences associated with diagnostics and treatment [1–5]. The risk of infection of the exposed person (from a single needlestick injury—NSI, by a contaminated needle) is estimated to range between 10–30% for HBV [6], 1.8–10% for HCV [7], and 0.3% for HIV infection [8]. WHO reports in the World Health

Report 2002, that of the 35 million health-care workers, 2 million experience percutaneous exposure to infectious diseases each year. It further notes that 37.6% of Hepatitis B, 39% of Hepatitis C and 4.4% of HIV/AIDS in health care workers (HCWs) around the world are due to needlestick injuries (NSI) [9].

In Poland, there is no surveillance system regarding needlestick and sharp injuries (NSIs) but in the structure of infectious and parasitic occupational diseases among health care and social workers HBV, HCV, and Tuberculosis are the most common [10]. Tuberculosis is spread from person to person through the air but cases of blood-borne infection from NSI are also described [11]. It is important that in the epidemic chain HCW may be at risk of infection, but infected-HCW can be a source of infection for the patient [12]. Therefore, it is important to take all actions to prevent injuries to medical personnel. For this purpose, first in this manuscript, prevalence of NSIs and risk factors will be identified. Literature describes such NSIs risk factors as age, short work experience, long working hours and working in surgical or intensive care units [13]. Knowledge of the risk of infection, routes of transmission, and possible prevention is an important aspect in the development of appropriate behavior of HCWs in response to exposure to infectious material.

In psychology, the theories of reasoned action and planned behavior represent connect beliefs with behavior [14]. In accordance with the theory of reasoned action, the best basis for predicting planned behaviors is the attitudes of people towards a particular behavior and their subjective norms (SN), the behavioral intention and behavior are created from these two aspects. Subjective norms, that is, people's beliefs about how others, whose opinion matters, will react to this behavior, are a very important factor. If we want to make someone happy, we will do something even against our normal attitudes. To increase the prognostic power of the theory Ajzen introduced a ratio of perceived behavioral control as a third determinants of behavior intentions. The theory of planned behavior assumes that perceived behavioral control is an entity's ease or difficulty in achieving a particular behavior [15]. Understanding these three elements allows us to well predict the behavioral intentions of others that are highly correlated with their planned behaviors.

In this paper we do not study the actual psychological mechanisms leading to behaviors of HCWs, but we simply apply the random utility theory which is based on the hypothesis that every individual is a rational decision-maker, maximizing utility relative to his or her choices [16]. In our study, we described 4 improper or harmful behaviors of HCWs: taking off protective clothing (tc_i), no participation in trainings (nt_i), lack of NSIs reporting (lr_i), and recapping (re_i). Furthermore, we look for determinants of the following 4 HCWs attitudes to patients infected with blood-borne viruses: fear of infection (fs_i), long-term fear (fl_i), needs of introducing an information system about infected patients (is_i), and indifference (in_i).

A number of strategies are available for avoiding the disease burden associated with NSIs, including vaccination against HBV, post-exposure prophylaxis, reducing the number of injections and invasive procedures where appropriate, using safer devices and properly disposing of needles and other sharps [9]. Access to personal protective equipment, such as gloves, gowns, masks etc. and hand washing are non-specific methods of protection against many infectious diseases, and the described negligence in this area remind us of the constant need for training [17]. In our study we would like to draw attention to such negative behaviors as removing protective gloves while doing work at the patient, or putting on the covers for used needles.

The aim of the study was to analyze behaviors of HCWs in the field of needlestick injuries as well as to learn about their attitudes to patients infected with blood-borne viruses. We estimated the impact of knowledge on the behaviors and attitudes of HCWs. Additionally, we rated the frequency of contact of the HCWs with blood and other body fluids, circumstances that may have contributed to the injury (risk factors), and the NSIs reporting.

2. Materials and Methods

The present work is part of the study on exposure to infectious material of HCWs in Poland. In 2015, we sent inquiries - surveys to all hospitals in Poland ($N = 956$, as of 31 December 2014) to collect registry data on HCWs NSIs. As many as 252 hospitals sent us official register data (return index = 26.36%). Representing a total annual average of 28,051 physicians, 64,806 nurses/midwifes and 3449 paramedics. We selected 26 (10%) of these hospitals to which we sent a questionnaire in electronic form. It was a selection based on the accessibility of the respondents (courtesy, cooperation and interest of the management of hospitals). The survey was for volunteer HCWs so we did not calculate the return index. 487 completed questionnaires were returned correctly. Thus, the study was conducted in 26 selected hospitals in the period of October–December 2015 from which we obtained 487 surveys.

The hospitals were located in urban communes and in urban–rural communes. In Poland, the commune is the basic unit of local self-government. The urban commune is a community located in a city. The urban–rural commune consists of a city that is the seat of the commune authorities and the surrounding villages.

A self-administered questionnaire was designed to assess HCW's knowledge, behaviors and attitudes towards hand hygiene and needlestick injuries.

Regarding knowledge a short test was included focusing on five statements, to which possible answers were: "true", "false" or "I do not know". The following questions asked were:

Q1. Hand disinfection can be replaced by the use of protective gloves.
Q2. In an emergency situation, the disinfection of hands is not required.
Q3. Approximately 60% of HBV infections among adults in Poland are nosocomial.
Q4. In the case of a single puncture by used needle, it is easier to become infected with HIV than HBV.
Q5. Tuberculosis infection is possible only by droplets.

The answers to the above questions constitute five independent variables, which measure the level of HCW's knowledge. We also aggregated the results of knowledge that defined the overall knowledge variable classified as poor (less than 3 corrected answers), fair (3 corrected answers) and good (more than 3 corrected answers). In addition, we asked about the sources of knowledge and about participation in training on post-exposure proceedings.

Regarding behaviors, we asked how often personal protection equipment is used; has it happened that the HCW had removed protective clothing (e.g., gloves) to perform the operation "more easily" with the patient; we also asked about the recapping of used needles and the reporting of NSIs.

In terms of attitudes, we asked HCWs about the fear of infection in the workplace and also about changing their own behavior under the influence of awareness of care for an infected patient. We analyzed HCWs opinions on the obligation to provide information about infected patients. We also evaluated the feelings of HCWs after NSIs. In the questionnaire the variable "soon forgot about it" meant that the HCW who had been hurt was able to do his/her job further. And the variable "felt a long-lasting fear" meant that the HCW who had been hurt interrupted his/her work on the day of the risky event, "was paralyzed", and could not continue to "work" normally, s/he was thinking about a possible threat all the time.

To assess the frequency of exposure to infectious material in the workplace, we asked about the occupational exposure which occurred in the 12 months preceding the survey. Occupational exposure to blood-borne pathogens among HCWs includes percutaneous exposures to needles and other sharp objects, and mucocutaneous exposure (i.e., contact with intact or nonintact skin, and contact with mucous membranes) [18]. In this study "superficial wounds" were defined as "loss of epidermis only" and "deep cuts" were defined as "damage to deeper tissues like tendons, muscles, ligaments, nerves, blood vessels, or bones". In addition, we examined the circumstances that, according to the respondents, contributed to the injury.

The reliability and validity of the survey was assessed on the basis of previous studies [19].

In the present analysis, the following sociodemographic measures were taken into account: gender, job category, work experience (in years), and place of employment (urban commune or rural and urban commune).

Statistical Analysis

We assessed the degree of association between pairs of variables by presenting contingency tables in the first line, and we applied classical Fisher's Exact test for count data and Pearson's Chi-squared test of independence. Moreover, we used Goodman and Kruskal's gamma to measure the strength of association when both variables were measured at the ordinal scale, and for nominal variables, we calculated contingency coefficients.

The above mentioned behaviors (4 dependent variables) and attitudes (4 dependent variables) of HCWs were measured by simultaneous observation of dichotomous categorical variables received from the self-administered questionnaire. The values of each dependent variable falls into one of two categories, "Yes, I confirm this behavior/attitude" or "No, I do not confirm this behavior/attitude". To determine the main drivers (factors) of healthcare workers' behaviors and attitudes for each indicator variable we performed logistic regression with the following 6 explanatory (controls) variables: job category (jb_i with 3 categories: doctors, nurses or paramedics), gender (g_i), work experience (exp_i with 4 categories: less than 5, 6–15, 16–25, >25 years), and place of employment ($pemp_i$ with 2 categories: urban commune or rural and urban commune), personal situation (ps_i with 2 categories: I feel insecure at my workplace " or "I am professionally fulfilled") and the overall knowledge of worker (kn_i, with 3 categories poor, fair and good). For a given worker i, let y_i be a dichotomous variable describing his/her particular behavior or attitude i.e., $y_i \in \{tc_i, nt_i, lr_i, re_i\} \cup \{fs_i, fl_i, is_i, in_i\}$, and let U_{y_i} be the internal utility that worker i obtains from this behavior or attitude. The utility gains are given by $U_{y_i} = \beta_0 + \beta' x_i + \epsilon_i$ and depends on the above listed characteristics of the worker and her place of employment grouped into a vector $x_i = [jb_i, g_i, exp_i, kni, pemp_i, ps_{i,}]$, where the unobserved term, ϵ_i, is random shock with logistic distribution. The HCW i takes the attitude or behavior ($y_i = 1$) if $U_{y_i} > 0$ and do not if $U_{y_i} < 0$. The conditional probability of $y_i = 1$ is given by $Pr(y_i = 1|x_i) = \frac{1}{1+e^{-\beta_0 - \beta' x_i}}$.

To find the best model we performed the best subset regression algorithm and fitted a separate logistic regression for each possible combination of the $k = 1, 2, 3, 4, 5, 6$ predictors. We then look at all of the resulting models and identified the one that is best using the following rule: all predictors in the model are statistically significant and the value of the Akaike Information Criterion is minimized. To assess the influence of control variables on behaviors and attitudes we calculated the odds ratios.

The statistical computations were performed using R statistical software and Excel. The level of statistical significance was set at $p < 0.05$. The study protocol was approved by the Bioethics Committee of the Medical University of Lodz (Document No. RNN /163/14/KB of 11.02.2014).

3. Results

3.1. Characteristics of the Study Group

A total of 487 HCWs filled the questionnaire. About half of the study participants were female (56.9%), 44% of them were paramedics and 40% were nurses, and 31.4% had less than 5 years of employment. There was approximately an equal distribution among hospitals located in urban commune (44%) and rural/urban commune (55%), Table 1.

Table 1. Demographic characteristics of health care workers, N = 487 (%).

Demographic Characteristics		Number (%)
Gender	Male	210 (43.1)
	Female	277 (56.9)
Job Category	Doctors	76 (15.60)
	Nurses	196 (40.25)
	Paramedics	215 (44.15)
Work Experience (in years)	<5	153 (31.4)
	5–15	128 (26.3)
	16–25	89 (18.3)
	>25	117 (24.0)
Place of employment	Urban commune	215 (44.15)
	Rural and urban commune	272 (55.85)

3.2. Frequency and Circumstances of Injuries

During the 12 months preceding the study, most doctors, nurses and paramedics were in contact with the infectious material through intact skin. They had less contact through damaged skin, mucous membranes and splattering onto conjunctiva. Almost every second HCW (44.8%) suffered superficial wounds, and almost every fifth HCW (17.9%) had been cut deeply at least once. More often, both the superficial and deep injuries were among nurses (respectively to the second and every fourth) ($p < 0.05$), Table 2. The most frequent causes of injuries were: rush (31.4%), unpredictable patient behavior (29%), lack of attention (27%), stressful situation requiring urgent intervention such as sudden hemorrhage or collapse (16.3%), as well as too high workload (14.3%).

Table 2. Frequency of health care workers (HCWs) contacts with potentially infectious material within 12 months preceding the study.

Exposure Type	Job Category	Frequency of Exposure Within the Last 12 Months							
		Never		Once		At Least a Few Times		Statistical Significance	
		N	%	N	%	N	%	Chi^2	p-Value
Through intact skin	Doctors	18	23.7	16	21.1	42	55.2	14.394	0.072
	Nurses	56	28.6	20	10.2	120	61.2		
	Paramedics	57	26.5	34	15.8	124	57.7		
	Total	131	26.9	70	14.4	286	58.8		
Through damaged skin	Doctors	59	77.6	9	11.8	8	10.5	28.106	<0.05
	Nurses	119	60.7	21	10.7	56	28.5		
	Paramedics	153	71.2	26	12.1	36	16.7		
	Total	331	68.0	56	11.5	100	20.5		
Through mucous membranes	Doctors	57	75.0	7	9.2	12	15.8	14.894	0.061
	Nurses	118	60.2	17	8.7	61	31.1		
	Paramedics	144	67.0	23	10.7	48	22.3		
	Total	319	65.5	47	9.7	121	24.9		
Splattering onto conjunctiva	Doctors	45	59.2	17	22.4	14	18.4	33.216	<0.05
	Nurses	110	56.1	34	17.3	52	26.6		
	Paramedics	164	76.3	28	13.0	23	10.7		
	Total	319	65.5	79	16.2	89	18.3		
Superficial injury	Doctors	43	56.6	17	22.4	16	21.0	51.054	<0.05
	Nurses	90	45.9	39	19.9	67	34.3		
	Paramedics	136	63.3	60	27.9	19	8.9		
	Total	269	55.2	116	23.8	102	21.0		
Deep injury	Doctors	62	81.6	11	14.5	3	3.9	26.618	0.001
	Nurses	147	75.0	20	10.2	29	14.8		
	Paramedics	191	88.8	16	7.4	8	3.7		
	Total	400	82.1	47	9.7	40	8.2		

Chi^2—chi-square test of independence.

3.3. Knowledge, Behaviors, and Attitudes

The correct answers to all five questions from the knowledge test were given by 25 doctors (32.9%), 34 paramedics (15.8%) and 18 nurses (9.2%). The most common were 4 correct answers (doctors: $n = 31$, 40.8%, nurses: $n = 63$, 32.1%, paramedics: $n = 85$, 39.5%). We rated the level of knowledge as poor for 15% of HCWs, fair for 31% of HCWs, and good for 54% of HCWs.

The distribution of correct answers to individual questions is given in Table 3. The frequency of providing correct answers did not depend on the sex, seniority, or location of the hospital. Q3, Q4, and Q5 questions were more often answered correctly by doctors ($p < 0.05$), Table 3.

Table 3. Distribution of the responses provided by the HCWs during the test of knowledge.

Question	Correct answer *N* (%)									
	Doctors		Nurses		Paramedics		Total		Statistical Significance	
	N	%	*N*	%	*N*	%	*N*	%	Chi^2	*p*-Value
Q1. Can use of gloves replace disinfection of hands?	73	96.05	188	95.92	210	97.67	471	96.72	1.12	0.57
Q2. Is disinfection of hands necessary in emergency situations?	51	67.11	119	60.71	146	67.91	316	64.89	2.52	0.28
Q3. Do you agree that 60% of HBV infections in Poland is connected with health care?	56	73.68	112	57.14	143	66.51	311	63.86	7.66	0.02
Q4. Is it more likely to become infected with HIV than with HBV as a result of single needlestick injury with a contaminated needle?	71	93.42	154	78.57	169	78.61	394	80.90	9.13	0.01
Q5. Is infection with tubercule bacillus possible solely through droplet infection?	57	75	62	31.63	95	44.19	214	43.94	41.82	0.00

Chi^2—chi-square test of independence.

Among the 487 respondents, the majority of HCWs 79.5% ($n = 387$) felt the need to increase knowledge about the possibility of getting infected in the workplace. However, simultaneously as many as 82.1% of HCWs responded that their knowledge was gained during the basic training (school/study). 68.6% HCWs participated in various refresher courses, but only less than every second (45.6%) read scientific journals. Nurses most often participated in the trainings (chi^2 = 36.813, $p < 0.05$). For example, 25% of doctors, 22.8% of rescuers, and 10.2% of nurses never participated in the training on post-exposure proceedings.

Regarding behaviors, most HCWs used personal protective equipment such as clothes and protective gloves. Only 3.7% of employees answered that they never use protective gloves, 10.1% protective gowns, and 49.8% goggles or other face shields. However, it should be remembered that not all activities performed on the patient require the use of protective clothing. At the same time, a large number of respondents admitted that they took off protective clothing (e.g., gloves) to perform an activity "more easily" on the patient (doctors: $N = 33$, 43.4%; nurses: $n = 116$, 59.2%; paramedics: $N = 111$, 48.4%). This answer was the most common among nurses ($p = 0.036$).

On average, every tenth HCW (11.7%) was spotted for improper handling of used needles. Recapping concerned 15.5% of doctors ($n = 12$), 8.2% of nurses ($n = 16$) and 11.2% of paramedics

($n = 24$). Among them, when placing the cover on the contaminated needle, 2 doctors, 4 nurses and 4 paramedics were injured.

Most HCWs ($n = 440$, 90.3%) answered that they had always reported the fact of injury to the appropriate person responsible for keeping the register. Most often they were nurses (92.3%) and paramedics (93.5%) ($p < 0.01$). However, when asked about reporting the last NSIs that occurred in the last 12 months preceding the study, only 54.8% of HCWs reported this fact. The other half of incidents (45.2%) have not been reported anywhere. The main reason for not reporting the sharp injuries was the perception that there was no such need. The variables such as seniority, place of employment and knowledge did not have any significant impact on the attendance.

Regarding attitudes, every fourth HCWs (25.9%) feared infection in the workplace. Nurses had the most concerns (37.2%, $p < 0.01$), women (31.0%, $p < 0.01$), and HCWs with the shortest work experience (31.4%, $p < 0.01$). After the last injury, 35.2% of HCWs felt fear/anxiety but soon forgot about it. However, 16.3% of HCWs felt a long-term fear for their own health. Every third HCW (30.8%) did not feel anything special, arguing that NSIs are an inseparable part of the work of medical personnel. A small percentage of HCWs (5.3% doctors, 6.6% nurses and 1.4% paramedics) did not exercise greater caution in dealing with a patient known to be infected with HIV, HBV, or HCV. HCWs with shorter work experience mostly changed their behavior (83% from <5 years work experience and 78.9% HCWs from 6–15 years of work experience, $p = 0.002$). The HCWs from rural–urban communes changed their attitudes more often ($p = 0.052$). 93.4% of nurses, 89.5% of doctors and 87.0% of paramedics have never refused to perform the examination, surgery, or care of a patient with an infection. However, the others feared personal infection and they refused to help the infected patient at least once. Most HCWs (69.4%) would like patients to be required to inform medical personnel that they are infected with blood-borne viruses. Even more HCWs (78.2%) see the need to introduce in Poland an obligatory system of transmitting information about infected patients between different health care units (throughout the health care service system).

3.4. The Influence of Knowledge and Other Variables on Behaviors and Attitudes

Multivariate logistic regression analysis of the odds (OR) for behaviors and attitudes in relation to the potential risk factors listed above is presented in Table 4.

Regarding behaviors, taking off protective clothes to make it "easier" to take action with the patient was positively associated with long work experience (odds ratio (OR) 1.16, 95% confidence interval (95% CI): 0.995–1.36), and negatively associated with knowledge (OR 0.75, 95% CI: 0.58–0.96). Recapping was positively associated with knowledge (OR 7.74, 95% CI: 1.70–13.15), and negatively associated with job category (OR 0.15, 95% CI: 0.01–0.78) and place of employment (OR 0.21, 95% CI: 0.05-0.73). Males showed more than three times higher chance of not reporting injuries (OR 3.495, 95% CI: 1.65–7.49).

Regarding attitudes none of the variables significantly affected the possibility of refusing treatment/care to an infected patient. Concern about the possibility of getting infected in the workplace was positively associated with long work experience (OR 1.33, 95% CI: 0.99–1.78). Long-term fear after NSIs was also positively associated with knowledge (OR 2.28, 95% CI: 1.29–4.43). Males were less likely to experience such long-term fear (OR 0.38, 95% CI: 0.13–1.12).

Table 4. Multivariate logistic regression analysis of odds ratio (OR) for behaviors and attitudes of HCWs in relation to potential risk factors.

Variables	Odds Ratios with 95% Confidence Interval (CI) from Logistic Regression Models							
	Behaviors, OR (95% CI)				Attitudes, OR (95% CI)			
	No Participation in Trainings	Removing Protective Clothing to "Make It Easier" to Perform the Action at the Patient	Recapping	Lack of NSIs Reporting	Fear of Infection in the Workplace	After NSIs, I Did Not Feel Anything Special	Long-Term Fear for Their Own Health After NSIs	The Need to Introduce an Information System About Infected Patients
Job category (nurses)	0.465 ** (1) (0.22–1.01)	-	0.145 * (2) (0.01–0.78)	-	2.929 *** (1) (1.35–6.35)	-	4.040 * (1) (0.99–27.67)	-
Job category (paramedics)	0.585 ** (1) (0.31–1.14)	-	-	0.241 ***(2) (0.11–0.53)	2.639 ***(1) (1.28–5.41)	-	7.158 ** (1) (1.83–48.25)	2.849 *** (2) (1.78–4.68)
Gender (Male)	-	-	-	3.495 *** (1.65–7.49)	2.095 ** (1.08–4.09)	-	0.378 * (0.13–1.12)	-
Work experience (increasing seniority)	0.621 *** (0.46–0.82)	1.163 * (0.99–1.36)	-	-	1.327 * (0.99–1.78)	-	-	-
Place of employment (rural and urban commune)	-	-	0.209 ** (0.05–0.73)	-	-	-	-	0.679 * (0.43–1.06)
Personal situation (I am professionally fulfilled)	0.506 *** (0.309, 0.826)	-	-	-	0.482** (0.251, 0.878)	2.858 *** (1.485, 5.839)		
Knowledge (increasing level of knowledge)	-	0.747 ** (0.58–0.96)	7.74 ** (1.70–13.72)	-	-	0.717 * (0.48–1.06)	2.281 *** (1.29–4.43)	-

Note: * $p < 0.1$; ** $p < 0.05$; *** $p < 0.01$; (1) ref. = doctors; (2) ref. = others.

4. Discussion

Health care workers are at common risk of occupational exposure to blood and other potential infectious material. In the study Martins et al. 65% of employees of a selected hospital in Portugal reported having experienced at least one NSSI in the last 5 years [20]. Most of the events, similar to ours and other studies (Polish and international) [21–25] concerned nurses. It should be noted that nurses are the most numerous professional group among medical employees, they perform the most treatments and usually have direct contact with patients.

The risk of acquiring the blood-borne diseases through occupational exposure depends on the number of injuries, prevalence of BB infections in the patient population and probability of a percutaneous injury transmitting blood-borne viruses [26]. With increasing rate of national and international hepatitis B, hepatitis C, and HIV these are risks that HCWs cannot afford to take. In our study perceived causes of injury were: rush (31.4%), unpredictable patient's behavior (29%), and lack of attention (27%). In the study by Salzer et al. [27] time pressure and lack of experience were the most frequent causes of NSIs, while in other studies the main reason for occupational exposure was a sudden movement of the patient during the procedure [28]. The same reasons as in our study were obtained by Bećirević et al.: being in rush, patient's unpredictable reaction and decrease in concentration [29].

The knowledge of medical personnel should be considered insufficient. The level of knowledge of HCWs has been the subject of many studies but little is known about whether knowledge/lack of knowledge about the possible risk of infection can affect behaviors/attitudes [22,30]. In our study nurses showed the weakest knowledge. Interestingly, nurses most often participated in trainings and the least often presented negative behaviors in the recapping. At the same time, they usually took off their protective clothing to perform some procedures on the patient. Most often, they also reported NSIs. In our opinion, negative behavior may have resulted from the nature of the work rather than from lack of knowledge. Nurses have the most frequent contact with the patient, they are more likely to perform invasive procedures, so they will also have the biggest chance to remove protective clothing, e.g., protective gloves to "facilitate" their work. Such behaviors may result from excessive workload, in a hurry, and these HCWs risk factors have been indicated as the most common causes of injury. The training deals with the subject of recapping, and almost always reminds us of the obligation to report injuries. In this matter, knowledge influenced the improvement of behavior.

This study revealed that information on 45.2% of injuries was not entered into an official register. This is close to the results of some studies (i.e., 51% in the survey by Makary et al.) [31], but less than in others (i.e., 66.1% in the study by Cui et al. and 60.2% in the study by Jahangiri et al.) [32,33]. Most common reason for failure to report the incidents of NSIs were lack of time and heavy clinical schedule, as well as perception of low risk of infection [33,34] which is close to our results, in which part of HCWs in its own assessment did not see the need to report NSIs. This is still a gap for enhanced training. HCWs should be aware that reporting an injury is highly important and adjust their behavior accordingly.

Medical personnel suffer from anxiety and emotional distress following NSIs [35]. In our study, logistic regression showed that people with better knowledge are more afraid of their own health after being hurt and this fear lasted longer. The reason is unclear, but it may be related to the fact that people with better knowledge are aware of the possible dangers of wounds contaminated with a needle. However, the long-term fear was also positively correlated with the practice of nurse and rescuer, who at the same time showed lower knowledge in the knowledge test. In these cases, the fear may be due to the generally more frequent contacts of employees of these professions with infectious material. One should also take into account the possibility that the measurement of knowledge was imprecise because the test of knowledge covered only 5 questions. Probably fear for one's own health may affect better wound reporting in the paramedics and nurses group. Men in our study were less afraid, and at the same time reported less frequent incidents of injuries. Similarly, with doctors. It is quite understandable when we are not afraid of something, we do not see the need to report. In the research by Jahić et al. also physicians were significantly less likely to report exposure incidents than other staff [36]. The vast majority of HCWs are more cautious when dealing with an infected patient. Fortunately, the cases of refusal to provide assistance to patients infected with HBV, HCV, or HIV were rare, and were not subject to any risk factors. These are results similar to Ishimaru et al. in which the majority of nurses expressed a willingness to care for patients infected with HIV, HBV or HCV [37].

One of the major alarming observations in the current study is that most HCWs believed that patients with HIV should be required to inform physicians of their status. Moreover, they think that such information should be compulsorily transferred between different health institutions. In another Polish study, Gańczak et al. found insufficient knowledge of hospital staff in surgical wards, in which 40% of HCWs were in favor of moving away from performing surgical procedures if the HCW was infected with HBV or HCV, and 42.6% with respect to HIV infected HCWs. In the same research 16.2% HCWs stated that infected surgeons should disclose their HBV, HCV, or HIV serostatus [38]. HCWs should be aware of the risks, but above all they should have knowledge about prevention methods that effectively protect against infection. Although HBV infection can be prevented by vaccination, there is no effective vaccine for HCV and HIV. Before other infections, strict compliance with the universal precautions is important. In our study the vast majority of the HCWs were afraid of being infected during work, and almost all admitted that they performed medical procedures more carefully with patients they knew to be infected with HIV, HBV, or HCV. This may indicate a lack of awareness that absolutely every patient should be treated as a potential source of infection. The use of personal protective equipment for operations performed on the patient and carefully carrying out all procedures should not be dependent on the results of the patient's tests for markers of blood-borne virus infections, due to the possibility of patients being in the serological window or low sensitivity of the tests. The patient himself is not obliged to inform that he/she is infected; therefore, in a job where there is a possibility of contact with potentially infectious material, the same safety precautions must be used for all patients.

HCWs' knowledge about blood-borne infections and their prevention (hand hygiene) is insufficient but in our opinion, most behaviors and attitudes depended more on the type of profession than on knowledge. Better knowledge did not influence all behaviors; doctors showed better knowledge and this affected a smaller feeling of fear and less frequent NSIs reporting. Changing behavior and attitudes under the influence of the awareness of care for an infected patient is a sign of fear, which is also mentioned by the HCWs themselves. Knowledge did not significantly change these attitudes. Perhaps this is due to the fact of textbook teaching in the Polish education system. This justifies the poorer result of the knowledge test among nurses despite the relatively more frequent participation in training. Perhaps the courses and practical experience gained contribute to better nurse behavior, for example recapping. This issue requires more in-depth research. It can also imply for decision makers on medical education the need to move from theoretical instruction to the emphasis on practice. We look forward to wide participation in this discussion.

Limitations

Due to the number of surveys we have obtained, we can not generalize results for the whole country, and the entire population of hospital HCWs. Also the measure of knowledge may be imprecise due to the small number of questions in the test. This issue requires further research. For example, the test of knowledge could be extended with questions carefully checking whether the respondent knows what to do after the exposure, or whether he knows what health risks can result from this exposure.

5. Conclusions

The emphasis in the training of HCWs in the future should be on classes perfecting practical skills like paying more attention to reporting NSIs, improving occupational behaviors like avoiding needle recapping, and on the development of appropriate attitudes towards patients infected with HIV, HBV, or HCV in Poland, as elsewhere.

Author Contributions: A.G.-P. conceived and designed the study and developed a research tool; M.G. was responsible for the statistical analysis of the results; A.G.-P. analyzed the data, searched the literature and wrote the paper. All authors approved the final manuscript for publication.

Funding: This research received no external funding.

Acknowledgments: Work financed by Medical University of Łódź from the own activities of a scientific unit under No. 503/6-024-01/503-61-001-18. The authors wish to thank the Hospital Directors, Healthcare Workers and Mr Andrzej Olczyk for their help in the data collection.

Conflicts of Interest: The authors declare no conflict of interest.

References

1. Tarantola, A.; Abiteboul, D.; Rachline, A. Infection risks following accidental exposure to blood or body fluids in health care workers: A review of pathogens transmitted in published cases. *Am. J. Infect. Control.* **2006**, *34*, 367–375. [CrossRef]
2. Gómez-Moreno, A.; Garaigorta, U. Hepatitis B virus and DNA damage response: Interactions and consequences for the infection. *Viruses* **2017**, *9*, 304. [CrossRef] [PubMed]
3. Zoulim, F.; Chevallier, M.; Maynard, M.; Trepo, C. Clinical consequences of hepatitis C virus infection. *Rev. Med. Virol.* **2003**, *13*, 57–68. [CrossRef]
4. Taraphdar, P.; Guha, R.T.; Haldar, D.; Chatterjee, A.; Dasgupta, A.; Saha, B.; Mallik, S. Socioeconomic consequences of HIV/AIDS in the family system. *Niger. Med. J.* **2011**, *52*, 250–253. [CrossRef] [PubMed]
5. Saia, M.; Hofmann, F.; Sharman, J.; Abiteboul, D.; Campins, M.; Burkowitz, J.; Choe, Y.; Kavanagh, S. Needlestick injuries: Incidence and cost in the United States, United Kingdom, Germany, France, Italy, and Spain. *Biomed. Int.* **2010**, *1*, 41–49.
6. Mullan, R.J.; Baker, E.L.; Hughes, J.M.; Bell, D.M.; Jaffe, H.W.; Bond, W.W.; Kane, M.A., Jr.; Chamberland, M.C.; Marcus, R.; Favero, M.S.; et al. Centers for disease control and prevention: guidelines for prevention of transmission of human immunodeficiency virus and hepatitis B virus to health-care and public-safety workers. *MMWR Morb. Mortal. Wkly. Rep.* **1989**, *38*, 1–37.
7. Centers for Disease Control and Prevention. Recommendations for prevention and control of hepatitis C virus (HCV) infection and HCV-related chronic disease. *MMWR Morb. Mortal. Wkly. Rep.* **1998**, *47*, 1–39.
8. Beltrami, E.M.; Williams, I.T.; Shapiro, C.N.; Chamberland, M.E. Risk and management of blood-borne infections in health care workers. *Clin. Microbiol. Rev.* **2000**, *13*, 385–407. [CrossRef]
9. Rapiti, E.; Prüss-Üstün, A.; Hutin, Y. Sharps Injuries: Assessing the Burden of Disease from Sharps Injuries to Health-Care Workers at National and Local Levels. World Health Organization: Geneva, 2005. (WHO Environmental Burden of Disease Series, No. 11). Available online: https://www.who.int/quantifying_ehimpacts/publications/ebd11.pdf?ua=1 (accessed on 31 October 2018).
10. Świątkowska, B.; Hanke, W.; Szeszenia-Dąbrowska, N. *Occupational Diseases in Poland in 2016*; IMP: Lodz, Poland, 2017.
11. Karoney, M.J.; Kaumbuki, E.K.; Koech, M.K.; Lelei, L.K. Primary cutaneous tuberculosis in a 27-year-old medical intern from needle-stick injury: A case report. *Clin. Case Rep.* **2014**, *3*, 39–42. [CrossRef]
12. Jiang, L.; Ng, I.H.L.; Hou, Y.; Li, D.; Tan, L.W.L.; Ho, H.J.A.; Chen, M.I. Infectious disease transmission: Survey of contacts between hospital-based healthcare workers and working adults from the general population. *J. Hosp. Infect.* **2018**, *98*, 404–411. [CrossRef]
13. Ilhan, M.N.; Durukan, E.; Aras, E.; Türkçüoğlu, S.; Aygün, R. Long working hours increase the risk of sharp and needlestick injury in nurses: The need for new policy implication. *J. Adv. Nurs.* **2006**, *56*, 563–568. [CrossRef]
14. Ajzen, I. Martin Fishbein's legacy: The reasoned action approach. *Ann. Am. Acad. Political Soc. Sci.* **2012**, *640*, 11–27. [CrossRef]
15. Ajzen, I. The theory of planned behavior. *Organ. Behav. Hum. Decis. Process.* **1991**, *50*, 179–211. [CrossRef]
16. Kahneman, D. Thinking, Fast and Slow. Farrar, Straus and Giroux New York. 2011. Available online: http://codolc.com/books/Thinking,_Fast_and_Slow.pdf (accessed on 12 December 2018).
17. Wałaszek, M.; Kołpa, M.; Wolak, Z.; Różańska, A.; Wójkowska-Mach, J. Poor hand hygiene procedure compliance among polish medical students and physicians—The result of an ineffective education basis or the impact of organizational culture? *Int. J. Environ. Res. Public Health* **2017**, *14*, 1026. [CrossRef]

18. Pruss-Ustun, A.; Rapiti, E.; Hutin, Y. *Sharps Injuries: Global Burden of Disease from Sharps Injuries to Health-Care Workers. World Health Organization (WHO) Environmental Burden of Disease Series, No. 3*; WHO Document Production Services: Geneva, Switzerland, 2003; ISBN 9241562463.
19. Garus-Pakowska, A.; Górajski, M.; Szatko, F. Awareness of the risk of exposure to infectious material and the behaviors of Polish paramedics with respect to the hazards from blood-borne pathogens—A nationwide study. *Int. J. Environ. Res. Public Health* **2017**, *14*, 843. [CrossRef]
20. Martins, A.; Coelho, A.C.; Vieira, M.; Matos, M.; Pinto, M.L. Age and years in practice as factors associated with needlestick and sharps injuries among health care workers in a Portuguese hospital. *Accid. Anal. Prev.* **2012**, *47*, 11–15. [CrossRef]
21. Gholami, A.; Borji, A.; Lotfabadi, P.; Asghari, A. Risk factors of needlestick and sharps injuries among healthcare workers. *Int. J. Hosp. Res.* **2013**, *2*, 31–38. Available online: http://ijhr.iums.ac.ir/article_3875_bfedf23c9fdfaada895808b0a365191c.pdf (accessed on 14 June 2018).
22. Sharma, S.; Gupta, A.; Arora, A. Knowledge, attitude and practices on needle-stick and sharps injuries in tertiary care cardiac hospital: A survey. *Indian J. Med. Sci.* **2010**, *64*, 396–401. [CrossRef]
23. Szczypta, A.; Różańska, A.; Bulanda, M. Analysis of occupational exposure of healthcare workers in the years 1998-2013 for bloodborne pathogens on the example of the hospital of the surgical profile. *Med. Pracy* **2014**, *65*, 723–732. [CrossRef]
24. Kocur, E.; Śliwa-Rak, B.; Grosicki, S. Analysis of cases of occupational exposure to blood recorded in the city hospital in Zabrze in 2006–2015. *Przegl. Epidemiol.* **2016**, *70*, 603–615. Available online: www.przeglepidemiol.pzh.gov.pl/pobierz-artykul?id=2120 (accessed on 17 December 2018).
25. Garus-Pakowska, A.; Górajski, M.; Szatko, F. Did legal regulations change the reporting frequency of sharp injuries of medical personnel? Study from 36 hospitals in Łódź Province, Poland. *Int. J. Occup. Med. Environ. Health* **2018**, *31*, 37–46. [CrossRef]
26. Gańczak, M.; Szczeniowski, A.; Jurewicz, A.; Karakiewicz, B.; Szych, Z. Model-based estimates of the risk of HCV transmission from infected patients to gynaecologic and obstetric Staff. *Przegl. Epidemiol.* **2012**, *66*, 437–443.
27. Salzer, H.J.F.; Hoenigl, M.; Kessler, H.H.; Stigler, F.L.; Raggam, R.B.; Rippel, K.E.; Langmann, H.; Sprenger, M.; Krause, R. Lack of risk-awareness and reporting behavior towards HIV infection through needlestick injury among European medical students. *Int. J. Hyg. Environ. Health* **2011**, *214*, 407–410. [CrossRef]
28. Motaarefi, H.; Mahmoudi, H.; Mohammadi, E.; Hasanpour-Dehkordi, A. Factors associated with needlestick injuries in health care occupations: A systematic review. *J. Clin. Diagn. Res.* **2016**, *10*, IE01–IE04. [CrossRef]
29. Bećirević, S.; Pranjić, N.; Sarajlić-Spahić, S.; Ahmetagić, S.; Huseinagić, S. Assessment of reporting, attitudes and knowledge about the stab incidents and professional risk of viral infection among health care professionals in primary health care. *Mater. Soc. Med.* **2013**, *25*, 113–117. [CrossRef]
30. Pavithran, V.K.; Murali, R.; Krishna, M.; Shamala, A.; Yalamalli, M.; Kumar, A.V. Knowledge, attitude, and practice of needle stick and sharps injuries among dental professionals of Bangalore, India. *J. Int. Soc. Prev. Community Dent.* **2015**, *5*, 406–412. [CrossRef]
31. Makary, M.A.; Al-Attar, A.; Holzmueller, C.G.; Sexton, J.B.; Syin, D.; Gilson, M.M.; Sulkowski, M.S.; Pronovost, P.J. Needlestick injuries among surgeons in training. *N. Engl. J. Med.* **2007**, *356*, 2693–2699. [CrossRef]
32. Cui, Z.; Zhu, J.; Zhang, X.; Wang, B.; Li, X. Sharp injuries: A cross-sectional study among health care workers in a provincial teaching hospital in China. *Environ. Health Prev. Med.* **2018**, *23*, 2. [CrossRef]
33. Jahangiri, M.; Rostamabadi, A.; Hoboubi, N.; Tadayon, N.; Soleimani, A. Needle stick injuries and their related safety measures among nurses in a University Hospital, Shiraz, Iran. *Saf. Health Work.* **2016**, *7*, 72–77. [CrossRef]
34. Rybacki, M.; Piekarska, A.; Wiszniewska, M.; Walusiak-Skorupa, J. Work safety among Polish health care workers in respect of exposure to bloodborne pathogens. *Med. Pracy* **2013**, *64*, 1–10. [CrossRef]
35. Lee, J.M.; Botteman, M.F.; Xanthakos, N.; Nicklasson, L. Needlestick injuries in the United States. Epidemiologic, economic, and quality of life issues. *AAOHN J.* **2005**, *53*, 117–133. [PubMed]
36. Jahic, R.; Piljic, D.; Porobic-Jahic, H.; Custović, A.; Petrovic, J.; Piljic, D. Epidemiological characteristics of the accidental exposures to blood-borne pathogens among workers in the hospital. *Med. Arch.* **2018**, *72*, 187–191. [CrossRef] [PubMed]

37. Ishimaru, T.; Wada, K.; Hoang, H.T.X.; Bui, A.T.M.; Nguyen, H.D.; Le, H.; Smith, D.R. Nurses' willingness to care for patients infected with HIV or Hepatitis B/C in Vietnam. *Environ. Health Prev. Med.* **2017**, *22*, 9. [CrossRef] [PubMed]
38. Gańczak, M.; Szych, Z.; Szczeniowski, A.; Dmytrzyk-Danilów, G. Attitudes of medical specialists toward HBV, HCV or HIV infected surgical staff and a sero-survey among staff members. *Med. Pracy* **2013**, *64*, 639–647. [CrossRef]

International Journal of
Environmental Research and Public Health

MDPI

Article

Anger Suppression and Rumination Sequentially Mediates the Effect of Emotional Labor in Korean Nurses

Ji Eun Kim, Jeong Hoon Park and Soo Hyun Park *

Department of Psychology, Yonsei University, Seoul 03722, Korea; alalvh1004@hotmail.com (J.E.K.); jpark5664@naver.com (J.H.P.)
* Correspondence: parksoohyun@yonsei.ac.kr; Tel.: +82-2-2123-4880

Received: 30 January 2019; Accepted: 28 February 2019; Published: 5 March 2019

Abstract: The degree of emotional labor in nurses has been associated with negative physical and psychological health indices. The purpose of this study was to examine the relationship between emotional labor and depressive and anxiety symptoms in nurses. Specifically, the study addressed the question of whether anger suppression and anger rumination sequentially mediated the relationship. A total of 99 nurses was recruited from a university hospital in Korea. The questionnaires included instruments assessing emotional labor, anger suppression, anger rumination, as well as depressive and anxiety symptoms. Consistent with our hypothesis, there was a significant indirect effect of anger suppression and anger rumination on the relationship between emotional labor and depressive symptoms, as well as on the relationship between emotional labor and anxiety symptoms. The nurses' degree of emotional labor, anger suppression, and anger rumination was associated with psychological adjustment. Thus, the impact of nurses' negative affect needs to be adequately addressed, as inadequate resolution of anger may increase their vulnerability to experience depressive and anxiety symptoms. These findings may contribute to developing a strategy for enhancing nurses' psychological health.

Keywords: nurses; emotional labor; anger; depression; anxiety

1. Introduction

In recent years, the psychological adjustment of the emotional laborers has received a great deal of attention. The need for research on emotional labor experienced by nurses has become inevitable. Emotional labor demands the induction or suppression of feelings to maintain a particular outward appearance [1]. Also, the service provision and emotional expression of nurses needs to appear genuine for patients under circumstances where extreme or negative feelings have been triggered. Therefore, nursing involves emotional caring that requires a balance of emotional engagement and detachment, as hospitals are increasingly demanding emotional labor [2]. Nurses are likely to encounter difficulties in regulating their emotions due to emotional dissonance—a discrepancy between emotions they are actually experiencing and emotions they are required to express.

Korean nurses may struggle with difficulties in emotional labor due to the suppression of emotions in order to conform to patients' and organizational demands. Research suggests that Korean nurses report a greater degree of anger and stress than other professions. Among nurses who reported significant stress, 44.4% chose anger as the most frequently experienced emotion, and they suppressed anger more than they expressed anger [3]. It was concluded that nurses tend to experience negative emotions, in particular anger, and that the emotions are usually suppressed due to job demands.

In particular, anger suppression significantly affects psychological adjustment. Previous studies suggested that individuals who engage in greater anger suppression usually display a higher degree of depression and anxiety [4]. Cox, Van Velsor, and Hulgus also reported that women who cannot adequately express anger and opt to divert anger via avoidance of anger awareness or by using indirect means to cope with anger are more vulnerable to depression and anxiety than women who express anger [5]. From these findings, it can be assumed that nurses, who tend to experience frequent anger but also exhibit a tendency to suppress anger, may be particularly vulnerable to depressive and anxiety symptoms.

The suppression of negative emotions is associated with rumination, which may eventually cause, maintain, or increase depressive and anxiety symptoms [6]. The potential role of rumination in the context of emotional suppression is partially supported by research examining the relationship between rumination and thought suppression. These studies showed that consciously suppressing unwanted thoughts can ironically increase the availability of the suppressed thoughts [7]. Thus, it is possible that suppression may fuel rumination, which may subsequently increase susceptibility to experiencing depressive and anxiety symptoms.

Rumination is not only involved with a low activity mood, such as sadness, but it may also be involved with hyperactive mood states, such as anger. Rumination in this context has been termed "anger rumination". Anger rumination can be described as the tendency to persistently deliberate on past events that had triggered anger [8]. Although similar in concept, anger rumination has been suggested as an independent cognitive process which follows anger provocation, thereby maintaining or enhancing anger mood and anger-related behavior problems. In addition, higher use of rumination as a coping strategy in an anger-provoking situation contributes to depression and anxiety [8].

In summary, extant research indicates that in the process of emotional labor exerting influence on the degree of depressive and anxiety symptoms, the anger-related mechanism may play a significant role. Based on the assumption that there is an integrative causal association between emotional labor, anger suppression and rumination, as well as depressive and anxiety symptoms, the present study sought to empirically examine this possibility. In other words, nurses are required to suppress their anger evoked from emotional labor, and ruminating about anger-provoking incidents and anger mood may likely intensify the problem and possibly contribute to depressive and anxiety symptoms. The present study specifically addressed the question of whether anger suppression and anger rumination sequentially mediate the relationship in order to examine its causal relationship.

2. Materials and Methods

2.1. Study Design and Participants

The current study adopted a cross-sectional self-report survey design in order to examine the sequential mediating effect of anger suppression and anger rumination in the relationship between emotional labor and depressive and anxiety symptoms of nurses. The study protocol was approved by the Yonsei University Institutional Review Board (Approval No. 7001988-201612-SB-102-02).

The participants in the study were 99 nurses who worked for at least six months at a university hospital in the Republic of Korea. They were recruited during January of 2017. Data were collected via the distribution of self-report questionnaires given to all nurses in the hospital who expressed interest in participating in the study. Of the 110 surveys distributed, 99 surveys were returned. All 99 surveys were usable for further data analysis without problems concerning missing data or multiple responses. Of the 99 respondents, the mean age was 30 years (standard deviation (SD) = 7.17) and 98.0% were women. The majority of participants were staff nurses (n = 90, 90.9%) who had been working in their current position between 12 and 60 months (n = 51, 51.5%). Their work pattern consisted mostly of triple shifts (n = 89, 89.9%), whereas nine participants (9.1%) reported a non-shifting work schedule (Table 1). The work shifts consisted of a day shift (7:30–15:00), an evening shift (15:00–22:00), and a night shift (22:00–7:30).

Table 1. Summary of demographic characteristics (*N* = 99).

Characteristics	*n* (%)
Age (years)	
≤29	65 (65.7)
30–39	23 (23.3)
≥40	11 (11.0)
Education level	
Associate degree	21 (21.2)
Bachelor degree	63 (63.7)
Attending graduate school	4 (4.0)
Master or doctorate degree	10 (10.1)
Other	1 (1.0)
Position department	
General ward	72 (72.7)
Intensive care unit	10 (10.1)
Other	17 (17.2)
Length of work experience in current position (months)	
<12	28 (28.3)
12–60	51 (51.5)
61–120	15 (15.1)
≥121	6 (6.1)
Work schedule	
Non-shift/day shift	9 (9.1)
Double shift	1 (1.0)
Triple shift	89 (89.9)
Current position	
Staff nurse	90 (90.9)
≥Charge nurse	9 (9.1)

2.2. Measures

Emotional Labor—The Korean-Emotional Labor Scale (K-ELS), developed and validated by Jang et al., and based on the characteristics of emotional labor in Korea, was used to measure emotional labor [9]. This tool was composed of 26 items with five subscales, and the total score was used in the present study. Sample items of the K-ELS are "I make efforts not to express negative feelings towards customers" and "I get hurt in the process of facing customers." The items were rated on a four-point Likert scale ranging from 1 (strongly disagree) to 4 (strongly agree). In the present study, the Cronbach's alpha coefficient for the K-ELS scale was 0.87.

Anger Suppression—The Korean State-Trait Anger Expression Inventory (STAXI-K) [10], which is a modified and validated version of the State-Trait Anger Expression Inventory (STAXI) [11], was used to measure anger suppression. This tool is composed of 10 items for each trait anger and state anger, and eight items for each anger-in, anger-out, and anger-control. The items are rated on a four-point Likert scale ranging from 1 (strongly disagree) to 4 (strongly agree). For this study's purpose, only the anger-in subscale from the state anger scale was used. Sample state anger scale items of the STAXI-K are "I am angry" and "I yell." A higher anger-in total score indicates more frequent anger suppression. In the present study, the Cronbach's alpha coefficient for the anger-in subscale was 0.79.

Anger Rumination—The Korean Anger Rumination Scale (K-ARS) [12], which is a modified and validated version of the Anger Rumination Scale (ARS) [13], was used to measure anger rumination. The items are rated on a four-point Likert scale ranging from 1 (almost never) to 4 (almost always in terms of how well the items resemble their beliefs about themselves; higher scores correspond to a greater degree of anger rumination. In the present study, the Cronbach's alpha coefficient for the K-ARS scale was 0.95.

Depressive Symptoms—Depressive symptoms were assessed using the Korean version of the Center for Epidemiologic Studies Depression Scale (CES-D) [14], originally developed by the National Institute of Mental Health [15]. This is a 20-item self-report questionnaire that measures the frequency and severity of depressive symptoms experienced within the last week. The items are rated on a four-point Likert scale ranging from 0 (very rare, i.e., less than one day during one week) to 3 (most of the time, i.e., more than five days during one week). In the present study, the Cronbach's alpha coefficient was 0.93.

Anxiety Symptoms—The State-Trait Anxiety Inventory (STAI), originally developed by Spielberger, Gorsuch, Lushene, Vagg, and Jacobs [16] and adapted for use in Korea [17], was used to measure anxiety symptoms. It measures state anxiety (20 items) and trait anxiety (20 items), where state anxiety represents anxiety that is temporary and changing, and trait anxiety represents anxiety that is permanent and stable. For the purpose of this study, only 20 items measuring trait anxiety were used. The items are rated on a four-point Likert scale ranging from 1 (not at all) to 4 (very much). In the present study, the Cronbach's alpha coefficient for trait anxiety was 0.91.

2.3. Data Analysis

The sequential multiple mediation analysis suggested by Hayes was conducted using PROCESS Macro for SPSS (IBM Corp., Armonk, NY, USA) [18]. The significance of all the possible indirect effects from the study's model were examined using the bootstrapping method of 5000 resamples. The 95% confidence intervals that did not include zero indicated a significant indirect effect. Previous research suggested that work shift pattern, length of work experience, and job position may influence nurses' degree of depressive symptoms [19,20]. Therefore, these demographic variables were controlled as covariates in the statistical analyses.

3. Results

3.1. Descriptive Statistics and Intercorrelations between Variables

Table 2 presents descriptive statistics and intercorrelations between the study variables. Emotional labor was positively correlated with both anger suppression ($r = 0.43$, $p < 0.001$) and anger rumination ($r = 0.30$, $p = 0.003$). Anger suppression demonstrated significant positive correlations with depressive ($r = 0.30$, $p = 0.003$) and anxiety ($r = 0.24$, $p = 0.020$) symptoms. Anger rumination was also positively associated with depressive ($r = 0.42$, $p < 0.001$) and anxiety ($r = 0.35$, $p = 0.001$) symptoms. However, the degree of emotional labor did not show significant correlations with either depressive ($r = 0.13$, $p = 0.215$) or anxiety ($r = 0.11$, $p = 0.289$) symptoms.

Table 2. Summary of intercorrelations, means, and standard deviations for study variables.

Measure	1	2	3	4	5	Mean	*SD*
	r (*p*)						
1. AngerSup	1					14.21	3.90
2. KARS	0.59 (<0.001)	1				29.99	9.26
3. CES-D	0.30 (0.003)	0.42 (<0.001)	1			18.67	9.81
4. STAI	0.24 (0.020)	0.35 (0.001)	0.84 (<0.001)	1		47.48	9.29
5. K-ELS	0.43 (<0.001)	0.30 (0.003)	0.13 (0.215)	0.11 (0.289)	1	69.31	9.07

Note: Anger suppression (AngerSup); Korean version of the Center for Epidemiologic Studies Depression Scale (CES-D); Korean Anger Rumination Scale (KARS); Korean-Emotional Labor Scale (K-ELS); Korean State-Trait Anxiety Inventory (STAI).

3.2. Sequential Mediation Analysis

Sequential mediation analyses were conducted after controlling for the work shift pattern, the length of work experience, and the job position as aforementioned (Table 3).

Table 3. Sequential mediation effect of anger suppression and anger rumination in the relationship between emotional labor and depression/anxiety.

Dependent Variables		Effect	SE	t	p	LLCI	ULCI
Depression (Y)	Total effect	0.10	0.11	0.85	0.396	−0.13	0.32
	Total indirect effect	0.16	0.07			0.05	0.33
	Indirect paths						
	X→M1→Y	0.01	0.07			−0.12	0.14
	X→M2→Y	0.04	0.05			−0.03	0.18
	X→M1→M2→Y	0.12	0.06			0.04	0.26
	Direct effect	−0.07	0.11	−0.63	0.531	−0.29	0.15
Anxiety (Y)	Total effect	0.09	0.11	0.86	0.790	−0.12	0.30
	Total indirect effect	0.12	0.06			0.02	0.27
	Indirect paths						
	X→M1→Y	−0.02	0.06			−0.14	0.12
	X→M2→Y	0.04	0.04			−0.02	0.16
	X→M1→M2→Y	0.09	0.05			0.02	0.22
	Direct effect	−0.03	0.11	−0.27	0.790	−0.24	0.19

Note: Emotional labor (X); anger suppression (M1); anger rumination (M2); lower levels for 95% confidence interval (LLCI); upper levels for 95% confidence interval (ULCI).

Depression—There was a significant total indirect effect, which was the sum of all possible indirect effects in the model between emotional labor and depressive symptoms (effect = 0.16; confidence interval (CI): from 0.05 to 0.33), but a non-significant direct effect (effect = −0.07, $t = -0.63$, $p = 0.531$). Regarding each indirect effect, there was a significant indirect effect indicating that the path from anger suppression to anger rumination sequentially mediated the relationship between emotional labor and depressive symptoms (X→M1→M2→Y: effect = 0.12; CI: from 0.04 to 0.26). The indirect effects from emotional labor to anger suppression to depressive symptoms (X→M1→Y: effect = 0.01; CI: from −0.12 to 0.14) and from emotional labor to anger rumination to depressive symptoms (X→M2→Y: effect = 0.04; CI: from −0.03 to0.18) were not significant. The coefficients and standard error (SE) for each path are presented in Figure 1.

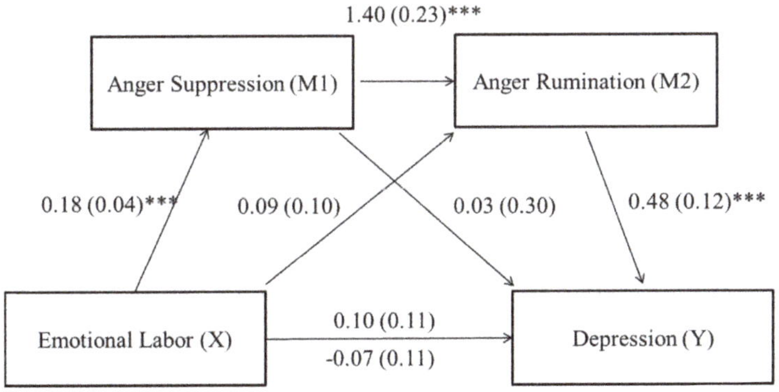

Figure 1. Sequential mediation model for emotional labor and depression via anger suppression and anger rumination. Unstandardized path coefficients and SE indicated above. The coefficient appearing above the line connecting emotional labor and depression represents the total effect and the coefficient below the line represents the direct effect. *** $p < 0.001$.

Anxiety—The total indirect effect was significant (effect = 0.12; CI: from 0.02 to 0.27), but there was a non-significant direct effect (b = −0.03, t = −0.27, p = 0.790). Regarding each indirect effect, there was a significant indirect effect of emotional labor on anxiety through anger suppression and anger rumination, again indicating sequential mediation (X→M1→M2→Y: effect = 0.09; CI: from 0.02 to 0.22). The indirect effects from emotional labor to anger suppression to anxiety (X→M1→Y: effect = −0.02; CI: from −0.14 to 0.12) and the indirect effect from emotional labor to anger rumination to anxiety (X→M2→Y: effect = 0.04; CI: from −0.02 to 0.16) were not significant. The coefficients and SE for each path are presented in Figure 2.

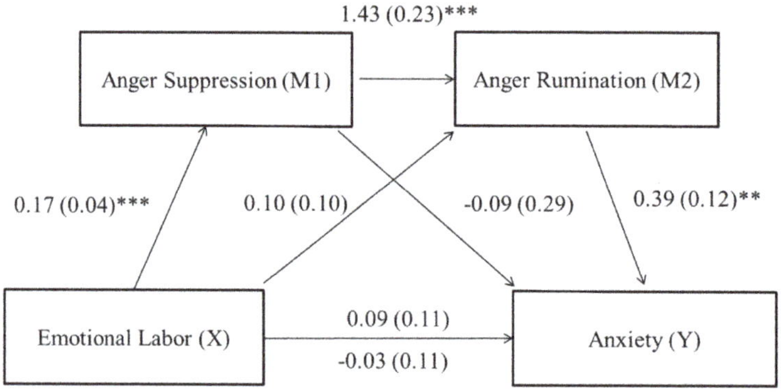

Figure 2. Sequential mediation model for emotional labor and anxiety via anger suppression and anger rumination. The unstandardized path coefficients and SE are indicated above. The coefficient appearing above the line connecting emotional labor and anxiety represents the total effect and the coefficient below the line represents the direct effect. ** $p < 0.01$, *** $p < 0.001$.

4. Discussion

Consistent with our hypothesis, the results indicated that emotional labor had an indirect sequential effect on depressive and anxiety symptoms through anger suppression and anger rumination, and the direct effect of emotional labor on depression and anxiety was not significant after controlling for anger suppression and anger rumination. Hence, the nurses' emotional labor itself may not serve as a risk factor per se for psychological maladjustment. In addition, anger suppression or rumination may not lead to emotional problems. The results of the present study indicate that nurses who experience a high degree of emotional labor, who tended to suppress anger and who also ruminated about the causes and effects of anger-provoking situations, may maintain or intensify anger mood, which ultimately increased their vulnerability to experience depressive and anxiety symptoms.

Interestingly, the indirect effect of anger suppression alone was not significant. Specifically, emotional labor was associated with anger suppression, but the pathway from anger suppression to depressive and anxiety symptoms was not significant. It is still an ongoing discussion as to whether emotional suppression always demonstrates a negative effect on psychological adjustment. There are results from meta-analytic studies which suggest that emotional suppression exhibits a negative impact on an individual's psychological health, but at the same time, there have also been studies that have reported on adaptive aspects of emotional suppression [21,22]. Thus, it cannot be assumed that simply suppressing negative emotions always leads to psychological maladjustment. Moreover, the indirect effect of anger rumination on the path from emotional labor to depressive and anxiety symptoms was not significant. Specifically, anger rumination had a significant effect on depressive and anxiety symptoms, but the path from emotional labor to anger rumination was not significant. Based on our results, the cognitive process of repetitively recalling anger-provoking situations (rumination) may have a significant impact in aggravating depressive and anxiety symptoms, especially when anger is suppressed.

In spite of the results from previous studies which reported that emotional labor has a negative effect on psychological adjustment [23], emotional labor and depressive and anxiety symptoms were not significantly correlated in the current study. This result may be related to the characteristic of emotional labor. The two main emotion regulation strategies used by emotional laborers are surface acting, (i.e., displaying nongenuine desired emotions) and deep acting, (i.e., modifying their genuine emotions to actually feel the desired and situationally required emotions) [1]. According to Drach-Zahavy, Yagil, and Cohen, surface acting requires constant effort to suppress negative emotion, which leads to the depletion of psychological resources and as a result impedes one's well-being [24]. On the other hand, deep acting may work as a protective factor in psychological adjustment, since it also involves efforts to maintain a positive view in negative or stressful situations. Empirical research has also demonstrated that this kind of cognitive effort may have a positive effect. In addition, in social interactions, deep acting may assist in the formation of relatively positive relationships and increase the opportunity to receive positive feedback from others by presenting authentic emotions during interactions [25]. If this effect is applied to nurses, deep acting may contribute to the formation of relatively positive interactions with patients, and nurses may also experience job satisfaction through potential positive feedback. These opposite possibilities may simultaneously affect depressive and anxiety symptoms.

The present study may provide valuable information for constructing a specific intervention strategy to protect nurses' psychological adjustment. More specifically, training in the use of different kinds of adaptive emotional regulation strategies other than anger suppression and anger rumination may be needed. For example, cognitive reappraisal was found to be more effective at reducing and handling anger than efforts to suppress anger [26]. Furthermore, positive reappraisal (i.e., searching for positive aspects or meaning instead of ruminating about anger-provoking events) and positive refocusing (i.e., focusing on pleasant and positive experiences unrelated to the experienced negative events) may be effectively utilized [27]. Supplementing clinically validated effective interventions for depressive and anxiety disorders, such as cognitive behavior therapy (CBT), with such emotion regulation training components may further effectively reduce nurses' psychological discomfort such as anger and depressive and anxiety symptoms.

5. Limitations and Future Directions

As reported in the meta-analysis results of Hülsheger and Schewe, there may be a significant moderating effect of cultural differences in the relationship between emotional labor and psychological distress [28]. Eastern cultures are characterized as an interdependent culture that values conformity, and the suppression of emotional expression for the sake of group harmony is frequently demanded [29]. Thus, there may exist a mediating effect of cultural differences on the sequential mediating effect of anger suppression and anger rumination found in the present study. Hence, the results of the current study need to be replicated through cross-cultural research. If differences are found, research identifying the cultural factors that contribute to the differences also needs to be conducted.

There is a possibility that the university hospital worked as a protective factor compared to other work environments. According to previous studies, work organization, structure, and policy have a significant impact on employees' anger [30]. University hospitals have relatively well-established organizational support and a protective system that may work in some degree as a protective factor for the nurses' anger [10]. Thus, examining the organizational characteristics of nurses working at private hospitals and other emotional laborers that may influence the result is suggested for further research.

Also, since the current study was conducted using cross-sectional data, we cannot confirm long-term variation trends in anger suppression and rumination and subsequent depression and anxiety. It is uncertain whether it is a temporary or a long-term effect that anger suppression and rumination have on depressive and anxiety symptoms. A study by Takebe et al. longitudinally examined the relationship between anger suppression and anger rumination [9]. Thus, future studies that examine the long-term effects on depressive and anxiety symptoms are suggested, based on our finding that these variables are significantly associated.

6. Conclusions

The present study suggested the existence of a potential mechanism by which anger that is evoked from emotional labor may be related to depressive and anxiety symptoms. Thus, hospitals should acknowledge that it is critical to manage nurses' anger through the construction of a specific intervention strategy to protect nurses' psychological adjustment.

Author Contributions: The conception and design of the study, or acquisition of data: J.E.K., J.H.P., and S.H.P. The drafting the article or revising it critically for important intellectual content: J.E.K., J.H.P., and S.H.P. The final approval of the version to be submitted: J.E.K., J.H.P., and S.H.P.

Funding: This work was supported by the National Research Foundation of Korea (NRF) (grant number NRF-2016-11-1385) and the Basic Science Research Program of the National Research Foundation of Korea funded by the Ministry of Science (grant number NRF-2015R1A2A2A04006136).

Acknowledgments: All the procedures performed in the studies involving human participants were in accordance with the ethical standards of the institutional and/or national research committee and with the 1964 Helsinki declaration and its later amendments or comparable ethical standards.

Conflicts of Interest: On behalf of all authors, the corresponding author states that there is no conflict of interest.

References

1. Hochschild, A.R. *The Managed Heart: Commercialization of Human Feeling*, 3rd ed.; University of California Press: Berkeley, CA, USA, 2012.
2. Kim, M.; Lee, S.; Song, J.; Yu, J.; Youn, J. Concept analysis of nurses' emotional labor. *Glob. Health Nurs.* **2014**, *4*, 78–87.
3. Han, J.; Kim, M. The convergence study of interpersonal caring behaviors on anger, job stress and social support in nurses. *J. Korean Converg. Soc.* **2016**, *7*, 87–98. [CrossRef]
4. Versella, M.V.; Piccirillo, M.L.; Potter, C.M.; Olino, T.M.; Heimberg, R.G. Anger profiles in social anxiety disorder. *J. Anxiety Disord.* **2016**, *37*, 21–29. [CrossRef] [PubMed]
5. Cox, D.; Velsor, P.V.; Hulgus, J. Who me, angry? Patterns of anger diversion in women. *Health Care Women Int.* **2004**, *25*, 872–893. [CrossRef] [PubMed]
6. Liverant, G.I.; Kamholz, B.W.; Sloan, D.M.; Brown, T.A. Rumination in clinical depression: A type of emotional suppression? *Cogn. Res.* **2010**, *35*, 253–265. [CrossRef]
7. Ryckman, N.A.; Lambert, A.J. Unsuccessful suppression is associated with increased neuroticism, intrusive thoughts, and rumination. *Personal. Individ. Differ.* **2015**, *73*, 88–91. [CrossRef]
8. Takebe, M.; Takahashi, F.; Sato, H. Anger rumination as a risk factor for trait anger and anger-in: A longitudinal study. *Personal. Individ. Differ.* **2016**, *101*, 451–455. [CrossRef]
9. Jang, S.; Kang, D.; Kang, H.; Kim, S.; Kim, I.; Kim, J. Development of Korean Emotional Labor Scale. 2013. Available online: https://oshri.kosha.or.kr (accessed on 10 June 2015).
10. Chon, K.; Hahn, D.; Lee, C.; Spielberger, C.D. Korean adaptation of the state-trait anger expression inventory: Anger and blood pressure. *Korean J. Health Psychol.* **1997**, *2*, 60–78.
11. Spielberger, C.D.; Krasner, S.S.; Solomon, E.P. The experience, expression, and control of anger. In *Health Psychology: Individual Differences and Stress*; Janisse, M.P., Ed.; Springer-Verlag: New York, NY, USA, 1988; pp. 89–108.
12. Lee, K.; Cho, H. Validation study of the Korean version of the anger rumination scale. *J. Emot. Behav. Disord.* **2008**, *24*, 1–22.
13. Sukhodolsky, D.G.; Golub, A.; Cromwell, E.N. Development and validation of the anger rumination scale. *Personal. Individ. Differ.* **2001**, *31*, 689–700. [CrossRef]
14. Chon, K.; Choi, S.; Yang, B. Integrated adaptation of CES-D in Korea. *Korean J. Health Psychol.* **2001**, *6*, 59–76.
15. Radloff, L.S. The CES-D scale a self-report depression scale for research in the general population. *Appl. Psychol. Meas.* **1977**, *1*, 385–401. [CrossRef]

16. Spielberger, C.D.; Gorsuch, R.L.; Lushene, R.; Vagg, P.R.; Jacobs, G.A. *Manual for the State-Trait Anxiety Inventory*; Consulting Psychologists Press: Palo Alto, CA, USA, 1983.
17. Kim, J.; Shin, D. A study based on the standardization of the STAI for Korea. *New Med. J.* **1978**, *21*, 69–75.
18. Hayes, A.F. *Introduction to Mediation, Moderation, and Conditional Process Analysis: A Regression-Based Approach*; The Guilford Press: New York, NY, USA, 2013.
19. Shariat, A.; Tamrin, S.B.M.; Daneshjoo, A.; Sadeghi, H. The adverse health effects of shift work in relation to risk of illness/disease: A review. *Acta Med. Bulg.* **2015**, *42*, 63–72. [CrossRef]
20. Yoon, S.; Kim, J. Job-related stress, emotional labor, and depressive symptoms among Korean nurses. *J. Nurs. Sch.* **2013**, *45*, 169–176. [CrossRef] [PubMed]
21. Aldao, A.; Nolen-Hoeksema, S.; Schweizer, S. Emotion-regulation strategies across psychopathology: A meta-analytic review. *Clin. Psychol. Rev.* **2010**, *30*, 217–237. [CrossRef] [PubMed]
22. Georges, J.M. Evidence of the unspeakable: Biopower, compassion, and nursing. *Adv. Nurs. Sci.* **2011**, *34*, 130–135. [CrossRef] [PubMed]
23. Holman, D.; Chissick, C.; Totterdell, P. The effects of performance monitoring on emotional labor and well-being in call centers. *Motiv. Emot.* **2002**, *26*, 57–81. [CrossRef]
24. Drach-Zahavy, A.; Yagil, D.; Cohen, I. Social model of emotional labor and client satisfaction: Exploring inter- and intrapersonal characteristics of the client-provider encounter. *Work Stress* **2017**, *31*, 182–208. [CrossRef]
25. Cote, S.A. Social Interaction Model Of The Effects Of Emotion Regulation On Work Strain. *Acad. Manag. Rev.* **2005**, *30*, 509–530. [CrossRef]
26. Szasz, P.L.; Szentagotai, A.; Hofmann, S.G. The effect of emotion regulation strategies on anger. *Behav. Res.* **2011**, *49*, 114–119. [CrossRef] [PubMed]
27. Hu, T.; Zhang, D.; Wang, J.; Mistry, R.; Ran, G.; Wang, X. Relation between emotion regulation and mental health: A meta-analysis review. *Psychol. Rep.* **2014**, *114*, 341–362. [CrossRef] [PubMed]
28. Hülsheger, U.R.; Schewe, A.F. On the costs and benefits of emotional labor: A meta-analysis of three decades of research. *J. Occup. Health Psychol.* **2011**, *16*, 361–389. [CrossRef] [PubMed]
29. Allen, J.A.; Diefendorff, J.M.; Ma, Y. Differences in emotional labor across cultures: A comparison of Chinese and U.S. service workers. *J. Bus. Psychol.* **2014**, *29*, 21–35. [CrossRef]
30. Moura, K.; Troth, A.C.; Jordan, P.J. Crossing the impropriety threshold: A study of experiences of excessive anger. In *Research on Emotion in Rganizations*; Hartel, C.E.J., Zerbe, W.J., Ashkanasy, N.M., Eds.; Emerald Group Publishing Limited: London, UK, 2015; pp. 369–395.

International Journal of
Environmental Research and Public Health

MDPI

Article

Risk Assessment for Musculoskeletal Disorders in Forestry: A Comparison between RULA and REBA in the Manual Feeding of a Wood-Chipper

Margherita Micheletti Cremasco [1], Ambra Giustetto [1], Federica Caffaro [2], Andrea Colantoni [3], Eugenio Cavallo [2,*] and Stefano Grigolato [4]

1 Department of Life Sciences and Systems Biology, University of Torino, Via Accademia Albertina 13, 10123 Torino, Italy; margherita.micheletti@unito.it (M.M.C.); ambra.giustetto@unito.it (A.G.)
2 Institute for Agricultural and Earthmoving Machines (IMAMOTER), National Research Council of Italy (CNR), Strada delle Cacce, 73, 10135 Torino, Italy; f.caffaro@ima.to.cnr.it
3 Department of Agriculture and Forest Sciences (DAFNE), Tuscia University, Via San Camillo de Lellis, 01100 Viterbo, Italy; colantoni@unitus.it
4 Department of Land, Environment, Agriculture and Forestry, Università degli Studi di Padova, Viale dell'Università 16, 35040 Padova, Italy; stefano.grigolato@unipd.it
* Correspondence: eugenio.cavallo@cnr.it; Tel.: +39-011-39-77-724

Received: 10 December 2018; Accepted: 27 February 2019; Published: 5 March 2019

Abstract: The analysis of the postural attitude of workers during the interaction with workstation's elements and working environment is essential in the evaluation and prevention of biomechanical overload risk in workplaces. RULA (Rapid Upper Limb Assessment) and REBA (Rapid Entire Body Assessment) are the two easiest methods for postural risk assessment in the workplace. Few studies investigated postural risk in forestry sector with regard to human–machine interaction, in particular manually fed wood-chippers. The aim of this study was to evaluate the postures assumed by an operator during the manual feeding of a wood-chipper, and to compare RULA and REBA, in order to identify the more effective and appropriate method for the assessment of the risk of biomechanical postural overload. The results pointed out several postural issues of the upper limbs, and showed that RULA is a more precautionary method to protect operator's health during the targeted tasks. Implications to improve the human–wood-chipper interaction are discussed.

Keywords: ergonomics; forestry; postural risk assessment; RULA; REBA; wood-chipper

1. Introduction

The analysis of the postural attitude of the worker during the interaction with workstation's elements and working environment is essential in the evaluation and prevention of biomechanical overload risks in workplaces [1]. Awkward working postures may decrease the workers' concentration and increase accidents frequency and biomechanical overload [2–6], giving rise to musculoskeletal disorders in the different body regions involved, as at the main limb joints level and the vertebral column [7].

Some standards [8–10] dealing with the biomechanical overload caused by incongruous static and dynamic postures have been developed to define the risk assessment methods to evaluate postural load referable to activity and workstation characteristics and to human–machine interaction. They are referenced in international [11] and national [12] legislations aimed at protecting workers' health and safety.

RULA (Rapid Upper Limb Assessment) [13] and REBA (Rapid Entire Body Assessment) [14] are two easy methods for occupational postural risk assessment. Indeed, previous studies [15,16] showed that observational methods are considered effective in the assessment of biomechanical work-related overload, having the advantage of being more versatile and less expensive in terms of time and resources required compared to objective laboratory measures. Both RULA and REBA allow to obtain a numerical index that represents the quantitative value of the risk at which the worker is exposed during the targeted work activity and to derive the priority level of intervention and the actions needed. The RULA method is suggested for the identification of postural disorders of the upper limbs, of the neck and of the back in relation to the muscular action and external loads applied to the body. The REBA method is applied to identify postural disorders of the whole body, in relation to the muscular action, to the external loads applied to the body and to the type of grip. They are referenced in the international standard for occupational risk assessment [9] and cited among the selected tools for Work-related Musculoskeletal Disorders (WMSDs) prevention according to International Ergonomics Association (IEA) and World Health Organization (WHO) [17]. These methods are also widely applied in several working contexts, mainly industrial work activities (secondary sector) and those producing services and goods (tertiary sector), characterized by a precise standardization of tasks, geometries, gestures and relative execution frequencies that allow a systematic and controlled forecasting and quantification of the biomechanical overload risk. Furthermore, the two methods have been combined and compared to assess postural risk in industry [18–20], construction [21], supermarkets [22], hospital and dental sector [23], work with video terminals [24], waste collection activity [25], for firefighters and emergency medical technicians [26], and artisans [27–29] and sawmill activities [30].

RULA and REBA have been adopted a few times in the agricultural [31,32] and forestry sectors [33,34] because the evaluation of the biomechanical overload risk in the primary sector activities is more difficult; due to the large variability of the tasks the operators have to perform, depending on crops, operations (seeding, weeding, pruning, harvesting, etc.), the machinery and tools adopted, the, sometimes extreme, weather conditions they have to be carried out with, and the daily and seasonal exposure, as well as the lack of a strict standardization of the work in general [35,36]. Interaction with machines, tools and environments in agriculture, and particularly in forestry, requires therefore a particular attention in the application of risk assessment methods conceived for other contexts, or the formulation of specific methods that consider the distinctive characteristics of these activities [37].

Kundu and Gaur [38] compared RULA and REBA in a study addressed at investigating how much these techniques were appropriate for evaluating the postures assumed by agricultural workers. They highlighted some shortfalls in using these techniques to study risk factors associated with agricultural field operations and suggested to add some factors as posture duration, field condition, environmental factors and nutritional status to better assess the occupational risks and possible remedies, especially for agricultural work in the fields.

Besides RULA and REBA, other methods have been used to assess the postural risk in manual agricultural activities. For example, Kong et al. [39] compared RULA, REBA, OWAS (Ovako Working Posture Analyzing System [40]) and ALLA (Agricultural Lower Limb Assessment [41]) for various agricultural tasks. They found that ALLA better estimated the risk because it identifies critical issues that the other methods do not analyse and, therefore, it always returns a higher level of risk, compared to the other methods. Ojha and Kwatra [42] combined REBA and VAS (Visual Analog Scale) methods in rice cultivation manual operations. REBA indicated postural load and suggested interesting corrective measures. However, in both studies [39,42], the object of the analysis was a manual activity, while, in developed countries, most of the farming operations require the use of machinery and workers spend many hours in interacting with them, making the investigation of the human–machine interaction more relevant [43].

Among the studies specifically dealing with the human–machine interaction in agriculture, RULA is the most frequently adopted method. Vyavahare and Kallurkar [44] used RULA to assess postures assumed during the interaction with agricultural machines such as maize dehusker-sheller. The study analysed and evaluated the risk of various key postures, such as squat, forward/lateral bending, hands flexion/extension, wrist/spine twisting. Putri et al. [45] used RULA to study the use of thresher machines for threshing rice plants. In the first study, RULA helped to optimize a digital human manikin posture, resulting in precise risk assessment and better designed and widely accepted products and workplaces, while, in the second study, RULA provided indications to redesign the machine to reduce injuries and musculoskeletal overload caused by the mismatch between the dimensions of the engine and farmers' postures and dimensions.

In the forestry sector, the studies report postural risk evaluation mainly referred to manual tools. Gallo and Mazzetto [34] applied different methods including REBA and OWAS to evaluate the postural risks from the cutting operations with chainsaw, showing their good applicability for the assessment of WMSD in forestry. The comparison between OWAS and REBA showed that REBA has a higher level of detail of assessment because it considers the angles between body segments and extremities as the wrist, the neck, the elbow and the shoulders (parameters that are not considered by OWAS method) for both sides of the body and, furthermore, it assesses the type of handle coupling and the characteristics of the performed activities. REBA results to be suitable for suggesting interventions to be performed to decrease musculoskeletal overload, even though it has not been developed specifically for forestry operations and it presents some weaknesses during the assessment, as the lack of coded postures as the kneeling posture.

Forestry is recognized as a highly hazardous industry [46] and working postures are one of the most investigated risk factors for workers' safety, even though the postural aspects in the human–machine interaction have been under investigated in this sector [47,48]. With regard to machinery, manually fed wood-chippers are one of the most widely used machines in forestry, agricultural, landscaping and urban tree maintenance to reduce the volume of woods for following disposal or re-use in bio-energy production [47]. The attention to this machine is rising because of the significant increasing interest in biomass production as biofuel [49] and because they are often involved in fatal and non-fatal injuries [50]. Data on the occurrence of accidents provide an objective index of the danger of machinery as well as a valid reason for identifying the most critical features of these machines.

In the United States, between 1992 and 2002, Struttman [50] reported 31 fatal and 2042 non-fatal accidents involving wood-chippers. The estimated social cost of these fatal accidents were estimated in 2003 to US$28.5 million; furthermore, an in-depth analysis disclosed that 58% of these fatal accidents involved groundskeepers and machinery operators in the forestry and agricultural sectors [50]. Analyses of the non-fatal accidents showed that 60% of the accidents caused immediate injury or amputation of parts of the upper-body limbs. For 25% of these injuries, the victims were unable to return to work for periods of up to 30 work days [51]. Further studies indicated that more than one-third of these accident victims had less than 11 months of experience in that particular job [50].

In the further period between 2008 and 2018, statistics from the United States Occupational Safety and Health Administration of Department of Labor [52] reported 56 incidents during chipping operations: 64% of the accidents dealt with feeding operations and 36% of them were fatal for the operators. From the same statistics, the accidents not related with feeding operations of wood-chippers had a lower rate, 16%, of fatal accidents.

Accurate statistics about accidents with wood-chippers are not available from most of the European Union countries [53]. Only the French Ministry of Agriculture, Agrifood, and Forestry reported that at least one severe accident related to the use of wood-chippers occurs every year in France and that, in most of the cases, the operators involved were young apprentices [54], one of the category of users for which warnings to eliminate hazardous behaviours when intrinsically safe machine are used, are less effective [55,56].

Based on the literature review, the aim of this study was to identify the more effective and appropriate method between RULA and REBA for the assessment of the risk of biomechanical postural overload, evaluating the postures assumed by an operator during the manual load of a wood-chipper, in a controlled experimental setting. The study further discusses which of the two methods is more precautionary in evaluating postural risk and reports higher risk indices, for the specific activity considered.

For the present study, a small manually fed wood-chipper has been selected since: (1) small-size wood-chippers are widespread among forestry, agricultural and urban green maintenance operators; (2) similar types of wood-chippers are used for occasional and accessory operations to the main activity [47]; (3) often experienced, but not specialized, operators are involved in the wood-chipping operations and this category of operators are known to be the most exposed to safety risks [57]. As a consequence, the manual feeding seems to be critical both in terms of safety and health risks for the operators [58,59].

2. Materials and Methods

2.1. The Wood-Chipper

The manually fed wood-chippers generally consist of a feeding system, a chipping units based on rotating knives (drum or disc mounted) and on a discharge system. Alternative solutions for the comminution devices are available for production of quality wood chips for fuel [60]. In the case of manually-fed wood-chippers, the operators feed small trees, part of trees and/or branches into the infeed chute by hand with a following risk of biomechanical postural overload, which is typical of manually-loaded wood machines [61].

The study was carried out with a manually fed wood-chipper model Tirex, made available by the manufacturer Peruzzo (Peruzzo Srl, Curtarolo, Italy). The machine was connected to the rear three-point hitch of a 55 kW tractor and was powered by the rear Power Take-Off (PTO) (Figure 1). The feeding system consists of a feeding hopper with an infeed chute above 600 mm from the ground level and with a width of 1200 mm at the external edge. The feeding system consists of two horizontal rollers electro-hydraulically controlled by a load-limiting mechanism and located at the end of the infeed chute at a distance of 1200 mm from the external infeed chute limit, in accordance with EN 13,525:2005 + A2:2009 [62]. The machine is equipped with an electro-hydraulic feed control bar fixed on the bottom and along the two sides of the infeed chute. The chipping unit consists of a flywheel (diameter 620 mm, mm thickness 30 mm) rotating at 1500 rpm and with a torque of about 33 Nm. The flywheel is equipped with four knives (thickness 25 mm and length 200 mm) while an anvil is fixed to the frame of the machine. The manufacturer claims the machine is able to chip wood stems with a diameter up to 180–200 mm.

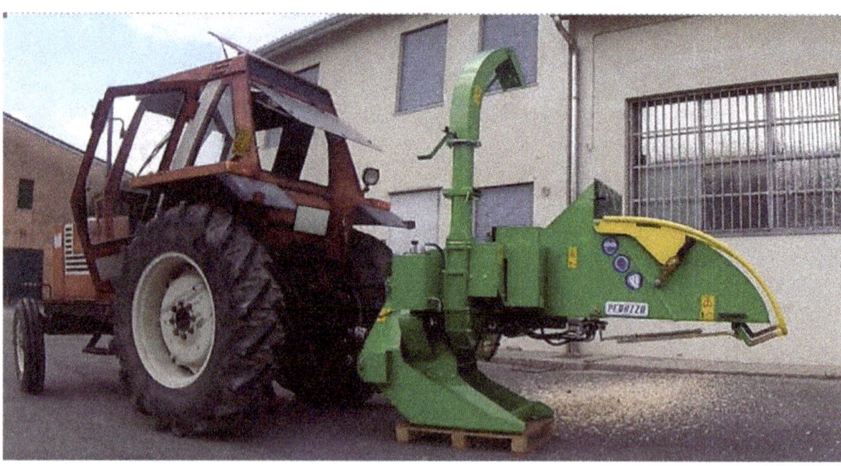

Figure 1. The manually fed wood-chipper used during the test.

2.2. Research Design

The study was conducted at the Azienda agraria sperimentale "L. Toniolo" of the Università degli Studi di Padova (Padova, Italy). Since we were interested in controlling as many variables as possible to better compare RULA and REBA, the evaluation of the differences in risk levels between the two methods was carried out by keeping the machine and participant characteristics constant, while changing the log size. To reduce the inter-individual variability in the adoption of the targeted postures, one single participant was involved in the study. He was a not-specialized operator, with no previous history of either occupational accidents or musculoskeletal disorders. Specific measures were defined for the logs to be used in the tests, with regard to log length and diameter, and an acceptable mass, ranging between 2 and 10 kg, to be manually handled by the operator (Figure 2).

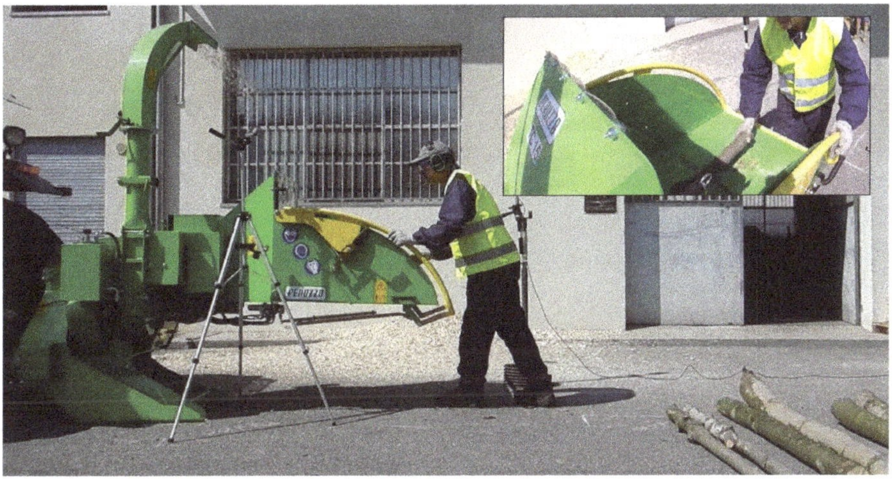

Figure 2. Example of tasks to be performed during the tests.

Plane-tree wood was used for the tests, preparing both logs of different length and diameters, and branches of more variable dimensions, in order to observe if and how much the size of the wood induced different postures and gestures, which may be associated with different levels of postural risk. The logs were prepared in three different lengths (1 m, 1.5 m, 2 m) and two diameters (65 mm and 135 mm). For each length/diameter combination and for the branches, three elements were prepared to perform three repeated tests. Therefore, six tasks involving logs plus one task regarding branches were performed. The operator performed each task three times to evaluate any intra-individual difference in postures and gestures with respect to the manipulated element. Thus, overall seven tasks were performed for a total of 21 loadings (six tasks for the logs, each repeated three times, and one task for the branch repeated three times). The 21 loadings were randomly performed.

The research protocol was approved by the Research Advisory Group of the Institute for Agricultural and Earthmoving Machines (IMAMOTER) of the National Research Council of Italy (CNR) on 28 February 2018.

2.3. Video Recording

The operator was video recorded and photographed while feeding the machine. One video camera was placed in front of the infeed chute while a second one recorded images from the side of the infeed chute. During the analysis of the recorded videos, every time a log or a branch was loaded, the frame-by-frame vision was carried out until the most critical position was detected. The video analysis was performed with Kinovea software, an open-access video analysis software available online reproducing the video in slow-motion. Kinovea is a valid and reliable method to perform motion and postural analysis [63]. It allows for detecting body and its districts' angles during the single posture observations: angles were measured according to the reference axes reported in RULA and REBA methods to obtain the corresponding score.

2.4. Assessment Methods of Applied Biomechanical Risk

The study investigated the human–chipper interaction comparing two observational methods of biomechanical overload postural risk: RULA method [13] and REBA method [14].

In RULA method [13], the body is divided into different parts gathered into two groups, A and B: group A includes arm, forearm and wrist of the right and left limb; group B includes the neck, the trunk and the feet. The method consists in assigning a score to each segment depending on the posture taken and it allows to obtain two distinct scores (Scores A and B) through the use of numerical tables or spreadsheets; these scores represent the level of postural load of the musculoskeletal system, determined by the combination of the postures of the whole body. Muscle use and force scores are then added to Scores A and B to obtain two new scores (Scores C and D) that, through a third table or a spreadsheet, allow for obtaining the final score, or Grand Score.

Based on the appropriate combination of scores, the final score can range between 1 and 7. The final score is related to four levels of action and four levels of risk. Scores, actions and risk levels for RULA are summarized in Table 1:

- Action level 1: Low risk level. A score of 1 or 2 indicates that posture is acceptable if it is not maintained or repeated for long periods.
- Action level 2: Medium risk level. A score of 3 or 4 indicates that further investigation is needed and changes may be required.
- Action level 3: High risk level. A score of 5 or 6 indicates that investigation and changes are required soon.
- Action level 4: Very high risk level. A score of 7 indicates that investigation and changes are required immediately.

Table 1. RULA and REBA scores with the respective action level.

RULA Score	Action Level	REBA Score	Action Level	Risk Level
		1	0	Negligible
1–2	1	2–3	1	Low
3–4	2	4–7	2	Medium
5–6	3	8–10	3	High
7	4	11–15	4	Very High

RULA: Rapid Upper Limb Assessment; REBA: Rapid Entire Body Assessment.

In REBA method [14], the body is divided into different segments divided into two groups: the first one includes neck, torso and legs; the second group is composed by arm, forearm and wrist without distinction from the right or the left one. The method consists in assigning a score to each segment of the body according to the posture taken and, using numerical tables or spreadsheet, it allows for obtaining two different scores that represent the level of postural load of the musculoskeletal system determined from the combination of the whole body postures. The two scores should be respectively added to the grip score and to the load and strength score to get two new scores (Scores A and B). From the use of a third table or spreadsheet, it is possible to obtain Score C, which, added to the activity score, allows for obtaining the final score, or Grand Score. The final score can range between 1 and 15 and it is related to five levels of action and five levels of risk. Table 1 reports scores, actions and risk levels for REBA:

- Action level 0: The risk is negligible so no action is required.

- Action level 1: Low risk level. The final score between 2 and 3 indicates that changes may be required.
- Action level 2: Medium risk level. The final score from 4 to 7 indicates the need for measures and further analysis.
- Action level 3: High risk level. The final score between 8 and 10 indicates the need for an intervention and a change in a short time.
- Action level 4: Very high risk level. The final score from 11 to 15 indicates that an action is immediately required.

2.5. Data Analysis

For each task, three risk indices were obtained for each of the two methods, RULA and REBA.

The goal was to analyze the highest level of risk calculated, considering the variability of the execution of the gesture, evaluated three times separately. Among the results obtained, the highest value, among the three for each task, and then the highest between the right and left side was selected.

The results of the two scores calculated for each task with RULA and REBA were compared to highlight any tendency of any of the two methods to over or underestimate the risk. This was done both on the basis of risks category, considering the action level—color code (Table 1), and the values of normalized indices.

In order to compare the differences between REBA and RULA scores, it was necessary to normalize the absolute values as the two methods are based on different scales: RULA has four risk levels that categorize scores from 1 to 7, while REBA is based on five levels of risk that categorize scores from 1 to 15. The use of standardized scores to compare different methods for postural risk assessment has been adopted previously in similar analyses [64,65], thus we normalized the score values ranging from 0 to 1, applying the following formula to each worst value obtained for each task by the two methods:

$$\text{normalized value} = [\text{score obs} - \text{score value min}]/[\text{score value max} - \text{score value min}].$$

3. Results

The risk assessment carried out by applying RULA and REBA (Table 2) showed a medium-high level of risk for all the tasks. None of the tasks reported a score referable to a negligible or low risk as well as a very high risk level that would require an immediate intervention.

Table 2. Comparison between RULA and REBA risk evaluation (worst case for each task calculated with each method) for the seven tasks considered with details of the dimensional characteristics of the manipulated wooden elements.

Task [1]	Object Length (m)	Object Diameter (mm)	Object Mass (kg)	RULA Worst Case	REBA Worst Case	Action Level
1	1	65	2–10	5	8	both 3
2	1	135	2–10	7	11	both 4
3	1.5	65	2–10	5	5	3 with RULA 2 with REBA
4	1.5	135	2–10	6	10	both 3
5	2	65	2–10	4	5	both 2
6	2	135	>10	5	8	both 3
7		Branches		3	5	both 2

[1] Note. Tasks 1–6 represent the loading of logs with three different lengths (1 m, 1.5 m, 2 m) and 2 diameters (65 mm and 135 mm); Task 7 represents the loading of branches.

Regarding the differences between the risk indices of each task, it can be seen that, based on the dimensional differences of the handled logs, the risk level is limited in the case of logs with longer length and smaller diameter. This could be due to the posture induced by small length logs which could cause a higher postural overload because of the greater proximity to the machine that could determine worse joint angles. The highest indices were observed in the manipulation of short and larger diameter logs (Task 2), while the lower levels of risk indices occurred in the manipulation of the branches (Task 7). The comparison between the results obtained with RULA and REBA, based on the resulting action level, highlighted a good overlapping between the two methods, with the exception of Task 3, related to wooden elements of an intermediate size (1.5 m) and small diameter (65 mm). In this case, the RULA carried out a more precautionary assessment as it gave an index that fell into a higher action level compared to the corresponding level calculated with REBA. In the comparison of the normalized numerical indices, all of the RULA scores were higher than the corresponding REBA scores for all of the tasks (Table 3). The application of RULA showed to be more precautionary than REBA for all the tasks, as it returned a higher score value in each loading.

Table 3. Comparison between the normalized scores of RULA and REBA indices for the seven tasks.

Task [1]	RULA	REBA
1	0.67	0.50
2	1.00	0.71
3	0.67	0.29
4	0.83	0.64
5	0.50	0.29
6	0.67	0.50
7	0.33	0.29

[1] Note. Tasks 1–6 represent the loading of logs with different lengths and diameters; Task 7 represents the loading of branches.

4. Discussion

The present study showed that RULA and REBA are two effective methods for assessing the postural overload determined by incongruous postures adopted in the act of manually loading the wood-chipper with logs of various diameters and lengths. The two methods appeared to be both effective and suitable for the identification and quantification of the level of postural risk using a manually fed wood-chipper, as they highlighted similar levels of urgency of intervention, analysis and modification actions. The high congruence between RULA and REBA evaluations confirmed similar results from other investigations in the industrial context [66]. However, the present study showed that RULA tended to be more precautionary, giving a higher risk index, for all the tasks, consistent with previous studies comparing the two methods in the industrial sector [18]. This underestimation by REBA was also found in KOSHA's research [67] in different sectors like ship building, automotive, electronics, general manufacturing, and service industries.

Comparing the action level in which the calculated indices fall, and, therefore, the corresponding severity and urgency of intervention, RULA and REBA suggested an almost identical level and, in only one case (Task 3, intermediate size and small diameter wooden elements), RULA returned a higher action level than REBA (Table 2). Task 3 is also the one which reported the highest difference between normalized RULA and REBA scores. Comparing normalized scores, RULA always resulted in being more precautionary as it returned higher values for all the tasks. The evaluation of the branches' manipulation task presented the most contained difference between the two normalized values, but also in this case the risk estimated by RULA, even if slightly, prevailed. RULA appeared to be constantly more precautionary in the risk assessment for all of the tasks considered, both in medium or high risk conditions. RULA also seemed to be more precise as it better highlighted the differences in the level of risk exposure between the manipulation of logs and branches. This could be due to the presence of different postural issues of the upper limbs, such as radial or ulnar deviation of the wrist, rotation of the wrist and movements performed across the body or out to the side, which play an important role in the postural risk assessment of these tasks and are not considered by REBA. About the branches loading, RULA normalized score returned a value of 0.33, which was the lowest of all tasks. REBA did not seem to be influenced by these differences among logs and branches manipulation.

The minimum normalized REBA score was 0.29, and it was the same value for both the manipulation of the branches (Task 7) and for the manipulation of logs of Tasks 3 and 5.

RULA highlighted how biomechanical workload in the interaction with the wood-chipper is limited to the upper part of the body and it determines an important involvement especially of the wrist and forearm, and on the rachis due to flexion of the chest and postural asymmetries. REBA scores, obtained evaluating the lower limb biomechanical risk in greater detail, had no higher values than RULA in all the tasks, confirming the absence of serious criticalities for the lower limbs in wood-chipper manual feeding.

According to the results of the present study—even though they were obtained by observing one single operator and should not therefore be considered as conclusive—RULA is more precautionary, probably because of the more precise workload evaluation of the upper limbs and trunk. RULA considers in a much more limited way the postural and workload conditions of the lower limbs compared to REBA, but, nevertheless, in the present investigation, REBA did not give higher risk estimation values, which means that, during the loading of the wood-chipper, there was not any evidence of risk to the lower limbs (otherwise, REBA would have highlighted it with a higher risk index). Therefore, RULA may be a more adequate method for the assessment of postural risk of interaction with the machinery when exposure to risk of the lower limbs is less relevant. This consideration confirms results from previous studies which reported the effectiveness of RULA in evaluating the interaction with agricultural machines [44].

The analysis pointed out different RULA scores due to the different lengths and diameters of logs, with shorter ones determining incongruous postures. This consideration opens new perspectives for the analysis of human–wood-chipper interaction stressing the importance of avoiding short logs during the cutting operations, when they are intended to be chipped. In this way, a postural disadvantage occurs even if the mass is reduced. Future investigation should be addressed at investigating a larger number of operators regarding how much log mass, besides the length, determines incongruous postures (high RULA score) and physical effort (applied force and perceived fatigue). The results of such studies could provide suggestions about an "optimal" cutting length for logs, determining a better postural conditions for operators of manually fed wood-chippers. Indeed, in ergonomics, it is not enough to concentrate on the design of the machine, but it is important to intervene in the different components of human–machine interaction through a holistic approach, as widely documented in the literature and recommended by international standards [68–71].

Besides the attention paid to safety and technical characteristics of the forestry machine, this study highlighted the importance to inform and train the operators to perform gestures, postures and activities in accordance with the ergonomic principles. In this way, in addition to optimize the human–machine interaction, it can be possible to intervene on the organization and management of the whole activity. This integrated approach may contribute to risk reduction and enhance the system productivity and operator's wellbeing.

5. Conclusions

Agricultural and forestry operators interact with a variety of tasks and machinery, which can require ad hoc methods for the assessment of postural risk. The present investigation showed that the RULA method is suitable for the evaluation of postural overload in the human–machine interaction related to a manually fed wood-chipper, more than the REBA method, because it showed indices that corresponded to a higher level of risk for all the tasks observed, independently of the shape, size, mass of the wooden material and, therefore, it would be a more precautionary method to protect operator's health. Further considerations about the postural risk of manually-loaded wood-chippers should focus not only on the posture of the operators, but also on the safety standards imposed by the safety regulations (for instance, the former EN 13,525:2005 + A2:2009 [62]). The extended application of RULA in real and differentiated agro-forestry conditions will allow for assessing postural risks and physical effort to improve human–machine interaction and operators' wellbeing in the wood-chipping activity.

Author Contributions: M.M.C., A.G., F.C., A.C., E.C. and S.G. conceived and designed the study; A.C. and S.G. collected the data; M.M.C. and A.G. analyzed the data; M.M.C., A.G., F.C., A.C. and S.G. interpreted the data; M.M.C., A.G. and F.C. wrote the paper; A.C., E.C. and S.G. critically reviewed the paper; M.M.C., A.G., F.C., A.C., E.C. and S.G. gave final approval.

Funding: This study was supported by the "Protection of agricultural machinery operators from crush, entanglement, shearing" (PROMOSIC) project, funded by INAIL, the Italian National Institute for Insurance against Accidents at Work.

Acknowledgments: This research did not receive any specific grant from funding agencies in the public, commercial or not-for-profit sector.

Conflicts of Interest: The authors declare no conflict of interest.

References

1. Joan Burton. *Healthy Workplace Framework and Model: Background and Supporting Literature and Practices*; World Health Organization: Geneva, Switzerland, 2010; pp. 1–131.
2. Caffaro, F.; Lundqvist, P.; Micheletti Cremasco, M.; Nilsson, K.; Pinzke, S.; Cavallo, E. Machinery-Related Perceived Risks and Safety Attitudes in Senior Swedish Farmers. *J. Agromed.* **2018**, *23*, 78–91. [CrossRef] [PubMed]
3. Caffaro, F.; Preti, C.; Micheletti Cremasco, M.; Cavallo, E. Three-axial evaluation of whole-body vibration in agricultural telehandlers: The effects of an active cab-suspension system. *J. Occup. Environ. Hyg.* **2017**, *14*, 758–770. [CrossRef] [PubMed]
4. Hallbeck, M.S.; Bosch, T.; Gu Van Rhijn, J.W.; Krause, F.; De Looze, M.P.; Vink, P. A tool for early workstation design for small and medium enterprises evaluated in five cases. *Hum. Factors Ergon. Manuf.* **2010**, *20*, 300–315. [CrossRef]
5. Lee, S.; Yu, S.; Choi, J.; Han, C. A methodology to quantitatively evaluate the safety of a glazing robot. *Appl. Ergon.* **2011**, *42*, 445–454. [CrossRef] [PubMed]
6. Caffaro, F.; Micheletti Cremasco, M.; Preti, C.; Cavallo, E. Ergonomic analysis of the effect of a telehandler active suspended cab on whole body vibration level and operator comfort. *Int J. Ind. Erg.* **2016**, *53*, 19–26. [CrossRef]
7. Devereux, J.; Buckle, P. Musculoskeletal Disorders in Europe: Definitions and Statistics. Eurogrip. 2007. Available online: https://www.etui.org/Topics/Health-Safety-working-conditions/Musculoskeletal-disorders/What-are-MSDs (accessed on 8 January 2019).
8. ISO 11226:2000. *Ergonomics—Evaluation of Static Working Postures*; International Organization for Standardization: Geneva, Switzerland, 2000.
9. ISO 11228-3:2007. *Ergonomics—Manual handling—Part 3: Handling of Low Loads at High Frequency*; International Organization for Standardization: Geneva, Switzerland, 2007.
10. UNI EN 1005-4:2009. *Sicurezza del Macchinario—Prestazione Fisica umana—Parte 4: Valutazione delle Posture e dei Movimenti Lavorativi in Relazione al Macchinario*; UNI Ente Italiano di Normazione: Milan, Italy, 2009. (In Italian)
11. EEC Directive 90/269/EEC. Council Directive of 29 May 1990 on the Minimum Health and Safety Requirements for the Manual Handling of Loads Where There Is a Risk Particularly of Back Injury to Workers (Fourth Individual Directive within the Meaning of Article 16 (1) of Directive 89/391/EEC). 1990. Available online: https://eur-lex.europa.eu (accessed on 8 January 2019).
12. Decreto Legislativo 81:2008. Testo unico sulla Salute e Sicurezza sul Lavoro. Available online: http://www.lavoro.gov.it/documenti-e-norme/studi-e-statistiche/Documents/Testo%20Unico%20sulla%20Salute%20e%20Sicurezza%20sul%20Lavoro/Testo-Unico-81-08-Edizione-Giugno%202016.pdf (accessed on 8 January 2019). (In Italian)
13. McAtamney, L.; Nigel Corlett, E. RULA: A survey method for the investigation of work-related upper limb disorders. *Appl. Ergon.* **1993**, *24*, 91–99. [CrossRef]
14. Hignett, S.; McAtamney, L. Rapid Entire Body Assessment (REBA). *Appl. Ergon.* **2000**, *31*, 201–205. [CrossRef]
15. David, G.C. Ergonomic methods for assessing exposure to risk factors for work-related musculoskeletal disorders. *Occup. Med.* **2005**, *55*, 190–199. [CrossRef] [PubMed]
16. Zare, M.; Biau, S.; Croq, M.; Roquelaure, Y. Development of a biomechanical method for ergonomic evaluation: Comparison with observational methods. *Int. J. Soc. Manag. Econ. Bus. Eng.* **2014**, *8*, 223–227.

17. Occhipinti, E.; Colombini, D. IEA/WHO toolkit for WMSDs prevention: Criteria and practical tools for a step by step approach. *Work* **2012**, *41*, 3937–3944. [PubMed]
18. Kee, D.; Karwowski, W. A Comparison of Three Observational Techniques for Assessing Postural Loads in Industry. *Int. J. Occup. Saf. Ergon.* **2007**, *13*, 3–14. [CrossRef] [PubMed]
19. Labbafinejad, Y.; Imanizade, Z.; Danesh, H. Ergonomic Risk Factors and Their Association with Lower Back and Neck Pain among Pharmaceutical Employees in Iran. *Work. Health Saf.* **2016**, *64*, 586–595. [CrossRef] [PubMed]
20. Lasota, A.M. A REBA-based analysis of packers workload: A case study. *Sci. J. Logist.* **2014**, *10*, 87–95.
21. Kulkarni, V.S.; Devalkar, R.V. Postural analysis of building construction workers using ergonomics. *Int. J. Constr. Manag.* **2018**. [CrossRef]
22. Coyle, A. Comparison of the Rapid Entire Body Assessment and the New Zealand Manual Handling 'Hazard Control Record', for assessment of manual handling hazards in the supermarket industry. *Work* **2005**, *24*, 111–116. [PubMed]
23. Janowitz, I.L.; Gillen, M.; Ryan, G.; Rempel, D.; Trupin, L.; Swig, L.; Mullen, K.; Rugulies, R.; Blanc, P.D. Measuring the physical demands of work in hospital settings: Design and implementation of an ergonomics assessment. *Appl. Ergon.* **2006**, *37*, 641–658. [CrossRef] [PubMed]
24. Mirmohammadi, S.J.; Mehrparvar, A.H.; Olia, M.B.; Mirmohammadi, M. Effects of training intervention on non-ergonomic positions among video display terminals (VDT) users. *Work* **2012**, *42*, 429–433. [PubMed]
25. Ncube, F.; Ncube, E.; Kuku, V. Postural Analysis of a Developing Country's Municipal Solid Waste Handlers and a Reference Group of Hospital General Hands using the RULA Method. *Glob. J. Health Sci.* **2017**, *9*, 194. [CrossRef]
26. Gentzler, M.; Stader, S. Posture stress on firefighters and emergency medical technicians (EMTs) associated with repetitive reaching, bending, lifting, and pulling tasks. *Work* **2010**, *37*, 227–239. [PubMed]
27. Mukhopadhyay, P.; Srivastava, S. Evaluating ergonomic risk factors in non-regulated stone carving units of Jaipur. *Work* **2010**, *35*, 87–99. [PubMed]
28. Sahu, S.; Moitra, S.; Maity, S.; Pandit, A.K.; Roy, B. A comparative ergonomics postural assessment of potters and sculptors in the unorganized sector in West Bengal, India. *Int. J. Occup. Saf. Ergon.* **2013**, *19*, 455–462. [CrossRef] [PubMed]
29. Upasana; Vinay, D. Work posture assessment of tailors by RULA and REBA Analysis. *Int. J. Sci. Environ. Technol.* **2017**, *6*, 2469–2474.
30. Jones, T.; Kumar, S. Comparison of ergonomic risk assessment output in a repetitive sawmill occupation: Trim-saw operator. *Work* **2008**, *31*, 367–376. [PubMed]
31. Mokhtar, M.M.; Deros, B.M.; Sukadarin, E.H. Evaluation of Musculoskeletal Disorders Prevalence during Oil Palm Fresh Fruit Bunches Harvesting Using RULA. *Adv. Eng. Forum* **2013**, *10*, 110–115. [CrossRef]
32. Taghavi, S.M.; Mokarami, H.; Ahmadi, O.; Stallones, L.; Abbaspour, A.; Marioryad, H. Risk Factors for Developing Work-Related Musculoskeletal Disorders during Dairy Farming. *Int. J. Occup. Environ. Med.* **2017**, *8*, 39–45. [CrossRef] [PubMed]
33. Cheţa, M.; Marcu, M.V.; Borz, S.A. Workload, exposure to noise, and risk of musculoskeletal disorders: A case study of motor-manual tree feeling and processing in poplar clear cuts. *Forests* **2018**, *9*, 300. [CrossRef]
34. Gallo, R.; Mazzetto, F. Ergonomic analysis for the assessment of the risk of work-related musculoskeletal disorder in forestry operations. *J. Agric.* **2013**, *44*, 730–735. [CrossRef]
35. Proto, A.R.; Zimbalatti, G. Risk assessment of repetitive movements in olive growing: Analysis of annual exposure level assessment models with the OCRA checklist. *J. Agric. Saf. Health* **2015**, *21*, 241–253. [PubMed]
36. Proto, A.R.; Zimbalatti, G. Risk assessment of repetitive movements in the citrus fruit industry. *J. Agric. Saf. Health* **2010**, *16*, 219–228. [CrossRef] [PubMed]
37. European Commission. *A Non-Binding Guide to Best Practice with a View to Improving the Application of Related Directives on Protecting Health and Safety of Workers in Agriculture, Livestock Farming, Horticulture and Forestry*; EU Law and Publications: Brussels, Belgium, 2011.
38. Kundu, A.; Gaur, R. Validation of RULA, REBA in agriculture works in Indian context. In Proceedings of the 9th Triennial Congress of the IEA, Melbourne, Australia, 9–14 August 2015; pp. 1–8.
39. Kong, Y.K.; Lee, S.; Lee, K.S.; Kim, D.M. Comparisons of ergonomic evaluation tools (ALLA, RULA, REBA and OWAS) for farm work. *Int. J. Occup. Saf. Ergon.* **2018**, *24*, 218–223. [CrossRef] [PubMed]

40. Karhu, O.; Kansi, P.; Kuorinka, I. Correcting working postures in industry: A practical method for analysis. *Appl. Ergon.* **1977**, *8*, 199–201. [CrossRef]
41. Kong, Y.K.; Han, J.-G.; Kim, D.M. Development of an Ergonomic Checklist for the Investigation of Work-related Lower Limb Disorders in Farming—ALLA: Agricultural Lower-Limb Assessment. *J. Ergon. Soc. Korea* **2010**, *29*, 933–942. [CrossRef]
42. Ojha, P.; Kwatra, S. An ergonomic study on the assessment of work related musculoskeletal disorder risks among agriculture workers of Uttarakhand, India. *Int. J. Sci. Eng. Res.* **2014**, *5*, 188–191.
43. Mayton, A.G.; Kittusamy, N.K.; Ambrose, D.H.; Jobes, C.C.; Legault, M.L. Jarring/jolting exposure and musculoskeletal symptoms among farm equipment operators. *Int. J. Ind. Ergon.* **2008**, *38*, 758–766. [CrossRef]
44. Vyavahare, R.T.; Kallurkar, S.P. Ergonomic Evaluation of Maize Sheller cum Dehusker. *Int. J. Curr. Eng. Technol.* **2015**, *5*, 1881–1886.
45. Putri, N.T.; Susanti, L.; Tito, A.; Sutanto, A. Redesign of thresher machine for farmers using rapid upper limb assessment (RULA) method. *IEEE Int. Conf. Ind. Eng. Eng. Manag.* **2016**, 1304–1309.
46. International Labour Organization (ILO), Sectoral Activities Programme. Guidelines for Labour Inspection in Forestry. 2005. Available online: http://www2.ilo.org/wcmsp5/groups/public/---ed_protect/---protrav/---safework/documents/normativeinstrument/wcms_107610.pdf (accessed on 23 January 2019).
47. Bagagiolo, G.; Laurendi, V.; Cavallo, E. Safety Improvements on Wood Chippers Currently in Use: A Study on Feasibility in the Italian Context. *Agriculture* **2017**, *7*, 98. [CrossRef]
48. Potočnik, I.; Poje, A. Forestry Ergonomics and Occupational Safety in High Ranking Scientific Journals from 2005–2016. *Croat. J. For. Eng.* **2017**, *38*, 291–310.
49. Schaufler, D.H.; Yoder, A.M.; Murphy, D.J.; Schwab, C.V.; Dehart, A.F. Safety and Health in On-Farm Biomass Production and Processing. *J. Agric. Saf. Health* **2014**, *20*, 283–299.
50. Struttmann, T.W. Fatal and nonfatal occupational injuries involving wood chippers–United States, 1992-2002. *MMWR Morb Mortal Wkly Rep.* **2004**, *53*, 1130–1131.
51. Marsh, S.M.; Fosbroke, D.E. Trends of occupational fatalities involving machines, United States, 1992–2010. *Am. J. Ind. Med.* **2015**, *58*, 1160–1173. [CrossRef] [PubMed]
52. Occupational Safety and Health Administration (OSHA). Fatality and Catastrophe Investigation Summaries. Available online: htps://www.osha.gov/pls/imis/accidentsearch.html (accessed on 22 January 2019).
53. Colantoni, A.; Mazzocchi, F.; Laurendi, V.; Grigolato, S.; Monarca, F.; Monarca, D.; Cecchini, M. Innovative Solution for Reducing the Run-Down Time of the Chipper Disc Using a Brake Clamp Device. *Agriculture* **2017**, *7*, 71. [CrossRef]
54. Al-bassit, L.; Tricot, N. *Amelioration de la Securite de la Dechiqueteuse Forestiere Etude de Reconception*; Irstea Report; IRSTEA: Antony Cedex, France, 2015.
55. Center for Disease Control and Prevention (CDC), Department of Health and Human Services, the United States. Preventing Wood Chipper Fatalities. Available online: https://blogs.cdc.gov/niosh-science-blog/2015/12/17/wood-chippers/. (accessed on 23 January 2019).
56. Caffaro, F.; Mirisola, A.; Cavallo, E. Safety signs on agricultural machinery: Pictorials do not always successfully convey their messages to target users. *Appl. Ergon.* **2017**, *58*, 156–166. [CrossRef] [PubMed]
57. Caffaro, F.; Roccato, M.; Micheletti Cremasco, M.; Cavallo, E. Part-time farmers and accidents with agricultural machinery: A moderated mediated model on the role played by frequency of use and unsafe beliefs. *J. Occup. Health* **2018**, *60*, 80–84. [CrossRef] [PubMed]
58. Brickman, D.B. On the safety of infeeding commercial tree chippers. In *Engineering Technology Management*; ASME: New York, NY, USA, 2003; pp. 31–38.
59. Moore, P.H.; Casini, V.J. Injury associated with working near or operating wood chippers. *Appl. Occup. Environ. Hyg.* **2001**, *16*, 649–651.
60. Spinelli, R.; Cavallo, E.; Facello, A. A new comminution device for high-quality chip production. *Fuel Process. Technol.* **2012**, *99*, 69–74. [CrossRef]
61. Spinelli, R.; Aminti, G.; Magagnotti, N.; De Francesco, F. Postural risk assessment of small-scale debarkers for wooden postproduction. *Forests* **2018**, *9*, 111. [CrossRef]
62. EN 13525:2005+A2:2009. *Forestry Machinery—Wood Chippers—Safety*; European Committee for Standardization: Bruxelles, Belgium, 2009.
63. Elwardany, S.H.; El-Sayed, W.H.; Ali, M.F. Reliability of Kinovea Computer Program in Measuring Cervical Range of Motion in Sagittal Plane. *OALib J.* **2015**, *2*, 1–10. [CrossRef]

64. Kee, D.; Karwowski, W. LUBA: An assessment technique for postural loading on the upper body based on joint motion discomfort and maximum holding time. *Appl. Ergon.* **2001**, *32*, 357–366. [CrossRef]
65. Boulila, A.; Ayadi, M.; Mrabet, K. Ergonomics study and analysis of workstations in Tunisian mechanical manufacturing. *Hum. Factors Ergon. Manuf.* **2018**, 166–185. [CrossRef]
66. Chiasson, M.E.; Imbeau, D.; Aubry, K.; Delisle, A. Comparing the results of eight methods used to evaluate risk factors associated with musculoskeletal disorders. *Int. J. Ind. Ergon.* **2012**, *42*, 478–488. [CrossRef]
67. KOSHA (Korea Occupational Safety and Health Agency). *Status of Musculoskeletal Disorders-Related Risky Tasks*; KOSHA: Seoul, Korea, 2005.
68. ISO 6385:2016. *Ergonomics Principles in the Design of Work Systems*; International Organization for Standardization: Geneva, Switzerland, 2016.
69. Manuaba, A. A total approach in ergonomics is a must to attain humane, competitive and sustainable work systems and products. *J. Hum. Ergol.* **2007**, *36*, 23–30.
70. Meyer, A.; Fourie, I. Collaborative information seeking environments benefiting from holistic ergonomics. *Libr. Hi Tech* **2015**, *33*, 439–459. [CrossRef]
71. Dempsey, P.; Kocher, L.; Nasarwanji, M.; Pollard, J.; Whitson, A. Emerging ergonomics issues and opportunities in mining. *Int. J. Environ. Res. Public Health* **2018**, *15*, 2449. [CrossRef] [PubMed]

International Journal of
Environmental Research and Public Health

MDPI

Article

Warning against Critical Slopes in Agriculture: Comprehension of Targeted Safety Signs in a Group of Machinery Operators in Italy

Lucia Vigoroso, Federica Caffaro * and Eugenio Cavallo

Institute for Agricultural and Earthmoving Machines (IMAMOTER), National Research Council of Italy (CNR), Strada delle Cacce, 73–10135 Torino, Italy; l.vigoroso@ima.to.cnr.it (L.V.); eugenio.cavallo@cnr.it (E.C.)
* Correspondence: f.caffaro@ima.to.cnr.it; Tel.: +39-011-39-77-720

Received: 18 December 2018; Accepted: 17 February 2019; Published: 20 February 2019

Abstract: Steep slopes are the main cause of rollover incidents in agriculture. Targeted safety signs have been developed to warn machinery operators against risky slopes. However, machinery user's manuals and road signs report information regarding slope steepness in two different ways, by using the tilt angle in degrees and the slope percentage, respectively. In this study, we investigated the comprehension of safety signs depicting critical slopes, either in degrees or as percent values in a group of Italian agricultural machinery operators while considering the possible influence of previous experience with agricultural machinery, previous incidents, and on-farm occupation. Eighteen tractor and self-propelled machinery operators were administered graphical representations of seven slope angles in a randomized order and then were asked to estimate the slope steepness as both a tilt angle and a slope percentage. The participants tended to overestimate slope steepness in degrees, whereas the opposite was true for percentages. Farmers who were previously involved in a machinery-related incident were more accurate in their estimates. The present results raise some considerations regarding the need to redesign safety communication and to promote targeted training interventions.

Keywords: agriculture; injury risk; occupational safety; road sign comprehension; slope angle; warning sign

1. Introduction

Agriculture is one of the most dangerous industries, with an incident rate that is nearly triple that of other sectors, both in the United States and in the European Union [1,2]. Nearly 80% of all incidents are caused by farm machinery, and tractors are involved in most of the fatalities [3,4], with rollovers predominating [5]. The National Institute of Occupational Safety and Health (NIOSH) reported approximately 130 tractor rollover incidents per year in the United States [6]; Darçın and Darçın [7] reported that, in Bilecik, Turkey, 58 out of 80 tractor fatalities between 2005 and 2015 were due to rollovers, whereas Kogler et al. [8] and Pessina and Facchinetti [9] showed that tractor rollover resulted in many fatal injuries in Austria and in Italy in 2015 and 2017, respectively. In Italy, in particular, approximately 90 of 120 fatalities involving tractors in 2016 were fatal rollovers [10]. In addition to tractors, many other off-road self-propelled machines with a ride-on operator (driver) adopted in farming, such as harvesters [11] or handling machinery [12], or farm-like (lawnmowers, All Terrain Vehicles (ATV) and Side-by-Side) [13] operations are exposed to the risk of rolling or tipping over. According to Abubakar et al. [5] driving a vehicle downhill, crossing a steep slope, and climbing uphill represent the main reasons for machine rollovers. Previous studies showed also that agricultural machinery operators often disregard the steepness of terrain [13–15] and they tend to be inaccurate when estimating slopes [5,14]. This may lead to driving in hazardous conditions, thereby increasing the risk of a rollover incident [16].

To ensure the health and safety of workers, a five-step hierarchy of controls should be applied to the design of machinery and equipment [17,18]. The first three steps, i.e., elimination (step 1), substitution (step 2) and engineering controls (step 3), in particular, are the preferable methods to avoid a worker's exposure to dangerous situations, since they remove the hazards at the source. Regarding machinery rollover, some studies have commented on possible solutions (step 1 and step 2) to improve tractor stability [19]. However, it is difficult to completely eliminate the hazard and to guarantee the comprehensive stability of the vehicle, since the risk of overturning is the result of the interaction between different factors, including the slope steepness [5,20]. Therefore, different technical protective measures can be adopted to prevent injuries (step 3) in the case of a rollover: the combined use of a Roll-Over Protective Structures (ROPS) and a seatbelt is the most effective way to prevent fatal injuries during rollover incidents [6,21–23]. The effectiveness of such features has been investigated and recognized for many years, and they have been required to be fitted to tractors since the '80s in the markets of developed countries [24–26]. Retrofitting programmes to implement ROPS on tractors that were originally sold without a ROPS and a seatbelt have been recently implemented both in the United States and in the European Union to extend the benefits of these devices to a larger number of units [21,27]. Although "eliminating hazards is the most effective way to make the workplace safer [...] this is not always practical" [28]. Thus, there is a need to focus on the work activity and to push towards the correct use of safety tools. To that end, the fourth step of the hierarchy of controls, i.e., administrative controls, includes training and the installation of signs, warning labels, and pictograms to inform users about the residual risks that could not be eliminated either by design or by adopting technical solutions [16,17].

The comprehension of safety signs in agriculture has been previously investigated with regard to pesticides [29,30], machinery-related risks [31], and the use of Personal Protective Equipment [32], and the research has often highlighted poor comprehensibility and a positive relation with the expertise of the target audience [33,34]. For instance, Caffaro, Schmidt, Murphy, and Cavallo [34] showed that years of experience with agricultural machinery significantly increased users' comprehension of the meaning of safety pictograms that were affixed to agricultural machinery.

However, the comprehensibility of safety signs on slopes has not been investigated yet. Increasing knowledge about this issue is even more relevant if we consider that international standards and user manuals for safe operation of machinery do not adopt a unique graphical solution to depict critical steepness. On the one hand, the international standard ISO 16231-2 [35] for the assessment of stability of self-propelled agricultural machinery defines the maximum slope on which a machine is intended to work as a percentage; on the other hand, in OECD Code 6 [36], for the testing of front-mounted ROPS fitted on tractors and in the American National Standard ANSI/ROHVA 1-2016 [37] for determining the maximum steepness to operate ATVs, the slopes are described in degrees. Furthermore, the user manuals of different agricultural machinery display information regarding the maximum slope to operate a vehicle as a percentage [38,39], whereas the safety labels that were affixed to machinery give the same information in degrees [21]. Finally, in the Vienna Convention on Road Signs and Signals [40], the well-known road sign warning against a dangerous slope depicts the slope in terms of a percent value.

Based on these previous considerations, the present study investigated which kind of graphical representation of slope steepness, i.e., the tilt angle in degrees or a slope percentage, in a safety sign that was administered to a group of agricultural machinery operators was more comprehensible.

Furthermore, the study investigated the role that is played by the driving experience of agricultural machinery, the on-farm occupation, and the previous history of incidents in the comprehension of the safety sign. Experience with machinery was considered because of its known significant influence on the comprehension of safety signs [41], whereas we were interested in exploring the role of the other two variables based on previous evidence regarding their relevance in the field of risk perception and exposure in agriculture.

Concerning on-farm occupation, Day et al. [42] observed that farmworkers and contractors reported increased injury risk when compared with farmers. Whereas farmers spent longer daily working hours on farms [43], farmworkers and contractors interacted with many hazardous tools and equipment that could increase their risk exposure [42]. Concerning operators' previous history of incidents, contrasting results are reported in the literature. McLaughlin and Sprufera [44] showed that operators who are involved at least once in an incident without negative consequences feel more confident in their interaction with machinery, thereby increasing their exposure to risky situations; on the other hand, in a study that was conducted by Caffaro et al. [45], operators who survived incidents with farm machinery developed a positive attitude towards safety and increased risk perception.

By analysing which kind of graphical representation of slopes (i.e., degrees or percentages) on safety signs was better comprehended and which variables affected the comprehension, this study aimed to provide useful suggestions in terms of the re-design of safety signs on slopes and/or targeted training activities to improve safety communication.

2. Materials and Methods

2.1. Participants

The investigation was performed in Italy because of the high number of machinery rollover-related fatalities [46] in this country. Eighteen Italian operators of tractors and self-propelled agricultural machinery (17 males, one female) from Northern Italy participated in the study. The participants were recruited from different agricultural holdings near Torino, Piedmont region, North western Italy. To obtain more comparable data, only participants who were familiar with agricultural machinery, i.e., with at least five years of operating experience (cutoff for experts, as in Kumar et al. [47]), were involved in the study. The study was conducted in accordance with the Declaration of Helsinki and the protocol was approved by the Research Advisory Group of the Institute for Agricultural and Earthmoving Machines (IMAMOTER) of the National Research Council of Italy (CNR) on February 16, 2018.

2.2. Material and Procedure

Seven different levels of slope steepness were chosen for the investigation. Based on the study that was conducted by Abubakar et al. [5] and Murphy et al. [19] regarding the stability limits for different farm tractors, five tilt angles were chosen: 5°, 10°, 15°, 20°, and 25°, which corresponded to slope percentages of 9%, 18%, 27%, 36%, and 47%, respectively. Two other angles were considered, as follows: 38°, corresponding to 78%, which is the angle of inclination that is used for tractors' preliminary lateral stability test conducted in accordance with OECD Code 6 [36], and 45°, with a corresponding percentage of 100%.

To investigate the above-indicated angles, we referred to a sign that warns against a steep slope, as designed in the Vienna Convention on Road Signs [40] and to the study that was conducted by Paniati [48], in which different alternatives of existing road signs were tested. The safety sign that was considered in this study is characterized by two elements: a black triangle that represents the slope and a slope percentage value above it. For the estimation of the slope steepness, two versions of the sign were designed with two different graphical indications to focus users' attention on the unit of measurement that had to be reported. For the estimation as a percentage, the element that represented the slope was underlined using a red line, with a percentage symbol (%) that was above this line. For the estimation in degrees, a small coloured arch that was used when dimensioning angles in a technical drawing was depicted to highlight the angle considered, and the degree symbol (°) replaced the percentage symbol adopted for the other version (see Figure 1). A total of fourteen signs (i.e., seven slopes to be expressed in degrees and seven as percentages) printed on 210 × 297 mm paper were presented in a random order to the participants. Participants were asked to indicate the degree of the tilt angle that was highlighted in red and the percentage of inclination of the red line with respect to the grey triangle's base. When a sign reporting the percentage symbol (%) was shown to the participant, the following instructions were given: "In your opinion, what is the slope percentage of the red line compared to the grey triangle's base?" Similarly, when a sign reporting the degree symbol (°) was shown, the participant was asked the following: "In your opinion, how many degrees is the red coloured angle in the picture?"

(**a**) (**b**)

Figure 1. Example of the two versions of the safety sign submitted to users' attention: (**a**) 36% slope and its corresponding (**b**) 20° angle.

The participants were not informed that each slope was shown to them twice, once with the percentage symbol (%) and once with the degree symbol (°), so as not to affect their answers.

Participants were individually shown the signs. All of the answers were verbally reported [49,50] and the interviewer recorded them. The instrument was pilot-tested before being used in the present investigation. A sociodemographic questionnaire assessing participants' occupation, years of experience with agricultural machinery, and history of previous incidents with agricultural machinery (dichotomous item, 0 = never involved and 1 = involved, as previously coded by Glasscock et al. [51]) closed the session.

Data Analysis

The answers that were reported by participants were classified according to the study conducted by Cavallo et al. [21], i.e., considering the limit for an acceptable estimation at ±2.5 degrees of the actual angle. In the absence of similar studies regarding percentages, the ±2.5 degrees limit was converted into a percentage value to use the same indicators to evaluate the users' estimation. Thus, the limit for the acceptable estimation of slopes expressed as percentages was set at ±4%. For descriptive statistics, the underestimations were coded as −1, correct answers were coded as 0, and overestimations were coded as +1.

For subsequent multivariate analyses, two different total scores, one for the answers in degrees and the other for the answers as percentages, were calculated as the sum of correct answers for each participant, recoding correct answers as 1 and both the over and underestimations as 0 (each total score ranged therefore between 0 and +7).

A multivariate analysis of co-variance (MANCOVA) was then performed to investigate the influence of previous experience, history of incidents, and on-farm occupation on the comprehension of the safety signs, with the total scores for degrees and percentages as dependent variables, on-farm occupation, and involvement in previous incidents as factors and years of experience as a covariate. The statistical analysis was performed with SPSS software v.24 (IBM Corp., Armonk, NY, USA).

3. Results

3.1. Characteristics of the Participants

The main sociodemographic characteristics of the participants are reported in Table 1. Regarding previous incidents, eight participants reported that they had previously overturned their tractor, whereas three other participants reported other kinds of incidents involving agricultural machinery (i.e., a rear-end collision and slipping from the stepladder).

Table 1. Sociodemographic characteristics of the participants.

Variable		N (%)
Gender	Male	17(94.5)
	Female	1 (5.5)
Occupation [1]	Farmer	7 (38.9)
	Farmworker	8 (44.4)
	Contractor	3 (16.7)
		Mean (SD)
Age (years)		38.9 (13.0)
Driving experience (years)		25.0 (13.0)

[1] Contractor = someone who is temporally hired jointly with specific equipment to perform farm work at a certain price or within a certain timeframe. For the subsequent analysis, this variable was re-categorized and coded as 1 = farmer and 0 = other to make group sizes more comparable.

3.2. Comprehension of Safety Signs: Tilt Angles in Degrees vs. Slope Percentages

When considering the answers expressed by all of the participants for the seven levels of slope steepness investigated, a total of 126 answers were collected for angles in degrees and 126 answers for slope percentages. The angles expressed in degrees that yielded the highest correct interpretations were the 5° and 45° angles, whereas the slope, as expressed as a percentage that yielded the highest number of correct interpretations, was 9% (see Table 2). Overall, the angles in degrees were mainly overestimated, whereas the slope percentages were mainly underestimated. As shown in Table 2, 85 out of 126 answers overestimated the actual tilt angle, whereas only 11 answers reported an underestimation. The opposite trend was found for slopes that were expressed in percentages: seventy-one out of 126 answers underestimated the slope, whereas 19 answers reported an overestimation. Interestingly, no participants gave a correct answer for all seven levels of slope steepness investigated, either as a degree or as a percent.

The MANCOVA showed that on-farm occupation and previous history of incidents had no significant main effect on the answers in degrees and percentages ($F (2, 12) = 2.306$, $p = 0.142$, and $F (2, 12) = 0.026$, $p = 0.974$, respectively). However, the analysis showed a significant Previous Incidents x On-farm Occupation effect ($F (2, 12) = 8.498$, $p = 0.005$): when having been previously involved in an incident, farmers were significantly more accurate in estimating the inclination angles in degrees, moving from a mean total score of 0.000 to 2.250. Years of experience with machinery showed no statistically significant effect ($F (2, 12) = 0.696$, $p = 0.518$) on the comprehension of safety signs.

Table 2. Answers reported for each angle investigated (both degrees and percentages).

Tilt Angle	Correct Answers *n* (%)	Overestimation *n* (%)	Underestimation *n* (%)	Min (°)	Max (°)	Slope Percentage	Correct Answers *n* (%)	Overestimation *n* (%)	Underestimation *n* (%)	Min (%)	Max (%)
5°	7 (38.8)	11 (61.1)	0 (0)	5	20	9%	14 (77.7)	1 (5.5)	3 (33.3)	2	15
10°	6 (33.3)	11 (55.5)	1 (5.5)	5	30	18%	5 (27.7)	4 (22.2)	9 (50.0)	5	31
15°	2 (11.1)	15 (77.7)	1 (5.5)	12	45	27%	5 (27.7)	4 (22.2)	9 (50.0)	8	50
20°	1 (5.5)	16 (83.3)	1 (5.5)	15	40	36%	6 (33.3)	2 (11.1)	10 (55.5)	13	50
25°	2 (11.1)	14 (72.2)	2 (11.1)	20	60	47%	2 (11.1)	5 (27.7)	11 (61.1)	15	80
38°	5 (27.7)	10 (50)	3 (16.6)	35	50	78%	2 (11.1)	3 (16.6)	13 (72.2)	20	100
45°	7 (38.8)	8 (44.4)	3 (16.6)	30	70	100%	2 (11.1)	0 (0)	16 (88.8)	35	100

4. Discussion

Previous research has reported a high rate of tractor rollover incidents in agriculture that are caused by a steep slope [1], and safety signs play a key role in warning users against these hazards [52]. In this study, the comprehension of two different graphical representations of slope steepness, in degrees and percent values, was investigated, while also considering the possible effects of previous experience with machinery, history of incidents, and on-farm occupation. Overall, the number of correct estimations was similar between degrees and percentages; however, incorrect answers tended to overestimate the slope when expressed in degrees and to underestimate the slope when it was expressed in percent values. Being a farmer that was previously exposed to a machinery-related incident significantly enhanced the estimation accuracy for tilt angles expressed in degrees.

Drivers' accuracy in slope angle estimation is an important component of avoiding vehicle rollovers [14], which is one of the most common and dangerous types of tractor incidents, and the overestimation of a slope expressed in degrees can be considered to be a protective behaviour. In other words, even when operators were not accurate in slope estimation, when it was expressed in degrees, the error was in a protective direction, since they would presumably not operate the machinery on a slope that they think is steeper than it actually is. The present results on the overestimation of slopes expressed in degrees are consistent with those that were reported by Görücü et al. [15] and with other previous studies, in which, when the responses were orally reported, the participants tended to overestimate the investigated angles [50,53,54].

However, contrary to the results that were reported by Tillapaugh et al. [14], where "participants were less able to accurately estimate angle as slope became steeper" (p. 262), our results revealed an accurate and similar rate of correct estimations for both less steep angles (5° and 10°) and the steepest ones (38° and 45°), whereas the lowest rate of correct answers was reported for the intermediate angles (15°, 20°, and 25°). The results that were obtained for these latter values are even more critical if we consider that the user's manual and warning labels on machinery recommend to not operate the machine above these slope limits [13], since it would threaten the stability of the machine or compromise the efficiency of the braking system.

Contrary to the results of other studies, years of experience in driving agricultural machinery, previous history of incidents, and on-farm occupation did not affect the estimation of slope steepness per se. However, a significant interaction effect between on-farm occupation and a history of incidents with agricultural machinery was found. The analysis showed that farmers who had reported a previous incident with agricultural machinery were more accurate in slope estimations when reporting in degree values. As regards the role that is played by operators' previous experience of incidents, Chan and Ng [41], found similar results, in which the injury experience during working hours significantly enhanced individual performance regarding the comprehension of safety signs. This result is consistent with those of Caffaro et al. [55], in which participants who survived an incident developed a higher risk perception and more careful behaviour. With regard to this, a possible development of the present research could be to investigate the probability of adopting correct and precautionary driving behaviours in agricultural machinery operators with different exposures to previous incidents. Focused training activities and high engagement in safety training are considered to be useful tools in improving the comprehension of safety communication and safety awareness [56] to reduce fatal injuries. This holds true, not only for operators with lower rates of safety sign comprehension, but also for other operators, since, as reported by Chan and Ng [41], " ... even people who perform relatively well in guessing, such as those with safety incident experience, will also benefit from such training [...]" (p. 695).

The issue of the most appropriate method of communication about slopes is worthy of further investigation with a larger sample of operators for more reliable results, when comparing, for instance, expert and novice drivers and/or older and younger operators. An additional future development of the research could also address differences in the estimation of slope steepness between male and female agricultural operators in gender-balanced samples. A participatory approach [57] that is based on the iterative and interactive involvement of users throughout the design process of communication regarding slopes could be adopted to better account for tractor and self-propelled machinery operators' informative needs and to increase the level of comprehension of safety information regarding slopes, which may help to maximize operators' preventive behaviours. Future developments of the study could also address the relationship between configuration of, comprehension of, and compliance with safety signs, based on previous evidence regarding the association between signs' configuration and drivers' behaviour in reducing vehicle speeds in highway work zones [58–60]. The behaviour of agricultural machinery drivers after being exposed to different types of safety signs on critical slopes could be observed using a stability simulator, as was seen in Cavallo et al. [13].

5. Conclusions

According to the hierarchy of controls, hazards in the use of machinery should be eliminated or controlled through design and engineering solutions. In the case of residual hazards, such as slope steepness for tractor rollovers, safety signs warn operators, and help them to develop safe behaviours. Thus, they are designed to be easily comprehended by users. However, adopting different methods to visually communicate information regarding slope steepness could cause confusion and reasonably lead operators to perform incorrect behaviours while driving the machines. The present results, despite the small number of participants that are involved in the study, highlight some critical aspects that may deserve further attention in future investigations. Expressing slope steepness in degrees appeared to be more protective for operators when compared to percentages; indeed, the steepness was often overestimated in the case of tilt angles expressed in degrees, whereas slope percentages were mainly underestimated. Even though operators might be expected to be more comfortable with this latter unit of measurement, since road signs report slopes as a percentage grade, this investigation showed that this might not always be the case for agricultural machinery operators, highlighting the importance of assessing target users' knowledge. Moreover, the significant interaction between having been previously involved in machinery-related incidents and on-farm occupation on safety sign comprehension raises some considerations regarding the possibility of designing targeted training interventions to promote the early detection of hazards and risks. Overall, the findings of the present study indicate that the quality of the interaction between individual variables and processes and sign features should be taken into consideration during the design process of safety signs regarding slopes to ensure that safety communications are more comprehensible and possibly more effective.

Author Contributions: Conceptualization, L.V., F.C. and E.C.; Data curation, L.V.; Formal analysis, L.V. and F.C.; Investigation, F.C.; Methodology, E.C.; Project administration, E.C.; Writing—original draft, L.V.; Writing—review & editing, F.C. and E.C.

Funding: This research received no external funding.

Acknowledgments: This research did not receive any specific grant from funding agencies in the public, commercial or not-for-profit sector.

Conflicts of Interest: The authors declare no conflict of interest.

References

1. International Labour of Organization. Agriculture: A Hazardous Work. Available online: http://www.ilo.org/safework/areasofwork/hazardous-work/WCMS_110188/lang--en/index.htm (accessed on 1 June 2018).
2. Donham, K.J.; Yoder, A.; Grafft, L. Acute Injuries in Agriculture. In *Agricultural Medicine: Rural Occupational and Environmental Health, Safety, and Prevention*; Donham, K.J., Thelin, A., Eds.; John Wiley & Sons, Inc.: Hoboken, NJ, USA, 2016; p. 573.
3. European Commission. *The Magnitude and Spectrum of Farm Injuries in the European Union Countries*; Center for Research and Prevention of Injuries (CE.RE.PR.I): Athens, Greece, 2004; Available online: https://ec.europa.eu/health/archive/ph_projects/2002/injury/fp_injury_2002_frep_02_en.pdf (accessed on 9 January 2019).

4. Farm Injury–Resource Center. Eighty Percent of Farm Deaths Associated with Machines. 2017. Available online: http://farminjuryresource.com/2017/03/02/eighty-percent-farm-deaths-associated-machines/ (accessed on 11 January 2019).
5. Abubakar, M.S.; Ahmad, D.; Akande, F.B. A Review of Farm Tractor Overturning Accidents and Safety. *Pertanika J. Sci. Technol.* **2010**, *18*, 377–385.
6. Northeast Organic Dairy Producers Alliance (NODPA). Rollover Protection for Farm Tractor Operators. 2016. Available online: http://www.nodpa.com/in_rollover-protection-091316.shtml (accessed on 9 January 2019).
7. Darçın, E.S.; Darçın, M. Fatal tractor injuries between 2005 and 2015 in Bilecik, Turkey. *Biomed. Res.* **2017**, *28*, 549–555.
8. Kogler, R.; Quendler, E.; Boxberger, J. Occupational Accidents with Agricultural Machinery in Austria. *J. Agromed.* **2015**, *21*, 61–70. [CrossRef] [PubMed]
9. Pessina, D.; Facchinetti, D. A Survey on Fatal Accidents for Overturning of Agricultural Tractors in Italy. *Chem. Eng. Trans.* **2017**, *58*, 79–84.
10. Fargnoli, M.; Lombarbi, M.; Haber, N.; Puri, D. The Impact of Human Error in the Use of Agricultural Tractors: A Case Study Research in Vineyard Cultivation in Italy. *Agriculture* **2018**, *8*, 21. [CrossRef]
11. Molari, G.; Badodi, M.; Guarnieri, A.; Mattetti, M. Structural strength Evaluation of driver's protective structures for self-propelled agricultural machines. *J. Agric. Saf. Health* **2014**, *20*, 165–174.
12. Caffaro, F.; Cremasco, M.M.; Preti, C.; Cavallo, E. Ergonomic analysis of the effect of a telehandler active suspended cab on whole body vibration level and operator comfort. *Int. J. Ind. Ergon.* **2016**, *53*, 19–26. [CrossRef]
13. Cavallo, E.; Görücü, S.; Murphy, D. Perception of side rollover hazards in a Pennsylvania rural population while operating an all-terrain vehicle (ATV). *Work* **2015**, *51*, 281–288. [CrossRef]
14. Tillapaugh, J.A.; Murphy, D.J.; Sommer, I.J.; Garvey, P.M. Operator assessment of tractor roll angle with and without a tractor stability visual feedback device. *J. Agric. Saf. Health* **2010**, *16*, 249–264. [CrossRef]
15. Görücü, S.; Cavallo, E.; Murphy, D. Perceptions of Tilt Angles of an Agricultural Tractor. *J. Agromed.* **2014**, *19*, 5–14. [CrossRef]
16. Ayres, T.; Wood, C.; Schmidt, R.; Young, D.; Park, M.; Angeles, L. Affordance percepion and safety intervention. In Proceedings of the IEA 200/HFSE 2000 Congress, San Diego, CA, USA, 30 July–4 August 2000; pp. 6–51.
17. Purschwitz, M.A. Personal Protective Equipment and Safety Engineering of Machinery. In *Agricultural Medicine*; Lessenger, J.E., Ed.; Springer: New York, NY, USA; Berlin/Heidelberg, Germany, 2006; pp. 53–69.
18. Occupational Safty and Health Administration (OSHA). Recommended Practices for Safty and Health Programs-Hazard Prevention and Control. Available online: https://www.osha.gov/shpguidelines/hazard-prevention.html (accessed on 11 January 2019).
19. Zong, C.; Zhu, T.; Wang, C.; Liu, H. Multi-objective stability control algorithm of heavy tractor semi-trailer based on differential braking. *Chin. J. Mech. Eng.* **2012**, *25*, 88–97. [CrossRef]
20. Murphy, D.J.; Beppler, D.C.; Sommer, H.J. Tractor stability indicator. *Appl. Ergon.* **1985**, *16*, 187–191. [CrossRef]
21. Cavallo, E.; Langle, T.; Bueno, D.; Tsukamoto, S.; Görücü, S.; Murphy, D. Rollover Protective Structure (ROPS) Retrofitting on Agricultural Tractors: Goals and Approaches in Different Countries. *J. Agromed.* **2014**, *19*, 208–209. [CrossRef]
22. Aherin, R.A.; Arcury, T. *Tractor Safety. For the Landscaping and Horticultural Services Industry*; K-State Research and Extension: Manhattan, KS, USA, 2006; Available online: http://nasdonline.org/1919/d001874/tractor-safety.html (accessed on 21 January 2019).
23. Molari, G.; Rondelli, V. Evaluation criteria for the anchorage resistance of safety belts on agricultural tractors. *Biosyst. Eng.* **2007**, *97*, 163–169. [CrossRef]
24. Cavallo, E.; Ferrari, E.; Coccia, M. Likely technological trajectories in agricultural tractors by analysing innovative attitudes of farmers. *Int. J. Technol. Policy Manag.* **2015**, *15*, 158–177. [CrossRef]
25. Springfeldt, B. Rollover of tractors—International experiences. *Saf. Sci.* **1996**, *24*, 95–110. [CrossRef]
26. Ayers, P.; Khorsandi, F.; John, Y.; Whitaker, G. Development and evaluation of a computer-based ROPS design program (CRDP). *J. Agric. Saf. Health* **2016**, *22*, 247–260.

27. Tinc, P.J.; Ayers, P.; May, J.J.; Purschwitz, M.A.; Park, S.; Bayes, B.; Sorensen, J. Implementing a National Tractor Safety Program: Using "Whole System in a Room" to Mobilize Partners and Implement Solutions. *J. Agromed.* **2016**, *21*, 127–131. [CrossRef]
28. WorkCover. Manual Handling Hierarchy of Controls. Available online: https://web.archive.org/web/20141222123533/http://www.workcover.nsw.gov.au/formspublications/publications/Documents/hierarchy_of_controls_5620.pdf (accessed on 11 January 2019).
29. Vijay Kautilya, D.; Shruti Pravhat, H.; Chendrashekaran, P.; Khatijia, B. A Cross-Sectional Survey on the Awareness of Pesticide Labels and Pesticide Safety Pictograms among Paddy Farming in South India. *J. Health Sci. Surveill. Syst.* **2016**, *4*, 158–166.
30. Kapeleka, J.; Mwaseba, D.L. Effectiveness of Pesticide Labels as A Communication Tool for Smallholder Farmers on Pesticides Handling. *Int. J. Sci. Technol. Res.* **2017**, *6*, 50–60.
31. Caffaro, F.; Mirisola, A.; Cavallo, E. Safety signs on agricultural machinery: Pictorials do not always successfully convey their messages to target users. *Appl. Ergon.* **2017**, *58*, 156–166. [CrossRef] [PubMed]
32. Boelhouwer, E.; Davis, J.; Franco-Watkins, A.; Dorris, N.; Lungu, C. Comprehension of hazard communication: Effects of pictograms on safety data sheets and labels. *J. Saf. Res.* **2013**, *46*, 145–155. [CrossRef] [PubMed]
33. Chan, K.; Chan, A.H.S. Understanding industrial safety signs: Implications for occupational safety management. *Ind. Manag. Data Syst.* **2011**, *111*, 1481–1510. [CrossRef]
34. Caffaro, F.; Schmidt, S.; Murphy, D.J.; Cavallo, E. Comprehension rates of safety pictorials affixed to agricultural machinery among Pennsylvania rural population. *Saf. Sci.* **2018**, *103*, 162–171. [CrossRef]
35. International Standard Organization (ISO). *ISO 16231-2—Self-Propelled Agricultural Machinery—Assessment of Stability—Part 2: Determination of Static Stability and Test Procedures*; International Standard Organization: Geneva, Switzerland, 2015.
36. Organisation for Economic Co-Operation and Development (OECD). *Code 6—OECD Standard Code for the Official Testing of Front Mounted Roll-Over Protective Structures on Narrow-Track Wheeled Agricultural and Forestry Tractors*; Forestry: Paris, France, 2017.
37. American National Standard ANSI/ROHVA 1-2016. *American National Standard for Recreational Off-Highway Vehicles*; Recreational Off-Highway Vehicle Association: California, CA, USA, 2016.
38. Trelleborg. Technical Manual. Available online: https://www.trelleborg.com/wheels/~{}/media/wheels-uk/technical--info--uk/trelleborgtechnicalmanual_eng_uk.pdf%0A (accessed on 17 January 2019).
39. National Agricultural Safety Database (NASD). Tractor Safety. Available online: http://nasdonline.org/1919/d001874/tractor-safety.html (accessed on 9 January 2019).
40. Vienna Convention on Road Signs and Signals. Vienna Convention on Road Signs and Signal—United Nations Publication. 1968. Available online: https://www.unece.org/fileadmin/DAM/trans/conventn/Conv_road_signs_2006v_EN.pdf (accessed on 11 January 2019).
41. Chan, A.H.S.; Ng, A.W.Y. Investigation of guessability of industrial safety signs: Effects of prospective-user factors and cognitive sign features. *Int. J. Ind. Ergon.* **2010**, *40*, 689–697. [CrossRef]
42. Day, L.; Voaklander, D.; Sim, M.; Wolfe, R.; Langley, J.; Dosman, J.; Hagel, L.; Ozanne-Smith, J. Risk factors for work-related injury among male farmers. *Occup. Environ. Med.* **2008**, *66*, 312–318. [CrossRef] [PubMed]
43. Torén, A.; Oberg, K.; Lembke, B.; Enlund, K.; Rask-andersen, A. Tractor-driving hours and their relation to self-reported low-back and hip symptoms. *Appl. Ergon.* **2002**, *33*, 139–146. [CrossRef]
44. Mclaughlin, A.C.; Sprufera, J.F. Aging Farmers Are at High Risk for Injuries and Fatalities: How Human-Factors Research and Application Can Help. *N. C. Med. J.* **2011**, *72*, 481–483.
45. Caffaro, F.; Micheletti Cremasco, M.; Roccato, M.; Cavallo, E. It does not occur by chance: A mediation model of the influence of workers' characteristics, work environment factors, and near misses on agricultural machinery-related accidents. *Int. J. Occup. Environ. Health* **2017**, *23*, 52–59. [CrossRef]
46. FederUnacoma. Incidenti col Trattore: Un Problema "Generazionale". 2014. Available online: https://agronotizie.imagelinenetwork.com/agrimeccanica/2014/11/17/incidenti-col-trattore-un-problema-ldquogenerazionalerdquo/40804 (accessed on 14 January 2019).
47. Kumar, A.; Mahajan, P.; Mohan, D.; Varghese, M. IT-Information Technology and the Human Interface: Tractor vibration severity and driver health: A study from rural India. *J. Agric. Eng. Res.* **2001**, *80*, 313–328. [CrossRef]

48. Paniati, J.F. Redesign and Evaluation of Selected Work Zone Sign Symbols. *Transp. Res. Rec.* **1989**, *1213*, 47–55.
49. Bhalla, M.; Proffitt, D.R. Visual-motor recalibration in geographical slant perception. *J. Exp. Psychol. Hum. Percept. Perform.* **1999**, *25*, 1076–1096. [CrossRef] [PubMed]
50. Feresin, C.; Agostini, T. Perception of visual inclination in a real and simulated urban environment. *Perception* **2007**, *36*, 258–267. [CrossRef] [PubMed]
51. Glasscock, D.J.; Rasmussen, K.; Carstensen, O.; Hansen, O.N. Psychosocial factors and safety behaviour as predictors of accidental work injuries in farming. *Work Stress* **2006**, *20*, 173–189. [CrossRef]
52. Wogalter, M.S.; Dejoy, D.M.; Laughery, K.R. *Warnings and Risk Communication*; Taylor & Francis: Philadelphia, PA, USA, 1999; 374p.
53. Chiu, E.; Quan, J.; Bridgeman, B. Treading a Slippery Slope: Slant Perception in Near and Far Space. In *European Perspectives on Cognitive Science*; Kokinov, B., Karmiloff-Smith, A., Nersessian, N.J., Eds.; New Bulgarian University Press: Sophia, Bulgaria, 2011; p. 3235.
54. Proffitt, D.R.; Creem, S.H.; Zosh, W.D. Seeing mountains in Mole Hills: Geographical-Slant Perception. *Psychol. Sci.* **2001**, *12*, 418–423. [CrossRef]
55. Caffaro, F.; Lundqvist, P.; Micheletti Cremasco, M.; Nilsson, K.; Pinzke, S.; Cavallo, E. Machinery-related perceived risks and safety attitudes in senior Swedish farmers. *J. Agromed.* **2017**, *23*, 78–91. [CrossRef]
56. Burke, M.J.; Salvador, R.O.; Smith-Crowe, K.; Chan-Serafin, S.; Smith, A.; Shirley, S. The dread factor: How hazards and safety training influence learning and performance. *J. Appl. Psychol.* **2011**, *96*, 46–70. [CrossRef]
57. Menger, L.M.; Rosecrance, J.; Stallones, L.; Roman-Muniz, I.N. A Guide to the Design of Occupational Safety and Health Training for immigrant, Latino/a Dairy workers. *Front. Public Health* **2016**, *4*, 282. [CrossRef]
58. Bai, Y.; Finger, K.; Li, Y. Analyzing motorists' responses to temporary signage in highway work zones. *Saf. Sci.* **2010**, *48*, 215–221. [CrossRef]
59. Huang, Y.; Bai, Y. Effectiveness of graphic-aided portable changeable message signs in reducing vehicle speeds in highway work zones. *Transp. Res. Part C* **2014**, *48*, 311–321. [CrossRef]
60. Rahman, M.; Strawderman, L.; Garrison, T.; Eakin, D.; Williams, C.C. Work zone sign design for increased driver compliance and worker safety. *Accid. Anal. Prev.* **2017**, *106*, 67–75. [CrossRef] [PubMed]

International Journal of
Environmental Research and Public Health

MDPI

Article

Development of the Fatigue Risk Assessment and Management in High-Risk Environments (FRAME) Survey: A Participatory Approach

Ashley E. Shortz [1], Ranjana K. Mehta [2,*], S. Camille Peres [1], Mark E. Benden [1] and Qi Zheng [3]

1 Department of Environmental and Occupational Health, Texas A&M University, College Station, TX 77843, USA; aeshortz@tamu.edu (A.E.S.); peres@tamu.edu (S.C.P.); mbenden@sph.tamhsc.edu (M.E.B.)
2 Department of Industrial and Systems Engineering, Texas A&M University, College Station, TX 77843, USA
3 Department of Epidemiology and Biostatistics, Texas A&M University, College Station, TX 77843, USA; qzheng@sph.tamhsc.edu
* Correspondence: rmehta@tamu.edu; Tel.: +1-979-458-2369

Received: 20 December 2018; Accepted: 10 February 2019; Published: 13 February 2019

Abstract: Existing risk assessment tools are not effective or sustainable in identifying Oil and Gas Extraction (OGE) workers at high risk of fatigue-related injuries or incidents. We developed a comprehensive Fatigue Risk Assessment and Management in high-risk Environments (FRAME) survey through an industry-academic participatory approach. The FRAME survey was developed through: (1) systematic gathering of existing fatigue scales; (2) refining the inventory using the Delphi Consensus technique; and (3) further refinement through employee/worker focus groups. The participatory approach resulted in a final FRAME survey across four fatigue dimensions—sleep, shiftwork, physical, and mental fatigue, and was composed of 26 items. The FRAME survey was founded on occupational fatigue science and refined and tailored to the OGE industry, through rigorous industry stakeholder input, for safer, effective, practical, and sustainable fatigue assessment and management efforts.

Keywords: oil and gas; overexertion; sleep; shift; workload; questionnaire

1. Introduction

Fatigue plays a vast role in all industries in terms of performance, safety, and productivity and is continually ranked among the top five human factors issues year after year [1]. It is estimated that fatigue costs more than $18 billion per year in lost productivity alone, of which 84% is due to reduced performance at work, rather than absenteeism [2]. Fatigue in oil and gas operations specifically can have detrimental and catastrophic effects. An example is the BP Texas City Incident of 2005, which resulted in the deaths of 15 workers, 180 injuries, and a loss of at least $1.5 billion [3]. Fatigue was identified as a contributing factor as some operators had been working 12-h shifts for as many as 29 consecutive days. Another major incident was the Piper Alpha oil platform disaster that resulted in the deaths of 167 workers [4]. It was determined that poor communication at the shift turnover was a contributing factor. Currently, due to the lack of consistent, sufficient, and effective incident reporting methods, it is difficult to estimate the extent to which fatigue has contributed to oil and gas extraction (OGE) incidents and injuries [5–7]. However, it is estimated that up to 80% of industrial accidents and incidents are due to human errors, for which fatigue was often partly responsible [5].

While the OGE sector is one of the most regulated sectors in terms of safety standards and regulations [8], fatalities in OGE are still alarmingly high, especially when compared to all other U.S. workers. The fatalities rate in this sector is about seven times greater [9]. This could be due to the dynamic environment surrounding OGE operations, including high physical and mental workload, coupled with long work periods and shiftwork and prolonged social isolation [10]. The disproportionate fatality rate in this industry could be due to the complex combination and interaction of these factors contributing to high levels of fatigue. For example, OGE workers are typically working in remote locations for a 2–3 weeks' deployment and these locations are among the most demanding in terms of the technology used in daily operations and workforce demands [10]. Usually work schedules in OGE operations are 12-h periods in two shifts (day and night). While it has been established that 12-h shifts are not necessarily unfavorable, when they are coupled with long work weeks and night work, which are common practices in OGE operations, concomitant adverse events have been observed [11]. In addition to long work periods and shiftwork, OGE workers, especially drillers, are confronted with extreme cognitive demands. Drillers are responsible for the day-to-day operations on the rig. This includes monitoring and maintaining well control (i.e., to avoid blowout), organizing and leading work on the rig floor, as well as ensuring safety of the team [12]. Such high cognitive demands, paired with long work days and rotating schedules could potentially compound fatigue levels, thus increasing the risk of an adverse event.

Due to the multidimensional nature of fatigue, effective fatigue assessment is a critical challenge, particularly when considering the complex OGE working environment. While there is no gold standard for measuring comprehensive fatigue, several objective and subjective fatigue assessment methods exist that have been employed in different occupational sectors. The method for assessing fatigue is typically tailored to the environment and setting in which fatigue is being evaluated and can be considered as research-oriented (i.e., neuroimaging techniques and electrocardiogram) [13,14] and/or practice oriented in nature (i.e., performance test and subjective assessments) [15,16]. For example, within the transportation sector, there is an abundance of literature that demonstrates utility of different assessment methods to measure driver fatigue. Traditional lab-based studies have used methods that include brain activity via electroencephalography (EEG), eye movements using electrooculography, cardiovascular responses, biochemical markers, psychomotor tests, and subjective responses [17–19], while onboard devices exist that use EEG, which monitor and detect changes in drivers' states [20]. In the aviation sector, there is a trend of using performance tests such as the psychomotor vigilance test as a primary measure of fatigue rather than traditional lab-based methods [21], whereas subjective surveys are typically used within the healthcare industry [22,23].

A recent study employed real-time physiological monitoring in order to assess shiftwork in a 3-week offshore operation [24,25]. While valuable information was gained from physiological monitoring, the authors argued that this fatigue assessment approach was not sustainable or feasible for the OGE environment. Due to the hazardous and volatile environment of offshore operations, introducing sensors into this environment may create additional safety risks. This presents a challenge of identifying workers with high-risk fatigue levels. Without effective assessment methods, fatigue management practices that are targeted and effective in reducing fatigue-related incidents in the OGE industry are likely to be ineffective.

A potential safe and sustainable solution could be a non-intrusive, industry-specific subjective assessments tool for assessing fatigue in high-risk environments. Indeed, research within the OGE domain has traditionally assessed fatigue using subjective surveys and questionnaires [26–30]. However, the question remains whether these subjective research tools can be practically adopted in everyday OGE operations to assess worker fatigue. Mehta et al. [25] augmented physiological monitoring in their offshore shiftwork investigation with existing subjective methods to assess fatigue. The surveys included some of the more occupationally used fatigue scales, such as the Swedish Occupation Fatigue Inventory and the Occupational Fatigue Exhaustion Recovery [26–28]. They found that none of these surveys were comprehensive, relevant, and feasible for the OGE workforce. For example, compliance for completing these surveys declined over time due to the time-intensive nature of completing the surveys. On average, it took workers approximately 45 min to complete all the surveys used in this study. Additionally, the workers reported that some of the questions were not clear and they had trouble understanding certain terms (e.g., some were unsure what "palpitations" meant). Because the SOFI was developed for the healthcare domain, the descriptions included medical terminology that nurses and caregivers are familiar with. As such, Mehta et al. [25] highlighted a critical gap in OGE fatigue assessment research and practice. Thus, feasible and sustainable fatigue assessment surveys need to be developed for the OGE sector that address user needs and education levels or utilize stakeholder feedback in OGE-specific hazardous work environment.

One methodology that holds strong potential to address tool development disconnect between research and practice is the Delphi consensus technique. The Delphi consensus technique is an iterative process that typically involves three to four rounds of questionnaires until consensus is reached regarding a specific topic. This technique has been employed successfully toward the development of human factors risk quantification in oil and gas drilling operations [31], fatigue surveys [32], as well as medical checklists used for safe surgical practices [33,34], and forecasting and issue identification, and framework development [35,36]. Since the Delphi consensus technique has been successfully applied in the OGE sector for human factors and in the use of other fatigue survey development, this technique provides a method that would be ideal for the development of an OGE specific fatigue survey.

The purpose of this study was to develop a comprehensive fatigue assessment tool specific for OGE operations utilizing the Delphi Consensus technique with participation from several OGE industry stakeholder groups, such as safety managers, consultants, researchers, and workers. To our knowledge, this was one of the first collaborations integrating user feedback from the OGE stakeholders and workers as well as occupational health and safety researchers. This effort will increase the likelihood that the new fatigue assessment tool will be adopted by the OGE industry, thus increasing its sustainability [37].

2. Materials and Methods

This study adopted a qualitative approach to develop a fatigue assessment inventory. A critical component in the development of this method was the integration of end user, i.e., OGE industry, inputs and expertise throughout the development process. This was completed in three phases. Phase 1 included a systematic gathering of existing fatigue survey based on predetermined criteria to develop a preliminary fatigue inventory. Phase 2 included the refinement of the inventory for content validation, conciseness, and relevance to OGE operations through industry stakeholders (i.e., safety managers from major OGE companies) and health and safety researchers (i.e., current doctoral students, post-doctoral researchers, and faculty from Department of Environmental and Occupational Health at Texas A&M University) using the Delphi consensus technique. Phase 3 involved further refinement of the inventory by OGE workers, who are the intended end-users. The inventory was refined for language and relevance to daily OGE work in this phase.

2.1. Fatigue Inventory Development (Phase 1)

Before the development of any assessment technique, the construct needs to be clearly defined and operationalized for the specific domain. In this study, fatigue in the OGE environment was operationally defined as a physiological state of reduced mental or physical performance capability resulting from sleep loss, disrupted circadian phase, and high workload (physical and mental). This definition was borrowed from the comprehensive definition of fatigue in aviation [38].

Potential items under consideration for developing the fatigue inventory were obtained from a systematic gathering of articles published from 1970 to 2016 and indexed in the Scopus database. Scopus was chosen for its thorough coverage of more than 22,800 titles with subject areas ranging from social sciences (psychology, economics, and business: 8698 titles), health sciences (100% MEDLINE, nursing, and dentistry: 7133 titles), physical sciences (chemistry, engineering, and physics: 7441 titles) and life sciences (neuroscience, pharmacology, and biology: 4601 articles). The criteria for inclusion was determined as: (1) ability to identify distinct fatigue symptoms, (2) applicability to health workforce, (3) sensitivity to a range of fatigue levels, and 4) English language. The search was completed in

April 2016. Search terms included: fatigue, physical demand, cognitive demand, psychosocial demand, stress, sleep, shiftwork, staff, adult, worker, employee, healthy, scale, assessment, and survey.

2.2. Fatigue Inventory Refinement (Phases 2 and 3)

Phase 2 included the refinement of the preliminary inventory for content validation, brevity, and relevance to OGE operations using two Delphi Consensus panels [39]. The size of Delphi panels varies widely. However, most studies using the Delphi Consensus method use panels of 15 to 35 people [40]. The Delphi consensus method used for this study was composed of 13 OGE stakeholders, with representation from researchers, consultants, and practitioners. Upon informed consent, the Delphi panel was presented with the preliminary fatigue inventory and instructed to exclude items based on the following criteria: (1) too general at describing a symptom of fatigue, (2) redundant of previous item, and (3) not relevant to OGE operation. Each item was vetted and discussed and then voted on whether to keep or remove the item. Items with a score of less than 80% consensus were removed. In Phase 3, focus groups were conducted with OGE workers, who are the intended end-user. OGE workers were provided with the refined inventory from the two Delphi consensus conducted in Phase 2. The inventory was further refined for language and relevance to OGE work.

2.3. Participants

Participants were recruited for Phases 2 and 3. Participant demographics are shown in Table 1. For Phase 2, OGE stakeholders, health and safety researchers and practitioners, were recruited to participate in the Delphi consensus study to refine the preliminary fatigue inventory. Industry stakeholders (from major energy companies based in Houston, TX; 61,000–75,000 employees) were invited for the Mary Kay O'Connor Process Safety Center at Texas A&M University. For Phase 3, one focus group was formed, with OGE workers across different job categories from a medium-sized (Houston, TX; 5000 employees) well-servicing company. Their role was to further refine inventory based on the language and relevance to OGE operations. Participants across both phases provided their informed consent approved through the Texas A&M Institutional Review Board (IRB2016-0676M).

Table 1. Participant Demographics.

	Delphi Panel 1 (n = 8)	Delphi Panel 2 (n = 5)	Worker Focus Group (n = 11)
Gender			
Male	6	4	100%
Female	2	1	
Age (Years)	38.57 (12.45)	38.40 (17.47)	44.36 (3.98)
Race			
American Indian	0%	0%	18.2%
Black or African American	0%	0%	9.1%
White	62.5%	60%	18.2%
More than one race	12.5%	0%	8.3%
Unknown or not reported	25%	30%	41.7%
Ethnicity			
Hispanic or Latino	12.5%	0%	54.6%
Not Hispanic or Latino	87.5%	100%	27.3%
Unknown or not reported	0%	0%	18.2%
Education			
Some High School	0%	0%	18.2%
HS Graduate or Equivalent	0%	0%	54.6%
Some College	100%	100%	9.1%
Unknown or not reported	0%	0%	18.2%
Experience (Years)	8.71 (11.22)	11.70 (11.29)	16.11 (4.36)

3. Results

3.1. Fatigue Inventory Development (Phase 1)

Figure 1 illustrates the flowchart for number of articles identified in each of the steps described above. Ultimately, 14 peer-reviewed articles were included and reviewed, which yielded 12 widely used surveys, scales, or questionnaires (2 surveys were duplicated) [12,23,32,41–49]. This resulted in 230 question items. These questions were directly used with their accompanying instructions and scales in Phase 2.

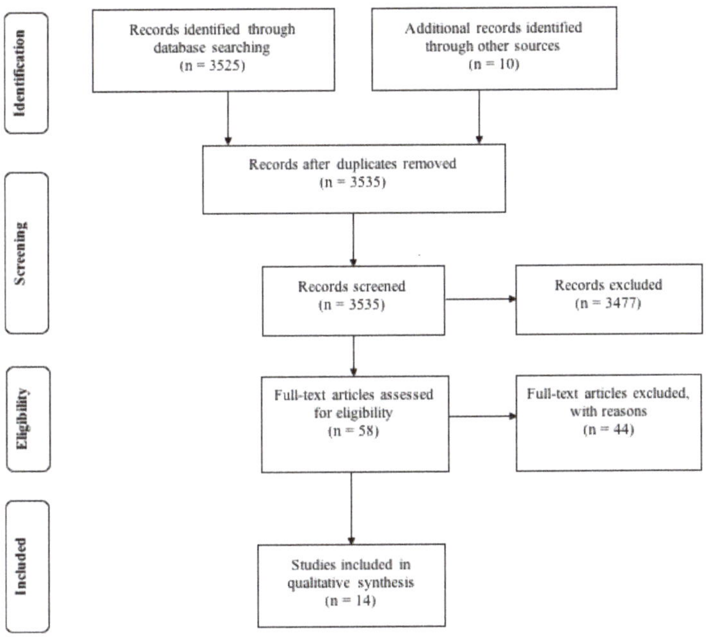

Figure 1. Flowchart of articles gathered.

3.2. Fatigue Inventory Refinement (Phase 2)

This phase was completed in two steps utilizing two different Delphi Consensus panels. The first panel (Table 1) was provided the initial inventory, created in Phase 1. The panel was instructed to refine the inventory by improving grammar and language, and by eliminating redundant items. Two hundred and thirty items were discussed and the consensus technique led to a reduced 50-item inventory. Some examples of items that were removed due to vagueness of description included: (1) *"I feel tired"* (2) *"Thinking required effort"* and (3) *"I feel weak,"* Another example for an item that was removed due to redundancy (e.g., *"My thoughts easily wonder"*) was similar to a previous item (e.g., *"I have trouble concentrating"*). Items such as *"I don't do much during the day"* and *"I think I do a lot during the day"* were removed as the panel argued that truthful responses will be difficult to obtain as responders might be afraid to lose their job or human resources might interfere. An example of an item that was included after rewording the description was *"I use my days off recovering from work"* from the original *"I use a lot of my spare time recovering from work"*. Another example was *"Vision is blurred"* was changed to *"Vision is blurred or distorted."* This was revised to combine two items on the preliminary inventory.

The panel was also required to reach consensus regarding how far the worker need to reflect (e.g., right now, past 24 h, or past week) to provide their responses on the fatigue symptoms. All panel members felt that a time frame (i.e., right now vs. previous week vs. three months ago) for the instructions of the inventory needed to be established. A majority of the panelists stated that asking "*right now*" would not only reflect the most accurate symptom response from the worker, but also provide supervisors real-time valuable feedback from the workers necessary for implementing quick fatigue mitigation strategies (e.g., reallocation/rescheduling of personnel and work tasks).

In step 2, 5 OGE stakeholders refined the inventory for OGE relevance and/or utility of the responses on the items to guide management strategies. This reduced the inventory to 38 items. However, the panel added a question they felt was important regarding assessing cognitive fatigue. The added item was "*Fatigue interferes with my mental functioning*" which was developed from "*Fatigue interferes with my physical functioning.*" Two items were removed based on the panel's suggestion that responses would not be accurate due to the respondent being afraid of losing job or to the Human Resources tending to interfere. These items included "*I frequently dozed off during break period*" and "*I feel no desire to do anything.*" Some examples of items removed due to redundancy included: (1) "*I can concentrate well*" and (2) "*Having tremors in limbs.*" This brought the total items to 39 items at the end of Phase 2.

The panel gave similar feedback about the importance of inventory instructions. The panel suggested that all items began with the same phrase of either "*To what extent...*" or "*To what degree ...* " but "*To what degree ...* " was favored. Additionally, a timeframe of "*right now*" or "*during the last shift*" was determined as the most critical and valuable for fatigue management.

3.3. Fatigue Inventory Refinement Through OGE Worker Focus Group (Phase 3)

Eleven OGE workers refined the inventory for OGE relevance and language. In this phase, all 39 items were kept. Feedback from the focus group was used to reword questions for better comprehension, which is expected to allow workers to accurately respond to questions. The workers agreed that all 39 items were relevant to OGE operations. However, they suggested that a few items be reworded. For example, the item "*To what degree do your joints (e.g., knee or elbow) feel achy?*" was changed to "*To what extent do your joints (e.g., knee or elbow) feel stiff or achy?*" Another example included changing the item "*To what degree do you experience tense muscles?*" to "*To what extent do you experience stiff muscles?*"

Additionally, workers gave their input on the type of scale they would prefer to respond to (i.e., 1 (*none*) to 7 (*a lot*) vs. 0 (*Not at all*)-10 (*Extremely*)). Of the 11 workers, 9 preferred the 0 (*not at all*) to 10 (*extremely*), and the other two did not have any comments regarding the response scale. A majority of the workers stated that it was natural for them to perceive zero as "*nothing*" or "*not at all*", while 1 meant a little bit or slightly more than zero. Additionally, workers expressed that they preferred "*to what extent ...* " rather than "*to what degree ...* ". The workers also suggested that having a Spanish version of the final inventory would be critical for implementation and translation to sustainable practice. Over 50% of workers spoke Spanish as their first language. They expressed that while they understood the English version, it would be easier for them to understand and respond accurately and quickly with a translated inventory.

3.4. Final Fatigue Inventory (FRAME)

After health and safety researchers, OGE stakeholders, and OGE workers reviewed the preliminary inventory of 230 items, the final inventory decreased to 39 items. The 39 items were further reviewed by the study research team to verify that all dimensions of fatigue (e.g., physical, mental, sleep, and shift-related) were represented. In this review, the research team identified 13 items that would not offer sufficient value to the organization (e.g., supervisors, safety managers, etc.) for implementing effective fatigue management practices, but that could provide a better understanding of workers' personal strategies to manage fatigue. Because the original purpose of the fatigue inventory was to help organizations develop effective and sustainable fatigue mitigation strategies, these items were removed to enhance ease of use of the new tool. Examples of the removed items included: (1) "*To what extent do you worry about issues at home making it hard to relax?*" (2) "*To what extent do you use alcohol to help you sleep?"* (3) *"To what extent are you concerned for how long you can keep going at your work?"* and (4) *"To what extent would you work overtime or an extra shift when you are sleepy or fatigue in you needed extra money?"* It should be noted that the mentioned items were discussed extensively in Phase 1 and Phase 2. Participants from both the Delphi Panels and Employee focus groups suggested that these were interesting items and hence were ultimately kept in the inventory, but unsure how responses could be used for fatigue management programs. Ultimately, 26 items were selected for final fatigue inventory (Figure 2). Figure 2 also lists the number of items that were classified within each dimension of fatigue (physical, mental, sleep or shift-related) in each phase. It should be noted that items can be classified as more than one dimension. An example of this is the item *"fatigue interferes with carrying out certain duties and responsibilities."* This item could be classified as all four dimensions.

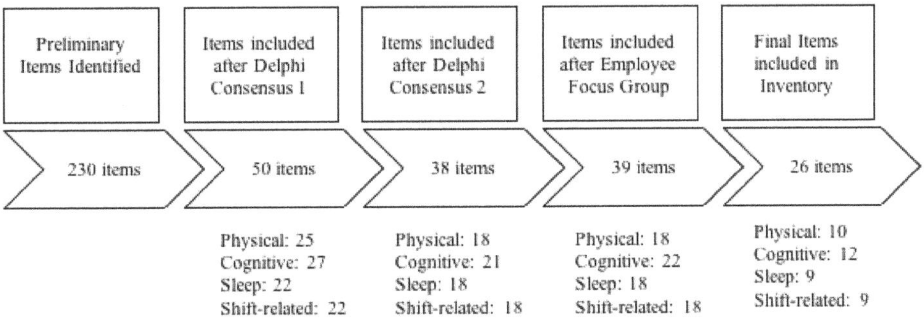

Figure 2. Summary of Inventory Item Reduction.

The final fatigue inventory recommended by the research team along with when the question should be asked (pre-shift or post-shift) is shown in Table 2.

Table 2. Final Fatigue Inventory Questions.

Item	Administered		Dimension of Fatigue			
	Pre-Shift	Post-Shift	Physical	Mental	Sleep	Shift-Related
To what extent are you having to re-do or repeat tasks?	X	X	X	X	X	X
To what extent are you experiencing eye strain?	X	X		X	X	X
To what extent do your legs feel tired or heavy?	X	X	X			
To what extent are your joints (e.g., knee or elbow) feeling achy or stiff?	X	X	X			
To what extent are you experiencing stiff muscles?	X	X	X			
To what extent are you having trouble concentrating?	X	X		X		
To what extent are you having trouble paying attention (e.g., like during meetings or briefs)?	X	X		X		
To what extent has your sleepiness interfered with your work?	X	X			X	X
To what extent are you still tired even after waking up from sleep?	X				X	X
To what extent did you recover between shifts?	X				X	X
To what extent did you have trouble sleeping?	X				X	X
To what extent did you feel exhausted?		X	X	X	X	X
To what extent did you experience cramps in your muscles?		X	X			
To what extent did you experience rapid heartbeats?		X	X			
To what extent did your legs feel numb?		X	X			
To what extent did your arms, hands, and/or fingers feel numb?		X	X			
To what extent did fatigue interferes with your physical functioning.		X	X			
To what extend did fatigue interferes with your mental functioning.		X		X		
To what extent did you experience blurred or distorted vision?		X		X		
To what extent did you daydream during work duties?		X		X		
To what extent did you have trouble remembering work-related things (i.e., instructions or procedures)?		X		X		
To what extent did you find it difficult to pay attention to someone, even when you were being spoken to directly?		X		X		
To what extent did you find it easy to keep track of everything was going on around you?		X		X		
To what extent did you have trouble getting back into work after an interruption?		X		X		
To what extent did you experience difficulty staying awake during work?		X			X	X
To what extent did you feel drowsy during your shift?		X			X	X
Total	11	20	10	12	9	9

4. Discussion

The aim of this study was to develop a comprehensive fatigue assessment inventory specific for OGE operations through involvement of OGE stakeholder input. The resulting survey instrument, named Fatigue Risk Assessment for high-Risk Environments (FRAME) survey has a total of 26 items encompassing four dimensions of fatigue. It should be noted that this survey was developed by obtaining input from the OGE industry, and as such its application to other high risk industries, such as mining, need to be evaluated.

A recent study comparing objective and subjective fatigue assessment in offshore work used five different surveys to capture comprehensive operator fatigue over the course of a hitch [25]. An average worker needs approximately 45 min to complete all the surveys as the wordings were not clear difficult to understand. As a result, compliance was low as time progress over the hitch. Moreover, lengthy surveys are at risk of resulting in participant response fatigue, implying that questions asked later in a long survey are typically prone to increased error and untruthful and unreliable responses [50]. Pilot studies have found the FRAME survey, developed here, takes no longer than 10 min to complete, simply due to the reduced number of times [51]. This would allow for compliance to be greater and additionally recovery time between shifts, as operators will not spend a great amount of time completing surveys. Sustained use of the FRAME survey could help to facilitate the successful implementation of effective fatigue management practices outline in the API Recommended Practice 755: Fatigue Risk Management System [52].

Fatigue-related incidents have been continually identified as one of the most dangerous risk factors in high-risk industrial setting [27]. When workers were asked to define fatigue, most simply said it's when they are "tired" or "exhausted". Fatigue is typically described as tiredness, overexertion and strenuous movements [27]. Overexertion injuries were the third leading cause for days away from work in 2007 behind being struck by an object or caught in object, equipment, or material [53]. Currently, the most common method for assessing physical fatigue in OGE sector is surveys and questionnaires [26,29,30,54]. Regarding physical workload, the FRAME survey has 10 items to gauge physical fatigue, ensuring that this important dimension of fatigue is assessed through the new tool.

Not only does physical workload affect fatigue-related performance and safety outcomes, intense mental workload associated in specific operations, specifically drilling and well control scenarios, can contribute significantly to fatigue development. In both onshore and offshore operations alike, drillers are responsible for maintaining and ensuring rig safety, in addition to performing day-to-day tasks required for rig performance. The day-to-day tasks are outlined by a well operation plan [55]. The well operation plan is an overview of the drilling parameters that must be monitored and maintained. In addition to following the well operation plan, drillers are also responsible for providing well control if necessary. This means that in the case of an adverse event such as a kick or loss of circulation, they are required to intervene to avoid blowout [55]. Performance on daily operations relies heavily on cognitive dexterity [12]. Similar to physical fatigue assessments, the most common method that is currently used to assessing cognitive fatigue in OGE is surveys and questionnaires such as the Swedish Occupational Fatigue Inventory and Work Ability Index [26–28]. However, none of these surveys were designed specifically use for OGE operation. Since the FRAME survey was developed with OGE input and consideration, it is better suited than current surveys being used for cognitive fatigue assessment. To assess cognitive fatigue, the FRAME survey has 12 items. It might be argued that workers may tend to respond to some questions based on their awareness rather than their experience (for e.g., question item 18 in Table 2). Future testing (such as reliability analysis) may help identify questions whose responses could potentially be biased by awareness rather than actual experiences.

In OGE operations, insufficient sleep and changing shift pattern are the primary cause of fatigue [11]. Traditional work schedules are typically 7–14-day tour, with sequential 12-h shifts and shift changes. Evidence suggests that 12-h shift are not necessarily detrimental, but when coupled with extended workdays (i.e., beyond 4 days) and/or night work, there are many adverse effects on worker performance, safety and health [11]. As sleep and shift-related factors are a common source of fatigue, the FRAME survey has nine items to effectively assess these factors. A common practice in OGE operations is the use of a swing shift (i.e., switching from a night shift to a day shift or from a day to night shift). Swing shifts are used to allow workers to become adapted to day schedule for them to return home after a hitch [56]. It has been observed that workers can physiologically adapt to 12-h night shift but their internal circadian cycle is desynchronized for at least the first 4-5 days [57]. But those who start with a day-shift then switch to night shift do not adequately adapt [57]. The common practice of switching shifts in the middle of a hitch could potentially introduce several health and safety. The responses from sleep and shift-related questions could help to test effectiveness or implications of a swing shift. In addition to understanding the implications of swing swifts, responses on the shift and sleep-related questions could explain or allow for better interpretation of other responses for other questions within the FRAME survey. For example, if a worker has reported a low score (i.e., did not recover between shifts) to the item *"To what extent did you recover completely between shifts"*, it should be taken into account if they report a high score (i.e., found it extremely difficult to pay attention) to the item *"To what extent did you find it difficult to pay attention to someone, even when being spoken to directly."* By understanding the cause and consequence of fatigue, effective mitigation strategies can be designed, which ultimately may reduce fatigue-related injuries and incidents.

Valuable feedback has been received from employee focus groups regarding the survey content. It was suggested that a Spanish version of the FRAME survey would be highly beneficial. According to the BLS, 32.3% of workers within extraction are Hispanic or Latino, while the cross-industry average is merely 16.1% [58]. In 2011, 25% of OGE worker fatalities were Hispanic or Latino [53]. In addition to NIOSH identifying *"decrease-fatigue related injuries and fatalities in the oil and gas extraction industry"* as a top strategic goal for the Oil and Gas Extraction Program, *"reduce the incidence of injuries, illnesses, and fatalities among vulnerable workers in the oil and gas extraction industry such as contract workers, young and old workers, workers new to the industry, and immigrants"* has also been determined as a strategic goal. The addition of a Spanish version will allow for a greater number of workers to be properly assessed. However, future research would be needed to assess the readability of the FRAME survey with Spanish-speaking workers.

There are a few limitations that should be mentioned. First, the employee focus group was completed using only one onshore well-servicing company. However, the second Delphi Consensus Panel was composed of representatives from major energy companies. By using both small and major companies, considerations from different size companies were incorporated in the development of the FRAME survey. While subjective assessments only provide workers' perception of their fatigue, due to the dynamic working environment of OGE operations, an industry-specific survey that is feasible, sustainable, and non-intrusive appears to be a viable approach to improving our understanding of fatigue. However, objective assessments beyond physiological measures need to be explored for OGE operations. Future research is required to test the reliability and validity of the FRAME survey in onshore and offshore OGE operations against traditional fatigue assessment methods such as performance tests and physiological monitoring. In addition to testing the reliability and validity of the FRAME survey, the scoring method should also be evaluated. A potential scoring method could be to sum the response for each dimension individually. The sum score of each dimension may identify what aspect of fatigue the workers are at the greatest risk, which could help to identify mitigation practices. Finally, while the FRAME survey provides worker perceptions on the degree to which fatigue impacts their physical and cognitive capabilities, future work could investigate coupling the survey with quantifiable fatigue sources (e.g., weather, rig activity—that implicates physical and cognitive workload, shift lengths/durations) to provide better decision support to supervisors and schedulers for effective and guided fatigue management practices. It is possible that, while the Delphi panel added question items, the panel members were biased by the nature of questions in the existing surveys—which were largely focused on identifying and quantifying symptoms rather than identifying the role of work factors.

5. Conclusions

Fatigue is a critical work risk factor in the oil and gas industry and one of the barriers to effective fatigue management is its assessment. The present study adopted a participatory mixed-method approach to develop a 26-item survey to conduct fatigue risk assessment and management in high-risk environments (FRAME survey), that assessed fatigue across four major dimensions, namely, sleep, shiftwork, physical, and mental fatigue. Because the FRAME survey was founded on occupational fatigue science and refined and tailored to the oil and gas industry, through rigorous industry stakeholder input, it will facilitate safer, effective, practical, and sustainable fatigue assessment and management efforts.

Author Contributions: R.K.M. conceptualized, supervised, reviewed and edited, A.E.S. conceptualized, conducted, prepared original draft, S.C.P. supervised, reviewed and edited, M.E.B. and Q.Z., reviewed and edited.

Funding: Research reported in this publication was supported by the Gulf Research Program of the National Academies of Sciences, Engineering, and Medicine under Grant Agreement number [#2000007355].

Acknowledgments: We thank the industry members of the Mary K. O'Connor Process Safety Center at Texas A&M University who provided insights and feedback throughout the FRAME survey developmental process. The open access publishing fees for this article have been covered by the Texas A&M University Open Access to Knowledge Fund (OAKFund), supported by the University Libraries and the Office of the Vice President for Research.

Conflicts of Interest: The authors declare no conflict of interest. The funders had no role in the design of the study; in the collection, analyses, or interpretation of data; in the writing of the manuscript, or in the decision to publish the results.

References

1. Lerman, S.; Eskin, E.; Flower, D.; George, E.C.; Gerson, B.; Hartenbaum, N.; Hursh, S.R.; Moore-Ede, M. Fatigue risk management in the workplace. *J. Occup. Environ. Med.* **2012**, *54*, 231–258. [CrossRef] [PubMed]
2. Caruso, C.C. Negative impacts of shiftwork and long work hours. *Rehab. Nur.* **2014**, *39*, 16–25. [CrossRef] [PubMed]
3. Civil Service Bureau. *BP Texas City Final Investigation Report*; U.S. Chemical Safety and Hazard Investigation Board: Washington, DC, USA, 2007.
4. Cullen, W.D. *The Public Inquiry into the Piper Alpha Disaster*; Health and Safety Executive: Bootle, UK, 1990.
5. Theophilus, S.C.; Esenowo, V.N.; Arewa, A.O.; Ifelebuegu, A.O.; Nnadi, E.O.; Mbanaso, F.U. Human factors analysis and classification system for the oil and gas industry (HFACS-OGI). *Reliab. Eng. Syst. Saf.* **2017**, *167*, 168–176. [CrossRef]
6. Gordon, R.; Flin, R.; Mearns, K. Designing and evaluating a human factors investigation tool (HFIT) for accident analysis. *Saf. Sci.* **2005**, *43*, 147–171. [CrossRef]
7. Gordon, R.; Flin, R.; Mearns, K. Collecting human-factors data from accidents and incidents. *Old Product. Facil.* **2001**, *16*, 73–83. [CrossRef]
8. McLaughlin, P.A.; Sherouse, O. *The Impact of Federal Regulation on the 50 States*; George Mason University: Fairfax, VA, USA, 2016.
9. Bureau of Labor Statistics. *Number of Fatal Occupational Injuries by Selected Worker and Case Characteristics, 2014–2015*; Bureau of Labor Statistics: Washington, DC, USA, 2016.
10. Gardner, R. Overview and characteristics of some occupational exposures and health risks on offshore oil and gas installations. *Annals Occup. Hyg.* **2003**, *47*, 201–210.
11. Parkes, K.R. Shift schedules on North Sea oil/gas installations: A systematic review of their impact on performance, safety and health. *Saf. Sci.* **2012**, *7*, 1636–1651. [CrossRef]
12. Sneddon, A.; Mearns, K.; Flin, R. Stress, fatigue, situation awareness and safety in offshore drilling crews. *Saf. Sci.* **2013**, *56*, 80. [CrossRef]
13. DeLuca, J.; Genova, H.M.; Capili, E.J.; Wylie, G.R. Functional neuroimaging of fatigue. *Phys. Med. Rehab. Clin.* **2009**, *20*, 325–337. [CrossRef]
14. Christodoulou, C. The assessment and measurement of fatigue. In *Fatigue Window Brain*; MIT Press: Cambridge, MA, USA, 2005; pp. 19–35.

15. Thomas, M.; Sing, H.; Belenky, G.; Holcomb, H.; Mayberg, H.; Dannals, R.; Wagner, H., Jr.; Thorne, D.; Popp, K.; Rowland, L.; Welsh, A. Neural basis of alertness and cognitive performance impairments during sleepiness. I. effects of 24 h of sleep deprivation on waking human regional brain activity. *J. Sleep Res.* **2000**, *9*, 335–352. [CrossRef] [PubMed]
16. Aaronson, L.S.; Teel, C.S.; Cassmeyer, V.; Neuberger, G.B.; Pallikkathayil, L.; Pierce, J.; Press, A.N.; Williams, P.D.; Wingate, A. Defining and measuring fatigue. *J. Nurs. Scholars.* **1999**, *31*, 45–50. [CrossRef]
17. Lal, S.K.L.; Craig, A.A. Critical review of the psychophysiology of driver fatigue. *Biol. Psychol.* **2001**, *55*, 173–194. [CrossRef]
18. Dawson, D.; Searle, A.K.; Paterson, J.L. Look before you (s)leep: Evaluating the use of fatigue detection technologies within a fatigue risk management system for the road transport industry. *Sleep Med. Rev.* **2014**, *18*, 141. [CrossRef] [PubMed]
19. Borghini, G.; Astolfi, L.; Vecchiato, G.; Mattia, D.; Babiloni, F. Measuring neurophysiological signals in aircraft pilots and car drivers for the assessment of mental workload, fatigue and drowsiness. *Neurosci. Biobehav. Rev.* **2014**, *44*, 58–75. [CrossRef] [PubMed]
20. Lal, S.K.L.; Craig, A. Electroencephalography activity associated with driver fatigue. *J. Psychophysiol.* **2001**, *15*, 183–189. [CrossRef]
21. Lamond, N.; Dawson, D.; Roach, G.D. Fatigue assessment in the field: Validation of a hand-held electronic psychomotor vigilance task. *Aviat. Space Environ. Med.* **2005**, *76*, 486–489. [PubMed]
22. Barker, L.M.; Nussbaum, M.A. Fatigue, performance and the work environment: A survey of registered nurses. *J. Adv. Nurs.* **2011**, *67*, 1370–1382. [CrossRef]
23. Winwood, P.C.; Winefield, A.H.; Dawson, D.; Lushington, K. Development and validation of a scale to measure work-related fatigue and recovery: The occupational fatigue exhaustion/recovery scale (OFER). *J. Occup. Environ. Med.* **2005**, *47*, 594–606. [CrossRef]
24. Shortz, A.E.; Franke, M.; Kilic, E.S.; Peres, S.C.; Mehta, R.K. Evaluation of offshore shiftwork using heart rate variability. *Proc. Human Factors Ergon. Soc. Annu. Meeting.* **2017**, *61*, 1036–1039. [CrossRef]
25. Mehta, R.K.; Peres, S.C.; Kannan, P.; Rhee, J.; Shortz, A.E.; Sam Mannan, M. Comparison of objective and subjective operator fatigue assessment methods in offshore shiftwork. *J. Loss Prevent. Process Ind.* **2017**, *48*, 376–381. [CrossRef]
26. Adel, M.; Akbar, R.; Gabraeil, N.S.; Abbas, R.F. Work ability index (WAI) and its association with psychosocial factors in one of the petrochemical industries in Iran. *J. Occup. Health.* **2012**, *54*, 112–118.
27. Chan, M. Fatigue: The most critical accident risk in oil and gas construction. *Constr. Manag. Econ.* **2011**, *29*, 341–353. [CrossRef]
28. Hystad, S.W.; Saus, E.; Sætrevik, B.; Eid, J. Fatigue in seafarers working in the offshore oil and gas re-supply industry: Effects of safety climate, psychosocial work environment and shift arrangement. *Int. Marit. Health* **2013**, *64*, 72.
29. Ulleberg, P.; Rundmo, T. Job stress, social support, job satisfaction and absenteeism among offshore oil personnel. *Work Stress* **1997**, *11*, 215–228. [CrossRef]
30. Chen, W.Q.; Yu, I.; Wong, T.W. Impact of occupational stress and other psychosocial factors on musculoskeletal pain among Chinese offshore oil installation workers. *Occup. Environ. Med.* **2005**, *62*, 251–256. [CrossRef] [PubMed]
31. Quanmin, Z.; Hong, Z.; Jianchun, F. Human factor risk quantification for oil and gas drilling operation. *Procedia Eng.* **2011**, *18*, 312–317. [CrossRef]
32. Zhang, M.; Sparer, E.H.; Murphy, L.A.; Dennerlein, J.T.; Fang, D.; Katz, J.N.; Caban-Martinez, A.J. Development and validation of a fatigue assessment scale for U.S. construction workers. *Am. J. Indust. Med.* **2015**, *58*, 220–228. [CrossRef]
33. Abraham, O.; Jacob, F.B.; Jacob, O. A surgical safety checklist to reduce morbidity and mortality in a global population. *ANZ J. Surg.* **2007**, *77*, 621.
34. Pucher, P.; Brunt, L.; Fanelli, R.; Asbun, H.; Aggarwal, R. SAGES expert delphi consensus: Critical factors for safe surgical practice in laparoscopic cholecystectomy. *Surg. Endosc.* **2015**, *29*, 3074–3085. [CrossRef]
35. Hasson, F.; Keeney, S.; McKenna, H. Research guidelines for the delphi survey technique. *J. Adv. Nurs.* **2000**, *32*, 1008.
36. Okoli, C.; Pawlowski, S.D. The delphi method as a research tool: An example, design considerations and applications. *Inf. Manag.* **2004**, *42*, 15–29. [CrossRef]

37. Damodaran, L. User involvement in the systems design process-a practical guide for users. *Behav. Inf. Technol.* **1996**, *15*, 363–377. [CrossRef]
38. Avers, K.; Johnson, W.B. A review of federal aviation administration fatigue research. *Aviat. Psychol. Appl. Hum. Factors* **2011**, *1*, 87–98. [CrossRef]
39. Hsu, C.; Sandford, B.A. The delphi technique: Making sense of consensus. *Pract. Assess. Res. Eval.* **2007**, *12*, 1–8.
40. Gordon, T.J. The delphi method. *Futures Res. Methodol.* **1994**, *23*, 2007.
41. Beurskens, A.J.; Bultmann, U.; Kant, I.; Vercoulen, J.H.; Bleijenberg, G.; Swaen, G.M. Fatigue among working people: Validity of a questionnaire measure. *Occup. Environ. Med.* **2000**, *57*, 353–357. [CrossRef]
42. Ahsberg, E.; Gamberale, F.; Gustafsson, K. Perceived fatigue after mental work: An experimental evaluation of a fatigue inventory. *Ergonomics* **2000**, *43*, 252–268. [CrossRef]
43. Krupp, L.B.; LaRocca, N.G.; Muir-Nash, J.; Steinberg, A.D. The fatigue severity scale: Application to patients with multiple sclerosis and systemic lupus erythematosus. *Arch. Neurol.* **1989**, *46*, 1121–1123. [CrossRef]
44. Matthews, G.; Desmond, P.A. Personality and multiple dimensions of task-induced fatigue: A study of simulated driving. *Pers. Indiv. Differ.* **1998**, *25*, 443–458. [CrossRef]
45. Stein, K.D.; Martin, S.C.; Hann, D.M.; Jacobsen, P.B. A multidimensional measure of fatigue for use with cancer patients. *Cancer Pract.* **1998**, *6*, 143. [CrossRef] [PubMed]
46. Smets, E.M.A.; Garssen, B.; Bonke, B.; De Haes, J.C.J.M. The multidimensional fatigue inventory (MFI) psychometric qualities of an instrument to assess fatigue. *J. Psychosom. Res.* **1995**, *39*, 315–325. [CrossRef]
47. Carpenter, J.S.; Andrykowski, M.A. Psychometric evaluation of the Pittsburgh sleep quality index. *J. Psychosom. Res.* **1998**, *45*, 5–13. [CrossRef]
48. Kato, T. Development of the sleep quality questionnaire in healthy adults. *J. Health Psychol.* **2014**, *19*, 977–986. [CrossRef] [PubMed]
49. Patterson, P.D.; Buysse, D.J.; Weaver, M.D.; Suffoletto, B.P.; McManigle, K.L.; Callaway, C.W.; Yealy, D.M. Emergency healthcare worker sleep, fatigue, and alertness behavior survey (SFAB): Development and content validation of a survey tool. *Accid. Anal. Prev.* **2014**, *73*, 399–411. [CrossRef] [PubMed]
50. Egleston, B.L.; Miller, S.M.; Meropol, N.J. The impact of misclassification due to survey response fatigue on estimation and identifiability of treatment effects. *Stat. Med.* **2011**, *30*, 3560–3572. [CrossRef] [PubMed]
51. Shortz, A.E.; Hoyle, W.; Peres, S.C.; Mehta, R.K. Fatigue indicators of 12-h day and night shifts in simulated offshore well control scenarios. *Proc. Hum. Factors Ergonom. Soc. Annu. Meeting* **2018**, *62*, 897–899. [CrossRef]
52. API Industrial Hygiene TF Workshop. Fatigue Risk Management Systems for Personnel in the Refining and Petrochemical Industries. Available online: https://www.api.org/environment-health-and-safety/health-safety/process-safety-industry/industrial-hygiene-workshop/~{}/media/9e82dde5834d4abe915e5a8a9c5b74f5.ashx (accessed on 11 February 2019).
53. Bureau of Labor Statistics (BLS). *Fatality Data are from the Census of Fatal Occupational Injuries. Nonfatal Injury and Illness Data are from the Survey of Occupational Injuries and Illnesses*; Bureau of Labor Statistics: Washington, DC, USA, 2014.
54. Rundmo, T.; Hestad, H.; Ulleberg, P. Organizational factors, safety attitudes and workload among offshore oil personnel. *Saf. Sci.* **1998**, *29*, 75–87. [CrossRef]
55. Skogdalen, J.E.; Utne, I.B.; Vinnem, J.E. Developing safety indicators for preventing offshore oil and gas deepwater drilling blowouts. *Saf. Sci.* **2011**, *49*, 1187–1199. [CrossRef]
56. Ross, J.K. Offshore industry shift work-health and social considerations. *Occup. Med.* **2009**, *59*, 310–315. [CrossRef]
57. Gibbs, M.; Hampton, S.; Morgan, L.; Arendt, J. Adaptation of the circadian rhythm of 6-sulphatoxymelatonin to a shift schedule of seven nights followed by seven days in offshore oil installation workers. *Neurosci. Lett.* **2002**, *325*, 91–94. [CrossRef]
58. Bureau of Labor Statistics. *Hispanics and Latinos in Industries and Occupations: The Economics Daily*; U.S. Bureau of Labor Statistics: Washington, DC, USA, 2015.

International Journal of
Environmental Research and Public Health

MDPI

Article

Localization of Vehicle Back-Up Alarms by Users of Level-Dependent Hearing Protectors under Industrial Noise Conditions Generated at a Forge

Rafal Mlynski * and Emil Kozlowski

Department of Vibroacoustic Hazards, Central Institute for Labour Protection–National Research Institute, Czerniakowska 16, 00-701 Warsaw, Poland; emkoz@ciop.pl

* Correspondence: rmlynski@ciop.pl; Tel.: +48-22-623-3293

Received: 17 December 2018; Accepted: 29 January 2019; Published: 30 January 2019

Abstract: The use of hearing protectors in various noisy workplaces is often necessary. For safety reasons, auditory information may be required to correctly localize the direction of an auditory danger signal. The purpose of this study was to verify if the selection of a specific level-dependent hearing protector may be important for the ability to localize a vehicle back-up alarm signal. The laboratory conditions reflected industrial conditions, under which an impulse noise was emitted against a background of continuous noise. A passive mode and a level-dependent mode (maximum and incomplete amplification) were considered. Four different models of level-dependent earmuffs and one model of level-dependent earplugs were included in the tests. The tests enabled differentiation between the individual hearing protectors. The use of earplugs in level-dependent mode did not significantly affect the ability to correctly localize the back-up alarm signal. For the earmuffs, the global assessment of the impact of a mode change revealed that, depending on the model of the earmuffs, the impact may be insignificant, but may also result in considerable impairment of the ability to localize the back-up alarm signal.

Keywords: sound localization; level-dependent hearing protectors; back-up alarm; directivity of hearing; impulse noise; earmuffs; earplugs; auditory danger signal; warning signal; safety at work

1. Introduction

Noise is a physical factor that affects the hearing of people who have to be in places where it is emitted. Impulse noise is a particularly dangerous type of noise due to the sudden nature of its impact [1]. This type of noise may be present during military field exercises and in industrial conditions. Under industrial conditions, impulse noise occurs most often against a background of continuous noise. Noise reduction possibilities using technical means are limited [2]. Certain activities, such as metalworking, require manual handling close to the noise source so that physically separating a person's workplace from the noise source is impossible. The final solution, albeit the only one available, is the use of hearing protectors. Level-dependent hearing protectors are gaining in popularity and are being used more frequently. Their advantage over typical passive hearing protectors is that they do not reduce the relatively quiet sounds as much as sounds with a high sound pressure level [3]. This enables the perception of low pressure level sounds that are relevant for those using hearing protectors [4].

Level-dependent hearing protectors can be defined as a system consisting of a barrier that passively reduces the transmission of sound under these hearing protectors and from the sound transmission path in certain situations. The sound transmission path is created by means of an electronic system that reproduces the sound present in the user's environment through a speaker placed under a hearing protector. The electronic system must be designed so that the amplification in the sound transmission path decreases as the sound pressure level of the signal present outside the hearing protector increases. The sound under the hearing protectors must be transmitted so as to ensure safe noise conditions for the user of these devices. In this respect, hearing protectors should meet the requirements set out in relevant standards, which apply to both earmuffs [5] and earplugs [6].

Some studies have been conducted on the possibility of reducing impulse noise by means of level-dependent hearing protectors [7–9]. It was observed that, for hearing protectors with electronic systems used in military conditions, the provision of adequate hearing protection should not be considered the only problem. Detection, recognition, identification, localization, and communication were also found to play significant sound-related roles [10]. Thus, when using hearing protectors under industrial conditions, in addition to the protective properties of hearing protectors, using the information contained in auditory danger signals is also crucially important. The presence of an electronic system used to transmit the sound under the hearing protector affects the formation of the sound reaching the users of these devices. The use of these hearing protectors may impair the ability to localize sound, i.e., recognize the direction of the source of the sound [11–13]. For safety reasons, under industrial conditions, it is vital to be able to correctly localize the noise source, which particularly applies to vehicle back-up alarm signals. Localization enables the user to take action to avoid being hit by a vehicle. The problem with the perception of back-up alarm signals was deemed serious enough that a dedicated electronic system for earmuffs was designed and introduced. The system functions to support the detection of such signals during the use of earmuffs in noisy environments [14]. The ability to perceive back-up alarm signals when using hearing protectors was also assessed [15]. The results of the study cited showed, with some exceptions, that the ability of normal-hearing people to locate a vehicle's back-up alarm signal in the presence of pink noise did not improve when using level-dependent hearing protectors (one model of level-dependent earplugs and earmuffs) in comparison to using passive hearing protectors. In a different study [16], the authors checked the possibility of locating a back-up alarm signal in the presence of noise simulating quarry conditions using one specific model of hearing protector. The localization of the back-up alarm signal was found to be slightly worse when the protector was used in passive mode in comparison to when it was not used, and did not improve after the electronic system was switched on. Vaillancourt et al. [17] compared the effects of different types of signals used as a vehicle back-up alarm signal and concluded that, despite the specific advantages of a signal with broad frequency content, the use of passive hearing protectors more severely affected the detection thresholds when compared to a tonal alarm. Unfortunately, the study did not consider level-dependent hearing protectors.

The purpose of this study was to verify whether the selection of a specific level-dependent hearing protector could be important for the ability to localize the auditory danger signal, represented by a back-up alarm signal, under industrial conditions where impulse noise is generated against a background of continuous noise. We also aimed to examine the impact of changes in the amplification of the electronic system of level-dependent hearing protectors. The tests were carried out in the presence of ambient noise recorded under industrial conditions containing impulse components, which is in contrast to the previous study [11,13–15,17].

2. Materials and Methods

2.1. Ethics and Bioethics Commission

Prior to the commencement of this research, an application for the study was submitted to the Ethics and Bioethics Commission of the Cardinal Stefan Wyszyński University in Warsaw. The commission issued a positive review (No KEiB-22/2017) of the study, providing consent for the implementation and publication of the research results.

2.2. Hearing Protectors Included in the Tests

We considered commercially available level-dependent hearing protectors produced by different manufacturers including four models of earmuffs and one model of earplugs. The hearing protectors studied included: N1 (designation introduced for the purpose of this study and to retain the anonymity of the manufacturer), which were earmuffs designed for military applications, digitally controlled; N2, earmuffs designed for industrial applications, digitally controlled; N3, earmuffs designed for industrial applications, analogically controlled; N4, earmuffs designed for hunting, analogically controlled; and W, earplugs designed for industrial applications with polymer tips, digitally controlled. In the case of the earplugs, the subjects were provided two different sizes of tips. All hearing protectors carried the CE mark (means that specified European Union requirements relating to hearing protectors have been fulfilled), which is a mandatory requirement for a product to be considered as a personal protective device. The hearing protectors included in the study varied in terms of price. The most expensive was more than 11 times more expensive than the cheapest.

The tests were performed in three hearing protector operation modes: passive mode, with the level-dependent system switched off (labelled PASS); level-dependent mode, with maximum amplification in the sound transmission path (labelled LD-MAX); and level-dependent mode with the amplification set to incomplete (approximately half and labelled LD-MID).

2.3. Subjects

The test group consisted of 50 people. The group included an equal proportion of women and men. The age of the subjects ranged from 18 to 42 years old. The subjects qualified for the trial based on the condition of their hearing, which had to meet the requirements of EN 24869-1:1992 [18] regarding a subjective method for the measurement of sound attenuation. This standard requires that the hearing threshold should not be greater than 15 dB for frequencies up to 2000 Hz and no more than 25 dB for frequencies above 2000 Hz.

2.4. Back-Up Alarm

Vehicles used in Polish industrial plants are most often equipped with acoustic signaling devices to warn others about reverse driving, and they generate a tonal signal. Two types of signaling devices can be distinguished that differ in the location of the dominant spectral components of the signal generated. These can be in the 1/3-octave band with a center frequency of 1250 Hz or 3150 Hz. The dominant spectral components in the first type are within the range of 500 to 1500 Hz, as specified in ISO 7731:2003 [19], in reference to one of the conditions to be met by an auditory danger signal. In the tests, we used a vehicle's back-up alarm signal that met the required standards.

The system designed to reproduce the back-up alarm signal was based on eight M-Audio Bx5 D2 loudspeaker sets (inMusic Brands, Cumberland, RI, USA) that were placed at the height of a sitting person's head. The M-Audio loudspeaker sets were evenly distributed in eight directions, every 45°, where the first loudspeaker set was placed directly in front of the subject's face. This direction was marked as 0°. Figure 1 provides a graphic representation of the directions from which the back-up alarm signal was reproduced. The distance between the loudspeaker sets and the point determined by the center of the person's head was 1.8 m. The electrical signal was fed to the inputs of the M-Audio loudspeaker sets from a MOTU 24I/O audio interface (MOTU, Cambridge, MA, USA). The sampling frequency was 44,100 Hz. For the purpose of testing the perception of back-up alarm signals, 15 different sequences of these signals were prepared. The order of signal reproduction from individual directions was randomly determined. The test of each elementary measurement situation was performed based on a sequence of 24 instances of a back-up alarm signal, as this signal was reproduced from eight directions, and the measurement was repeated three times in each of the directions.

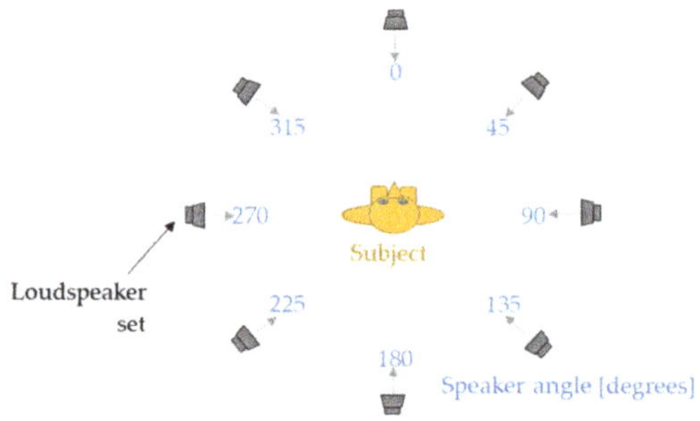

Figure 1. The directions from which the back-up alarm signal was reproduced and the location of the subject in the experimental setup.

2.5. Acquisition of the Direction Indications Provided by Subjects

The subjects indicated the directions from which a back-up alarm signal was received by pressing a button on a panel of eight push buttons arranged in a circle, reflecting the possible locations of the sound source. The response panel has been described in detail in a previous study [20].

2.6. Reflecting Industrial Noise Conditions

To reflect the presence of noise generated in industrial situations under laboratory conditions, a virtual acoustic environment using ambisonic technology was developed. The experimental setup was located in an acoustic chamber in the Tech-Safe-Bio CIOP-PIB Laboratory (Central Institute for Labour Protection—National Research Institute, Warsaw, Poland) [21]. The ambient noise obtained was reproduced in the experimental setup based on the recording of noise generated during metal processing at a forge. The ambient noise consisted of acoustic impulses generated by drop-forging hammers against a background of continuous noise. The recording was performed with the use of a Sennheiser AMBEO VR Mic ambisonic microphone (Sennheiser Electronic GmbH & CO KG, Wennebostel, Germany) connected to a Tascam DR-680 MkII recorder (TEAC Corporation, Tokyo, Japan).

A total of 17 Avantone MixCube loudspeakers (Avantone Pro, Tallman, NY, USA) were placed in the test room to reproduce ambient noise. The loudspeakers were located in a sphere with a 2-m radius in relation to the center of the seated person's (the subject's) head. Eight loudspeakers were placed circumferentially directly above the M-Audio BX5 D2 loudspeaker sets (inMusic Brands). Another four Avantone MixCube loudspeakers (Avantone Pro) were placed on the floor, and another four above the test subject (45 degrees upward in relation to the level of the subject's head). The 17th loudspeaker was placed directly above the subject's head. The sound reproduction system was supplemented with two sets of Nexo LS600/PS8 subwoofers (Nexo, Plailly, France). A photograph of the experimental setup during the tests is shown in Figure 2. The ambient noise was reproduced using a Rapture 3D Ambisonic Player (Blue Ripple Sound Limited, London, UK) at a sampling frequency of 48 kHz.

The A-weighted equivalent sound pressure level of the ambient noise reproduced on the experimental setup was 84.8 dB. The C-weighted peak sound pressure level was 111.8 dB. The values of the noise parameters were monitored before the beginning of each measurement session. The measurements were recorded at the location of the subject's head while the subject was absent by using a SVAN 979 Class 1 sound level meter (SVANTEK Sp. z o.o., Warsaw, Poland).

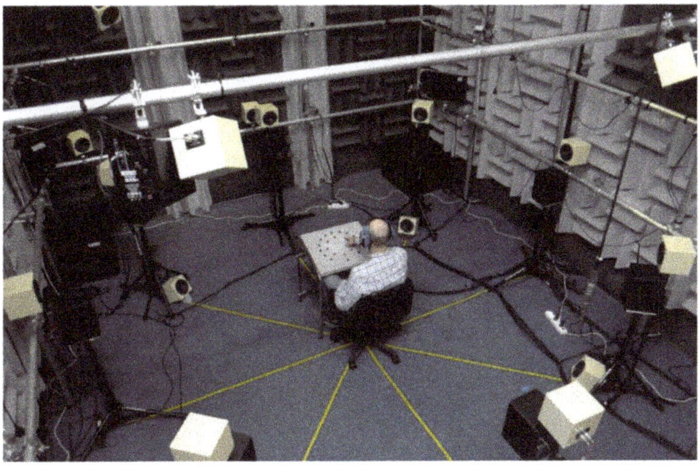

Figure 2. The experimental setup during the back-up alarm signal localization tests, performed with the participation of a subject wearing a level-dependent hearing protector.

2.7. Test Method

Before commencing the tests, each subject completed a training session. Each subject participated in the measurements for all five hearing protectors (listed in Section 2.2) in each of the three operation modes.

Industrial noise conditions were reflected during the tests. The ambient noise was reproduced according to the rules defined in Section 2.6. A back-up alarm signal was reproduced against the background of this noise according to randomly defined sequences (as described in Section 2.4). The task of the subject sitting in the center of the experimental setup was to indicate the direction of the back-up alarm signal by pressing the appropriate key on the panel (as described in Section 2.5). During the tests, each subject provided 360 indications (a sequence of 24 signals in each basic measurement situation for the three operation modes of each of the hearing protectors, for five different hearing protectors).

To analyze the obtained data, we created a direction recognition index for the back-up alarm signal. This index expresses, as a percentage, the ratio of the number of correct indications of the direction (or directions) in a given measurement situation to the number of all reproductions of the back-up alarm signal from the direction (or directions) considered in this situation.

2.8. Statistical Analysis

To determine which changes in the value of the direction recognition index between particular measurement situations should be considered significant, we completed a statistical analysis of the obtained data. For this purpose, a Wilcoxon test (equivalent to the Mann-Whitney *U* test) was used. The calculations were performed using MATLAB R2017b (version 9.3) with the Statistics and Machine Learning Toolbox (MathWorks Inc., Natick, MA, USA).

3. Results

3.1. Distribution of Indications between Individual Directions

The first step of the back-up alarm signal perception assessment involved analyzing how the indications of the subjects changed if the signal was reproduced from a specific direction. This analysis enabled the identification of the regularity of level-dependent earmuffs (N1–N4). In situations where the danger signal was reproduced from the 0° and 180° directions, in the majority of cases, a significant number of indications did not only reflect the direction from which the signal was played. Correct indications of the 0° direction were noted for 20–40%, 31–47%, and 25–45% of cases for earmuffs used in the PASS, LD-MAX, and LD-MID modes, respectively. Correct indications of the 180° direction were slightly more frequent and their numbers expressed as a percentage were 45–53%, 26–53%, and 26–67% for the PASS, LD-MAX, and LD-MID modes, respectively. In the case of these two back-up alarm signal reproduction directions, 0° and 180°, the most frequent errors were of the 'front–back' type. This means that the subjects had problems in determining whether the back-up alarm signal came from in front or from behind. This situation is represented by the example in Figure 3a, where, for the back-up alarm signal from the 0° direction, the indications of this direction given by all subjects accounted for 39% of all indications, whereas the indications of the 180° direction were only six percentage points lower, representing 33% of all indications. Indications for the other directions in any situation did not exceed 10% of the overall number of indications.

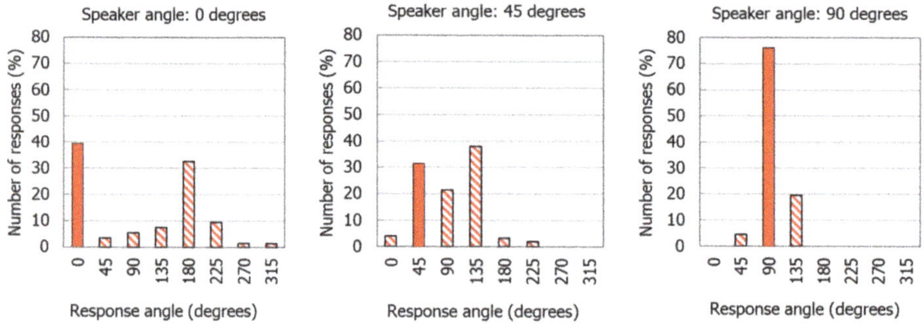

(a) (b) (c)

Figure 3. Distribution of the indications given by users of the N2 earmuffs in the LD-MAX mode when the back-up alarm signal was reproduced from a certain angle: (**a**) 0°, (**b**) 45°, and (**c**) 90°. LD-MAX—level-dependent mode, with maximum amplification in the sound transmission path.

An even worse situation occurred when the back-up alarm signal was reproduced from the directions at the angles of 45° and 315°. In these directions, the direction of the signal was reproduced was not the one that was indicated the most often. The subjects made errors in changing the direction from the front to the direction from the back of the person and indicated the directions of sound as adjacent to the directions from which the signal was played. An example of this situation is shown in Figure 3b, where, in the case of the back-up alarm signal coming from the 45° direction, the correct indications of this direction identified by all subjects were not the most frequent (31%). A larger number of indications, at 38%, was in the direction deviated from the axis crossing the person's ears by 45°; however, not from the front, but from beyond at 135°. Therefore, these were front–back type errors. A significant proportion of indications (21%) were in the direction adjacent (90°) to the direction from which the signal to be recognized was reproduced.

However, in the case of directions located to the side of the person, i.e., from directions at angles of 90° and 270°, the situation was different, since the majority of the indications of the subjects when the signals were reproduced from these directions were correct. Therefore, the correct indication of the 90° direction occurred in up to 81% of cases. This occurred when using the N3 earmuffs in LD-MAX mode. This was also the case for the 270° direction. In the case of these two directions (90° and 270°), the histograms were the slimmest. An example of this is shown in Figure 3c, where, in the case of the back-up alarm signal from the direction at the 90° angle (left side of the person), the correct indications of this direction given by all subjects were by far the most frequent, representing 76% of the total. For the other two directions of 45° and 135° (adjacent to direction 90°), 5% and 19% of indications were given, respectively.

The widest histogram distributions were obtained with the N4 earmuffs and indications regarding the reproduction of the back-up alarm signal from the directions at angles 0° and 180°. In such situations, the indications ranged over all eight directions. An example of this situation is shown in Figure 4a. For the earmuffs (N4), there were a significant number of front–back errors, which occurred for the back-up alarm signal reproduction directions at the angles of 45° and 315°. Then, in all operation modes of the N4 earmuffs, the majority of subjects responded that the signal came from the direction of 135° instead of 45° (as shown in Figure 4b) and similarly from the direction of 225° instead of 315°.

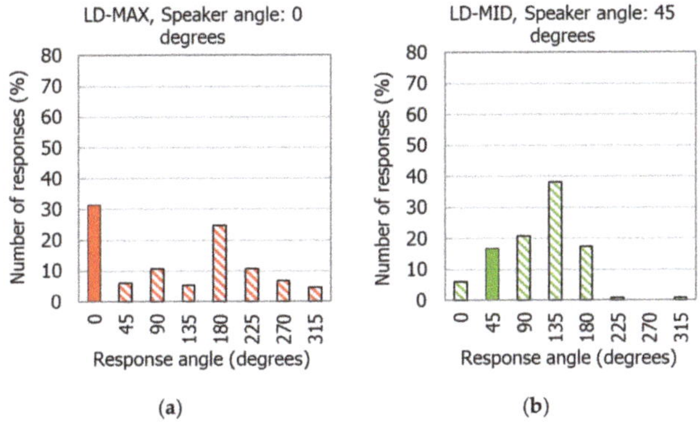

Figure 4. Distribution of the indications given by users of the N4 earmuffs, when the back-up alarm signal was reproduced from a certain angle: (**a**) 0° (earmuffs used in the LD-MAX mode) and (**b**) 45° (earmuffs used in the LD-MID mode). LD-MAX—level-dependent mode, with maximum amplification in the sound transmission path; LD-MID—level-dependent mode with the amplification set to incomplete (approximately half).

In the case of the W earplugs, the situation was different from the earmuffs. The direction most frequently indicated by the subject was almost always the direction from which the back-up alarm signal was reproduced. The histogram bar showing the direction from which the signal was reproduced was almost always (23 out of 24 histograms) the highest of the eight directions considered. For the directions from angles of 90° and 270° (at the side of the person), nearly 90% of the indications were correct, whereas the lowest frequency of correct direction recognition (37%) was for the angle of 0° when the earplugs were used in passive mode.

Similar direction recognition observations could be made when the signal came from the front/behind or from side of the person were also made in mean absolute error analysis. Mean absolute error was calculated as the mean angular distance between response and the direction from which signal was reproduced. The examples of error values are shown in Figure 5a,b, respectively, for N2 earmuffs and W earplugs. The greatest errors were observed for angles of 0° and 180°, regardless of the model of the level-dependent hearing protector. For angles of 90° and 270° mean error values were the smallest and they were approximately equal to the angular resolution used in the experiment (45°).

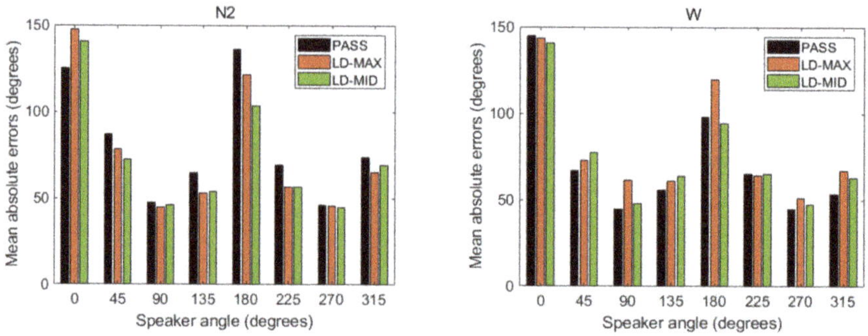

(a) (b)

Figure 5. Mean absolute errors calculated for the indications given by users of the N2 earmuffs (**a**); and W earplugs (**b**). PASS—with the level-dependent system switched off. LD-MAX—level-dependent mode, with maximum amplification in the sound transmission path; LD-MID—level-dependent mode with the amplification set to incomplete (approximately half).

3.2. Direction Recognition Index

3.2.1. Global Index Values

During the tests, all subjects provided a total of 18,000 indications; 8181 of which were correct, meaning the directions of the back-up alarm signal were correctly identified. Therefore, the global direction recognition index of the back-up alarm (as defined in Section 2.7) was 45.5%. For each of the hearing protectors, the subjects provided 3600 indications. The values of the direction recognition index determined for all results obtained for each hearing protector were: 41.6% (N1), 45.0% (N2), 45.9% (N3), 38.6% (N4), and 56.1% (W). The numbers indicate that the correct recognition of the direction of the back-up alarm signal is possible in more cases when level-dependent earplugs are used rather than level-dependent earmuffs.

3.2.2. Index Values Broken Down by the Different Modes of Using Hearing Protectors

To compare the influence of different modes of level-dependent hearing protectors on the ability to correctly recognize the direction of sound, the values of the direction recognition index were determined with a breakdown by these modes. The values obtained are shown in Figure 6. Every point in the chart was created based on the 1200 indications provided by the subjects. Overall, the use of earplugs enabled the correct localization of the back-up alarm signal in a greater number of cases than with earmuffs, regardless of the operation mode of the hearing protectors. Differences in the number of correct indications of the back-up alarm signal direction between the different operation modes of the hearing protectors was as low as 2.3 percentage points (N2 earmuffs). However, these differences could exceed 15 percentage points (N4 earmuffs).

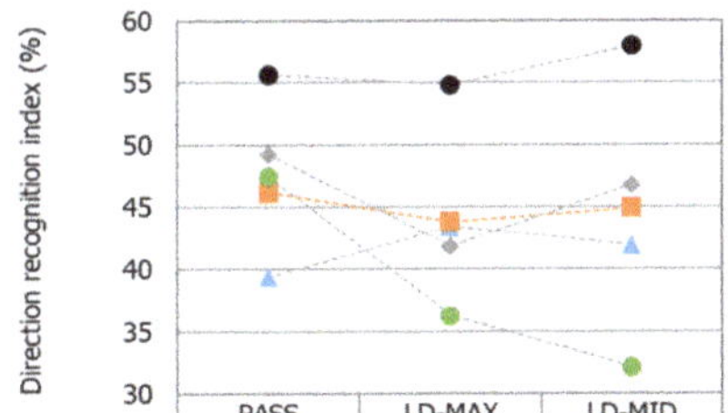

	PASS	LD-MAX	LD-MID
N1	39.3	43.4	41.9
N2	46.2	43.8	44.9
N3	49.3	41.8	46.8
N4	47.5	36.3	32.2
W	55.7	54.8	57.9

Figure 6. Values of the direction recognition index determined for all of the measurement data obtained for each of the hearing protectors with a breakdown by the operation mode of these protectors. PASS—with the level-dependent system switched off. LD-MAX—level-dependent mode, with maximum amplification in the sound transmission path; LD-MID—level-dependent mode with the amplification set to incomplete (approximately half).

3.2.3. Values of the Index Determined by Breakdown by Different Directions of Back-Up Alarm Signal Reproduction

The diagrams shown in Figures 7–9 present the results obtained in each of the three operation modes of the hearing protectors with a breakdown by the individual directions of the back-up alarm signal source. The results of the analysis, indicating which changes in the values of the direction recognition index should be deemed as significant, are presented in Table 1.

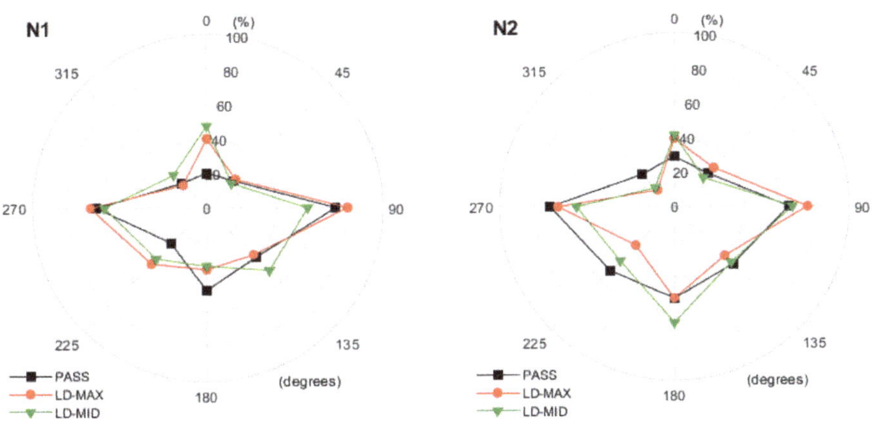

(a) (b)

Figure 7. The values of the direction recognition index determined for different directions when using earmuffs in different modes: (**a**) N1 and (**b**) N2. PASS—with the level-dependent system switched off. LD-MAX—level-dependent mode, with maximum amplification in the sound transmission path; LD-MID—level-dependent mode with the amplification set to incomplete (approximately half).

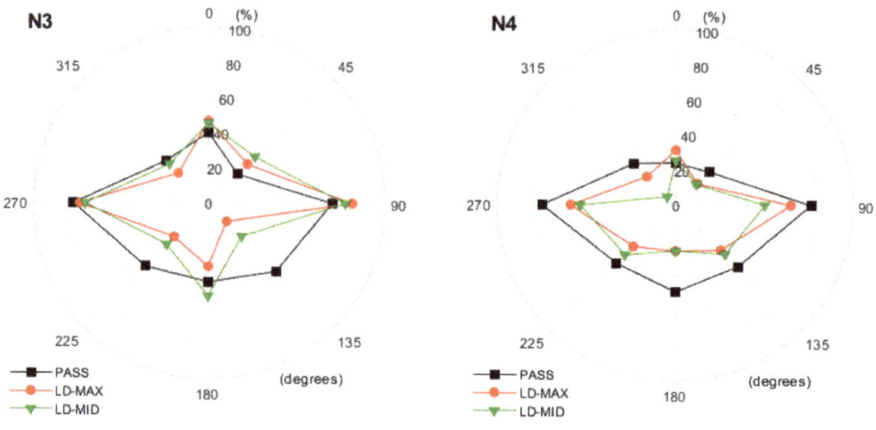

(**a**) (**b**)

Figure 8. The values of the direction recognition index determined for different directions when using earmuffs in different modes: (**a**) N3 and (**b**) N4. PASS—with the level-dependent system switched off. LD-MAX—level-dependent mode, with maximum amplification in the sound transmission path; LD-MID—level-dependent mode with the amplification set to incomplete (approximately half).

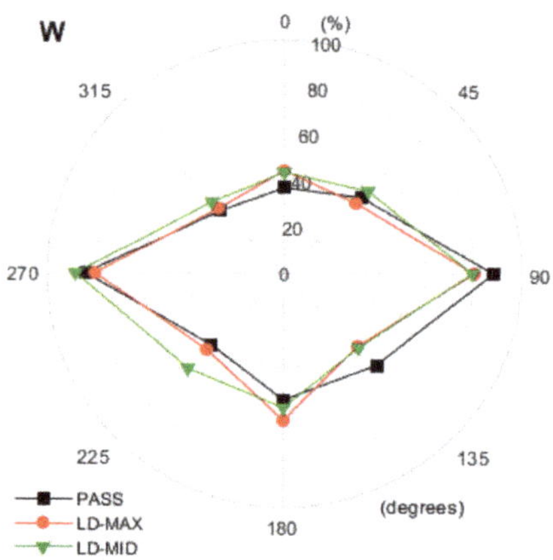

Figure 9. The values of the direction recognition index determined for different directions when using the W earplugs in different modes. PASS—with the level-dependent system switched off. LD-MAX—level-dependent mode, with maximum amplification in the sound transmission path; LD-MID—level-dependent mode with the amplification set to incomplete (approximately half).

Analyzing the data in Figures 7–9, we confirmed that users of level-dependent hearing protectors have the least difficulty in correctly indicating the direction of the back-up alarm signal when the signal is reproduced from the side of the person (angles 90° and 270°). The values of the direction recognition index were lower when the sound was played behind a person and the lowest when it came from directly in front of a person.

Table 1. Determined *p*-values for comparisons between different modes of using level-dependent hearing protectors for individual angles. PASS—with the level-dependent system switched off. LD-MAX—level-dependent mode, with maximum amplification in the sound transmission path; LD-MID—level-dependent mode with the amplification set to incomplete (approximately half).

Angle (°)	PASS –LD-MAX	PASS –LD-MID	LD-MAX –LD-MID	PASS –LD-MAX	PASS –LD-MID	LD-MAX –LD-MID
		N1 [1]			N2	
0	**<0.01** [2]	**<0.01**	0.20	0.05	**0.02**	0.73
45	0.78	0.67	0.48	0.37	0.51	0.12
90	0.17	**<0.01**	**<0.01**	**0.04**	0.72	0.10
135	0.72	0.06	**0.03**	0.25	0.82	0.35
180	**0.04**	**0.01**	0.72	1.00	**0.01**	**0.01**
225	**<0.01**	**0.02**	0.49	**<0.01**	0.17	**0.02**
270	0.55	0.41	0.15	0.38	**0.01**	0.06
315	0.77	0.17	0.10	**0.01**	**0.02**	0.62
		N3			N4	
0	0.25	0.35	0.82	0.16	0.79	0.25
45	0.12	**0.01**	0.28	0.05	**0.04**	0.88
90	**0.02**	0.15	0.39	**0.03**	**<0.01**	**0.01**
135	**<0.01**	**<0.01**	**0.01**	**0.02**	0.08	0.55
180	0.13	0.17	**<0.01**	**<0.01**	**<0.01**	1.00
225	**<0.01**	**<0.01**	0.26	**0.02**	0.25	0.23
270	0.51	0.19	0.52	**<0.01**	**<0.01**	0.35
315	0.06	0.62	0.16	**0.04**	**<0.01**	**<0.01**
		W				
0	0.20	0.24	0.91			
45	0.56	0.49	0.20			
90	0.06	**0.04**	0.89			
135	0.05	0.07	0.91			
180	0.13	0.56	0.35			
225	0.64	**0.02**	0.05			
270	0.37	0.32	0.06			
315	0.81	0.35	0.48			

[1] Hearing protector; [2] *p*-Values for comparisons that are significant ($p < 0.05$) are in bold font.

When using level-dependent hearing protectors, it is important to determine whether the change in the operation mode of the protector significantly affects the user's ability to correctly localize the back-up alarm signal. The data presented in Figures 7–9 indicate that, in many situations, a change in the mode of use of a hearing protector does not affect the direction recognition index. However, this is not a rule. For example, in the case of the N1 earmuffs (Figure 7a) and the 0° direction, the change from passive (PASS) to level-dependent mode led to a 27 percentage points and 20 percentage points increase in the number of correct indications for LD-MID and LD-MAX, respectively. These increases in the direction recognition index values, according to the data from Table 1, were statistically significant. Whereas, in the case of 90°, the change from the PASS to LD-MID mode resulted in a reduction in the number of correct indications by 16 percentage points, while at the angle of 180°, both variants of using the N1 earmuffs in level-dependent mode were less advantageous than in passive mode. This case was in contrast to the one observed for the angle of 225°. Here, in contrast to passive mode, both level-dependent modes were advantageous. The increase (statistically significant) was 13 percentage points (LD-MID) and 17 percentage points (LD-MAX). The results showed that the use of level-dependent mode relative to passive mode, depending on the specific angle at which the back-up alarm signal was received, resulted in an increase or decrease in the number of correct indications of the direction. In the case of the N1 earmuffs, statistically significant changes occurred in 7 out of 16 possible cases (eight related to the LD-MAX mode and eight to the LD-MID mode). An increase in the number of correct indications was observed in four cases and a decrease in three. A similar situation occurred in the case of the N2 earmuffs (Figure 7b), where statistically significant changes occurred in 7 out of 16 cases. In three of these cases, the number of correct indications increased, and in four cases, this number decreased. The use of the N3 earmuffs resulted in only 6 of 16 statistically significant increases (two cases) or decreases (four cases) in the number of correct indications. With the N3 earmuffs (Figure 8a), the reduction in the direction recognition index related to the operation in level-dependent mode in contrast to passive mode produced relatively high values ranging from 17 to 40 percentage points, observed for the angles of 135° and 225°. The values of the advantageous changes (increase in the value of the direction recognition index) were 14 (LD-MID, 45°) and 11 (LD-MAX, 90°) percentage points. For the N4 earmuffs (Figure 8b), a significant number of cases, 11 out of 16 possible, were identified where the impact of changing the earmuff's mode from the PASS to the LD-MAX or LD-MID was statically significant. All 11 changes were unfavorable; after activating the level-dependent mode, we observed that the number of correct indications of the back-up alarm signal direction decreased.

Results obtained during the use of W earplugs (Figure 9) indicate that a change in the mode of their use was of little significance. Statistically significant changes in the direction recognition index occurred only after the change from the PASS to LD-MID mode at the angles of 90° (decrease by 9 percentage points) and 225° (increase by 14 percentage points).

4. Discussion

The analysis of the changes in the indications of the 50 subjects between the individual eight directions shows that, for the 0° angle (straight in front of the person) and 180° (behind the person), in the majority of cases using level-dependent earmuffs, a considerable number of 'front–back' errors were observed. The people who participated in the study had problems in determining whether the back-up alarm signal came from the front or was possibly from behind. These types of errors (in addition to the indication of adjacent directions) were also frequent in the case of the directions of 45° and 315°. These situations were opposite to the cases when the back-up alarm signal was played from directions located at the sides of a person, i.e., from directions at the angles of 90° and 270°. The direction of signals reproduced from these directions was indicated correctly in the vast majority of cases.

These results provide the first significant differentiation between level-dependent earmuffs and earplugs. For the earplugs, in nearly all of the situations considered, the direction from which the signal was reproduced was indicated almost always more frequently than the remaining seven directions. For the earmuffs, this was not always true because, for the angles of 45° and 315°, the direction from which the signal to be recognized was reproduced was not indicated most frequently. The conclusions resulting from the distribution of indications for the individual directions are partly consistent with other studies, where the authors claimed that the problems in locating the sources of sound occurred particularly often on the front–back axis [22]. In addition, the back direction is indicated by the subjects less frequently when the sound comes from the front rather than the other way around [23]. In this study, the correct indications of the 180° direction were insignificantly more frequent than for the 0° direction. However, this pertained to different situations than the work mentioned above, i.e., during the use of hearing protectors.

Little data exist on sound direction recognition tests for level-dependent hearing protectors. However, the results obtained in this study can be referred, to a limited extent, to the data available. A study where the direction of sound reproduction of cocking an AK-47 (70 dB) in the presence of broadband masking noise (55 dB) was analyzed, presented the indications of 10 subjects with the reproduction of the test signal from directions 30° apart [13]. The analysis of the diagrams regarding the use of level-dependent earplugs (EB-15 earplugs and earplugs designed by the authors of the above-mentioned study) enabled the identification of a similar distribution of direction indications to the ones obtained in this paper. Despite of different test conditions, for the direction at the angle of 0°, a significant number of indications fell not only in this direction, but also at 180°. The same was true when the sound was reproduced from the direction of 180°. In addition, for the 30° direction, Brown et al. [13] reported the occurrence of front–back errors and the indication of adjacent directions, which is similar to the situation that occurred in this study when the back-up alarm signal was reproduced from the 45° direction. We observed that the relatively smallest diversity of indications in Brown et al. [13], where the test signal was reproduced from directions of 90° and 270°, corresponded to the slimmest shapes of the graphs in the histograms obtained in this study (Figure 3c).

In this study, we determined the direction recognition index for the back-up alarm signal. The values of this index, which were determined with a breakdown by hearing protector operation modes (i.e., set globally without dividing the individual directions of the alarm signal), showed that regardless of the mode of these protectors, it is possible to correctly localize the back-up alarm signal in a much larger number of cases when level-dependent earplugs are used compared to when level-dependent earmuffs are used. The average value of the index for the earplugs (with consideration of all three modes of operation) exceeded the average value for all four earmuffs and their modes of operation by more than 13 percentage points. The range of the direction recognition index values between the different operation modes of the hearing protectors was relatively small (two to four percentage points) for the N1 and N2 earmuffs and the W earplugs. Slightly greater differences in the direction recognition index between the modes were observed for the N3 earmuffs (seven percentage points). The largest span, exceeding 15 percentage points, was observed for the N4 earmuffs.

This global analysis of the results indicated that among the hearing protectors, the operation mode for some (N1, N2 earmuffs and W earplug) has an insignificant impact on the user's ability to localize the back-up alarm signal. The mode of use of the hearing protectors may also influence, to a certain extent, the ability to recognize the direction of a sound. This was the case with the N3 earmuffs, for which the level-dependent mode resulted in a noticeable deterioration in the ability to localize the back-up alarm signal. Additionally, the type of hearing protectors may significantly influence the possibility of recognizing the direction of back-up alarm signals. Hearing protectors may include those (N4) that significantly impair the user's ability to recognize the direction of the sound when switched from passive to level-dependent mode. This deterioration occurred with both the maximum and incomplete amplification in the level-dependent system of the N4 earmuffs, and amounted to above 11 and 15 percentage points in comparison to passive mode, respectively.

The results published in Alali and Casali [15] can be compared with the values of the direction recognition index measured as part of this study. In Alali and Casali [15], the correct recognition of the direction of the signal in the presence of pink noise with an A-weighted sound pressure level of 90 dB was 47.7% for the level-dependent earmuffs and 62.2% for the level-dependent earplugs. Within the framework of this study, for earmuffs, the direction recognition index (global values) ranged from 38.6% to 45.9%, and 56.1% for the earplugs. Considering the differences in the test conditions and the test facilities themselves, the results obtained can be regarded as comparable. In another study [11] where the recognition of sound directions, including the front–back, left-right, and up-down directions, was examined, the results from 20 subjects showed that the number of correct indications for level-dependent earplugs was about 42.5% and 31.5% for level-dependent earmuffs. Again, the test conditions (eight loudspeakers that were the source of the test signal with a 230 ms burst of wideband noise) or the models of the hearing protectors differed from those in this study, but the tendency of the relationship between the earplugs and the earmuffs is similar.

The determination of the direction recognition index for the back-up alarm signal, broken down by direction, enabled repeating the previous general observation that users of level-dependent hearing protectors have the least difficulty in correctly indicating the direction of the back-up alarm signal when it is reproduced from the side of a person (angles of 90° and 270°). The values of the direction recognition index were lower when the sound was played behind a person (180°) and the lowest when the source was directly in front of the person (0°). For the number of errors falling on the directions of 0° and 180°, and 90° and 270°, a similar distribution of results was obtained in the aforementioned study [13]. The root mean square error (RMSE), defining the mean angular distance of responses from the target angle, for the level-dependent EB-15 earplugs was about 38° and 55°, when the sound came from the front and back directions, respectively, and about 9° and 11° when the sound came from the right and left sides of a person, respectively. However, these results are not fully comparable with the results of our study as a different measure was applied to different models of test earplugs and different test conditions. Nevertheless, the ratio of the average number of incorrect indications of the front–back directions to incorrect indications of the left–right directions in both studies indicated the same trend, which was 3.1 in this study and 4.7 for the cited study [13].

Alali and Casali [15] demonstrated, with some exceptions, that the ability of normal-hearing people to locate a vehicle's back-up alarm signal in the presence of pink noise did not improve when using level-dependent hearing protectors (earplugs and earmuffs) in comparison to the use of passive hearing protectors. A similar finding was reported by Giguère et al. [16], where the situation did not improve after switching from passive mode to the electronic system mode. This conclusion was also reached in this study with regard to earplugs, where their operation mode had practically no impact on the measured values of the direction recognition index. For earmuffs, in this study and in certain cases, the change from passive mode to level-dependent mode (maximum or incomplete amplification in the level-dependent system) resulted in statically significant differences in the value of the direction recognition index. During the use of the N1 and N2 earmuffs, statistically significant changes occurred in 44% of cases; however, the number of changes resulting in increasing the direction recognition index value roughly balanced the number of changes resulting in a decrease in the index value. Using the N3 earmuffs in level-dependent mode resulted in a change in the direction recognition index in almost 38% of the cases, whereas the deterioration of the ability to recognize the direction was twice more often (four instances of decreases) than the improvement (two instances of increases) when compared to passive mode. A slightly different situation was observed for the N4 earmuffs, where there was a total of 69% of cases where the ability to correctly recognize the direction of sound was statistically significantly different from passive mode, but all of the changes were negative, meaning the changes resulted in a decrease in the value of the direction recognition index. The analysis of the use of earmuffs in level-dependent mode in comparison to passive mode, with a breakdown by different directions, demonstrated that in a certain number of cases (from 38% to 69%), the mode affected the ability of the users to localize the back-up alarm signal, which differed from the conclusion drawn in the cited study [15]. Notably, the authors [15] used different ambient noise (pink noise with A-weighted sound pressure levels of 60 dB and 90 dB), a different back-up alarm signal, and included hearing protectors (one model of a specific type of hearing protector) other than the ones used in this study.

This issue is important from the perspective of ensuring safety in a workplace. The methodology used in this study can be used to assess the ability of workers using level-dependent hearing protectors to recognize the direction of an auditory danger signal. Test results indicate that the model of a level-dependent hearing protector available to a worker will significantly affect their ability to localize the vehicle's back-up alarm signal. However, the tests carried out under laboratory conditions cannot fully replicate the conditions encountered in an industrial facility. The localization of auditory danger signals by users of level-dependent hearing protectors may be, to some degree, worse in real-life conditions than in experiments conducted in a laboratory because the attention of the subjects who participated in the experiment was entirely focused on the task of sound localization. In real industrial conditions, however, the workers are focused on their jobs.

5. Conclusions

The tests enabled the differentiation of the level-dependent hearing protectors in terms of the ability to assess the direction of an auditory danger signal, represented by a back-up alarm signal, by the user of these protectors under industrial conditions where impulse noise is generated against a background of continuous noise.

We found that the operation mode of level-dependent earplugs, i.e., passive or level-dependent, did not significantly affect the ability to correctly indicate the direction of a back-up alarm signal.

The assessment of the earmuffs was complicated. The analysis of a breakdown by the individual directions indicated that, in a significant number of cases, there was a change in the operation mode result depending on the direction of the back-up alarm signal, either by an increase or decrease in the ability to properly recognize this direction. The global assessment showed that depending on the model of the earmuffs, the impact of switching on level-dependent mode may be insignificant, but it may be clearly noticeable, or even result in a significant deterioration of the ability to recognize the direction of the back-up alarm signal.

The above conclusions on level-dependent earplugs and earmuffs mean that, in workplaces where it is important for the safety of a worker using hearing protection to correctly recognize the direction of a back-up alarm signal, the choice of a specific model of these protectors is of crucial importance.

Author Contributions: Conceptualization, R.M. and E.K.; Formal analysis, R.M.; Investigation, R.M. and E.K.; Methodology, R.M. and E.K.; Project administration, R.M.; Visualization, R.M.; Writing—original draft, R.M.; Writing—review & editing, R.M. and E.K.

Funding: This paper is based on the results of a research task carried out within the scope of the fourth stage of the National Program "Improvement of safety and working conditions" partly supported in 2017–2019—within the scope of research and development—by the Ministry of Science and Higher Education/National Centre for Research and Development. The Central Institute for Labour Protection, National Research Institute is the Program's main coordinator.

Conflicts of Interest: The authors declare no conflict of interest.

References

1. Mrena, R.; Savolainen, S.; Pirvola, U.; Ylikoski, J. Characteristics of acute acoustical trauma in the Finnish Defense Forces. *Int. J. Audiol.* **2004**, *43*, 177–181. [CrossRef] [PubMed]
2. Mlynski, R.; Kozlowski, E.; Adamczyk, J. Assessment of impulse noise hazard and the use of hearing protection devices in workplaces where forging hammers are used. *Arch. Acoust.* **2014**, *39*, 73–79. [CrossRef]
3. Tufts, J.B.; Hamilton, M.A.; Ucci, A.J.; Rubas, J. Evaluation by industrial workers of passive and level-dependent hearing protection devices. *Noise Health* **2011**, *13*, 26–36. [CrossRef]
4. McKinley, R.L.; Gallagher, H.L.; Theis, M.; Murphy, W.J. Continuous and impulsive noise attenuation performance of passive level dependent earplugs. *J. Acoust. Soc. Am.* **2012**, 132. [CrossRef]
5. EN 352-4:2001 Hearing Protectors. *General Requirements Part 4: Level-Dependent Ear-Muffs*; European Committee for Standardization: Brussels, Belgium, 2001.
6. EN 352-7:2002 Hearing Protectors. *General Requirements Part 7: Level-Dependent Ear-Plugs*; European Committee for Standardization: Brussels, Belgium, 2002.
7. Murphy, W.J.; Flamme, G.A.; Meinke, D.K.; Sondergaard, J.; Finan, D.S.; Lankford, J.E.; Khan, A.; Vernon, J.; Stewart, M. Measurement of impulse peak insertion loss for four hearing protection devices in field conditions. *Int. J. Audiol.* **2012**, *51* (Suppl. 1), 31–42. [CrossRef]
8. Murphy, W.J.; Fackler, C.J.; Berger, E.H.; Shaw, P.B.; Stergar, M. Measurement of impulse peak insertion loss from two acoustic test fixtures and four hearing protector conditions with an acoustic shock tube. *Noise Health* **2015**, *17*, 364–373. [CrossRef] [PubMed]
9. Fackler, C.J.; Berger, E.H.; Murphy, W.J.; Stergara, M.E. Spectral analysis of hearing protector impulsive insertion loss. *Int. J. Audiol.* **2017**, *56* (Suppl. 1), 13–21. [CrossRef]
10. Lee, K.; Casali, J.G. Development of an auditory situation awareness test battery for advanced hearing protectors and TCAPS: Detection subtest of DRILCOM (detection-recognition/identification-localization-communication). *Int. J. Audiol.* **2017**, *56* (Suppl. 1), 22–33. [CrossRef]
11. Zimpfer, V.; Sarafian, D. Impact of hearing protection devices on sound localization performance. *Front. Neurosci.* **2014**, *8*, 135. [CrossRef] [PubMed]
12. Casali, J.G.; Robinette, M.B. Effects of user training with electronically-modulated sound transmission hearing protectors and the open ear on horizontal localization ability. *Int. J. Audiol.* **2015**, *54* (Suppl. 1), 37–45. [CrossRef]
13. Brown, A.D.; Beemer, B.T.; Greene, N.T.; Argo IV, T.; Meegan, G.D.; Tollin, D.J. Effects of Active and Passive Hearing Protection Devices on Sound Source Localization, Speech Recognition, and Tone Detection. *PLoS ONE* **2015**, *10*, e0136568. [CrossRef] [PubMed]

14. Bernstein, E.R.; Brammer, A.J.; Yu, G. Augmented warning sound detection for hearing protectors. *J. Acoust. Soc. Am.* **2014**, *135*, EL29–EL34. [CrossRef] [PubMed]
15. Alali, K.A.; Casali, J.G. The challenge of localizing vehicle backup alarms: Effects of passive and electronic hearing protectors, ambient noise level, and backup alarm spectral content. *Noise Health* **2011**, *13*, 99–112. [CrossRef] [PubMed]
16. Giguère, C.; Laroche, C.; Vaillancourt, V.; Shmigol, E.; Vaillancourt, T.; Chiasson, J.; Rozon-Gauthier, V. A multidimensional evaluation of auditory performance in one powered electronic level-dependent hearing protector. In Proceedings of the 19th International Congress on Sound and Vibration 2012, Vilnius, Lithuania, 8–12 July 2012.
17. Vaillancourt, V.; Nélisse, H.; Laroche, C.; Giguère, C.; Boutin, J.; Laferrière, P. Comparison of sound propagation and perception of three types of backup alarms with regards to worker safety. *Noise Health* **2013**, *15*, 420–436. [CrossRef] [PubMed]
18. EN 24869-1:1992. *Acoustics—Hearing Protectors—Subjective Method for the Measurement of Sound Attenuation*; European Committee for Standardization: Brussels, Belgium, 1992.
19. ISO 7731:2003. *Ergonomics—Danger Signals for Public and Work Areas—Auditory Danger Signals*; International Organization for Standardization: Geneva, Switzerland, 2003.
20. Mlynski, R.; Kozlowski, E. Examination of recognition of the direction from which an industrial truck auditory danger signal was coming. *Meas. Autom. Monit.* **2017**, *63*, 6–9.
21. Morzynski, L.; Pleban, D.; Szczepanski, G.; Mlynski, R. Laboratory for testing sound perception in virtual acoustic working environment, In Proceedings of the 48st Spanish Congress on Acoustics, TecniAcustica 2017, A Coruna, Spain, 3–6 October 2017.
22. Ovcharenko, A.; Cho, S.J.; Chong, U.P. Front–back confusion resolution in three-dimensional sound localization using databases built with a dummy head. *J. Acoust. Soc. Am.* **2007**, *122*, 489–495. [CrossRef] [PubMed]
23. Hill, P.A.; Nelson, P.A.; Kirkeby, O.; Hamada, H. Resolution of front-back confusion in virtual acoustic imaging systems. *J. Acoust. Soc. Am.* **2000**, *108*, 2901–2910. [CrossRef] [PubMed]

International Journal of
Environmental Research and Public Health

MDPI

Article

Living the 14/14 Schedule: Qualitative Analysis of the Challenges and Coping Strategies among Families of Offshore Wind Workers

Janika Mette *, Swantje Robelski, Maria Kirchhöfer, Volker Harth and Stefanie Mache

Institute for Occupational and Maritime Medicine, University Medical Centre Hamburg-Eppendorf, 20459 Hamburg, Germany; s.robelski@uke.de (S.R.); maria.kirchhoefer@googlemail.com (M.K.); harth@uke.de (V.H.); s.mache@uke.de (S.M.)

* Correspondence: j.mette@uke.de; Tel.: +49-40-428-37-4256

Received: 14 December 2018; Accepted: 12 January 2019; Published: 16 January 2019

Abstract: Offshore wind workers in Germany usually spend 14 days offshore, alternating with 14 days of spare time at home. The offshore lifestyle may considerably affect offshore workers' partners and families. However, there is a lack of evidence regarding the psychosocial adaptation among offshore wind couples living the 14/14 schedule. The present study intended to offer a contemporary view on the topic from the perspective of the women of offshore workers. Our aim was (1) to examine the perceived features of living the 14/14 schedule, (2) explore women's coping strategies, and (3) investigate their views on the reconciliation of offshore work and partnership/family life. The women reported differentiated views on the benefits and costs associated with their living situation, and stated various coping strategies that facilitated psychosocial adaptation. Despite some burdens, overall, most of the women seemed to have adapted relatively favourably to their lifestyle. This was particularly eased by recent sociological and technological advances, e.g., improved communication technologies.

Keywords: offshore wind industry; reconciliation of offshore work and family life/partnership; coping strategies; psychosocial adaptation; qualitative analysis

1. Introduction

In Germany, coastal areas of the Northern and Baltic Sea offer possibilities for the construction of offshore wind parks. The growth of the German offshore wind industry as part of the green energy revolution is shown by recent figures: in the first six months of 2018, 62 new wind energy convectors were taken into operation [1]. All in all, there were 20 German offshore wind parks by the end of June 2018, generating about 5.300 megawatt (MW) [2]. This development goes along with an increase in employment figures in the branch. Recent estimates indicate that approximately 27,200 workers, most of them men, are currently employed in the German offshore wind industry along the value chain [3].

Offshore wind jobs are associated with many hardships, as well as physical and psychological demands for their employees [4–7]. A key element of working in the German offshore wind branch is the 14/14 work schedule that is applied: offshore wind workers usually spend 14 days offshore, where they work in 12-h-shifts and live on platforms, ships, or neighboring islands. These periods of leave alternate with 14 days of spare time the workers spend at home. From a psychosocial viewpoint, this schedule implies that the workers are confronted with a phase of absolute separation from their families and social environment, followed by an intensive free time period spent together. The 14/14 work schedule is unique and qualitatively different from other work patterns, e.g., work schedules of shift workers or employees with on-call-work. While the latter jobs still allow off-duty time at home each day, offshore workers spend entire weeks away [8]. The 14/14 schedule of workers in the offshore wind industry also deviates considerably from the schedules of other commute workers: the periods of absence of offshore workers are longer than those of commuters coming home for the weekend, but shorter than those of, e.g., seafarers in the maritime sector spending months away from home.

It has recently been noted that the recurrent absences from home represent a job demand for many offshore wind workers, leading to difficulties in reconciling offshore work and family life [5,6,9]. However, the specific lifestyle of the offshore personnel does not only influence the workers themselves, but may also affect their partners and families at home who must deal with the repeated partings, reunions, and phases of intermittent absence. For example, female partners of offshore workers may find it challenging to manage all domestic and parenting tasks alone, to deal with the disruption to shared family activities, and to establish routines in their daily life. Likewise, there could be certain features of the 14/14 schedule that may potentially enhance family life, e.g., the chance to continuously spend intensive time together on a regular basis.

The notion of women experiencing difficulties in dealing with the intermittent absences of their partners is supported by studies carried out in branches with extended periods away from home, e.g., the offshore oil and gas branch and mining industries [8,10–12]. Research from the offshore oil and gas sector has indicated that partners staying at home experience various demands on their own [8], being condensed within the statement of "living two lives". Moreover, early research on the intermittent presence and absence of offshore oil and gas workers has differentiated between three perceived phases for the couples: her single life at home, his offshore life, and their common life together [11]. Specific demands for the women, as revealed in previous studies, consisted of experienced negative emotions, as well as difficulties related to role allocation and family structures [8,13].

Similar to offshore branches, mining industries are also characterized by long distance commuting and specific rosters. They are often referred to as fly-in fly-out (FIFO) branches. The presence of the partner at home is also rather frequent and extended in the FIFO branches in comparison to other industries with prolonged absences. It has been proposed that the living situation of FIFO couples may be described as a cycle with the stages reunion, time commonly spend together, parting, and time alone [12]. In this cycle, every stage was associated with certain demands, adjustments, and negotiations to be made by the couples, and with a range of perceived emotions attached to the transitions.

Although the offshore lifestyle was found to be related to specific demands, an early study among so-called offshore wives did not find differences between the mental and physical health of offshore and onshore wives [14]. Likewise, recent research results suggest a healthy functioning range for psychological wellbeing, relationship satisfaction, and perceptions of family function in FIFO workers and their partners [15]. Further research on the health of FIFO families showed a generally high level of family cohesion, healthy flexibility, and a general contentment with regard to family satisfaction and communication [10].

The ability to deal with the challenges encountered by partners of commute workers may partly depend on the coping strategies being applied. According to the transactional approach of Folkman and Lazarus [16,17], coping can be defined as the cognitive and behavioral efforts made to master, tolerate, or reduce external and internal demands, as well as conflicts among them. Coping efforts may either concern the management of the stress-inducing problem (problem-focused coping) or the regulation of emotions or distresses (emotion-focused coping) related to the situation encountered [16,17]. Research among FIFO families has, for example, indicated the existence of different coping strategies of the couples to deal with the difficulties they have encountered. As described in an interview study, such strategies encompassed maintaining open communication, parting on good terms and without major arguments or conflicts, and generally maintaining a positive attitude towards the situation [12].

Despite existing research studies in FIFO and offshore oil and gas industries, there is a lack of evidence regarding the situation of offshore wind couples living the specific 14/14 schedule. Findings for couples in the oil and gas and FIFO branches are not directly applicable to the situation of couples in the offshore wind industry, since the work schedules in the branches can differ considerably, and employees in the afore mentioned branches usually do not follow the 14/14 work pattern as applied in the German offshore wind branch. Moreover, there are further differences between the branches, e.g., regarding specific regulations, work areas, and work tasks [4,6,18].

In addition, much of the existing research on offshore couples dealing with intermittent absences was conducted in the 80's, 90's, and early 00's, indicating a need for an updated view. Within the last decades, profound organizational, technological, and sociological changes have taken place which pertain to offshore industries [8]. For example, the extension of means of communication provides couples with further possibilities to keep in regular contact. Changes in society have also occurred in terms of women's qualifications and employment rates, making it more likely that women of offshore workers are engaged in paid work. Finally, as a corollary of social changes, women's role models and aspirations have evolved: nowadays, women tend to have stronger expectations as to their husband's involvement in childcare and housekeeping [8]. Such recent changes could have either beneficial or detrimental impacts on the living situation of couples dealing with intermittent absences, which has not yet been empirically explored.

Since a further increase in the offshore wind workforce is to be expected, more couples and families will have to deal with the particularities of living the 14/14 schedule. Therefore, it is crucial to conduct up-to-date research and generate new knowledge on the specific features of this lifestyle. This study intended to offer a contemporary view on the psychosocial adaptation of offshore wind families against the background of the modern society and working world.

The aim of our study was to examine how women of male offshore wind workers perceive the specific features of living the 14/14 schedule. In adherence to the approach by Parkes and colleagues [8], we focused on the different phases of women's daily life, including aspects of being home alone and time spent together as a couple. Moreover, our purpose was to investigate the coping strategies of the women and the couples to deal with the specific living situation. Furthermore, we aimed to explore the women's perceptions of the reconciliation of offshore work and partnership/family life.

We proposed the following research questions:

1. What are the advantages and disadvantages of living the 14/14 schedule as perceived by the women of offshore wind workers, particularly regarding the following phases:
    (1) life without offshore partner;
    (2) life together as a couple/family;
    (3) transition phases (reunion/parting)?
2. What coping strategies are employed by the women and couples to deal with the specific features of living the 14/14 schedule?
3. How do the women judge the reconciliation of offshore work and partnership/family life, including aspects of organizational support?

2. Materials and Methods

2.1. Study Design and Participants

We conducted 14 semi-structured telephone interviews with female partners of German offshore wind workers from January to March 2017. The interviews were carried out by two female psychologists working as researchers in occupational health psychology at the time of the study. We applied purposeful sampling and recruited interviewees of different ages, with and without children, and with offshore partners working in different companies. Participants were eligible if they were female, fluent in the German language, and at least 18 years old. Moreover, the females' partners had to have worked for at least six months in the offshore wind industry, and had to have experiences with the 14/14 work schedule. To recruit suitable participants, we sent invitation mails, emails, and leaflets to German offshore wind workers from different companies who had already participated in a prior interview study conducted at the research institute [5,6]. Moreover, we posted the study information on online platforms and forums for German offshore wind workers. We asked the workers to inform their female partners, who then contacted us directly via mail or telephone. Study participation was voluntary. Prior to the interviews, participants were asked to sign a declaration of informed consent. All participants were in a position to understand and consent to the study requirements, and provided written informed consent. The interviews were conducted until no new themes were identified, i.e., data saturation was reached. They were conducted in German and were tape recorded. Interview length was from 28 to 54 min. Participants were able to terminate the interviews at any time. No non-participants were present during the interviews. No repeat interviews were carried out. Field notes were made immediately after each interview.

2.2. Interview Guideline

A semi-structured interview guideline was developed within the framework of the empirical and theoretical background. The interview topic list is depicted in Table 1. A pre-test interview was performed in order to receive feedback from research colleagues and improve the interview guideline.

Table 1. Interview topic list.

1	Introduction	Study information, confidentiality, informed consent
2	Socio-demographics	*Interviewee*: age, marital status, occupation, work schedule, duration of partnership with offshore partner, shared household, children *Offshore partner*: offshore experience, occupation, work schedule
3	Phase 1: Single life without offshore partner	Advantages and disadvantages of the phase, contact opportunities while partner is offshore
4	Phase 2: Daily life with offshore partner	Advantages and disadvantages of the phase, associated behavior patterns and feelings
5	Phase 3: Transition phase	Associated behavior patterns and feelings, needs and expectations upon the partner's arrival
6	Coping strategies	Strategies of the interviewee and the couple
7	Reconciliation of offshore work and family life/partnership	Reconciliation of offshore work with family life/partnership; wishes for a facilitated reconciliation

2.3. Analysis

All audio recordings were transcribed verbatim. The transcripts of the interviews were anonymized and analyzed in a deductive-inductive process according to Mayring's qualitative content analysis [19] by means of the software MAXQDA Analytics Pro, version 12 (VERBI Software GmbH, Berlin, Germany) [20]. An iterative process was applied in which the authors identified and refined codes, categories, and sub-categories. The coding was mutually checked for accuracy and was thoroughly discussed until consensus regarding the final coding system was reached. The final coding system was summarized in a separate document in which the material was further reduced and compacted. During the course of analysis, reflexivity and transparency regarding the potential influence of the researchers' objectives and preconceptions on the results and interpretations were encouraged. Transcripts and results were not returned to the interviewees. All quotes that were used for publication purposes were translated into English.

3. Results

3.1. Sample Characteristics

As illustrated in Tables 2 and 3, seven women were aged between 31 and 40 years old; 10 women were married; seven women reported to work full-time, two worked part-time, and five were currently on maternity or parental leave; and eight women were mothers of children living in the household at the time of the study. The partners of 10 women had worked offshore from the beginning of their partnership. Furthermore, 12 offshore partners were currently working in a regular 14/14 work schedule, and two partners were working in a different schedule at the time of the interview but did have experience with the 14/14 schedule. Additionally, seven partners had at least three years of offshore work experience.

3.2. Single Life without the Offshore Partner

3.2.1. Advantages

As a major advantage of living the single life, many women found themselves to be more independent and self-reliant in their scheduling of activities and appointments. This was also reported regarding duties and routines within the household and parenting:

> *"Very simple things, like, for example, when to make purchases, what to buy, when to clean certain things (…)." (Interviewee #8)*

Table 2. Participant characteristics.

Interviewee	*n*
Gender	
female	14
Age	
20–30 years	4
31–40 years	7
41–50 years	3
Marital status	
not married	4
married	10
Work schedule	
full-time	7
part-time	2
currently in maternity or parental leave	5
Duration of partnership	
1–5 years	6
6–10 years	4
11–20 years	2
>20 years	2
Partnership with partner working offshore from the start	
yes	4
no	10
Children	
yes and living in household	8
expecting	4
no	2
Offshore partner	*n*
Work schedule	
14 days offshore/14 days onshore	12
other	2
Offshore experience	
<1 year	1
1–2 years	6
3–4 years	3
>4 years	4

Table 3. Participant characteristics (in detail).

ID	Age *	Marital Status	Occupation	Work Schedule	Duration of Partnership *	Partnership with Partner Offshore *	Shared Household *	Children (in Household)	Occupation	Offshore Experience *	Work Schedule **
Interviewee									**Offshore partner**		
1	28	married	not specified (currently on parental leave)	full-time	10	6	9, 5	1 (1)	service technician	6	14/14
2	33	not married	not specified	full-time	3	3	2, 5	0 (0)	technical project management	6	irregular
3	35	married	office management	full-time apprenticeship	10	2, 5	10	2 (2)	quality management	2, 5	14/14 **
4	32	married	social worker (currently on maternity leave)	full-time	5, 5	1, 5	5	0 (0)	health and safety	1, 5	14/14
5	29	married	florist	full-time	2, 5	2, 5	2, 5	1 (1)	service technician	5	8/4
6	39	married	administrative official	part-time	15	5	12	2 (2)	operations manager	5	14/14 **
7	29	married	architect (currently on maternity leave)		10	2	9	0 (0)	offshore medic	2	14/14
8	25	married	maritime sector	full-time	8	0, 5	6	0 (0)	platform master/	0, 5	14/14 **
9	46	married	teacher	full-time	27	3	25	2 (2)	service technician	3	14/14
10	31	married	tailoress (currently on maternity leave)	part-time	5	1, 5	4, 5	0 (0)	nautical officer	1, 5	14/14
11	35	married	health insurance	part-time	13	2	11	1 (1)	service technician	2	14/14
12	34	not married	occupational therapist (currently on maternity leave)	full-time	3, 5	3, 5	0, 5	0 (0)	service technician		14/14
13	42	not married	tailoress	full-time	2, 5	2, 5	1, 5	2 (2)	electrician	3	14/14
14	50	married	house economics	full-time	30	2	28	1 (1)	service technician	2	14/14

* in years ** in turns with office weeks for specific trainings.

A further advantage of the time spent alone was that the women pursued their own interests to a greater extent and were able to become engaged in several leisure activities:

> *"Advantages, perhaps, that one deals with being alone and tries to find strategies to better cope with it. You do not rely on the fact that there is always someone there, but you put more thoughts in your own leisure activities." (Interviewee #4)*

Meeting friends and family, doing sports, and following diverse hobbies were stressed by the women as important leisure activities in this phase.

3.2.2. Disadvantages

An important disadvantage of living the single life was reported to consist of the management and organization of daily life without the partner's general support. Spare time was described to be affected by the partner's absence in such way that the women perceived being forced to spend big parts of their social life alone:

> *"A disadvantage is, of course, that you can only maintain your social contacts alone. If there are invitations or birthday parties, or if you just want to spend a nice evening with friends, this doesn't work." (Interviewee #13)*

During their time alone, there were moments in which the women especially missed their partners. These often concerned moments that both partners usually shared, in particular regarding time during the evenings or weekends. Difficult situations such as sickness, problems at work, or issues with childcare were also mentioned. Moreover, the partner's being missing on special occasions, e.g., weddings or special moments in the children's development, was emphasized. Some interviewees indicated emotional changes, e.g., feeling lonely or more tense than usual:

> *"I realize that I'm not feeling well when he's not there. Sometimes I do not sleep for nights because I cannot stand it." (Interviewee #5)*

Another disadvantage consisted of perceived insecurities related to child care and parenting. Some interviewees described that they considered themselves as single mothers when their partners were offshore:

> *"Well, more or less, I am a single parent for two weeks." (Interviewee #9)*

The perceived unpredictability, e.g., regarding the exact time of the partner's arrival back home, was also seen as disadvantageous. Moreover, the awareness of constraints in reachability when the partner was offshore—especially in cases of emergency—was highlighted as burdening.

Many women spoke about changes in their work routines when their partners were away. They described often working overtime during this phase in order to be able to work less or leave on time when the partner was at home:

> *"Of course, when my husband is not there, I work more. When he's at home, I scale that back a bit, so that we have more time for each other." (Interviewee #9)*

Especially women with children found themselves to be less flexible and more constrained in their work times when they were alone, e.g., due to their children's schedules. Some mothers also described that their children's ill-health seemed to be connected to the absence of their father:

> *"It also happens that the children get sick if he is not there for a long time."*
>
> *(Interviewee #6)*

3.2.3. Communication and Contact Styles

Staying in contact with the partner during his offshore assignments was reported to be crucial for the women. Most of them described being able to contact their partners on a daily basis. The scheduling of contact was stated to depend on the shifts and workloads of the partner:

> *"During his shift, I can write him and if he reads it in between, he can also answer me. But we rather talk on the phone during his free shifts." (Interviewee #12)*

Certain difficulties and restrictions to make contact were also described by some women; however, contact that could be initiated by both partners was reported to be the rule. The usage of several media (phone, messenger services, video telephony) was mentioned by the majority of the women. In particular, improved communication technologies were stated to enable more intensive contact and direct exchange. All in all, the majority of the women stated being satisfied with both the frequency and regularity of contact. Reasons for dissatisfaction were related to the time of contact and the general notion that technology-mediated contacts were not comparable to personal contacts.

3.3. Life as a Couple

3.3.1. Advantages

Advantages of the 14/14 work schedule were often attributed to the time spent together as a couple during the partners' free turn. This time was stated to provide the couple with much time for joint activities and family life. The family life was perceived as being even more intensive due to the previous phase of separation, providing the couple with an opportunity to miss and look forward to seeing each other again. This was indicated to contribute to the liveliness of the relationship:

> *"It's also good for our relationship, it's good to have such a short break (...). That brings in a certain freshness." (Interviewee #6)*

The presence of the offshore partner at home was reported to allow for a higher quality of communication through face-to-face talks. A further advantage of the time spent together was that the partner could be involved in the child care and housekeeping. Family fathers were also able to follow their children's development more closely during their free time at home.

More generally, some women described time-wise benefits of the daily living together, such as a greater flexibility for the couple in terms of planning short vacations or having breakfast together during the week. Financial benefits of the offshore job (e.g., in the form of good salaries) that contributed to family life were also mentioned.

3.3.2. Disadvantages

A main disadvantage of the daily living together in the 14/14 schedule concerned the lack of habitualness and missing daily routine which could not be established in the course of two weeks:

> *"We are all habitual people and habits can be very difficult at 2 weeks/2 weeks, I think." (Interviewee #11)*

A few interviewees described feeling an increased need to talk to their partners and to plan appointments when they were home. Some women even described a perceived pressure to get all everyday things—for which they normally had four weeks of time—done during the two weeks together:

> *"You always have the feeling that you must put everything into these two weeks, because afterwards, your time together is over. Need for action, discussion needs ... what you just can't always hold on the phone." (Interviewee #9)*

In terms of their work, many women described their own job as meaningful to them, regardless of the presence or absence of their partners. However, some women found it harder to go to work with their partners being at home and preferred staying at home with them, e.g., because they experienced feelings of guilt for leaving the partner alone.

In addition, some women reported that the situation was especially disadvantageous for their partners: their free turns could be rather unsatisfactory, since the time they were able to spend with their families and friends was restricted due to other people's normal work routines:

> *"It was not satisfactory for him either. He was not socializing as much as he had wished. The days are long when all people around you work full time." (Interviewee #11)*

Other interviewees explained that their partners struggled to find a balance in terms of the time spent with the family and with friends outside home. This was due to the fact that the workers were solicited a lot during their onshore turns, in particular on the weekends:

> *"The time on the two weekends becomes very, very scarce. When there should be time for the partnership, but also for family, friends, and your own interests." (Interviewee #4)*

Several women described that their partners absolved work tasks and were contacted for professional purposes during their free turns onshore. Talking about offshore work and being contacted by colleagues were associated with greater difficulties for the partners to mentally detach and recover from work. Therefore, many interviewees disapproved of this behavior.

3.3.3. Conflicts and Compromises

When asked about conflicts and compromises due to the specific living situation, about half of the women stated not noticing any specific conflicts. The non-existence of conflicts was attributed to the couple's mutual understanding and awareness of their limited time together:

> *"Because we are separated again and again, you appreciate it (the time spent together) very much. And that makes us both feel that we are not arguing so fast and so much." (Interviewee #10)*

The other women reported that minor conflicts or discussions attributable to their specific living situation sometimes occurred. Conflicts, for example, emerged when the partner refused to get involved in housekeeping, or when he dedicated too much time to his work during his free turn. Further discussions were described to relate to planning difficulties of the couple due to the partners' offshore work. Moreover, minor discussions between the offshore partner and the children were reported to occur. In addition, it was stated that 'offshore couples' sometimes had to deal with a lack of understanding from their friends, who did not comprehend the amount of time the couple needed for themselves.

The majority of the interviewees thought that they had to make more compromises compared to couples living a 'normal life'. They expressed that more agreements and consultations were necessary to suitably plan living together. Compromises were, for example, described in terms of the parenting, since the children had to live without their father for a while. Moreover, planning difficulties were a central concern, since all appointments had to be made in accordance with the partner's offshore schedule:

> *"We have to direct our everyday life according to these offshore trips. He never knows when the trips will be —they are not set at the beginning of the year—so we just cannot plan at all." (Interviewee #5)*

3.4. Transition Phase

3.4.1. Reunion with the Partner

The women described varying feelings, e.g., increasing anticipation and excitement, upon their partners' arrival back home. Typical behavior patterns were tidying up the house and avoiding other appointments:

> *"Then I just run from A to B and check that everything is neat (...). That the food is ready and that no more laundry is lying around. That there are no disruptive factors in order for us to simply enjoy this moment together." (Interviewee #5)*

Only a few interviewees stated that they did not perceive a certain transition phase when their partners arrived back home. The majority declared that they needed a familiarization phase in which they had to adapt to their partner and the two adult household again:

> *"At the beginning, you often need some time to get close again, because you have not seen the other person for so long." (Interviewee #7)*

The transition phase was generally described to last between one and four days. Women described that the arrival of the partner could upset the whole household, and that the habits and routines of the women at home were suddenly turned around:

> *"You develop different habits—your own habits—when the partner is not there. And as soon as he comes back, it's all jumbled up." (Interviewee #8)*

In households with children, it was pronounced that the children behaved more actively and turned up during the father's arrival, demanding more attention than usual:

> *"When he comes back, the children are usually there, and then the alarm goes from 0 to 100 in the booth." (Interviewee #13)*

3.4.2. Needs and Expectations upon the Partners' Arrival

Needs and expectations of the women regarding the time as a couple consisted of spending as much time together as possible and following social activities. Some women particularly highlighted their expectation that the partner should get involved in housekeeping and other duties at home:

> *"I indeed expect that he will also take care of the household and of the things that happened while he was not there." (Interviewee #13)*

In contrast, expectations of the offshore partners stated by the women included that the women should await them at home upon their arrival and that the couple should share a good meal together on the first evening. A relevant need of the partner consisted of physical closeness to the women.

Some interviewees believed that their needs and expectations corresponded well with those of their partners; for example, when both partners wished for physical closeness, calmness, and time spent together. In contrast, other women perceived discrepancies, which were especially related to the women's "work situation" versus the partners' "free time situation": while the women had to continue their daily work routine, the offshore partners found themselves to be in a holiday mood:

> *"I get up at the same time in the morning, go to work, and come back in the evening. And then my partner took the time as a vacation, but I was still in the working cycle." (Interviewee #4)*

3.4.3. Parting

The interviewees described that the time spent together as a couple usually passed rapidly. Some women described that during the last days before their partners' departure, the workers started to mentally prepare themselves for their offshore assignments. The departure was termed as a difficult situation by some women, provoking feelings of sadness. Some women also reported that their children's behavior changed during their father's departure. For example, they could demonstrate their displeasure by crying or working themselves up.

Figure 1 gives an overview of the specific features, advantages, and disadvantages of living the 14/14 schedule as related to the different phases of daily life.

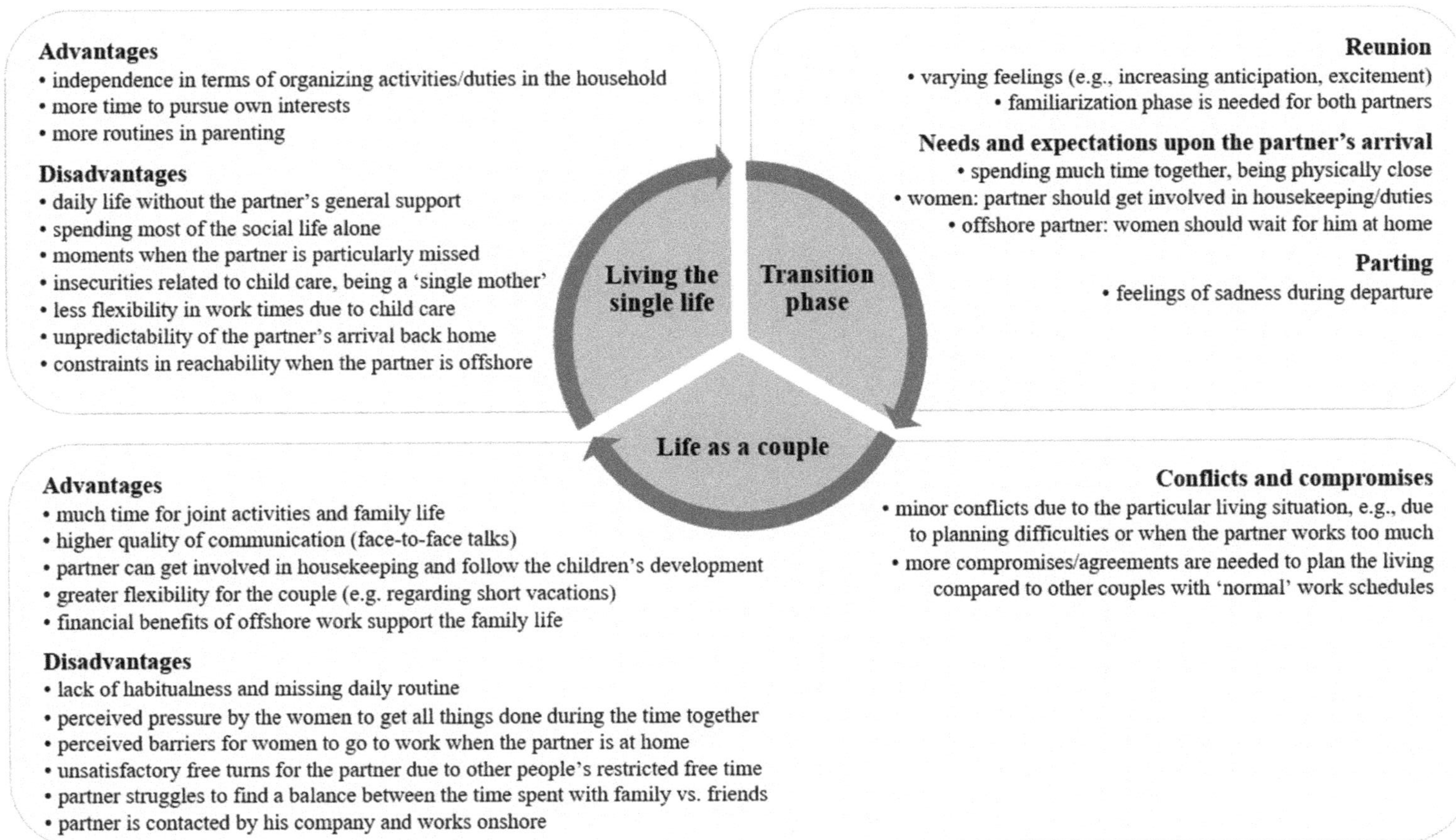

Figure 1. Specific features of living the 14/14 schedule related to the phases of daily life.

3.5. Coping Strategies

3.5.1. Strategies of the Women

When asked about strategies to cope with the absence of their partners, many women described that actively searching for the support of families and friends played an important role:

> *"I think that you rely more on the social network around you. That you particularly promote your network. You simply intensify other social contacts, family, friends." (Interviewee #4)*

In general, pursuing an active lifestyle was described as a coping strategy by many women. This included, for example, doing sports or meeting friends. Further ways to cope with the situation were stated to consist of adapting oneself to the schedule, focusing on the time spent together as a couple, and staying in regular contact during periods of separation:

> *"For me, this is already somewhat normal. And we talk on the phone in the evenings and write each other during the evenings when he has enough time." (Interviewee #12)*

Some interviewees stated that they coped with the situation by structuring their time in an organized manner, while others reported that they coped by keeping their expectations low regarding the time spent together. Some women reported that they did not apply any coping efforts.

When being asked about sustaining exchange with other women living in a similar situation, most interviewees responded that they had not made contact with other women of offshore workers, although some found such an exchange to be desirable. A few others, in contrast, described having irregular contact with other partners of offshore workers. These contacts were reported to be organized autonomously and without the offshore companies' support.

3.5.2. Strategies of the Couples

In terms of coping strategies applied by the couples, many women emphasized the meaning of communication and structure for dealing with the phases of separation:

> *"This always means a lot of exchange with each other, and a lot of talking and communicating. Then it works. But those who do not have this ability will find it difficult." (Interviewee #9)*

The importance of adhering to fixed and regular contact times was stressed. Additionally, spending time as a family/couple when the partner was onshore was underlined, explaining that other obligations or appointments were avoided in order to create more family-time:

> *"Certain rituals are that, when he's at home, (…) the last weekend before he leaves, or at least 1 or 2 days, that you have these days completely to yourself. And then accept no appointments." (Interviewee #10)*

Mutual understanding and trust were also highlighted as important. Still, there were couples who did not apply any coping strategies or rituals to deal with the specific situation.

Table 4 summarizes the coping strategies applied by the women and couples.

Table 4. Coping strategies of the women and the couples.

Coping Strategies of the Women	Coping Strategies of the Couples
Seeking support of families and friends	Adhering to fixed contact times
Pursuing an active lifestyle	Mutual understanding and trust
Structuring time in an organized manner	Spending an intensive time together
Adapting oneself to the living situation	
Focusing on time spent together as a couple	
Keeping expectations low	
Contact with other women in the same situation	

3.6. Reconciliation of Offshore Work and Family Life/Partnership

3.6.1. Opinions on Reconciliation

The women's views on whether or not they considered offshore work and family life to be reconcilable differed. There were some interviewees who described offshore work as being sufficiently family-friendly, especially when the children were already older in age. The primary reason for the family-friendliness was that fathers were able to spend intensive periods of time at home:

"Which father of a family can say that he is completely at home for 2 weeks, from morning to night?" (Interviewee #10)

In contrast, other women did not consider offshore work to be family-friendly due to the several named disadvantages implied by the 14/14 schedule. This was particularly pronounced by interviewees with smaller children, emphasizing that the partner would miss out on too much of their development:

"I just think that the men miss too much. Especially when a child is born. In the first year, our son actually had only me, his dad was always a bit of a rival." (Interviewee #5)

A dividedness regarding interviewees' opinions was also apparent with regard to the reconciliation of offshore work and partnership. Some women believed that offshore work was partnership-friendly and that it helped in keeping the partnership alive. Living with the periodical absences of the partner was reported to be practicable without children:

"Without a child, I'd say, it works. Then you can deal with it, even without noticing a negative impact on the relationship." (Interviewee #4)

However, other interviewees stated that the 14/14 schedule imposed heavy demands on the relationship, and that they personally perceived the situation as burdensome:

"The big disadvantage is that the private life suffers greatly, that one must cut back on the partnership because the contact is missing." (Interviewee #5)

The appraisal of whether or not offshore work was partnership-/family-friendly was stated to depend on the couples' expectations (e.g., the amount of time the couple wanted to spend together and the desired frequency of contact). Moreover, the amount of support from external sources (e.g., parents, friends) played a role in the women's judgement:

"If you do not have family support, then it is not necessarily family-friendly. So I think that the environment still plays a big role." (Interviewee #7)

3.6.2. Needs and Wishes for Improving Reconciliation

When asked about wishes for improving the reconciliation of offshore work and family life/partnership, some women stated that they did not have any specific wishes, or explained that they did not think that any measures for improvement could be taken due to the unchangeable 14/14 schedule. Others, however, described wishes regarding their partners' work schedule (e.g., other days of arrival and departure, longer offshore or onshore stays). The wish for greater regularity and predictability of the offshore assignments was also expressed:

"These are my concerns, reliability and predictability." (Interviewee #6)

Furthermore, it was proposed that the workers should get more free time offshore in order to increase chances for communication with the families and to strengthen the workers' recovery from work. A few women also wished to get to know their partners places of work to develop a better understanding of the work situation offshore.

3.6.3. Support from Offshore Companies

The women mostly described that they did not know about specific offers provided by their partners' companies to facilitate the reconciliation of offshore work and family life/partnership. However, they described single offers provided by the companies that they considered to be helpful, e.g., flights back home at short-notice in case of emergencies:

"Of course, if there was a death in the family or something, definitely. Or now with the child's birth, I could call him anytime and would try to get him off the platform." (Interviewee #10)

Some women said that company events were organized for the whole family, and that parental leave for fathers was an option. Further offers consisted of the free use of a telephone and internet connection on the offshore platforms, allowing the couples to stay in contact:

"That's a good option, I think, that companies put a lot of emphasis on enabling the workers to have regular contact with their families at home." (Interviewee #10)

4. Discussion

By conducting our interview study, we were able to gain important insights into the challenges, advantages, and disadvantages, as well as the psychosocial adaptation, associated with living the 14/14 schedule from the perspective of women of offshore wind workers.

We generally found the proposed differentiation between the three distinct social realities for offshore couples (her single life at home, a phase of transition, and the couple's common life together), as suggested by Solheim [11], to be similarly described in our study. Moreover, our results seem to be in line with the FIFO cycle proposed by Gallegos [12] for both offshore employees and their partners. For example, the occurrence of mixed emotions during transition phases, as identified in previous research [12,15], was also prevalent for the women in our sample.

Overall, despite some burdens, the women in our sample seemed to have adapted relatively favorably to the challenges and demands of living the 14/14 schedule. Although minor difficulties and problems related to the partnership and family life were stated, most women seemed to be able to cope with the challenges associated with the 14/14 work schedule. When contrasting our findings with those of earlier research studies in the offshore oil and gas branch, we found previous research to illustrate a slightly more negative picture regarding the psychosocial adaptation of offshore families [21]. However, the situation seems to have improved over the last decades. For example, Parkes and colleagues [8] noted a positive trend, and our study further supports this development.

4.1. Single Life without the Offshore Partner

As regards the single life of the women, we found the main advantage to consist of the greater self-reliance and independence women perceived in their daily living. This is in line with previous results showing that women were able to enjoy their independence and freedom [21,22], and that they could benefit from their partners' absences in developing greater personal confidence [8]. However, in general, we found that the women in our study reported more disadvantages than advantages of their single life. Negative aspects, such as perceptions of loneliness when the partner was away, have been similarly revealed in previous studies [8,12]. For example, in an interview study, two thirds of the spouses of offshore oil and gas workers reported loneliness to be a problem "sometimes" or "often" [8].

In contrast to earlier studies in which women reported experiencing social isolation due to their partners' absences [8,13,22], our interviewees did not describe difficulties in fully participating in social life during this phase. This difference could be related to the fact that the women in our study did not seem to center their social lives strictly around their partners; in contrast, many of them stated that they actively engaged in social life when their partners were away. In earlier studies, women were found to deliberately restrict their social lives when their partners were away [8,22].

An important finding of our study relates to the use and impact of new ways of communication as a result of technological advances. We found the women in our study to positively highlight their chances for communication via the use of diverse social media. While earlier studies declared problems in communication due to the—back then—existing communication systems [13], today's offshore women may draw on several communication systems which allow them to keep in contact with their partners. The importance of improved telecommunications in facilitating adjustment and maintaining family connectedness has also been noted for offshore and FIFO families [8,10,22]. One study, for example, found that women who could initiate calls to contact their offshore partners had less difficulty in adjusting to the absence compared to women who were unable to do so [8].

Our results indicate an intrinsic work motivation among the women in our sample: becoming engaged in work was identified to be important, helping them to fill the days when their partner was offshore. In contrast to an earlier study in which women's employment tended to increase family strain [23], we did not find this to be the case in our study. This discrepancy should be interpreted in view of the specific sample: six out of 14 women did not have children in the household, thereby potentially increasing their chances to engage in paid work. Furthermore, the result may also be attributable to sociocultural changes that have occurred during the last decades: nowadays, it is more common and socially accepted for women to build their own careers. The trend of increased employment rates among women is also reflected in our sample, in which all women were employed (despite five women currently being on parental or maternity leave). In contrast, in earlier samples of offshore wives, only one third [23] and two thirds of the women [8] respectively, were engaged in paid work. Similarly, only two women in our study were in part-time employment, whereas more than half of the women in the study of Parkes and colleagues [8] worked part-time, which was found to be influenced by the demands of childcare. The fact that most women in our study worked full-time may also be related to currently increasing options for child care, e.g., provided by day care centers and kindergartens.

4.2. Life as a Couple

With respect to life as a couple, the women in our study had differentiated views on the costs and benefits of the 14/14 schedule for their living situation. A major advantage related to the 14/14 schedule was seen in the workers' rest periods onshore, allowing an increased duration of presence at home and favoring family life. This advantage was also noted in earlier studies [8,12,13,21].

As previously identified [11,12,24], we found that both partners initially needed a familiarization phase to readjust to having another adult in the household. Similar to our results, it was previously found that reunions and partings are the most difficult times emotionally for couples and families [10,12]. Moreover, in accordance with previous findings [12], women in our study reported that their routines could become less structured when their partners returned home.

In terms of the children's behavior, some women described their children's conduct as varying and depending on the phase of absence, presence, or transition. Gallegos [12] has similarly described that the behavior of children of FIFO workers could become clingy, and that it could take some time for the children to feel comfortable upon their father's return.

Notably, there were only a few conflicts described as having occurred during the time spent together, although conflicts seemed to be a stressor for couples in previous studies [21–23], especially during the first days spent together [21]. In contrast to previous research highlighting women's increased responsibilities as a potential source of conflict [13,15], conflicts described by our sample seemed to emerge from the partners' behaviors at home, e.g., their reluctance to get involved in housekeeping. In earlier times, housework did not represent a source of conflict for offshore oil and gas couples [21]; the major responsibility for domestic work remained with the wives, which was attributed to the more traditional views on household division back then [21]. In contrast, our results support the notion that women's aspirations and role models have changed [8], since women in our sample reported distinct expectations regarding the workers' engagement in the household.

The fact that conflicts among the couples were described to occur rather seldom could also be related to the coping strategies that were applied, which may be effective in reducing potential conflicts.

Moreover, the women in our study seemed to be aware of existing differences compared to non-offshore families; for example, they acknowledged that more compromises had to be made in contrast to other couples. It has been noted previously that such an awareness may increase the implementation of strategies to support family functioning [15].

4.3. Coping Strategies

We found the women in our study to apply several coping strategies for dealing with their situation, such as seeking support, thinking positively, and regulating adverse emotions. Thereby, our results undermine previous findings indicating that many offshore women actively pursue some form of coping, e.g., engaging in an active lifestyle or utilizing social support [8,12,22,23]. In earlier studies, women of offshore oil and gas workers were found to use coping strategies to mitigate loneliness when the partner was offshore (e.g., keeping busy, keeping in touch with the family, and taking part in recreational activities [8]). Similarly, FIFO workers were found to engage in social networks providing them with assistance and companionship while the workers were away [12]. Still, there is a need for further investigation of the women's coping strategies. Aspects such as work schedules (full-time, part-time) and childcare may require different coping strategies that should be examined by further research.

An important strategy of the couples was reported to consist of staying in regular contact, which was also of importance for oil and gas, as well as FIFO, families [8,10,12]. In studies among FIFO families, regular effective communication was the most important strategy to protect family cohesiveness [12], and was found to be strongly associated with family satisfaction [10].

4.4. Reconciliation of Offshore Work and Family Life/Partnership

Women's views regarding the reconciliation of offshore work and family life/partnership seemed to partly depend on their availability of external sources, such as support from friends and family, as well as on the couples' own expectations. This agrees with the notion that a stronger accordance between perceptions and expectations of partners, e.g., regarding family satisfaction, could lead to less family conflicts [10] and less critical family structures [13].

A support offer provided by offshore companies was named in terms of the flexibility of shifts in cases of emergency. This has also been noted by women of offshore oil and gas workers, who were confident that their partners could be flown home in a family emergency [8]. However, in sum, the women in our study did not report an intensive bandwidth of offers provided by offshore companies to facilitate the reconciliation of offshore work and family life. This finding might either indicate a need for the companies to improve their offers, or to make existing offers more visible for offshore families. In contrast, in FIFO, as well as oil and gas industries, more company support has become evident, e.g., consisting of counseling services, peer-programs, organized family events, or visits to the site for families [8,12]. Such offers may also add to the reconciliation for couples and families in the offshore wind industry.

4.5. Strengths and Limitations

A strength of our study is the fact that we recruited women with varying sociodemographic characteristics, e.g., different ages and family status. This enabled us to establish a more complete picture of the situation of offshore women with varying backgrounds. To increase the trustworthiness of our findings, we employed rich descriptions of our results and displayed many direct quotes from the interviewees [25]. Moreover, we discussed our results profoundly within the group of researchers, and contrasted them with empirical references.

However, it should be noted that our findings are based on a convenience sample which was partly achieved via a snowballing technique, thereby increasing the risk of self-selection among the participants. For example, women with a greater interest in the topic might have been more prone to participate, and may not be representative of other female partners of offshore workers. Moreover, our sample is likely to represent a self-selected group of 'survivors', as it has been noted for other samples of offshore women [8,21]. There are several indications for this assumption: for example, interviewees' partners were currently working offshore, and many of them had already worked offshore for several years. It can be assumed that offshore workers are more likely to continue with their work when their women are also able to adjust to the offshore lifestyle [8]. Our sample, therefore, likely represents a survivor group of women that have responded rather positively to this lifestyle and experienced less difficulties in adjustment. Moreover, it should be kept in mind that 10 out of 14 workers were already involved in offshore work at the beginning of the relationship, meaning that most couples did not have to deal with a disrupt change of their living situation during the course of the relationship.

Further methodological limitations concern the fact that we conducted telephone interviews instead of face-to-face interviews, implying an asynchronous communication of place by telephone and a reduction of social clues [26,27].

Another limitation of our study may be seen in the relatively small sample size. However, the size of interviews in our study appeared to be sufficient to achieve data saturation. In support of this, it has been concluded that data saturation usually occurs within the first twelve interviews [28]. In any case, generalizations of our results are impeded by the nature of our qualitative research design.

Further research studies with larger sample sizes are needed. In such studies, it would be interesting to conduct interviews with couples in order to incorporate both the views of offshore workers and their female partners. Moreover, quantitative research studies should be conducted to statistically explore the antecedents, moderators, and outcomes of psychosocial adaptation among offshore couples. Previous research has, for example, suggested that role expectations, the presence of dependent children at home, and the quality of communication in the relationship may influence the effects of stressors on psychosocial adaptation [10]. Moreover, since our sample likely represents a survivor group of couples living the 14/14 schedule, it seems worthwhile to compare their situation with the situation of families where workers decided to leave offshore work.

5. Conclusions

The present study expanded upon the current scientific evidence and provided an up-to-date perspective on the situation of offshore wind couples and families living the 14/14 work schedule. The women in our study reported differentiated views as to the benefits and costs associated with their particular lifestyle. Various coping strategies were stated by the women, which could facilitate psychosocial adaptation. Despite experiencing certain burdens, most of the women in our sample seemed to have adapted relatively favorably to their living situation. Our results suggest that certain sociological and technological advances within the last decades, e.g., changes in women's role models and improved communication technologies, may ease psychosocial adaptation among offshore families.

Author Contributions: Conceptualization, J.M., S.R., M.K., V.H., and S.M.; methodology, J.M., M.K., and S.M.; recruitment of participants and conduct of interviews, J.M. and M.K.; data curation and analysis, J.M. and S.R.; writing—original draft preparation, J.M. and S.R.; writing—review and editing, M.K., V.H., and S.M.; visualization, J.M.; supervision, S.M. and V.H.

Funding: This research received no external funding.

Acknowledgments: We would like to thank all women who participated in the interview study. We would also like to acknowledge Johanna Bertram for her help in data preparation.

Conflicts of Interest: The authors declare no conflict of interest.

Data availability: The data analyzed during the current study are not publicly available due to German national data protection regulations. They are available on individual request from the corresponding author.

References

1. Stiftung Offshore Windenergie. Status des Offshore-Windenergie-Ausbaus in Deutschland. Available online: https://www.offshore-stiftung.de/sites/offshorelink.de/files/documents/Factsheet_Status_Offshore-Windenergieausbau_1._Halbjahr_2018_20180731_0.pdf (accessed on 13 December 2018).

2. Internationales Wirtschaftsforum Regenerative Energien. Windparks in Deutschland. Available online: http://www.offshore-windindustrie.de/windparks/deutschland (accessed on 11 December 2018).
3. O'Sullivan, M.; Edler, D.; Lehr, U. *Ökonomische Indikatoren des Energiesystems. Methode, Abgrenzung und Ergebnisse für den Zeitraum 2000–2016*; GWS Research Report 2018/01; GWS mbH Osnabrück: Osnabrück, Germany, 2018.
4. Velasco Garrido, M.; Mette, J.; Mache, S.; Harth, V.; Preisser, A.M. A cross-sectional survey of physical strains among offshore wind farm workers in the German exclusive economic zone. *BMJ Open* **2018**, *8*, e020157. [CrossRef] [PubMed]
5. Mette, J.; Velasco Garrido, M.; Harth, V.; Preisser, A.M.; Mache, S. Healthy offshore workforce? A qualitative study on offshore wind employees' occupational strain, health, and coping. *BMC Public Health* **2018**, *18*, 172. [CrossRef] [PubMed]
6. Mette, J.; Velasco Garrido, M.; Harth, V.; Preisser, A.M.; Mache, S. "It's still a great adventure"—Exploring offshore employees' working conditions in a qualitative study. *J. Occup. Med. Toxicol.* **2017**, *12*, 35. [CrossRef] [PubMed]
7. Mette, J.; Velasco Garrido, M.; Preisser, A.M.; Harth, V.; Mache, S. Linking quantitative demands to offshore wind workers' stress: Do personal and job resources matter? A structural equation modelling approach. *BMC Public Health* **2018**, *18*, 934. [CrossRef] [PubMed]
8. Parkes, K.R.; Carnell, S.C.; Farmer, E.L. 'Living two lives': Perceptions, attitudes and experiences of spouses of UK offshore workers. *Community Work Fam.* **2005**, *8*, 413–437. [CrossRef]
9. Kirchhoefer, M.; Mache, S.; Harth, V.; Mette, J. Vereinbarkeit von Berufs- und Familienleben bei Offshore-Beschäftigten–eine Übersicht. *Zbl. Arbeitsmed.* **2018**, *68*, 54–58. [CrossRef]
10. Taylor, J.C.; Simmonds, J.G. Family Stress and Coping in the Fly-in Fly-out Workforce. *Aust. Community Psychol.* **2009**, *21*, 23–36.
11. Solheim, J. Coming Home to Work. In *Women, Work and Family in the British, Canadian and Norwegian Offshore Oilfields*; Lewis, J., Porter, M., Shrimpton, M., Eds.; Palgrave McMillan: London, UK, 1988; pp. 140–162.
12. Gallegos, D. Fly-In Fly-Out Employment: Managing the Parenting Transitions. Available online: http://researchrepository.murdoch.edu.au/id/eprint/10916/1/aeroplanes.pdf (accessed on 13 December 2018).
13. Forsyth, C.J.; Gauthier, D.K. Families of offshore oil workers: Adaptations to cyclical father absence/presence. *Sociol. Spectr.* **1991**, *11*, 177–201. [CrossRef]
14. Taylor, R.; Morrice, K.; Clark, D.; McCann, K. The psycho-social consequences of intermittent husband absence: An epidemiological study. *Soc. Sci. Med.* **1985**, *20*, 877–885. [CrossRef]
15. Sibbel, A.M. Living FIFO: The Experiences and Psychosocial Wellbeing of Western Australian Fly-In/Fly-Out Employees and Partners. Ph.D. Dissertation, Edith Cowan University, Joondalup, Australia, 2010. Available online: http://ro.ecu.edu.au/theses/132 (accessed on 14 December 2018).
16. Folkman, S.; Lazarus, R.S. An Analysis of Coping in a Middle-Aged Community Sample. *J. Health Soc. Behav.* **1980**, *21*, 219–239. [CrossRef] [PubMed]
17. Folkman, S.; Lazarus, R.S.; Gruen, R.J.; DeLongis, A. Appraisal, coping, health status, and psychological symptoms. *J. Pers. Soc. Psychol.* **1986**, *50*, 571. [CrossRef] [PubMed]
18. Puskeppeleit, M. Medizin im Offshore-Bereich. In *Maritime Medizin: Praxiswissen für Schiffsärzte und Ärzte im Offshore-Bereich*; Ottoman, C., Seidenstücker, K.H., Eds.; Springer: Berlin/Heidelberg, Germany, 2015; pp. 35–47.
19. Mayring, P. Qualitative Inhaltsanalyse. Available online: http://www.qualitative-research.net/index.php/fqs/article/view/1089/2383 (accessed on 16 January 2019).
20. VERBI Software Consult Sozialforschung GmbH. MAXQDA 12: Reference Manual. Available online: http://www.maxqda.com/download/manuals/MAX12_manual_eng.pdf (accessed on 13 December 2018).
21. Clark, D.; McCann, K.; Morrice, K.; Taylor, R. Work and Marriage in the Offshore Oil Industry. *Int. J. Soc. Econ.* **1985**, *12*, 36–47. [CrossRef]
22. Lewis, J.; Shrimpton, M.; Storey, K. Family Members' Experience of Offshore Oil Work in Newfoundland. In *Women, Work and Family in the British, Canadian and Norwegian Offshore Oilfields*; Lewis, J., Porter, M., Shrimpton, M., Eds.; Palgrave McMillan: London, UK, 1988; pp. 163–189.
23. Clark, D.; Taylor, R. Partings and Reunions: Marriage and Offshore Employment in the British North Sea. In *Women, Work and Family in the British, Canadian and Norwegian Offshore Oilfields*; Lewis, J., Porter, M., Shrimpton, M., Eds.; Palgrave McMillan: London, UK, 1988; pp. 112–139.

24. Rodrigues, V.F.; Fischer, F.M.; Brito, M.J. Shift work at a modern offshore drilling rig. *J. Hum. Ergol. (Tokyo)* **2001**, *30*, 167–172. [CrossRef]
25. Van Nes, F.; Abma, T.; Jonsson, H.; Deeg, D. Language differences in qualitative research: Is meaning lost in translation? *Eur. J. Ageing* **2010**, *7*, 313–316. [CrossRef] [PubMed]
26. Opdenakker, R.J.G. Advantages and Disadvantages of Four Interview Techniques in Qualitative Research. Available online: http://www.qualitative-research.net/index.php/fqs/article/view/175/391 (accessed on 15 January 2019).
27. Novick, G. Is there a bias against telephone interviews in qualitative research? *Res. Nurs. Health* **2008**, *31*, 391–398. [CrossRef] [PubMed]
28. Guest, G.; Bunce, A.; Johnson, L. How many interviews are enough? An experiment with data saturation and variability. *Field Methods* **2006**, *18*, 59–82. [CrossRef]

International Journal of
Environmental Research and Public Health

MDPI

Article

Trends in Workplace Injuries in Slovak Forest Enterprises

Miloš Gejdoš [1], Mária Vlčková [1,*], Zuzana Allmanová [1] and Žaneta Balážová [2]

[1] Department of Forest Harvesting, Logistics and Ameliorations, Faculty of Forestry, Technical University in Zvolen, 960 01 Zvolen, Slovakia; gejdos@tuzvo.sk (M.G.); zuzana.allmanova@tuzvo.sk (Z.A.)
[2] Institute of Foreign Languages, Technical University in Zvolen, 960 01 Zvolen, Slovakia; zaneta.balazova@tuzvo.sk
* Correspondence: vlckova@tuzvo.sk; Tel.: +421-45-5206-269

Received: 26 November 2018; Accepted: 24 December 2018; Published: 7 January 2019

Abstract: The aim of the paper is to analyse the effect of key factors affecting the risk of workplace injuries and to identify the most common workplace accidents regarding injured body parts with respect to anthropometric data measurements of the population. Data associated with workplace accidents over the years 2000–2016 were drawn from the records of the state enterprise Forests of the Slovak Republic, situated in Banská Bystrica. Gathered data were processed and entered into the database complemented by the data on accidents of the self-employed working in the forestry industry. A total of 1874 workplace accidents in the state enterprise were recorded and statistically evaluated during the analysis period. A method for contingency table was used to analyse correlation between qualitative (categorical) variables in the dataset. A Poisson regression model was used to determine the injury rate. Forest harvesting is considered the most risky phase of the process of harvesting, processing, and transport. The highest number of workplace accidents (31.8% of all recorded workplace accidents) occurred during the forest harvesting phase during the analysis period. Timber skidding, with 16% of recorded accidents, was the second highest-risk phase. The workplace injury rate in the forest industry in Slovakia decreased over the course of the years 2000–2016. Head and facial injuries were those with the highest rate (67.1% injuries of these body parts) during the phase of harvesting and skidding.

Keywords: workplace injuries; work safety; health and safety; work errors forestry; injury rate

---

1. Introduction

The scope of human physical and mental abilities is limited. Long-term uncomfortable or painful feelings can cause damage to organisms due to a significant weakening in performance, with a higher injury risk [1]. The forestry sector is one of the industries of the national economy with the highest injury risk. The specific working conditions in forests, involving the type of terrain, weather conditions, and the use of power tools and heavy machinery, make work hazardous, with a certain risk of serious injuries [1–4]. The risk of work-related injuries is very high in forestry jobs in general [5,6]. In order to create healthy and safe working environments, processes, and conditions, accident investigations can reveal information about causation that can be used to develop injury prevention and protection programmes.

In order to create health and safe working environment, real accidents have to be analysed and subsequently, a system of preventive measures has to be developed. Methods to protect health are constantly evolving. Forestry generates many jobs, which are offered mostly by private companies in the case of Slovakia. Several activities carried out on forest estates are managed by private enterprises that underestimate the risks to health and safety that can arise. When health and safety legislation and requirements are not met, the health and lives of workers are endangered. Work-related health issues in small enterprises are recorded in many countries, both developing and developed. Some examples include South Africa, Sweden, Slovakia, and Croatia [7–10].

Many previous studies have focused on injury incidence and prevalence to underscore the need for great safety in the workplace. The authors of [11,12] state that an analysis of injury rate can provide complete information about changes in injury rate depending on a specific prognostic variable. Further results can be gathered using Poisson regression models.

Employees in forestry, especially those exposed to harmful factors for at least six years, appear to suffer from work-related injuries. Noise, vibration, extreme temperatures, dust, exhaust fumes (especially carbon monoxide), and fixed or constrained body positions are considered to be harmful to health. [13]. Working with chainsaws, the most commonly used tool by forest workers in Slovakia, can be considered one of the most dangerous activities in forestry.

The aim of the paper is to analyse work phases in forestry that may be associated with risk of injury. Moreover, the research is focused on determining the significant factors affecting the risk of damage to the health in the forestry sector.

2. Materials and Methods

2.1. Data Collection and Processing

Data associated with workplace injuries were drawn from the records of the state enterprise Forests of the Slovak Republic situated in Banská Bystrica. Gathered data were processed and entered into the database, complemented by data on injuries of the self-employed working in forestry. Questionnaires about the accidents were delivered to various forest enterprises in order to gather relevant information about circumstances and causes of workplace accidents. Workplace accidents were identified with accordance with "European Statistics on Accidents at Work" (ESAW) [14] in order to create a dataset. Circumstances and causes of workplace accidents in Slovakia were determined using the authors' classification based on the Decree of Ministry of Labour, Social Affairs and Family of the Slovak Republic No. 500/2006 Coll. on establishment of a template for reported occupational accident in accordance with the unified statistical reporting system in the European Union [15]. A dataset of workplace accidents was created over the years 2000–2016. During the analysis period, 1874 workplace accidents in forest enterprises in Slovakia were recorded.

2.2. Contingency Tables

A method for contingency tables was used to analyse the correlation between qualitative (categorical) variables in a dataset consisting of workplace injuries.

Investigation of the correlation between two variables is based, similarly to a one-dimensional statistical dataset, on finding frequencies mentioned in contingency tables. The research methodology follows that of several works [16–18].

For the case of the two categorical variables A and B, where the classes of variable A are A_1, A_2, A_3, … A_k and the classes of variable B are B_1, B_2, B_3 … B_m, a $k \times m$ contingency table as illustrated in Table 1 is formed.

Table 1. Template of contingency table.

Variable B		Classes of Variable B						Total
Variable A		B_1	B_2	...	B_J	...	B_m	
Classes of Variable A	A_1	n_{11}	n_{12}	...	...	...	n_{1m}	n_{1A}
	A_2	n_{21}	n_{22}	...	...	...	n_{2m}	n_{2A}
	.	.	.		.		.	.
	A_i	n_{i1}	n_{i2}	...	n_{iJ}	...	n_{im}	n_{JA}
	.	.	.		.		.	.
	A_k	n_{K1}	n_{K2}		n_{KJ}		n_{Km}	n_{kA}
Total		n_{B1}	n_{B2}	...	n_{BJ}	...	n_{Bm}	N

Source: Authors' compilation.

The degree of correlation between two categorical variables A and B is measured following the comparison of the observed frequencies in individual classes of the contingency table n_{ij} to the expected frequencies n'_{ij}, when the variables are independent. The expected variables are calculated using Formula (1):

$$n'_{ij} = \frac{n_i \cdot n_j}{n} \tag{1}$$

They are calculated as the product of the corresponding frequencies (n_i for the variable A and n_j for the variable B) divided by the size of dataset n.

The chi-squared test of independence was used to determine whether the occurrence of serious workplace accidents during the phase of harvesting and skidding is statistically significant.

Testing the hypothesis on the significance of expected dependence is based on the calculation of χ^2 (chi-squared) defined by Formula (2):

$$\chi^2 = \sum_{i=1}^{k} \sum_{j=1}^{m} \frac{(n_{ij} - n'_{ij})^2}{n'_{ij}} \tag{2}$$

χ^2 is calculated in the contingency table, where besides observed frequencies n_{ij} (cell of the table), the calculated expected frequencies n'_{ij}, and even the differences $(n_{ij} - n'_{ij})$ are displayed.

Expected frequencies (n'_{ij}) must be calculated for cells of the table without observed frequencies. The value of these frequencies is χ^2 (Equation (3)):

$$n'_{ij} = \frac{(n_{ij} - n'_{ij})^2}{n'_{ij}} \tag{3}$$

The results gathered using the formula are relevant when the size of dataset is $n > 40$. In case that $20 < n < 40$ and some of expected frequencies n'_{ij} are less than 5, the class with the mentioned frequency must be combined with two or more adjacent classes of variable A or B. The mentioned method cannot be used in the case of the size of dataset is $n < 20$.

Testing the null hypothesis (H_0) on the independence of variables A and B follows χ^2:

$$H_0 \; : \; n_{ij} - n'_{ij} = 0, \; or \; \sum_{i=1}^{k} \sum_{j=1}^{m} (n_{ij} - n'_{ij}) = 0 \tag{4}$$

Small values of χ^2 confirm H_0; on the other hand, large values of χ^2 reject it.

The test statistics have an approximately χ^2 distribution only if less than 20% of $n'_{ij} < 5 \; \forall \; i, j$. If $\chi^2 > \chi^2_{\,(k-1)\,(m-1)}\,(\alpha)$, the hypothesis on the independence of variables A, B is rejected.

Critical values $(k - 1)\,(m - 1)\,(\alpha)$ are percentage points, and $(k - 1)\,(m - 1)$ is the number of degrees of freedom.

Sometimes χ^2 is called the likelihood ratio. The value of χ^2 provides information whether correlation between variables A and B can be considered to be statistically significant or not. However, it does not provide information on the degree of dependence of the variables. The degree of dependence can be measured using the coefficient of association of two categorical variables A and B. It is calculated using the Formula (5) [18]:

$$r_{AB} = \sqrt{\frac{\chi^2}{n\sqrt{(k-1)\cdot(m-1)}}} \tag{5}$$

2.3. Injury Rate Analyses

The aim of the injury rate analysis is to make decision about the effect of the commonly used prognostic variables on the injury rate. Moreover, the association between the prognostic variables and injury rate is studied as well [19]. The analysis is carried out using the Poisson regression model. The model is often used to analyse the data related to age group in epidemiology [20–23] and it is mentioned in several works [19,24,25].

Statistical models provide a possible solution to the problem. Poisson regression models provide a standard framework for more complex statistical analyses of injury rate. However, a detailed insight into the impacts of many variables is possible as well. The injury rate is estimated with regard to the number of accidents (*d*) divided by the amount of produced wood (1000 m^3) (*N*),

$$\text{injury rate} = d/N, \text{(number of accidents/1000 m}^3\text{)} \tag{6}$$

Data gathered in the year 2017 could not be included in the analysis because data associated with the wood produced by the Slovak forest industry in that year were not available. Data associated with wood production over the previous years were drawn from the Green report issued by the Ministry of Agriculture and Rural Development of the Slovak Republic [26].

The number of injuries is predicted using the Poisson distribution with the mean $\mu_d = N \times \lambda$, where λ is the incident injury rate. The average number of injuries, injury rate is expressed by parametric function of prognostic variables. As the Poisson distribution assumes that the meaningful value in distribution is greater than zero, this function of prognostic variables is often limited by values of a function greater than zero. The following logarithmic-linear model is usually used to model the injury rate λ as a function of a set of prognostic variables $X_1, \ldots X_p$:

$$\log(\lambda) = \log(\mu_d/N) = \beta_0 + \beta_1 X_1 + \ldots + \beta_p X_p \tag{7a}$$

or

$$\log(\mu_d) = \beta_0 + \beta_1 X_1 + \ldots + \beta_p X_p + \log(N) \tag{7b}$$

where β is a regression coefficient of average number of injuries of *i-th* prognostic variable X ($i = 1 \ldots n$). Thus, the log (of rate) is a linear function of prognostic variables. In the language of generalised linear models (GLMs), the usual specification of the linear component is due to the inclusion of the term log (*N*). This term is called the "offset" [27,28]. In the log function (Formula 7b) the average number of injuries is expressed using the linear combination of prognostic variables, while log (*N*) is expressed by fixed-value coefficient. The analyses relate to the amount of produced wood. The number of employees (full-time as well as part-time workers) can be used as an alternative to the produced wood (1000 m^3).

If the variance and the mean are equal, this is the condition to select the Poisson distribution for the number of injuries (*d*). Multiple linear regression with homogeneity of variances is based on the Poisson distribution.

If the variance and the mean are not equal, standard errors relating to parameter proposal are incorrect. The condition is usually broken when the variance is larger than the mean, the so-called over-variance. Methods dealing with over-variance are mentioned in the work [28]. The relevancy test for Poisson regression models of both the variance and the mean is determined in the χ^2 distribution used to compare the observed and expected frequencies [27]. A comparison of statistical models based on measuring the model discrepancy and variance is also used for qualitative evaluation of model adequacy. If the variance and the degrees of freedom are approximately equal, the model is considered to be adequate.

Many important aspects have to be taken into consideration when the models are used, for example, whether models are specified correctly, the determination of prognostic variables, and appropriate methods for distribution. Additional analyses have to be carried out in order to determine the suitability of the regression model for making predictions. Moreover, the data quality must be evaluated (reliability, accuracy, etc ...) as well as random factors related to the analyses of injury rate resulting from the various source of data.

3. Results

3.1. Injuries in Forestry Operations

Timber harvesting is the most risky phase of the process of harvesting, processing, and transport (Figure 1). The highest number of workplace accidents (31.8% of all recorded workplace accidents) occurred during the mentioned phase in the analysis period, due to motor-assisted technology with chainsaws in the timber harvesting phase. Timber skidding, with 16% of recorded accidents, was the second highest-risk phase. The timber harvesting phase is the riskiest phase. Forty-eight percent of fatal injuries and 26% of serious injuries leading to permanent damage to health were recorded in the forest industry during the analysis period. Seventy-five percent of all serious or fatal injuries and 48% of all workplace accidents mentioned in the database occurred during the phase of harvesting and skidding.

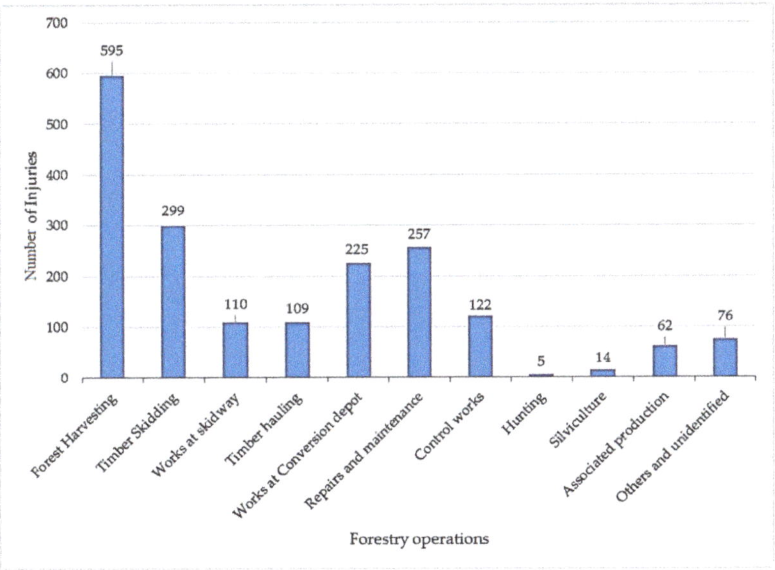

Figure 1. Workplace injuries in Slovak forestry over the years 2000–2016.

Observed and expected frequencies related to fatal injuries and serious workplace injuries leading to permanent damage to health during the phase of harvesting and skidding and also during other phases and activities with recorded workplace injuries are shown in a contingency table (Table 2). The null hypothesis was tested:

Hypothesis 1. *The difference in the occurrence of fatal injuries and serious workplace injuries leading to permanent damage to health during the phase of harvesting and skidding and also during other phases and activities is not statistically significant.*

Table 2. Contingency table for the occurrence of fatal injuries (A-injuries) and serious injuries (B-injuries) in forest harvesting and timber skidding operations.

Phase	Injuries/Abundance	A-Injuries	B-Injuries	Σ
Forest harvesting + timber skidding	Real injuries	96	126	222
	Expected abundance	63	159	
Other	Real injuries	32	199	231
	Expected abundance	65	166	
Σ		128	325	453

Source: Authors' compilation.

- $\chi^2 = 47.4400$
- Degree of freedom (DF): 1

At the level of significance $\alpha = 0.05$ with the degree of freedom 1, the value of chi-squared is 3.8. The calculated χ^2 is bigger than $\chi^2{}_{1(0.05)}$ and the null hypothesis can be rejected with 95% confidence. The difference in the occurrence of fatal injuries and serious workplace injuries leading to permanent damage to health during the phase of harvesting and skidding and also during other phases and activities is statistically significant. More fatal injuries than the "expected dependence" occurred during the phase of harvesting and skidding. The risk of fatal injuries recorded in the mentioned phases is higher than in all other phases and activities in the forest industry.

Due to the coefficient of association of $r_{AB} = 0.32$, there is a low positive relationship.

3.2. Injury Rate

The injury rate in the forest industry over the years 2000–2016 was decreasing. The trend in the injury rate for the forest industry on 1000 m^3 of produced wood in the years 2000–2016 is illustrated in the graph (Figure 2).

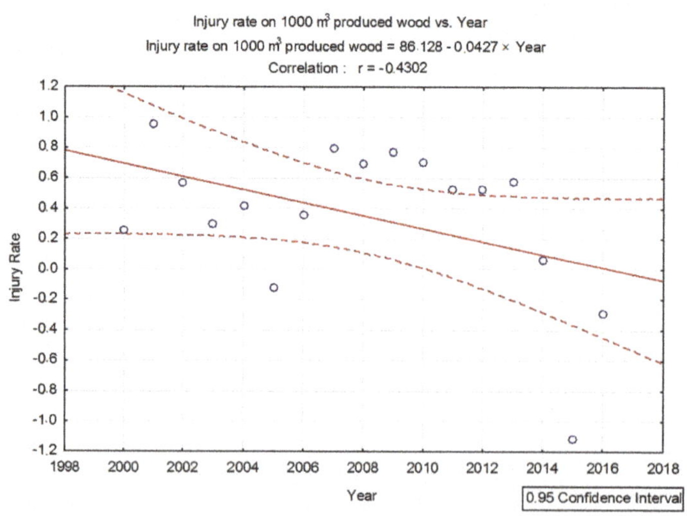

Figure 2. Trend in the injury rate on 1000 m^3 in the Slovak forestry sector over the years 2000–2016.

A simple one-dimensional Poisson regression model can be used to analyse whether the trend in the injury rate is a function of one hypothetical variable—the calendar year. The number of workplace injuries and the amount of produced wood in the Slovak forest industry in 1000 m^3 were primary data in the first model. The effect of other prognostic variables was not taken into consideration. It is expressed using the formula:

$$\ln(\lambda_{year}) = b_0 + b_1(year) \quad (8)$$

where λ_{year} is an injury rate or each year.

A regression model (Figure 3) described using Formula (8) (hereinafter Model (8)), means that ln (injury rate) should be dependent on the year (b_1). Results of the regression analysis are mentioned in Table 3.

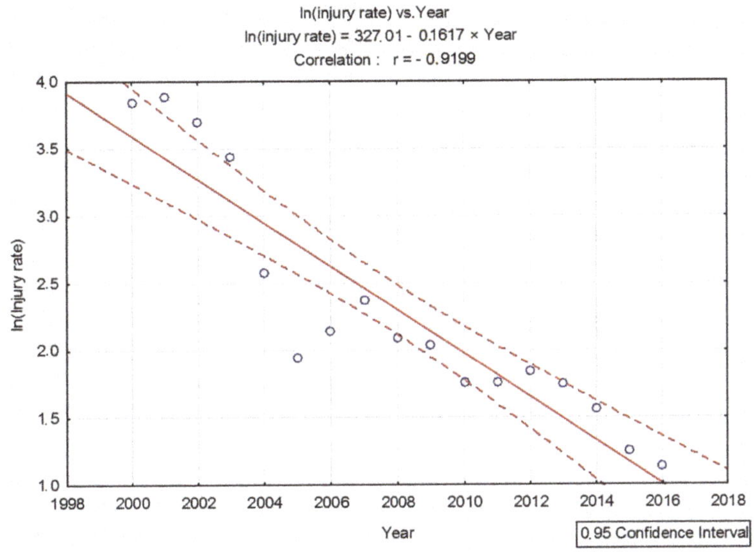

Figure 3. Trend in the injury rate in the Slovak forestry sector over the years 2000–2016 after calculation with Model (8).

Table 3. Simple regression results with dependence variable (injury rate in forestry).

Simple Regression Results with Dependence Variable: C (Injury Rate) R = 0.9199, R^2 = 0.8463, Edited R^2 = 0.8360, F (1,15) = 82.5660, *p*						
***N* = 17**	**B**	**Standard Error from *b***	***b***	**Standard Error from *b***	***T* (15)**	***p*-value**
Absolute term			327.0145	35.7358	9.1509	0.0000
Year	−0.9199	0.1012	−0.1617	0.0178	−9.0865	0.0000

Source: Authors' compilation.

Coefficients used in Model (8) were b_0 = 327.0145 and b_1 = −0.1617, with the standard error of s.e.$_{(b0)}$ = 35.7358 and s.e.$_{(b1)}$ = 0.0178. As is shown in the model, the injury rate decreases by 0.16 units per year after logarithmic transformation. Expected change in the number of injuries was exp (−0.1617) = 0.8510 from year to year. Therefore, the injury rate decreases approximately by 14.9% (= 100 × (1 − 0.8510)%) annually. An approximate 95% confidence interval for the parameter which is changed yearly is −0.1617 ± 1.96 (0.0178) = (−0.1264; −0.1969). Seeing that b_1 = 0 is not in this interval, a significant change in the primary observed injury rate per year is expected.

3.3. Injured Body Parts

Forestry jobs have a risk of permanent damage to health or ability to perform manual tasks. Therefore, an analysis of injured body parts has to be carried out. According to many authors, the anthropometric parameters of the Slovak adult population have been increasing to date [29–31]. That is why the risk of workplace accidents in several forest operations has been affected as well. The overview of the number of injuries related to individual body parts occurring in forest industry in the years 2000–2016 is shown in Figure 4.

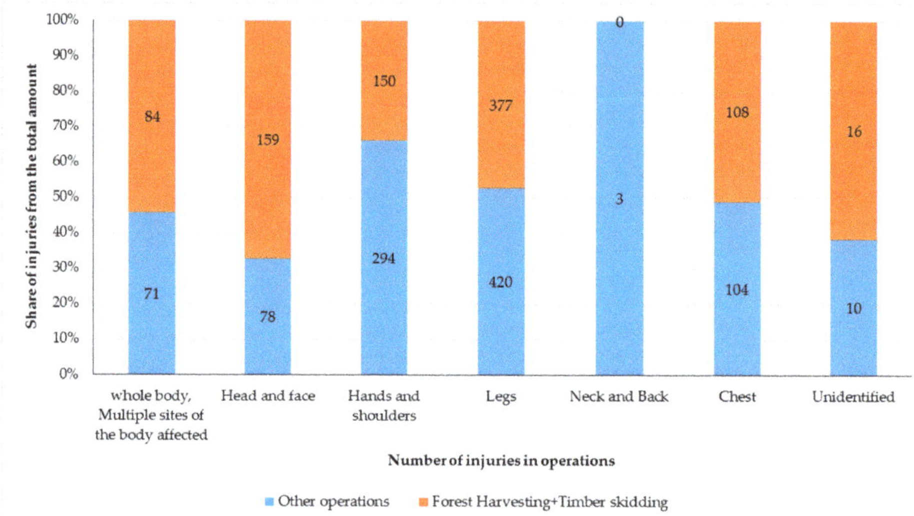

Figure 4. Injured body parts due to forestry operations in Slovak forestry over the years 2000–2016.

The most common parts of the body affected by workplace accidents are legs—all parts of legs (42.5% of all injuries). Leg injuries are not usually life-threatening. Head and facial injuries are those with the highest rate (67.1% injuries of these body parts) during the phase of harvesting and skidding. Moreover, these injuries can result in life-threatening damage. Injuries of the whole body or several body parts at the same time occur most often (54.2%) in the phase of harvesting and skidding. The mentioned results correspond to the high rate of fatal injuries in the phase of forest harvesting and timber skidding (3.1), as injuries to these body parts are most often life-threatening.

4. Discussion

A non-significant decrease in the injury rate over the years 2000–2016 was determined in the analysis of the workplace injury rate in the Slovak forest sector. Grzywinski et al. [32] analysed workplace accidents in Szczecinek (NW Poland) legally administered by the Regional Directorate of State Forests in the years 1990–2009. A total of 10,420 workplace accidents and an injury rate of almost 15 injuries per 1000 employees were recorded. Following the analysis, it seems the privatisation in the forestry industry did not affect the number of workplace accidents significantly.

Benavides et al. [33] carried out an analysis in Spain, finding that the injury rate of full-time workers (44.9 per 1000 employees in the year 2002) was lower than the injury rate of seasonal workers (120.6 per 1000 employees in the year 2002). This is influenced by the quality of professional training as well as the work experience of full-time workers. In [34], a decrease in fatal injury rate in agriculture, game keeping, and forestry in Arkhangelsk region from 43.9 per 1000 employees in the year 1996 to 20.8 per 1000 employees in the year 2007 is mentioned. The authors of [35] compared the fatal injury rates in Australia and the United States over the years 1989–1992 and in New Zealand over the years

1985–1994. The average fatal injury rate in New Zealand was 4.9/100,000, while in Australia it was 3.8/100,000, and in the United States it was 3.2/100,000. In the course of the years 1975–1984, the death rate of forest workers in New Zealand was 8.0 per 100,000 employees per year.

Suchomel [36] carried out the analysis of workplace accidents in the process of forest harvesting over the years 1984–1993. The position of individual phases in the process of harvesting, processing and transport was as follows: forest harvesting—32%, timber skidding—29%, work on the skidway—9%, timber hauling—8%, work at the conversion depot—6%, repairs and maintenance—15%, and internal control—1%. Following the overview, almost the same order of the phases as during the analysis period 2000–2016 can be seen. Small differences result from subjective as well as objective factors. In the work [37] the analysis of Sweden is carried out. The results show that serious workplace accidents are very common in Sweden and the death rate of self-employed in forestry is 7% of the total number of workers killed in work-related activities recorded by the employment office. Falling trees are the main cause of fatal or life-threatening injuries. Dangerous practises and procedures at work result in injuries when using work tools (e.g., portable chainsaws). Therefore, quality training as well as skill improvement must be offered to line workers to equip them to deliver health and safety to the workplace.

When evaluating specific injured body parts in the analysis of workplace accidents, the authors [37] found out that a knee is the most commonly injured part of the body in the process of forest harvesting. The results of our analysis show that leg injuries occurred most often during harvesting as well (258). This represents approximately 14% of all recorded injuries. An injury rate of 28% is mentioned in [38], a rate of 14% of all injuries in [36], and a rate of 19% (excluding foot and ankle injuries) in [1].

5. Conclusions

Forest harvesting and timber skidding represent operations with a high risk of injury. Working with chainsaws, the most commonly used tool by forest workers in Slovakia, can be considered one of the most dangerous activities in forestry. In order to create a healthy and safe working environment, real accidents have to be analysed and subsequently, a system of preventive measures has to be developed [39].

The self-employed must be the focus of attention. Making money is more important for them than following safety instructions and advice. Their equipment is not in accordance with regulations, and they do not wear protective clothing made for forestry workers seeking the best combination of safety and optimal ergonomics in daily work. They underestimate and break the general norms for ensuring the safety, health, and welfare of workers and do so intentionally. Minor injuries not threatening their lives or not leading to permanent damage to health are not recorded and the labour inspectorate is not informed about them. Forest jobs are also commonly offered to enterprises not putting equal emphasis on qualification, training, or skills. Workers have only poor information about doing enough to protect their health and keep them safe at work. The job of forest operators is a physically demanding job associated with health risk. The abovementioned facts are often ignored by the self-employed, who often work alone—for themselves. In case of workplace accidents there is nobody to arrange first aid or any other medical treatment they need on time. It is necessary to act and think quickly to avoid delayed treatment during an emergency, although this can be seen as ineffective or even harmful. Moreover, they often do not have health insurance coverage from commercial health insurance due to lack of finances and consequently, serious injury can result in severe financial hardship.

In practise, measures for prevention and control can be inspired by the results of the analysis. Following the analysis of the records related to workplace injuries and occupational diseases, the risk to health during the process of harvesting, processing, and transport can be evaluated. Changes in forest operations, especially in the phase of forest harvesting and timber skidding, aimed at technology innovation, environmentally-friendly procedures, and protection of the employees from workplace dangers need to be made. The education and training of forest operators should be focused on the safe use of a chainsaw, the proper use of personal protective equipment, and also on maintaining the good posture in order to prevent workplace injuries caused by fatigue. Mechanical and physical risk prevention must be supported in small and medium-sized enterprises (there are currently very weak prevention measures). In the case of a decrease in workplace injuries, the social insurance contribution paid by an enterprise should be lower. This is a method to motivate employers to follow requirements in order to provide a safer environment in the workplace. In order to cope better with health and safety issues for the self-employed, further safety legislation and laws must be implemented.

Even though the results of the analysis show a decrease in injury rate considering an increase in forest production, misinterpretation is a common problem when using statistical information, especially data related to the self-employed. Due to a high number of fatal and serious injuries in the process of forest harvesting and timber skidding, there is widespread recognition of the importance of good education and training of forest operators. Great emphasis must be placed on the use of proper equipment and technology as well as safety processes and procedures to minimise the risk of injury in the workplace.

Author Contributions: M.V. conceived and designed the experiments; M.V., Z.A. and M.G. analysed the data; M.G. and Ž.B. wrote the paper.

Funding: The research described in this paper was financed jointly by APVV-16-0297 (Update of the anthropometric database of the Slovak population) and VEGA Number. 1/0031/18 (Optimization of technological and work processes and risk assessment in the production of forest biomass for energy purposes). The APC was funded by (APVV-16-0297).

Conflicts of Interest: The authors declare no conflict of interest.

References

1. Springer, Y.P.; Lucas, D.L.; Castrodale, L.J.; McLaughlin, J.B. Work-related injuries in the Alaska logging industry, 1991–2014. *Am. J. Ind. Med.* **2018**, *61*, 32–41. [CrossRef]
2. Tremblay, A.; Badri, A. A novel tool for evaluating occupational health and safety performance in small and medium-sized enterprises: The case of the Quebec forestry/pulp and paper industry. *Saf. Sci.* **2018**, *101*, 282–294. [CrossRef]
3. Danilovic, M.; Antonic, S.; Dordevic, Z.; Vojvodic, P. Forestry Work-Related Injuries in Forest Estate "Sremska Mitrovica" In Serbia. *Sumar. List* **2016**, *140*, 589–598.
4. Kogler, R.; Quendler, E.; Boxberger, J. Occupational Accidents with Agricultural Machinery in Austria. *J. Agromed.* **2016**, *21*, 61–70. [CrossRef]
5. Richard, S.; Oppliger, A. Zoonotic occupational diseases in forestry workers—Lyme borreliosis, tularemia and leptospirosis in Europe. *Ann. Agric. Environ. Med.* **2015**, *22*, 43–50. [CrossRef] [PubMed]
6. Suchomel, J.; Belanová, K.; Štollmann, V. Analysis of Occupational Diseases Occurring in Forestry and Wood Processing Industry in Slovakia. *Drvna Ind.* **2011**, *62*, 219–228. [CrossRef]
7. Pinzke, S.; Svennefelt, C.A.; Lundqvist, P. Occupational Injuries in Swedish Agriculture: Development and Preventive Actions. *J. Agric. Saf. Health.* **2018**, *24*, 193–211. [CrossRef]
8. Gejdoš, M.; Hitka, M.; Potkány, M.; Balážová, Ž. Analysis of Human Resources and Anthropometric Data Relating to Forestry Machine Operators in Slovakia. In *Innovation Management and Education Excellence Through Vision 2020*; Soliman, K., Ed.; Ibima Publishing: Milan, Italy, 2016; pp. 2256–2262.
9. Poje, A.; Potocnik, I.; Kosir, B.; Krc, J. Cutting patterns as a predictor of the odds of accident among professional fellers. *Saf. Sci.* **2016**, *89*, 158–166. [CrossRef]
10. Nkomo, H.; Niranjan, I.; Reddy, P. Effectiveness of Health and Safety Training in Reducing Occupational Injuries Among Harvesting Forestry Contractors in KwaZulu-Natal. *Workplace Health Saf.* **2018**, *66*, 499–507. [CrossRef]
11. Bailer, A.J.; Reed, L.D.; Stayner, L.T. Modeling Fatal Injury Rates Using Poisson Regression: A Case Study of Workers in Agriculture. Forestry, and Fishing. *J. Saf. Res.* **1997**, *28*, 177–186. [CrossRef]

12. Benavides, F.G.; Benach, J.; Martínez, J.M.; González, S. Description of fatal occupational injury rates in five selected European Union countries: Austria, Finland, France, Spain and Sweden. *Saf. Sci.* **2005**, *43*, 497–502. [CrossRef]
13. Vlčková, M. Analysis of Work Accidents and Occupational Diseases Development in Selected Forestry Subjects in Slovakia. Ph.D. Thesis, Technical University in Zvolen, Zvolen, Slovakia, 2004.
14. Eurostat. *European Statistics on Accidents at Work (ESAW)—Summary Methodology*; Eurostat: Luxembourg, 2013; ISBN 978-92-79-28419-9.
15. Edict Nr. 500/2006 The Ministry of Labour, Social Affairs and Family of the Slovak Republic. *Pattern of Record of Registered Work Injury*; Ministry of Labour, Social Affairs and Family of the Slovak Republic: Bratislava, Slovakia, 2006.
16. Nussbaum, E.B. *Contingency Tables the Chi-Square Test and Associated Effect Sizes*; Routledge: Oxford, UK, 2015; pp. 81–97.
17. Richardson, J.T.E. The analysis of 2 × 2 contingency tables-Yet again. *Stat. Med.* **2011**, *30*, 890. [CrossRef]
18. Šmelko, Š. *Štatistické Metódy v Lesníctve [Statistical Methods in Forestry]*; TU Zvolen: Zvolen, Slovakia, 1998; 276p, ISBN 80-228-0684-6.
19. Breslow, N.E.; Day, N.E. *Statistical Methods in Cancer Research Volume I—The Analysis of Case-Control Studies*; International Agency for Research on Cancer: Lyon, France, 1980; 338p, ISBN 978-9283201328.
20. Berry, G. The analysis of mortality by the subject-years method. *Biometrics* **1983**, *39*, 173–184. [CrossRef]
21. Frome, E.L. The analysis of rates using Poisson regression models. *Biometrics* **1983**, *39*, 665–674. [CrossRef] [PubMed]
22. Frome, E.L.; Checkoway, H. Epidemiologic Programs for Computers and Calculators—Use of Poisson Regression-Models in Estimating Incidence Rates and Ratios. *Am. J. Epidemiol.* **1985**, *121*, 309–323. [CrossRef] [PubMed]
23. Whittemore, A.S. Analyzing cohort mortality data. *Am. Stat.* **1985**, *39*, 437–441. [CrossRef]
24. Checkoway, H.; Pearce, N.E.; Crawford-Brown, D.J. *Research Methods in Occupational Epidemiology*; Oxford University Press: New York, NY, USA, 1989; ISBN-13 9780195092424.
25. Selvin, S. *Practical Biostatical Methods*; Duxbury Press: Belmont, CA, USA, 1995; ISBN 0-534-23802-5.
26. Anonymous. *Green Report*; Ministry of Agriculture and Rural Development of the Slovak Republic: Bratislava, Slovakia, 2017; 68p, ISBN 978-80-8093-235-0.
27. Dobson, A.J.; Barnett, A.G. *An Introduction to Generalized Linear Models*; CRC Press, Taylor & Francis Group: Boca Raton, FL, USA, 2008; ISBN 978-1-58488-950-2.
28. McCullagh, P.; Nelder, J.A. *Generalized Linear Models, Second Edition*; Chapman and Hall/CRC Press: Boca-Raton, FL, USA, 1989; ISBN 978-0-41231-760-6.
29. Gejdoš, M.; Vlčková, M. Analysis of Work Accidents in Timber Transport in Slovakia. In Proceedings of the 18th International Scientific Conference-Logi 2017, České Budějovice, Czech Republic, 18–19 May 2017. [CrossRef]
30. Hitka, M.; Mračková, E.; Sedmák, R. Changes of anthropometric characteristics of the adult population in Slovakia and their influence on material sources and work safety. *Adv. Mat. Res.* **2014**, *1001*, 401–406. [CrossRef]
31. Kampf, R.; Lorincová, S.; Hitka, M.; Stopka, O. Generational Differences in the Perception of Corporate Culture in European Transport Enterprises. *Sustainability* **2017**, *9*, 1561. [CrossRef]
32. Grzywinski, W.; Sawa, L.; Nowik, A.; Nowicki, G. Structure of work accidents in the Regional Directorate of the State Forests in Szczecinek in the years 1990–2009. *Sylwan* **2013**, *157*, 403–411.
33. Benavides, F.G.; Benach, J.; Muntaner, C.; Delclos, G.L.; Catot, N.; Amable, M. Associations between temporary employment and occupational injury: What are the mechanisms? *Occup. Environ. Med.* **2006**, *63*, 416–421. [CrossRef]
34. Varakina, Z.L.; Vyazmin, A.M.; Sannikov, A.L.; Nygard, C.H.; Grjibovski, A.M. Fatal occupational injuries in the Arkhangelsk region, Northwest Russia. *Occup. Med.-Oxf.* **2010**, *60*, 470–475. [CrossRef] [PubMed]
35. Feyer, A.M.; Wiliamson, A.M.; Stout, N.; Driscoll, T.; Usher, H.; Langley, J.D. Comparison of work related fatal injuries in the United States, Australia, and New Zealand: Method and overall findings. *Inj. Prev.* **2001**, *7*, 22–28. [CrossRef] [PubMed]
36. Suchomel, J. *Analysis of Selected Criteria and Methods for Modelling and Optimization of Harvesting Process*; Habilitation Work; Technical University in Zvole: Zvolen, Slovakia, 1999; p. 148.

37. Lindroos, O.; Burstrom, L. Accident rates and types among self-employed private forest owners. *Accid. Anal. Prev.* **2010**, *42*, 1729–1735. [CrossRef] [PubMed]
38. Lefort, A.J., Jr.; De Hoop, C.F.; Pine, J.C.; Marx, B.D. Characteristics of injuries in the logging industry of Louisiana, USA: 1986 to 1998. *Int. J. For. Eng.* **2003**, *14*, 75–89. [CrossRef]
39. Montorselli, N.B.; Lombardini, C.; Magagnotti, N.; Marchi, E.; Neri, F.; Picchi, G.; Spinelli, R. Relating safety, productivity and company type for motor- manual logging operations in the Italian Alps. *Accid. Anal. Prev.* **2010**, *42*, 2013–2017. [CrossRef] [PubMed]

International Journal of
Environmental Research and Public Health

MDPI

Article

Impact of Obesity on Employment and Wages among Young Adults: Observational Study with Panel Data

Hyeain Lee [1], Rosemary Ahn [1], Tae Hyun Kim [2,*] and Euna Han [3,*]

[1] College of Pharmacy, Yonsei University, Incheon 21983, Korea; hnlhailey@gmail.com (H.L.); ahn.rosemary@gmail.com (R.A.)

[2] Graduate School of Public Health and Institute of Health Services Research, Yonsei University, Seoul 03722, Korea

[3] College of Pharmacy, Institute of Pharmaceutical Sciences, Yonsei University, Incheon 21983, Korea

* Correspondence: thkim@yuhs.ac (T.H.K.); eunahan@yonsei.ac.kr (E.H.); Tel.: +82-2-2228-1521 (T.H.K.); +82-32-749-4511 (E.H.); Fax: +82-2-2392-7734 (T.H.K.); +82-32-749-4105 (E.H.)

Received: 12 December 2018; Accepted: 3 January 2019; Published: 7 January 2019

Abstract: This paper assesses the relationship between obesity and the job market by focusing on young adults early on in their careers, while considering the factor of gender and the individuals' job qualifications. This study extracted data on high school students for four years from the Korean Education and Employment Panel (from 2010 to 2013), a nationally representative dataset comprising of 2000 middle school students and 4000 high school seniors. The individual-level fixed effects were controlled using conditional logistic regression models and an ordinary least squares model. Obese and overweight men were 1.46 times more likely to be placed in professional jobs and had 13.9% higher monthly wages than their normal-weight counterparts. However, obese and overweight women were 0.33 times less likely to have service jobs, earned 9.0% lower monthly wages, and half as likely to have jobs with bonuses than that of their normal-weight counterparts. However, such penalty among women was found only when they had none of the assessed job market qualifications. Given that initial jobs and job conditions have lingering impacts in long-term job performance, the cumulative penalty for overweight or obesity could be more substantial for young adults in particular.

Keywords: obesity; labor market performance; job qualifications; young adults

1. Introduction

The prevalence of obesity has dramatically increased across the globe and has become a major public health concern [1]. From 1980 to 2013, an increase in obesity prevalence has been evaluated in developed countries from 28.8% to 36.9% for men, from 29.8% to 38.0% for women, from 16.2% to 22.6% for girls, and from 16.9% to 23.8% for boys [2]. This rise has also been observed in newly developed and developing countries where obesity had not been a concern [3]. South Korea is not exceptional in this regard, given that the number of those that are overweight or obese particularly among young adults in the 20s and 30s age group soared from 24.4% in 1998 to 43.8% in 2015 [4,5].

Obesity is a well-recognized risk factor for various illnesses, including cardiovascular diseases and cancer [6]. Being overweight or obese has negative implications in social aspects as well. Several previous studies signify appearance-based discrimination on obese and overweight persons to result in an overall negative effect [7]. For instance, slimness is considered a beauty norm, which accordingly leads obesity to be looked down upon in most modern societies [8,9]. In addition, for the reason that obesity is often controllable at the individual level, it results in the conception of having insufficient self-control and practicing unhealthy behaviors or having poor self-esteem and time management [10–12]. Furthermore, one's overweight or obesity status is visible.

Assuming that employers desire healthy workers with positive social characteristics, all these aspects of overweight or obesity place disadvantages on such individuals in the job market [13]. It has been reported that obese people earn less, are less likely to be hired, or are more likely to remain unemployed [14,15]. Further studies also indicate that obese individuals are less likely to be sorted into jobs that have socially desirable work profiles, such as earning a high salary, positioning in a professional or semi-professional sector, and receiving benefits of high quality in both monetary and non-monetary aspects [16].

The present study builds on previous literature and focuses on the labor market penalty for the obese in their early adulthood life, a period in which individuals are generally new to the labor market, and explored the association between overweight or obesity and job market performance varied by the respondents' job qualifications. While variables like education can be easily observed, studies find that the measure of the impact of these qualification variables regarding their careers take place after the firms gain access to more information on the productivity of their employees [17]. Likewise, given that young adults tend to be new in their jobs, they do not have the offsetting information that is needed to repel the stigma stemming from obesity [18]. Considering that disadvantage in the labor market early on in their careers may linger later in their career, overweight and obese young adults are more disposed to the negative effects of obesity in the job market [19,20]. Focusing on young adults also gives us leverage to partially mimic experimental settings, since the manifestation of any reverse impacts in job market activities on body mass have yet been realized [6].

There are certain features in a job profile that makes a job aspiring among young adults who are entering the labor market for the first time. The characteristics that comprise of a good job include social prestige, job security such as permanent status and labor union presence, monetary compensation, work contents, and fringe benefits [21]. Although remuneration is the core aspect of a good job, studies indicate that non-pecuniary characteristics also form important attributes that enhance the appeal of a job [21–24]. Thus, this study also addresses the correlation between overweight or obesity and job market performance by considering both a job's pecuniary as well as non-pecuniary aspects to comprehensively understand the relationship.

2. Materials and Methods

2.1. Data

The study obtained data from the Korean Education and Employment Panel (KEEP), a nationally representative dataset comprising of 2000 middle school students and 4000 high school seniors from general high schools and vocational schools. The data gathered via survey comprises of information on the respondents' education, employment, and household details since 2004, such as parents' socioeconomic status. This study extracted data on high school students for four years from the Korean Education and Employment Panel (from 2010 to 2013). The response rates of the annual survey during the period from 2010 to 2013 for this study were 76.5%, 75.8%, 76.4%, and 76.4%, respectively. Due to the potential non-randomness of the non-response to the survey, we applied weight on the non-response to adjust the gap between the actual responses and the objective responses. The following exclusion criteria was applied to a total of 9944 person-year observations: missing household information (17 observations), BMI under 10 (one observation) or over 40 (13 observations), and missing income information (40 observations). The final sample included 8340 person-year observations (4714 males and 3626 females), of which 4185 (1959 males and 2226 females) person-years were employed.

2.2. Variables

The dependent variable for this study is job performance, which is measured by: (1) employment status, (2) permanent status of one's job, (3) bonus provision, (4) presence of a labor union, (5) job sector (professional, semi-professional, sales, service, and blue-collar), and (6) monthly wage. Respondents who helped their family at least 18 h per week without payment were considered employed, whereas full-time students and students working as either teaching or research assistants were considered not employed. Temporary employment was defined as either having a job with a labor contract of less than one year or having daily jobs without contracts. Job sector, another measurement of job performance, was categorized based on the South Korean standard classification index (Korean Standard Industrial & Job Classification, 5th edition, 2000.1.7, Statistics Korea) into professional, semi-professional, sales, and service groups, with reference to the blue-collar sector, which comprises of other previously unlisted job classifications like skilled agricultural and fishery workers, installation technicians, and mechanics. Wages were measured on a monthly basis as a linear variable in units of 10,000 Korean Won (KRW). Each dependent variable excluding wage was represented by binary variables.

The key independent variable is obesity status. The study determined the independent variable using the individual's BMI, which is calculated by dividing the respondents' self-reported weight in kilograms by the square of the respondents' self-reported height in meters. Three dummy indicators were generated, representing a clinical classification of BMI: underweight (BMI < 18.5), overweight or obese (BMI ≥ 25), and normal weight (BMI between 18.5 and 25) as reference. Overweight and obesity were combined, considering that the World Health Organization Regional Office for the Western Pacific (WPRO) and Korea Center for Disease Control and Prevention [25] specified BMI ≥ 25 as obese for Asians [26,27]. This study also considered individual qualifications for the job market as independent variables, e.g., having foreign language and other special certificates, job training experiences, or internship experiences. All the qualifications were measured using dummy indicators, with non-experienced as the reference condition.

We controlled the following variables in all estimations as covariates: highest level of educational attainment (high school graduate or below, with reference to college graduate or above), demographic status (gender), health behaviors (cigarette and alcohol use and general health status), personal characteristics (decisiveness and self-restraint), experience of discrimination, and parents' socioeconomic profiles (employment status and highest education level attained). The ages of the respondents varied by a very small margin because the panel gathered data since the period in which respondents were in their senior year of high school. Furthermore, given that the sample population was in their late twenties, the respondents' marital status and number of children did not show much variations. Smoking was coded as a binary variable to denote whether the respondents were current smokers. Alcohol usage was measured as drink occasionally and drink frequently, with never drink as the reference. The respondents' general health statuses were also measured using a dummy variable that represents being healthy and feeling unhealthy, as the reference. Likewise, the respondents' practice of decisiveness and self-restraint were also measure with dummy indicators.

2.3. Estimation

The individual-level fixed effects were controlled using conditional logistic regression models for the dichotomous dependent variables and an ordinary least squares model for a linear measurement of the dependent variable (1):

$$Y_{it} = \beta_0 + \beta_1 BMI_{it} + \beta_2 Qualif_{it} + \beta_3 X_{it} + \mu_i + \varepsilon_{it} \quad (1)$$

where the subscripts i and t denote individual and year, respectively. Y indicates either linear log monthly wages or the following four binary dependent variables: employment, permanent status of the job, bonus provision of the job, and presence of a labor union. The β s indicate estimated parameters. BMI indicates either a linear measurement of BMI or a series of dummy indicators representing underweight and overweight or obese, with normal weight as the reference. $Qualif$ denotes dummy indicators for job qualifications including highest education attainment level, and obtainment of special certificates, job training or internship experiences. X is a vector of family information and individual demographic and socioeconomic variables. μ represents individual-level permanent observed and unobserved characteristics, and ε denotes time-varying error term. The unit of analysis was individual-year. For each dependent variable, two separate models were applied, one with a linear measurement of BMI and another wherein BMI was clinically classified into underweight and overweight or obesity (with normal weight as the reference). All estimations were run separately according to sex. Survey weights were applied in all analyses to adjust the unequal selection probability. All statistical analyses were performed using Stata 13.1 (StataCorp, College Station, TX, USA).

3. Results

Table 1 shows the distributional characteristics of the final sample by gender. The employment rate was 71.6% for women and 55.11% for men.

Table 1. Descriptive statistics.

Variables	Mean (Standard Deviation) (Minimum, Maximum)	
	Men (*N* = 4714)	Women (*N* = 3626)
Dependent variables		
Employed	0.5511	0.7168
Monthly wages (10,000 Korean Won) [a]	178.18 (76.89) (12, 1000)	163.38 (55.96) (15, 500)
Job sector classification [a]		
Professional/managerial	0.162	0.220
Semi-professional	0.078	0.193
Sales	0.104	0.084
Service	0.230	0.402
Others (reference)	0.423	0.101
Job Quality [a]		
Permanent position [b]	0.802	0.870
Having bonus [b]	0.619	0.587
With labor union [b]	0.216	0.164
Independent variable of interest		
BMI	23.31 (3.15) (13.36, 39.39)	20.20 (2.39) (14.52, 33.62)
BMI Group [c]		
Underweight	0.024	0.245
Normal weight (reference)	0.728	0.713
Overweight and Obese	0.248	0.042
Qualifications		
Job training [b]	0.046	0.054
Certificates [b]	0.101	0.087
Internship [b]	0.175	0.429
Own education level		
≤High School (reference)	0.616	0.240
College or higher	0.384	0.760
Other covariates		
Experience of discrimination based on physical appearance	0.058	0.084
Being Decisive [b]	0.600	0.492
Being Self-restrained [b]	0.593	0.495
Self-reported health status: healthy [b]	0.688	0.490
Currently smoking [b]	0.444	0.060
Drinking behavior		
Does not drink (reference)	0.196	0.234
Occasional drinker	0.708	0.718
Frequent drinker	0.098	0.051
Father's socioeconomic status		
High School graduate or lower education [b]	0.746	0.822
Employed [b]	0.946	0.937
Mother's socioeconomic status		
High School graduate or lower education [b]	0.891	0.927
Employed [b]	0.635	0.655

[a] Calculated only for the employed sample (1959 men and 2226 women). [b] Dummy indicator. [c] BMI groups include underweight (BMI < 25), overweight or obese (BMI ≥ 25), normal weight (18.5 < BMI ≤ 25) as references.

The higher employment rate among women possibly because of the national military service obligation for Korean men, which is approximately three years long and is usually fulfilled in their 20 s. The average monthly wages earned by men and women were 1,781,800 KRW (approximately 1537 USD) and 1,633,380 KRW (approximately 1415 USD), respectively. The majority of the employed had permanent jobs (80% of men and 87% of women). Approximately 61% of men and 58% of women were paid bonuses, but only 21% of men and 16% of women worked in companies with a labor union. There were also gender differences with regard to job qualifications. Women had a larger proportion of internship experiences (42%) than men did (17%), whereas it was the contrary when considering the attainment status of certificates (8% for women and 10% for men). The average BMIs of men and women were 23.31 and 20.20, respectively. Approximately, a quarter of men fell in the overweight or obese category, whereas roughly a quarter of women were in the underweight category. The proportion of women who have reported an experience in discrimination on physical appearance was higher than the proportion for men (8.4% for women versus 5.8% for men). Additionally, an estimate of 60% of men and 50% of women self-assessed that they were decisive or self-restrain in their daily lives.

Figure 1 shows an unadjusted distribution of monthly wages by units of one million KRW (approximately 1000 USD) over BMI. The figure illustrates a negative association between BMI and monthly wages among women, initially showing an ascending pattern up to the average BMI level, following a descending pattern as BMI increases past the average BMI. In the case of men, there was a positive relationship between BMI and monthly wages, showing a descending pattern in the underweight group and a gradual rise in the obese group. Figure 1 also shows the overall penalty in job quality of overweight or obese individuals. As illustrated, the tendency in which an individual has a permanent job, bonus, and assignment in a company that has a labor union dramatically decreases among both men and women with a BMI of 25 or more.

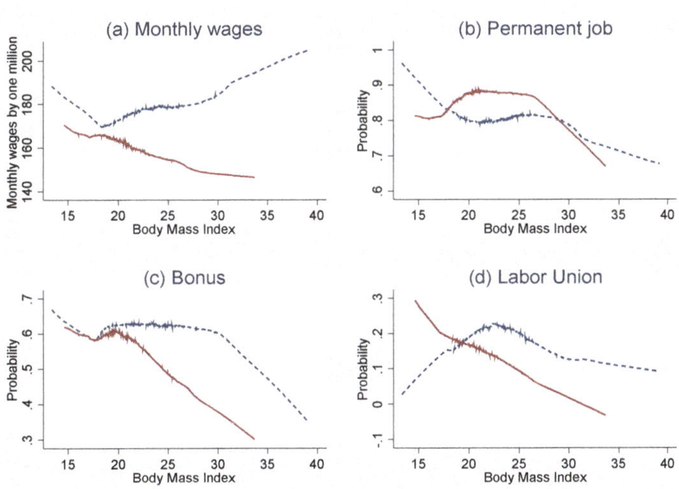

Figure 1. An unadjusted distribution of monthly wages in one million South Korean won and the probabilities of permanent job status, getting a bonus, and having labor union over BMI. Note: The X-axis represents body mass index, calculated as weight in kilograms divided by the square of height. The Y-axis represents one million Korean won (for monthly wages (**a**)) or probability (for having permanent job (**b**), bonus (**c**), and labor union (**d**)). In both the figures, the solid line is for women and the dotted line is for men.

The regression results as shown on Table 2 confirm no statistically significant association of BMI to overweight or obesity and the probability of employment for both genders. Subsequently, the study assessed the association of overweight or obesity with employment in specific job sectors, which consisted of professional, semi-professional, service, sales, and blue-collar sectors. A unit increase in BMI for men was associated with a higher likelihood of having professional jobs by 1.05 times, but a lower likelihood of having service jobs by 0.94 times. An alternative model with a clinical classification of BMI further revealed that there was a positive association between professional jobs and overweight or obese men (by 1.46 times) when compared to that of normal-weight men. On the contrary, men with higher BMI were less likely to belong to service jobs (by 0.94 times) and semi-professional jobs (by 0.50 times), compared to that of normal-weight men.

Table 2. Results from conditional logistic regression for the association between body mass status and overall employment and job sectors.

Key Independent Variables	Odds Ratio [b] (90% Confidence Interval):					
	Employed	Job Sector				
		Professional	Semi-Professional	Service	Sales	Blue-Collar
MEN						
Model 1						
BMI	0.988 (0.97, 1.00)	1.051 ** (1.01, 1.09)	0.982 (0.94, 1.03)	0.943 ** (0.90, 0.98)	1.015 (0.99, 1.05)	0.991 (0.97, 1.02)
Model 2						
Underweight [a]	1.033 (0.73, 1.46)	2.036 * (1.02, 4.07)	0.312 (0.06, 1.68)	1.281 (0.60, 2.74)	0.258 ** (0.09, 0.70)	1.453 (0.77, 2.17)
Overweight & Obese [a]	0.905 (0.63, 1.29)	1.469 ** (1.15, 1.87)	0.501 ** (0.42, 0.86)	0.983 (0.70, 1.25)	0.973 (0.79, 1.20)	0.955 (0.80, 1.14)
N	*4714*	*1959*	*1959*	*1959*	*1959*	*1959*
WOMEN						
Model 1						
BMI	0.996 (0.97, 1.02)	0.995 (0.96, 1.03)	0.983 (0.94, 1.02)	0.833 *** (0.78, 0.89)	1.019 (0.99, 1.05)	1.138 *** (1.08, 1.19)
Model 2						
Underweight [a]	1.111 (0.96, 1.28)	1.010 (0.82, 1.24)	1.100 (0.89, 1.36)	1.340 * (1.00, 1.79)	1.004 (0.84, 1.20)	0.523 *** (0.37, 0.74)
Overweight & Obese [a]	0.970 (0.70, 1.35)	0.220 (0.79, 1.89)	1.006 (0.62, 1.63)	0.333 ** (0.14, 0.80)	0.957 (0.66, 1.40)	1.450 (0.86, 2.44)
N	*3626*	*2226*	*2226*	*2226*	*2226*	*2226*

[a] BMI groups include underweight (BMI < 25), overweight or obese (BMI $\geq$ 25), normal weight (18.5 < BMI $\leq$ 25) as references. [b] * for p-value < 0.1, ** p-value < 0.05, *** for p-value < 0.01.

For women, there were statistically significant associations between the respondents' body mass status and the likelihood of having a service or sales job. Women with higher BMI were less likely to have service jobs (by 0.83 times), and the magnitude of the negative relationship between the two factors was more apparent for women in the overweight or obese category (by 0.33 times) compared to that of normal-weight women. In contrast, underweight women were nearly half as likely to have blue-collar jobs and were associated with a 13% higher probability of having a blue-collar job per unit increase in BMI (Table 2).

Table 3 shows the association between overweight or obesity and monthly wages. When controlling for time-invariant individual characteristics in a fixed-effect model, overweight or obesity among women was associated with lower monthly wages by 9.0%. Results among men were contrary to that of women, given that a unit increase in BMI was associated with higher monthly wages by 4.6%. An alternative model with a clinical classification of BMI also demonstrated that overweight or obese men had 13.9% higher monthly wages compared to the wages of their normal-weight counterparts (Table 3).

Table 3. Results from the individual-level fixed-effects model for the association between BMI and log monthly wages.

Key Independent Variable	Regression Coefficient [b] (Standard Error) on Log Monthly Wages	
	Women (*N* = 2226)	Men (*N* = 1959)
Model 1		
BMI	0.001 (0.007)	0.046 *** (0.009)
Model 2		
Underweight [a]	−0.003 (0.027)	0.025 (0.090)
Overweight & Obese [a]	−0.090 ** (0.040)	0.139 *** (0.044)

[a] BMI groups include underweight (BMI < 25), overweight or obese (BMI ≥ 25), normal weight (18.5 < BMI ≤ 25) as references. [b] ** *p*-value < 0.05, *** for *p*-value < 0.01.

There were statistically significant associations between overweight or obesity and job qualities, particularly among women. Underweight women were 1.57 times more likely to have a permanent job when compared to that of normal-weight women. Similarly, with each unit increase in BMI, women were 0.94 times less likely to have a job with a bonus provision, and overweight or obese women were only half as likely to have jobs with bonuses compared to that of normal-weight women. In addition, overweight or obese women were only 0.39 times likely to have a job in companies that have labor unions than that of their normal-weight counterparts. Such BMI penalties seen in job quality were marginally significant for employed men positioned in companies that have labor unions (Table 4).

Table 4. Results from conditional logistic regression models for the association between BMI and job quality.

Key Independent Variable	Odds Ratio [b] (90% Confidence Interval):		
	Having A Permanent Job	Getting Bonus in the Job	Having Job in a Company with a Labor Union
WOMEN			
Model 1			
BMI	1.043 (0.99, 1.09)	0.949 *** (0.92, 0.98)	0.905 *** (0.86, 0.95)
Model 2			
Underweight [a]	1.579 *** (1.25, 2.00)	1.010 (0.85, 1.20)	0.748 (0.60, 0.93)
Overweight & Obese [a]	1.125 (0.66, 1.92)	0.501 *** (0.34, 0.74)	0.390 ** (0.20, 0.74)
N	*2226*	*2226*	*2226*
MEN			
Model 1			
BMI	0.998 (0.96, 1.03)	0.982 (0.96, 1.01)	0.965 * (0.94, 0.99)
Model 2			
Underweight [a]	0.502 (0.23, 1.08)	1.032 (0.77, 2.19)	2.156 (0.97, 4.78)
Overweight & Obese [†a]	0.615 (0.28, 1.34)	1.305 (0.76, 2.23)	1.360 (0.60, 3.07)
N	*1959*	*1959*	*1959*

[a] BMI groups include underweight (BMI < 25), overweight or obese (BMI ≥ 25), normal weight (18.5 < BMI ≤ 25) as references. [b] * for *p*-value < 0.1, ** *p*-value < 0.05, *** for *p*-value < 0.01.

Table 5 exhibits the results obtained from subgroup analyses of two groups, where one group comprises of individuals with at the least one job qualification—the possession of foreign language or other special certificates, or experience in job training or internship—and the other group comprises of those without any of the three stated job qualifications. A part of the results revealed that, compared to having none of the three qualifications, having at the least one qualification alleviated penalty for those in the overweight or obesity category. When only considering women with none of the three qualifications, overweight or obesity was estimated to penalize the likelihood of having a permanent job (by 0.35 times compared to their normal-weight counterparts). Similarly, overweight or obese women were 0.33 times likely to have a job with a bonus provision than that of their counterparts. Women in the underweight category were estimated to have rewards for monthly wages in only the subgroup comprising of those without any of the three qualifications.

Table 5. Subgroup analyses by job qualification status for the association between BMI and job quality using conditional logistic regression or fixed-effects ordinary least squares.

Key Independent Variables	Odds Ratio [b] (90% Confidence Interval):			Regression Coefficient [b] (Standard Error):	
	Employed	**Permanent**	**Bonus**	**Labor Union**	**Wage**
MEN WITH AT THE LEAST ONE QUALIFICATION [c]					
BMI group					
Underweight †	1.196 (0.65, 2.21)	1.573 (0.40, 6.25)	0.486 (0.18, 1.26)	0.445 (0.12, 1.62)	0.061 (0.157)
Overweight & Obese †	0.988 (0.81, 1.21)	1.110 (0.77, 1.60)	1.144 (0.87, 1.50)	0.624 ** (0.46, 0.85)	0.087 (0.067)
N	*1912*	*920*	*920*	*920*	*920*
MEN WITHOUT ANY QUALIFICATION [c]					
BMI group					
Underweight †	0.896 (0.59, 1.37)	2.003 (0.80, 5.03)	0.854 (0.46, 1.60)	0.479 (0.17, 1.34)	−0.030 (0.127)
Overweight & Obese †	0.813 ** (0.69, 0.95)	1.316 (0.96, 1.81)	0.899 (0.70, 1.16)	0.597 ** (0.42, 0.84)	0.196 *** (0.065)
N	*2802*	*1039*	*1039*	*1039*	*1039*
WOMEN WITH AT THE LEAST ONE QUALIFICATION [c]					
BMI group					
Underweight †	0.772 ** (0.62, 0.96)	1.573 (0.40, 6.25)	1.082 (0.85, 1.37)	1.313 (0.98, 1.77)	−0.038 (0.083)
Overweight & Obese †	1.082 (0.65, 1.79)	1.110 (0.77, 1.60)	0.581 (0.36, 0.94)	0.290 (0.11, 1.79)	−0.076 (0.072)
N	*1881*	*1249*	*1249*	*1249*	*1249*
WOMEN WITHOUT ANY QUALIFICATION [c]					
BMI group					
Underweight †	1.015 (0.83, 1.24)	0.656 ** (0.47, 0.92)	0.873 (0.68, 1.13)	1.359 (0.99, 1.87)	0.109 *** (0.039)
Overweight & Obese †	0.741 (0.49, 1.13)	0.352 ** (0.18, 0.68)	0.332 *** (0.18, 0.61)	0.871 (0.38, 1.98)	−0.033 (0.071)
N	*1745*	*977*	*977*	*977*	*977*

† BMI groups include underweight (BMI < 25), overweight or obese (BMI ≥ 25), normal weight (18.5 < BMI ≤ 25) as references. [b] ** p-value < 0.05, *** for p-value < 0.01. [c] The following three qualifications were considered: having any certificates, job training, or internship.

Based on the analyses on men, overweight or obese men without any qualifications had a 0.81 times less chance of employment compared to that of their counterparts, whereas a statistically significant overweight or obesity penalty was not found for men with at the least one qualification. Overweight or obese men were less likely to have a job in companies that had a labor union compared to that of their counterparts, both in circumstances of having at the least one of the qualifications (by 0.62 times) and in having none of the qualifications (by 0.59 times). Higher monthly wages among overweight or obese men compared to that of their normal-weight counterparts were found only among men with none of the qualifications (Table 5).

4. Discussion

Our findings indicate that overweight or obesity had negative associations with labor market performance, particularly for women. The results are similar to those of previous studies showing penalties on overweight or obesity that affect job market performance, particularly among women [15,28–32], and highlight and confirm the existence of such penalties among young adults in their late 20s. Our findings also indicate that a penalty exists not only in the pecuniary aspect but also in other qualitative aspects of a job. For instance, overweight or obese women had job penalties in terms of not only monthly wage level but also job quality features, e.g., permanence status, bonus provision, and labor union presence. However, for men, overweight or obesity was associated with higher monthly wages and a higher likelihood of having professional jobs and enjoying other high quality features such as being part of a labor union.

The present study further explores the extent to which the impact of obesity on job performances is moderated by the level of individual job qualifications, which refers to stipulated abilities used to increase the chance of employment. Job qualifications play a significant role in making hiring decisions because it comprises of a crucial part of the restricted information that firms receive from their applicants. Therefore, firms tend to make judgments by basing off from the average performance for a given job qualification for comparison [33]. Young adults are new to the job market and are more likely to be more prone to the effect of job qualification due to the paucity of evidence of their job capabilities [33].

Education is a representative job qualification and is actively explored for its influence when signaling in the job market [34,35]. The present study expands the observation of job qualifications by adding features that require supplemental personal investments, such as the possession of any certificates, special training for a job, or the completion or presence of internships. This extension is particularly relevant in the context that young adults in South Korea have been substantially investing in extra qualifications other than in formal education, such as internships, foreign language certifications, or short-term coursework abroad—particularly resulting from the recent increase in unemployment rate [36]. The findings of the present study show that the job market penalty for overweight or obesity was mitigated to a certain extent by a boost in job qualifications among young adults. Previous studies also report that job qualifications could moderate poor achievements in the job market for overweight or obese individuals [6,28]. At the same time, other studies find that, regardless of previous experience in job training, obese women face a larger penalty in their job market performance, such as employment outcomes and monthly wages, compared to that of normal-weight women [6,37].

It is also important to acknowledge and address the limitations in the present study. First, since the data was gathered via written questionnaires, height and weight were self-reported. Considering that height is usually over-reported and weight is usually under-reported, the effect of overweight or obesity might be underestimated in this study [38,39]. The existence and extent of these errors cannot be ascertained from the data used in this study. Nevertheless, several studies report that adjusting the gap between the actual and self-reported numbers do not affect the overall estimation results [15,32]. Second, BMI has limited ability to measure actual obesity status particularly in the medical perspective because it does not effectively distinguish fat from fat-free mass such as muscle and bone [40]. Despite this limitation, BMI has several merits including handiness for measurement and high comparability to previous related studies due to its wide use, particularly in the social sciences field [41]. Since there is a limited number of studies that have used fat mass in assessing the impact of obesity on job performance [42], comparisons cannot be accurately constructed between this study and other related studies. BMI is also more affected by visible look than other obesity measurements such as % body fat, and thus, it is useful to assess the relationship between overweight/obesity and job market performance in terms of distaste on appearance in the job market. Third, there is also a potential of reverse causality in our estimations. For example, job performance may reversely influence one's body mass criteria. Any time-invariant mechanisms for reverse causality were controlled via individual-level, fixed-effect models for both linear and binary dependent variables related to job market performance. However, the presence of any remaining time-varying sources in the error term was not tested.

The study measured job market performance of young adults over a span of four consecutive years. Future studies must explore the evolution of the relationship between overweight or obesity and job market performance throughout their career path, to thoroughly understand the relationship between the two variables and their significance for the general population. Furthermore, comparative studies on the impact of obesity on the job market by different cultural and labor market contexts, both within and across continents, for young adults would also highlight the understanding of mechanisms that underlie in one's job market performance. Future studies should endeavor to compare differences in the relationship between obesity status and job market performance when obesity is measured based on look versus on actual body fat. Such comparisons will improve our understanding of the mechanism (via obesity-related health versus distaste related to appearance) behind this relationship.

5. Conclusions

In summary, this study builds on previous literature by demonstrating the persistence of an association between overweight or obesity and labor market performances in South Korea when holding young adults' job qualifications independent. Our results imply that the cumulative penalty for overweight or obesity could be more substantial for young adults in particular, given that it is likely of initial jobs and job conditions to have lingering impacts in long-term job performance. The obesity burden on individuals is likely to be spilled over to non-health areas such as the job market, and thus, more proactive public efforts will be needed to control obesity for the younger generations.

Author Contributions: Conceptualization, E.H.; Data curation, H.L.; Formal analysis, H.L.; Funding acquisition, E.H.; Investigation, R.A.; Methodology, T.H.K. and E.H.; Project administration, T.H.K.; Resources, H.L.; Software, E.H.; Supervision, E.H.; Validation, T.H.K.; Visualization, H.L.; Writing—original draft, H.L.; Writing—review & editing, R.A. and E.H.

Funding: This research was funded by the National Research Foundation of Korea grant number (2017R1A2B4003373). The content is solely the responsibility of the authors and does not necessarily represent the official view of the National Research Foundation of Korea. The National Research Foundation of Korea had no involvement in preparation and submission of this manuscript.

Conflicts of Interest: The authors declare no conflict of interest.

References

1. NCD Risk Factor Collaboration. Trends in adult body-mass index in 200 countries from 1975 to 2014: A pooled analysis of 1698 population-based measurement studies with 19·2 million participants. *Lancet* **2016**, *387*, 1377–1396. [CrossRef]
2. Morgen, C.S.; Sørensen, T.I. Obesity: Global trends in the prevalence of overweight and obesity. *Nat. Rev. Endocrinol.* **2014**, *10*, 513–514. [CrossRef] [PubMed]
3. Lin, S.-J. Examining the relationship between obesity and wages: Empirical evidence from Taiwan. *J. Dev. Areas* **2016**, *50*, 255–268. [CrossRef]
4. Korea Centers for Disease Control and Prevention. *National Health and Nutrition Examination Survey;* Korea Centers for Disease Control and Prevention: Soul, Korea, 1998–2015.

5. Rhee, S.Y.; Park, S.W.; Kim, D.J.; Woo, J. Gender disparity in the secular trends for obesity prevalence in Korea: Analyses based on the KNHANES 1998–2009. *Korean J. Intern. Med.* **2013**, *28*, 29–34. [CrossRef] [PubMed]
6. Caliendo, M.; Lee, W.-S. Fat chance! Obesity and the transition from unemployment to employment. *Econ. Hum. Biol.* **2013**, *11*, 121–133. [CrossRef]
7. Cavico, F.J.; Muffler, S.C.; Mujtaba, B.G. Appearance discrimination in employment. *Equal. Divers. Incl.* **2012**, *32*, 83–119. [CrossRef]
8. Wright, E.J.; Whitehead, T.L. Perceptions of body size and obesity: A selected review of the literature. *J. Community Health* **1987**, *12*, 117–129. [CrossRef]
9. Cachelin, F.M.; Rebeck, R.M.; Chung, G.H.; Pelayo, E. Does ethnicity influence body-size preference? A comparison of body image and body size. *Obesity Res.* **2002**, *10*, 158–166. [CrossRef]
10. Ruhm, C.J. Understanding overeating and obesity. *J. Health Econ.* **2012**, *31*, 781–796. [CrossRef]
11. Fan, M.; Jin, Y. Obesity and Self-control: Food Consumption, Physical Activity, and Weight-loss Intention. *Appl. Econ. Perspect. Policy* **2013**. [CrossRef]
12. Strauss, R.S. Childhood obesity and self-esteem. *Pediatrics* **2000**, *105*, e15. [CrossRef] [PubMed]
13. Caliendo, M.; Gehrsitz, M. Obesity and the labor market: A fresh look at the weight penalty. *Econ. Hum. Biol.* **2016**, *23*, 209–225. [CrossRef] [PubMed]
14. Chelcea, S.; Ivan, L. The "Aphrodite effect": Labor market discrimination based on attractiveness. *Psihol. Soc.* **2016**, *1*, 37–53.
15. Han, E.; Norton, E.C.; Stearns, S.C. Weight and wages: Fat versus lean paychecks. *Health Econ.* **2009**, *18*, 535–548. [CrossRef] [PubMed]
16. Han, E.; Kim, T.H. Body Mass Index and Self-employment in South Korea. *J. Biosoc. Sci.* **2016**, *49*, 463–477. [CrossRef]
17. Altonji, J.G.; Pierret, C.R. Employer learning and statistical discrimination. *Q. J. Econ.* **2001**, *116*, 313–350. [CrossRef]
18. Kim, T.H.; Han, E. Height premium for job performance. *Econ. Hum. Biol.* **2017**, *26*, 13–20. [CrossRef]
19. Oyer, P. Initial labor market conditions and long-term outcomes for economists. *J. Econ. Perspect.* **2006**, *20*, 143–160. [CrossRef]
20. Pinkston, J.C. The dynamic effects of obesity on the wages of young workers. *Econ. Hum. Biol.* **2017**, *27*, 154–166. [CrossRef]
21. Kim, T.H.; Han, E. Impact of body mass on job quality. *Econ. Hum. Biol.* **2015**, *17*, 75–85. [CrossRef]
22. Duncan, G.J.; Holmlund, B. Was Adam Smith Right After All? Another Test of the Theory of Compensating Wage Differentials. *J. Labor Econ.* **1983**, *1*, 366–379. [CrossRef]
23. Brown, C. Equalizing differences in the labor market. *Q. J. Econ.* **1980**, *94*, 113–134. [CrossRef]
24. Jencks, C.; Perman, L.; Rainwater, L. What is a good job? A new measure of labor-market success. *Am. J. Sociol.* **1988**, *93*, 1322–1357. [CrossRef]
25. Centers for Disease Control and Prevention in Korea. National Statistics for Health 2012. Available online: http://www.index.go.kr/potal/main/EachPage.do?mmenu=2&smenu=4 (accessed on 1 July 2017).
26. World Health Organization. *The Asia-Pacific Perspective: Redefining Obesity and Its Treatment*; Health Communications Australia: Sydney, Australia, 2000.
27. World Health Organization. Obesity and Overweight Fact Sheet N 311. March 2013. Available online: http://www.who.int/mediacentre/factsheets/fs311/en/em (accessed on 1 July 2017).
28. Morris, S. The impact of obesity on employment. *Labour Econ.* **2007**, *14*, 413–433. [CrossRef]
29. Roehling, M.V. Weight Discrimination in the American Workplace: Ethical Issues and Analysis. *J. Bus. Ethics* **2002**, *40*, 177–189. [CrossRef]
30. Flint, S.W.; Snook, J. Obesity and discrimination: The next 'big issue'? *Int. J. Discrimination Law* **2014**, *14*, 183–193. [CrossRef]
31. Kinge, J.M. Body mass index and employment status: A new look. *Econ. Hum. Biol.* **2016**, *22*, 117–125. [CrossRef]
32. Cawley, J. The Impact of Obesity on Wages. *J. Hum. Resour.* **2004**, *39*, 451–474. [CrossRef]
33. Lundberg, S.; Startz, R. Private Discrimination and Social Intervention in Competitive Labor Markets. *Am. Econ. Rev.* **1983**, *73*, 340–347.
34. Spence, M. Job Market Signaling. *Q. J. Econ.* **1973**, *87*, 355–374. [CrossRef]

35. Weiss, A. Human capital vs. signalling explanations of wages. *J. Econ. Perspect.* **1995**, *9*, 133–154. [CrossRef]
36. Cho, D.; Choi, K. A Study on the Time-varying Relationships between Korean Economic Growth and Unemployment. *J. Ind. Econ. Bus.* **2015**, *28*, 2329–2348.
37. Muenster, E.; Rueger, H.; Ochsmann, E.; Letzel, S.; Toschke, A.M. Association between overweight, obesity and self-perceived job insecurity in German employees. *BMC Public Health* **2011**, *11*, 162. [CrossRef] [PubMed]
38. Rowland, M.L.; Rowland, M.L. Self-reported weight and height. *Am. J. Clin. Nutr.* **1990**, *52*, 1125–1133. [CrossRef]
39. Dhaliwal, S.S.; Howat, P.; Bejoy, T.; Welborn, T.A. Self-reported weight and height for evaluating obesity control programs. *Am. J. Health Behav.* **2010**, *34*, 489–499. [CrossRef] [PubMed]
40. Garn, S.M.; Leonard, W.R.; Hawthorne, V.M. Three limitations of the body mass index. *Am. J. Clin. Nutr.* **1986**, *44*, 996–997. [CrossRef]
41. Burkhauser, R.V.; Cawley, J. Beyond BMI: The value of more accurate measures of fatness and obesity in social science research. *J. Health Econ.* **2008**, *27*, 519–529. [CrossRef]
42. Johansson, E.; Bockerman, P.; Kiiskinen, U.; Heliovaara, M. Obesity and labour market success in Finland: The difference between having a high BMI and being fat. *Econ. Hum. Biol.* **2009**, *7*, 36–45. [CrossRef]

International Journal of
Environmental Research and Public Health

MDPI

Article

Prevalence and Risk Factors of Depression, Anxiety, and Stress in a Cohort of Australian Nurses

Shamona Maharaj, Ty Lees and Sara Lal *

Neuroscience Research Unit, School of Life Sciences, University of Technology Sydney, 15 Broadway, Ultimo, Sydney, NSW 2007, Australia; shamona.maharaj@uts.edu.au (S.M.); ty.lees@uts.edu.au (T.L.)

* Correspondence: sara.lal@uts.edu.au

Received: 26 November 2018; Accepted: 23 December 2018; Published: 27 December 2018

Abstract: Nurses remain at the forefront of patient care. However, their heavy workload as a career can leave them overworked and stressed. The demanding nature of the occupation exposes nurses to a higher risk of developing negative mental states such as depression, anxiety, and stress. Hence, the current study aimed to assess the prevalence and risk factors of these mental states in a representative sample of Australian nurses. The Depression Anxiety Stress Scale was administered to 102 nurses. Information about demographic and work characteristics were obtained using lifestyle and in-house designed questionnaires. Prevalence rates of depression, anxiety, and stress were found to be 32.4%, 41.2%, and 41.2% respectively. Binominal logistic regressions for depression and stress were significant ($p = 0.007$, $p = 0.009$). Job dissatisfaction significantly predicted a higher risk of nurses developing symptoms of depression and stress respectively ($p = 0.009$, $p = 0.011$). Poor mental health among nurses may not only be detrimental to the individual but may also hinder professional performance and in turn, the quality of patient care provided. Further research in the area is required to identify support strategies and interventions that may improve the health and wellbeing of nursing professionals and hence the quality of care delivered.

Keywords: mental health; nursing; depression; anxiety; stress

1. Introduction

The health workforce in Australia is dominated by nurses, making them indispensable to the healthcare sector [1,2]. Nurses not only provide care and assistance to patients, but also participate in their rehabilitation, provide support to patients and their families, and advocate health education [3], playing an important role in improving and promoting health services in the community [4]. Their broad and multifaceted workload presents them with the largest amount of time spent with patients and allows them to cover all areas of the healthcare network [3]. Yet, the profession is invariably recognised as a stressful and demanding occupation.

Nurses regularly experience a variety of work-related stressors including but not limited to: long work hours, time constraints, meeting patients' needs, irregular schedules, and lack of professional support [2,5–7]. With such demanding occupations, the ongoing strain faced by healthcare professionals could have a severe impact on their mental health and quality of life [8,9]. Previous studies have shown that the ongoing stress faced by these professionals can have negative effects on their psychological well-being [10,11]. Poor mental health among health care providers may also hinder their professional performance and have a considerable effect on the quality of care they provide to patients [2,10] (inevitably impacting negatively on patients' health). Therefore, administrators and nursing managers are becoming increasingly interested in the health status of nurses.

Psychological indicators for distress include but are not limited to, low self-esteem, fatigue, and sleep/appetite disturbances [12]; while physical impacts may include the increased risk of cardiovascular disease, high blood pressure, decreased immunity, migraines, muscle aches, and chronic fatigue [13]. Additionally, high levels of stress may lead to or exacerbate maladaptive behaviours, such as smoking, over/under eating, excessive alcohol consumption, and substance abuse [14,15]. Depression and anxiety also remain two of the most prevalent mental disorders in Australia with 12-month prevalence rates of approximately 4% and 14% respectively [16]. Investigating depression, anxiety, and stress levels in nurses and identifying predictors for these mental states is crucial for future health systems to provide safer and more amenable workplaces while promoting the well-being of its employees.

The prevalence of depressive symptoms among nurses in the USA was between 35–41%, but another study reported it to be 18% [7,10], 11%–80% in Iranian nurses [17,18], 35% in Chinese nurses [19], 17% in Australian Midwives [20], and 51% in Brazilian nurses [21]. Additionally, approximately 33% of French nurse managers and 10% Canadian nurses were found to suffer from depressive symptoms as well [22,23]. A high incidence of anxiety in nursing professionals is also evident, with studies stating prevalence rates ranging from 20% in Australian Midwives [20] to 32–43% in Chinese nurses [11,19,24], 40–46% in Iranian nurses [4,25], 44–66% in Brazilian nurses [21,26], and 22–24% of American nurses who showed PTSD symptomology [27,28]. The level of stress among nurses can generally range from moderate to high [29,30] and the few prevalence rates that have been presented range from approximately 40–90% [31–34]. Predictive factors such as job satisfaction, high workloads, shift work, sleep disturbance, years of employment, and marital status [10,17–19,35] were commonly implicated with these mental disorders.

Hence, the current study aimed to

1. Assess the prevalence of depression, anxiety, and stress in a cohort of Australian nurses.
2. Determine demographic and work characteristics associated with each mental state.

2. Materials and Methods

2.1. Participants and Sampling

A cross-sectional study design was used to examine the prevalence and correlates of depression, anxiety, and stress symptoms in a cohort of Australian nurses. Data from 102 clinically active nurses were used in the current analysis. Prior to inclusion, all participants were screened for chronic disease/illness (including clinically diagnosed depression, anxiety, and other mental health issues), medication use, smoking habits (in excess of 10 cigarettes a day), and alcohol intake (in excess of 16 standard drinks a day) via an in-house designed lifestyle questionnaire. Participants were excluded if they answered yes to any of the screening questions above. All participants provided informed consent prior to the commencement of the study. At the commencement and conclusion of each session, the participant's blood pressure (BP) was measured three times with an automated blood pressure monitor (Omron IA1B, Kyoto, Japan), and then averaged to derive an average BP value to determine further inclusion into the study (requiring BP < 160/100 mmHg).

2.2. Data Collection/Measures

Demographic, lifestyle, and work-related data were collected using in-house designed questionnaires; developed to determine lifestyle risk factors/habits and determine inclusion/exclusion criteria for the study.

The 42-item Depression Anxiety Stress Scale (DASS) [36] was applied to assess symptom severity of each mental state. Together, each scale of the DASS assessed a comprehensive range of psychological distress symptoms to identifying psychological disturbances perceived by an individual ranging from situational anxiety, anhedonia, and dysphoria to levels of chronic non-specific arousal such as irritability and difficulty relaxing [36,37]. It can be noted that perceived job strain and control are commonly associated with self-reported mental health outcomes [38,39]. As the scale examines general mental health and is based on self-perception, it accounts for environmental and work-related factors that may influence how an individual is feeling.

2.3. Statistical Analysis

Data was initially subject to descriptive statistical analysis. Pearson's correlation analysis was conducted to assess associations between blood pressure and Depression, Anxiety, and Stress. Variables were then dichotomised to enable a good comparison of outcomes; participants with a cut-off score of $\geq$10 in depression, $\geq$8 in anxiety, and >15 in stress were considered as having these disorders as referenced by the DASS [36]. A forward-stepwise (conditional) binominal logistic regression was utilised to measure the strength of associations between variables and sought to identify significant predictors for the outcomes of interest to the study. The level of statistical significance was defined as $p < 0.05$. Statistical analysis was performed using SPSS Version 23.0 for the Windows platform (SPSS Inc.; Chicago, IL, USA).

3. Results

3.1. Demographics

Participants demographics are presented in Table 1. As seen in Table 1, a majority of the participants were females working as Assistants in Nursing (AIN's) and Registered nurses. A majority of the participants also worked in aged care and hospital environments, reflecting the large number of AIN's and registered nurses. Finally, most of the nurses assessed in the current study engaged in shiftwork.

Table 1. Demographics (n = 102).

Demographic/work factor	Mean ± SD or %
Age	30.91 ± 11.52
Gender (female)	79.41% (81F: 21M)
Position	
Assistant in Nursing	43.14% (44)
Enrolled nurse	15.69% (16)
Registered Nurse/Midwife	39.22% (40)
Other	1.96% (2)
Facility	
Aged care	33.33% (34)
Hospital	34.31% (35)
Multiple facilities	9.80% (10)
Other	5.88% (6)
Unspecified	16.67% (17)
Shift workers	78.43% (80)
Job satisfaction	
Yes	37.25% (38)
No	26.47% (27)
Unspecified	36.27 (37)

Mean DASS scores and prevalence for each mental state are displayed in Table 2. In the total sample, according to DASS scores, 32.4% of participants scored over the normal threshold for depression. Of those individuals, 21.57% fell into the mild/moderate categories while 4.9% showed sufficient scores for severe depression and 5.88% for extremely severe depression. However, though some individuals did not have scores over the normal threshold, 86.27% of the total cohort did report some level of depressive symptoms.

Similarly, 41.2% of participants scored over the normal threshold for anxiety. Of those individuals, 20.59% fell into the mild/moderate categories while 9.8% showed sufficient scores for severe anxiety and 10.78% for extremely severe anxiety. Though not all the scores were over the threshold, 91.18% of the total cohort did report some level of anxiety.

Finally, 41.2% of participants also scored over the normal threshold for stress. Of those individuals, 24.51% fell into the mild/moderate categories while 10.8% showed sufficient scores for severe stress and 5.88% for extremely severe stress. Once again, though some individuals did not score over the threshold, 95.10% of the total cohort did report some level of distress.

Table 2. Prevalence and Average scores for Depression, Anxiety, and Stress (n = 102).

	Normal Threshold	Cohort Mean ± SD	Interpretation	Prevalence (%)
Depression	<10	8.38 ± 8.81	Normal	32.4
Anxiety	<8	8.47 ± 7.86	Mild	41.2
Stress	<15	13.90 ± 9.94	Normal	41.2

As previously mentioned, blood pressure was assessed for inclusion criteria. Associations between blood pressure and depression, anxiety, and stress were non-significant, as seen in Table 3.

Table 3. Correlations between blood pressure and depression, anxiety, and stress.

	Pre Systolic	Pre Diastolic	Pre Heart Rate	Post Systolic	Post Diastolic	Post Heart Rate
Depression	r = 0.03, p = 0.849	r = 0.10, p = 0.493	r = −0.14, p = 0.346	r = 0.05, p = 0.758	r = −0.10, p = 0.540	r = −0.15, p = 0.330
Anxiety	r = 0.03, p = 0.848	r = 0.07, p = 0.646	r =−0.07, p = 0.632	r = 0.10, p = 0.492	r = −0.07, p = 0.647	r = 0.01, p = 0.931
Stress	r = 0.01, p = 0.929	r = 0.09, p = 0.537	r = 0.01, p = 0.959	r = 0.09, p = 0.554	r = −0.05, p = 0.728	r = −0.004, p = 0.979

3.2. Binary Logistic Regression Models

The logistic regression model for depression was significant (p = 0.007), explaining 14.2% (Nagelkerke R2) of the variance in depression, and correctly classified 67.7% of cases. Job dissatisfaction significantly predicted depression (S.E. = 0.538, Exp(B) = 4.07, df = 1, p = 0.009) with individuals who reported not being satisfied being more likely to present with depression.

The logistic regression model for anxiety was non-significant. The association between the study variables showed no significance between anxiety and the following: age, gender, facility, shift work, shift type, shift length, job satisfaction, physical issues, and registration level.

The logistic regression model for stress was significant (p = 0.009), explaining 13.2% (Nagelkerke R2) of the variance in stress, and correctly classified 66.2% of cases. Job dissatisfaction significantly predicted stress (S.E. = 0.53, Exp(B) = 3.85, df = 1, p = 0.011) with individuals who reported not being satisfied also being more likely to present with symptoms of distress.

4. Discussion

We assessed the status of depression, anxiety and stress symptomology in a representative sample of Australian nurses. Our study demonstrated that depressive symptoms were common in nurses with a prevalence rate of over 30%, compared to only 4% of the general Australian population [16]. Thus, the results suggested that more than a quarter of the current sample complied with DASS cut-off criteria for depression (scores of 10 and above). Notably, multiple had presented with severe depressive symptoms. Depression prevalence among nurses in our study was also within the ranges reported in previous literature around the world with depression rates ranging from approximately 18–53% [10,18–21]. Likewise, the prevalence of anxiety symptoms was common among the current sample, with a prevalence rate of over 40% compared to 14% of the general Australian population [16]. Again, more than a quarter of the current sample complied with the DASS cut off criteria for anxiety (8 and above) and among these individuals, over 10% had presented with severe anxiety. The prevalence of anxiety among nurses in our study also fell within the ranges commonly reported in the literature (ranging between 20–60%) [4,11,19–21,24,26,29]. Finally, levels of distress were high with over 40% of the current nursing sample complying with the DASS cut-off criteria for stress (scores of 15 and above) and once again multiple individuals presented with severe levels of distress while our prevalence rate was similar to those of other countries [32,34].

As previously mentioned, rates of depression, anxiety, and stress in the current cohort were much higher than population norms. Ignoring the signs of anguish and depression presented by nursing professionals may not only increase the amount of physical and emotional stress on the individual but may also result in low-quality patient care and higher work burdens on establishments [40]. Literature suggests that poor mental health may lead to a decrease in cognitive performance such as an individual's ability to focus and process information, in turn, resulting in inadequate performance [41,42]. Such consequences in the workplace can include decreased alertness and reduced job performance, which could endanger human lives and increase the risk of adverse medical events [43,44].

Australian state spending on mental health services has increased over the past few years, now costing approximately $9 billion [45] and more notably, the cost and number of workers' compensation claims associated with stress and stress-related mental disorders are noticeably higher in medicine and healthcare compared to other occupations [46,47]. Individuals who suffer from mental health issues also tend to have more days out of role, taking approximately five days off work and having 11 days of reduced productivity annually; adding billions of dollars lost to absenteeism and lost productivity [48,49]. Although the number of nurses in Australia has increased over the last decade [50], nurse shortages remain an ongoing issue [51]. High turnover, absenteeism, and lost productivity within the health workforce could amplify shortages and easily leave facilities understaffed and unable to meet patient demands, placing patients at risk [3,52]. Thus, as the prevalence of mental health disorders increases within the profession so too will the economic, social, and individual impacts of these disorders.

The current findings suggested that demographic and occupational factors associated with an increased incidence of developing symptoms of depression, anxiety, and stress were limited as only one occupational factor was associated with poor mental health outcomes. While job dissatisfaction was associated with an increased risk of distress and depression, no factors were found to significantly increase the likelihood of developing anxiety. Further, blood pressure parameters were similarly not associated with depression, anxiety, or stress. However, previous literature has implicated various demographic and work-related predictors for the relatively high prevalence of negative mental states among nurses. Previous studies have found common predictors such as age, job satisfaction, sleep disturbance, years of employment, and marital status [10,17–19,53] to increase the likelihood of developing stress, anxiety and depression. Associations between highly stressful work and its impact on mental wellbeing necessitate the consideration of interventions which aim to improve working conditions and reduce the personal and occupational stress of nurses in an aid to reduce and/or prevent symptoms of depression, stress, and anxiety [43].

Limitations (such as a small representative sample and cross-sectional study design) do exist in the current study, and hence further research may benefit from longitudinal study designs to fully determine predictors of stress, depression, and anxiety in nurses. As the current data was collected as part of a larger study, limited information was collected and available for analysis. A more comprehensive assessment of demographic, personal, and work-related factors that may be considered predictors for negative mental states may also be beneficial.

5. Conclusions

Nursing is an important role in our health care system, and patient care is heavily reliant upon their ability to work optimally and deliver the best care possible [54]. It is becoming increasingly recognised that nurses are affected by symptoms of stress, depression, and anxiety [9]. The prevalence of nurses affected by negative mental states in the current study was high, and it is possible that poor mental health can be detrimental to both the individual and the industry [2,10]. Further research is needed to help care for the well-being of nurses and minimize poor mental health in the workplace. Additionally, the development of short and long-term support strategies and interventions aimed at improving the mental health needs of nursing professionals should be a priority to combat the physical and psychological exhaustion associated with these mental states.

The stress, depression, and anxiety experienced by nursing professionals may not be entirely preventable but realising its prevalence in the workplace is considerably important [55]. A healthy workforce is essential in ensuring that both personal wellbeing and quality patient outcomes are achieved [55].

Author Contributions: Investigation, S.M.; Supervision, S.L.; Data Curation, X.X.; Writing-Original Draft Preparation, S.M.; Writing-Review & Editing, T.L.

Funding: This research is supported by an Australian Government Research Training Program Scholarship.

Acknowledgments: The authors would like to acknowledge the School of Life Sciences at the University of Technology Sydney, where this research was conducted and the participants for their time and interest.

Conflicts of Interest: All authors disclose no actual or potential conflicts of interest including any financial, personal, or other relationships with other people or organisations that could inappropriately influence (bias) their work.

References

1. Australian Institute of Health and Wellbeing. Nursing and Midwifery Workforce. 2015. Available online: https://www.aihw.gov.au/reports/workforce/nursing-and-midwifery-workforce-2015/contents/who-are-nurses-and-midwives (accessed on 15 May 2018).
2. Gong, Y.; Han, T.; Yin, X.; Yang, G.; Zhuang, R.; Chen, Y.; Lu, Z. Prevalence of depressive symptoms and work-related risk factors among nurses in public hospitals in southern China: A cross-sectional study. *Sci. Rep.* **2014**, *4*, 7109. [CrossRef] [PubMed]

3. DeLucia, P.R.; Ott, T.E.; Palmieri, P.A. Performance in Nursing. *Rev. Hum. Factors Ergon.* **2009**, *5*, 1–40. [CrossRef]
4. Ghods, A.A.; Sotodehasl, N.; Khalaf, M.E.; Mirmohamadkhani, M. Situational Anxiety among Nurses. *Middle East J. Rehabil. Health* **2017**, *4*. [CrossRef]
5. Pikó, B. Work-related stress among nurses: A challenge for health care institutions. *J. R. Soc. Promot. Health* **1999**, *119*, 156–162. [CrossRef]
6. Lim, J.; Bogossian, F.; Ahern, K. Stress and coping in Australian nurses: A systematic review. *Int. Nurs. Rev.* **2010**, *57*, 22–31. [CrossRef] [PubMed]
7. Letvak, S.; Ruhm, C.J.; McCoy, T. Depression in hospital-employed nurses. *Clin. Nurse Spec.* **2012**, *26*, 177–182. [CrossRef]
8. Stetz, M.C.; Thomas, M.L.; Russo, M.B.; Stetz, T.A.; Wildzunas, R.M.; McDonald, J.J.; Wiederhold, B.K.; Romano, J.A. Stress, mental health, and cognition: A brief review of relationships and countermeasures. *Aviat. Space Environ. Med.* **2007**, *78*, B252–B260. [PubMed]
9. Chiang, Y.-M.; Chang, Y. Stress, depression, and intention to leave among nurses in different medical units: Implications for healthcare management/nursing practice. *Health Policy* **2012**, *108*, 149–157. [CrossRef]
10. Welsh, D. Predictors of Depressive Symptoms in Female Medical-Surgical Hospital Nurses. *Issues Ment. Health Nurs.* **2009**, *30*, 320–326. [CrossRef]
11. Gao, Y.-Q.; Pan, B.-C.; Sun, W.; Wu, H.; Wang, J.-N.; Wang, L. Anxiety symptoms among Chinese nurses and the associated factors: A cross sectional study. *BMC Psychiatry* **2012**, *12*, 141. [CrossRef]
12. Dyrbye, L.N.; Thomas, M.R.; Shanafelt, T.D. Systematic Review of Depression, Anxiety, and Other Indicators of Psychological Distress Among U.S. and Canadian Medical Students. *Acad. Med.* **2006**, *81*, 354–373. [CrossRef] [PubMed]
13. Schneiderman, N.; Ironson, G.; Siegel, S.D. STRESS AND HEALTH: Psychological, Behavioral, and Biological Determinants. *Annu. Rev. Clin. Psychol.* **2005**, *1*, 607–628. [CrossRef] [PubMed]
14. Sinha, R. Chronic Stress, Drug Use, and Vulnerability to Addiction. *Ann. N. Y. Acad. Sci.* **2008**, *1141*, 105–130. [CrossRef] [PubMed]
15. Yau, Y.H.C.; Potenza, M.N. Stress and Eating Behaviors. *Minerva Endocrinol.* **2013**, *38*, 255–267. [PubMed]
16. Australian Bureau of Statistics (ABS) National Survey of Mental Health and Wellbeing: 2008 Summary of Results. Available online: http://www.abs.gov.au/ausstats/abs@.nsf/Latestproducts/4326.0Main%20Features32007 (accessed on 18 September 2018).
17. Tabrizi, K.N.; Kavari, S.H. P02-45—A study of depression prevalence in nurses and it's effective factors in shiraz namazi hospital. *Eur. Psychiatry* **2011**, *26*, 640. [CrossRef]
18. Ardekani, Z.Z.; Kakooei, H.; Ayattollahi, S.M.; Choobineh, A.; Seraji, G.N. Prevalence of mental disorders among shift work hospital nurses in Shiraz, Iran. *Pak. J. Biol. Sci.* **2008**, *11*, 1605–1609. [CrossRef] [PubMed]
19. Cheung, T.; Yip, P.S.F. Depression, Anxiety and Symptoms of Stress among Hong Kong Nurses: A Cross-sectional Study. *Int. J. Environ. Res. Public Health* **2015**, *12*, 11072–11100. [CrossRef] [PubMed]
20. Creedy, D.K.; Sidebotham, M.; Gamble, J.; Pallant, J.; Fenwick, J. Prevalence of burnout, depression, anxiety and stress in Australian midwives: A cross-sectional survey. *BMC Pregnancy Childbirth* **2017**, *17*, 13. [CrossRef]
21. Schmidt, D.R.C.; Dantas, R.A.S.; Marziale, M.H.P. Anxiety and depression among nursing professionals who work in surgical units. *Revista da Escola de Enfermagem da USP* **2011**, *45*, 487–493. [CrossRef]
22. Nourry, N.; Luc, A.; Lefebvre, F.; Sultan-Taïeb, H.; Béjean, S. Psychosocial and organizational work environment of nurse managers and self-reported depressive symptoms: Cross-sectional analysis from a cohort of nurse managers. *Int. J. Occup. Med. Environ. Health* **2014**, *27*, 252–269. [CrossRef] [PubMed]
23. Ohler, M.C.; Kerr, M.S.; Forbes, D.A. Depression in Nurses. *Can. J. Nurs. Res. Arch.* **2010**, *42*, 66–82.
24. Li, S.; Li, L.; Zhu, X.; Wang, Y.; Zhang, J.; Zhao, L.; Li, L.; Yang, Y. Comparison of characteristics of anxiety sensitivity across career stages and its relationship with nursing stress among female nurses in Hunan, China. *BMJ Open* **2016**, *6*, e010829. [CrossRef] [PubMed]
25. Nooryan, K.; Sasanpour, M.; Sharif, F.; Ghafarian Shirazi, H.R. Anxiety in Physicians and Nurses Working in Intensive Care Units in Yasuj's Hospitals/Iran. *Procedia Soc. Behav. Sci.* **2014**, *122*, 457–460. [CrossRef]
26. Veloso, L.U.P.; Laurindo, L.M.B. Prevalance of anxiety in nursing professionals of urgency medicine. *J. Nurs. UFPE* **2016**, *8*, 3969–3976. [CrossRef]

27. Mealer, M.L.; Shelton, A.; Berg, B.; Rothbaum, B.; Moss, M. Increased Prevalence of Post-traumatic Stress Disorder Symptoms in Critical Care Nurses. *Am. J. Respir. Crit. Care Med.* **2007**, *175*, 693–697. [CrossRef]
28. Mealer, M.; Burnham, E.L.; Goode, C.J.; Rothbaum, B.; Moss, M. The prevalence and impact of post traumatic stress disorder and burnout syndrome in nurses. *Depress. Anxiety* **2009**, *26*, 1118–1126. [CrossRef]
29. Opie, T.; Lenthall, S.; Wakerman, J.; Dollard, M.; Macleod, M.; Knight, S.; Rickard, G.; Dunn, S. Occupational stress in the Australian nursing workforce: A comparison between hospital-based nurses and nurses working in very remote communities. *Aust. J. Adv. Nurs.* **2011**, *28*, 36–43.
30. Subih, M.; Alamer, R.; Hadid, L.A.; Alsatari, M. Stressors Amongst Jordanian Nurses Working in Different Types of Hospitals and the Effect of Selected Demographic Factors: A Descriptive-Explorative Study. *Jordan Med. J.* **2012**, *45*, 331–340.
31. Al-Makhaita, H.M.; Sabra, A.A.; Hafez, A.S. Predictors of work-related stress among nurses working in primary and secondary health care levels in Dammam, Eastern Saudi Arabia. *J. Fam. Community Med.* **2014**, *21*, 79–84. [CrossRef]
32. Gheshlagh, R.G.; Parizad, N.; Dalvand, S.; Zarei, M.; Farajzadeh, M.; Karami, M.; Sayehmiri, K. The prevalence of job stress among nurses in Iran: A meta-analysis study. *Nurs. Midwifery Stud.* **2017**, *6*, 143–148. [CrossRef]
33. Khan, N.; Anwar, H.; Sayed, M. Prevalence of Stress Factors in Nurses in Leady Reading Hospital (LRH), Khyber Teaching Hospital (KTH) and Hayatabad Medical Complex (HMC) Hospitals, Peshawar, KPK. *Int. J. Innov. Res. Dev.* **2015**, *4*, 4.
34. Kibria, M.G. Prevalence of Stress and Coping Mechanism Among Staff Nurses of Intensive Care Unit in a Selected Hospital. *Int. J. Neurosurg.* **2018**, *2*, 8–12. [CrossRef]
35. Khodadadi, E.; Hosseinzadeh, M.; Azimzadeh, R.; Fooladi, M. The relation of depression, anxiety and stress with personal characteristics of nurses in hospitals of Tabriz, Iran. *Int. J. Med. Res. Health Sci.* **2016**, *5*, 140–148.
36. Lovibond, S.H.; Lovibond, P.F. *Manual for the Depression Anxiety Stress Scales*, 2nd ed.; Psychology Foundation: Sydney, Australia, 1995.
37. Crawford, J.; Henry, J. The Depression Anxiety Stress Scales (DASS): Normative data and latent structure in a large non-clinical sample. *Br. J. Clin. Psychol.* **2003**, *42*, 111–131. [CrossRef] [PubMed]
38. Karasek, R. Job demands, job decision latitude, and mental strain: Implications for job redesign. *Adm. Sci. Q.* **1979**, *24*, 285–308. [CrossRef]
39. De Jonge, J.; van Vegchel, N.; Shimazu, A.; Schaufeli, W.; Dormann, C. A longitudinal test of the demand-control model using specific job demands and specific job control. *Int. J. Behav. Med.* **2010**, *17*, 125–133. [CrossRef]
40. De Vargas, D.; Dias, A.P.V. Depression prevalence in Intensive Care Unit nursing workers: A study at hospitals in a northwestern city of São Paulo State. *Revista Latino-Americana de Enfermagem* **2011**, *19*, 1114–1121. [CrossRef]
41. Marazziti, D.; Consoli, G.; Picchetti, M.; Carlini, M.; Faravelli, L. Cognitive impairment in major depression. *Eur. J. Pharmacol.* **2010**, *626*, 83–86. [CrossRef]
42. Maharaj, S.; Lees, T.; Lal, S. Negative Mental States and Their Association to the Cognitive Function of Nurses. *J. Psychophysiol.* **2018**, 1–12. [CrossRef]
43. Johnson, J.; Hall, L.H.; Berzins, K.; Baker, J.; Melling, K.; Thompson, C. Mental healthcare staff well-being and burnout: A narrative review of trends, causes, implications, and recommendations for future interventions. *Int. J. Ment. Health Nurs.* **2018**, *27*, 20–32. [CrossRef]
44. Berland, A.; Natvig, G.K.; Gundersen, D. Patient safety and job-related stress: A focus group study. *Intensive Crit. Care Nurs.* **2008**, *24*, 90–97. [CrossRef] [PubMed]
45. Australian Institute of Health and Welfare. Mental Health Services in Australia, Expenditure on Mental Health-Related Services 2018. Available online: https://www.aihw.gov.au/reports/mental-health-services/mental-health-services-in-australia/report-contents/expenditure-on-mental-health-related-services (accessed on 15 May 2018).
46. Statistics Main Features—Doctors and Nurses. Available online: http://www.abs.gov.au/AUSSTATS/abs@.nsf/Lookup/4102.0Main+Features20April+2013 (accessed on 15 May 2018).

47. Australian Safety and Compensation Council. *Work-Related Mental Disorders in Australia—Report*; Australian Safety and Compensation Council, Australian Government: Canberra, Australia, 2006.
48. Safe Work Australia. *Incidence of Accepted Workers' Compensation Claims for Mental Stress in Australia*; Safe Work Australia: Canberra, Australia, 2013.
49. Slade, T.; Johnston, A.; Teesson, M.; Whiteford, H.; Burgess, P.; Pirkis, J.; Saw, S. *The Mental Health of Australians 2: Report on the 2007 National Survey of Mental Health and Wellbeing*; Department of Health and Ageing: Canberra, Australia, 2009.
50. Beyond Blue—Insure Workforce Report 2011. Available online: https://www.beyondblue.org.au/docs/default-source/policy-submissions/bw0088-policy-submission---insecure-work-in-australia.pdf?sfvrsn=ab4fa9e9_2 (accessed on 15 May 2018).
51. APH Nurse Shortages and the Impact on Health Services. 2004. Available online: https://www.aph.gov.au/Parliamentary_Business/Committees/Senate/Community_Affairs/Completed_inquiries/2002-04/nursing/report/c02 (accessed on 15 May 2018).
52. Tuckett, A.; Winters-Chang, P.; Bogossian, F.; Wood, M. "Why nurses are leaving the profession. Lack of support from managers": What nurses from an e-cohort study said. *Int. J. Nurs. Pract.* **2015**, *21*, 359–366. [CrossRef] [PubMed]
53. Ruggiero, J.S. Health, work variables, and job satisfaction among nurses. *J. Nurs. Adm.* **2005**, *35*, 254–263. [CrossRef] [PubMed]
54. Gatchel, R. The importance of the profession of nursing in health care: Current and future issues. *J. Appl. Biobehav. Res.* **2018**, *23*, e12127. [CrossRef]
55. Brandford, A.A.; Reed, D.B. Depression in Registered Nurses: A State of the Science. *Workplace Health Saf.* **2016**, *64*, 488–511. [CrossRef]

International Journal of
Environmental Research and Public Health

MDPI

Article

Six Years of Sick Leave Spells in a Group of University Civil Workers. Can Modern Work Bring Them a New Health Problem?

Adriano Dias [1], João Marcos Bernardes [1], Miriam Malacize Fantazia [1], Carlos Ruiz-Frutos [2,4,*] and Juan Gómez-Salgado [3,4]

1 Public Health Grade Program, Botucatu Medical School, Paulista State University, Botucatu, Sao Paulo 18618687, Brazil; dias.adriano@unesp.br (A.D.); jmbernardes@yahoo.com (J.M.B.); adrianodiass@hotmail.com (M.M.F.)
2 Department of Sociology, Social Work and Public Health, Universidad de Huelva, 21071 Huelva, Spain
3 Department of Nursing, Universidad de Huelva, 21071 Huelva, Spain; jgsalgad@gmail.com
4 Safety and Health Posgrade Program, Universidad Espíritu Santo, Samborondón, Guayaquil 091650, Ecuador
* Correspondence: frutos@uhu.es; Tel.: +34-656407861

Received: 1 November 2018; Accepted: 19 December 2018; Published: 21 December 2018

Abstract: The objective of this study is to analyse sick leave episodes of a university's collective of statutory workers in the State of São Paulo, between January 2010 and December 2015. For this, a descriptive study analysed 5776 registered spells of sick leave of four university units: agricultural sciences; human health, health and animal reproduction, and biological sciences; an administrative unit; and a university hospital. The medical expert assessment was carried out by general practitioners and psychiatrists who managed sick leave and return to work cases. Around 52% had up to three sick leave episodes, and 10% of the workers had 20 or more episodes. Each spell of sickness absence lasted a median of 30 days (IQR 8–60 days). Among all of sick leaves, 35% had as a primary cause mental or behavioural diseases, of which 30% were depressive disorders, followed by around 18% related to the musculoskeletal system and the connective tissues. In the medical reports, 80% of the workers reported pain and 30% reported psychological symptoms. The collective, seen as privileged by many for their job stability, has a high percentage of sick leave due to mental illness, with extended periods which affect the levels of disability and reduce possibilities of return.

Keywords: sickness absence; public workers; university; psychosocial work environment; occupational health; health workers

---

1. Introduction

Sickness absence is a complex phenomenon that is strongly influenced by factors other than health [1–3]. It has been suggested that many workers will attend work with conditions that others will be absent with, and that where there are high rates of absence there are also high rates of "presenteeism". Many EU governments have introduced programmes aimed at encouraging long term absentees getting back into the workforce [1].

In Brazil, civil servants may be statutory or public employees. The former are holders of public office and are subject to statutory regimes established by the federal, state and local governments. On the other hand, the latter are subject to the rules of the Consolidation of Labour Laws (CLT), the decree that governs labour relations in Brazil [4].

In Brazilian public universities, the same rule coexists. However, the workers are divided into two other categories, technical-administrative and professors. Also, there may additional differences between the weekly work time, which may be full or part-time, and the type of dedication, exclusive or not. Thus, Brazilian universities have a multiplicity of worker types, not to mention outsourced workers, who deserve a separate analysis.

As many as 12% of Brazilian workers are civil servants, a similar proportion to some Latin American countries, but far from the percentages found in developed countries, where the average is 21%, according to the Organization for Economic Co-operation and Development [5]. It is even further from some Scandinavian countries where more than a third of the economically active population is employed in the public service.

Even though working as a civil servant requires passing a civil service examination, it is highly desirable. This is due to the security and employment stability provided by the organisations, opportunities for professional formation and qualification, possibilities of professional advancement and salary increases through career plans and promotions, coverage of special pension regimes with higher pensions for lower contribution rates [6], while workers in the private sector tend to lead unemployment statistics. As a consequence of the higher level of education needed to be admitted to public service and its development during working years, more than half of civil servants have a higher education degree. On the other hand, in the private sector this percentage is 15% [7]. For example, more than 60% of the employees of a public university have a higher education degree, even though they occupy high school education level positions [8].

Although these benefits still exist or at least part of them, from the 1990s onwards and parallel to the transformations that occurred in business, the Government also reformed itself. It did so through a politico-ideological movement with economic roots, adopting management practices, until then typical of the private sector, and focusing on the search for quality and efficiency [9–13].

The changes in technical devices, management rules and the reorganisation of work environments resulted, for the workers, in an increase in qualification, workload and flexibility, in addition to the reduction of autonomy and remuneration. At the same time, this process accentuated competitive behaviours and disarticulated the capacity for social support, producing feelings of isolation and insecurity in employment [14,15]. In addition, the public service extinguished positions considered non-essential, allowing the hiring of outsourced workers (for a specific period of time, under different contract regimes and with unequal/lower salaries), of whom compliance with goals and an increase in pace and productivity was demanded [15].

A non-ideal work environment was generated as a result of all these changes, increasing psychosocial risk markers for workers' physical and mental health problems: excessive workloads, conflicting work demands, lack of clarity of function, lack of involvement in decision making and of influence on the way work is done, insecurity, ineffective communication and lack of social support from supervisors or colleagues [16,17]. These risk factors affected in quantity and intensity, what contrasts with the improvements in general health conditions of the world population in the same period [18] and, mainly, with the healthy worker effect [19].

The main indicator of workers' health problems is absenteeism [20], here defined as absence to work due to a disease and justified by a medical statement [21]. Studies on absenteeism in civil servants [22–27] indicate that the predominant disease is related to work activities and the professionals involved; and, also, that they are more frequent in female workers and in the age group between 30 and 45 years. Between 2003 and 2006, according to data from all civil servants employed by all departments and agencies related to the Government of São Paulo State (Southeast Brazil), nearly 200,000 sick leaves were granted each year, with mental disorders being responsible for almost 30% of these leaves [22].

In Brazil, official data [28] shows that mental disorders represent 10% of all pension benefits, being surpassed only by musculoskeletal disorders (20%) and external causes (25%). This is certainly resulting from the negative effects of these new work environments on workers' health.

In addition to the impact of absenteeism on productivity and interpersonal relationships at work, workers' illness often results in long-term sick leave. This implies difficulties in returning to work, mainly when it involves changes in job, function and the status derived from the limitations caused by the disease.

Thus, the objective of this study is to present an epidemiological profile of a university group of civil servants' sick leaves over a period of six years, as well as defining work characteristics and possible causes of sick leave.

2. Materials and Methods

2.1. Study Design and Setting

This is a descriptive study of sick leaves. Its population was composed of civil servants from a university located in inland São Paulo State, Brazil, that took sick leaves between the months of January 2010 and December 2015.

During the period that the information was collected by the University's Technical Section of Worker's Health, the university campus was composed by four academic units (agricultural sciences, human health, biological sciences and animal health and reproduction), an administration unit, and a university hospital.

2.2. Participants

The sum of the populations in these units, in the middle of the period (2012), was 4090 workers, among which about 60% were statutory civil servants, while the others were public employees subject to the CLT or outsourced public workers. The approximate proportional distribution of workers per unit, in the middle of the period, was: administration (5%), agricultural sciences (13%), human health and hospital (56%), animal health (11%), biological sciences (15%).

During the six years of the study, 965 workers were examined by physicians, resulting in 5776 episodes of sick leaves, which comprised the study sample. It should be noted that the estimates of the populations made available from each year were fluctuating, which made it difficult to establish precise annual denominators and imposed the need to analyse the data globally.

The institution has its own occupational medical service, who examines all statutory workers who request a sick leave with duration of two days or more. This service is composed by general practitioners, who evaluate sick leave applications due to non-psychiatric morbidity, and psychiatrists, who evaluate sick leave applications due to mental disorders. The service not only manages all sick leaves applications, since it is the only one that can grant or deny them, but also all cases of readaptation to work.

2.3. Variables and Data Sources

For the exploratory phase of the study, data was extracted from two institutional databases: (a) Integrated Occupational Management Software (IOM) (UNESP, São Paulo, Brazil), which identifies the worker and stores physician's evaluation data; (b) Healthcare Medical System (HMS) (UNESP, São Paulo, Brazil), which records information about cases of work readaptation.

It is important to highlight that the two databases were not integrated or built under the same computational architecture (neither for research purposes), nor did it allow searches or information filtering (in the case of the HMS), which made it necessary to evaluate one by one all cases of work readaptation already made by that service to make them coincide with the valuations of the period.

Then, after retrieving and organising the information, a database was built. It contained variables of the following types: sociodemographic (place of birth, sex, current age and age when hired by the university, marital status and coexistence with partner), job characteristics (position, work unit, rehabilitation history, working time in the institution and total work time), sick leave characteristics (duration of each episode, number of medical evaluations in the period, total duration of all episodes, reason of the leave classified by the International Classification of Diseases (ICD-10) and behaviour of repeated sick leaves) and work readaptation (if it happened, time passed until it happened and if it resulted in any limitations). The reason for each sick leave was defined as the first or main diagnosis pointed by the physician, since it could have multiple reasons. Thus, it was necessary to create data mining tools to search for the reason of each leave and for variables related to the physicians' evaluations (type of injury, affected part and presence of psychological symptoms) in the IOM, a textual qualitative record base.

2.4. Statistical Analysis

The variables were analysed using simple and cumulative percentage distributions and measures of central tendency and dispersion (for discrete and continuous variables, respectively), using IBM SPSS software, v.20.0 (IBM, Armonk, NY, USA).

2.5. Ethical and Legal Aspects

The research has been carried out with the consent and support of the Human Resources of the units involved and was approved by the Ethics Committee of the Botucatu Medical School (protocol 1.874.625, of 12/19/2016).

3. Results

A total of 5776 spells of sick leave, of two or more days, from 965 workers, were studied. Table 1 shows that workers who took a sick leave had been hired by the university at a young age (28.6 ± 6.7 years), but they had been in the institution for a long time (21.1 ± 7.6 years) before taking the first sick leave during the period studied.

Table 1. Sociodemographic and working characteristics of the study population (n = 965).

	Mean	SD	Min.	Max.	p25	Median	p75
Age started working at university	28.65	6.74	18.35	59.22	23.07	27.84	33.10
Time working at university	21.12	7.65	0.4	50.39	17.02	21.73	25.99

		n	%	C % *
Sex	Female	605	62.7	62.7
	Male	360	37.3	100.0
Marital status	Married	538	55.8	55.8
	Separated	232	24.0	79.8
	Divorced	132	13.7	93.5
	Single	57	5.9	99.4
	Widowed	6	0.6	100.0
Has a partner	Yes	538	55.8	55.8
	No	427	44.2	100.0
Origin	São Paulo	952	98.7	98.7
	Another state	13	1.3	100.0
Unit	Administration	41	4.2	4.2
	Agricultural sciences	61	6.3	10.6
	Human health	748	77.5	88.1
	Animal health	56	5.8	93.9
	Biological sciences	59	6.1	100.0
Position	Mid-level healthcare	374	38.8	38.8
	Administration	143	14.8	53.6
	Operational	119	12.3	65.9
	Academic support	72	7.5	73.4
	High-level healthcare	61	6.3	79.7
	Teaching	54	5.6	85.3
	Rural work	45	4.7	89.9
	Others high-level	22	2.3	92.2
	Supervision and reception	22	2.3	94.5
	Others mid-level	16	1.7	96.2
	Supervisor	15	1.6	97.7
	Radiotherapy	13	1.3	99.1
	Transport	9	0.9	100.0

* cumulative percentage.

The majority were women (62.7%), lived with a partner (55.8%) and born in the State of São Paulo (98.7%). The largest proportion of workers belonged to the Human Health university unit (77.5%) and occupied mid-level healthcare positions (38.8%).

Table 2 shows that the population had, on average, about 50 years of age when they took the sick leave and that the average total duration of the sick leave per worker was 564 days, varying between 15 to more than 6 thousand days, distributed in single (23.5%) and multiple (76.5%) leaves. It should be highlighted that 23.5% and 17% of the workers had had one and two spells of sick leave, respectively, and almost 80% of the workers had up to 10 episodes during the study period. 10% had 20 or more, reaching a maximum of 59. Each spell of sick leave (n = 5776) had a median length of absence of 30 days (IQR 8–60 days), with minimums and maximums of 2 and 1439 days, respectively.

Table 2. Characteristics of sick leaves.

	Mean	SD	Min.	Max.	p25	Median	p75
Age at the start of the process (n = 965) #	49.77	7.67	25.58	81.61	45.28	50.01	54.68
Total length of absence in days (n = 965)	564.47	1053.95	15.00	6077.00	79.00	147.00	351.00
Time until readaptation in days (n = 239)	343.24	684.99	2.00	5925.00	15.00	60.00	290.50
Each sick leave spell length of absence (n = 5776)	50.19	129.27	2.00	1439.00	8.00	30.00	60.00

		n	%	% cum.
Readaptation (n = 965)	No	714	74.0	74.0
	Yes	251	26.0	100.0
Readaptation with limitations (n = 251)	No	56	22.3	22.3
	Yes	195	77.7	100.0
Number of medical evaluations in the period (n = 965)	1	227	23.5	23.5
	2	162	16.8	40.3
	3	111	11.5	51.8
	4	73	7.6	59.4
	5	58	6.0	65.4
	6–10	140	14.5	79.9
	11–20	112	11.6	91.5
	21–59	82	8.5	100.0
ICD-10 chapter (n = 5776) *	I	130	2.3	2.3
	II	219	3.8	6.0
	III	13	0.2	6.3
	IV	83	1.4	7.7
	V	2022	35.0	42.7
	VI	131	2.3	45.0
	VII	215	3.7	48.7
	VIII	48	0.8	49.5
	IX	245	4.2	53.8
	X	182	3.2	56.9
	XI	189	3.3	60.2
	XII	96	1.7	61.9
	XIII	1031	17.8	79.7
	XIV	168	2.9	82.6
	XV	22	0.4	83.0
	XVI	1	0.0	83.0
	XVII	18	0.3	83.3
	XVIII	89	1.5	84.9
	XIX	362	6.3	91.1
	XX	25	0.4	91.6
	XXI	487	8.4	100.0
Injured body part (n = 1018) **	Trunk	228	22.4	22.4
	Hands	162	15.9	38.3
	Eyes	151	14.8	53.1
	Feet	130	12.8	65.9
	Arms	124	12.2	78.1
	Legs	99	9.7	87.8
	Head	87	8.5	96.4
	Fingers	37	3.6	100.0

Table 2. *Cont.*

	Mean	SD	Min.	Max.	p25	Median	p75
Type of injury (n = 1385) **			Pain		1112	80.3	80.3
			Fracture		141	10.2	90.5
			Contusion		55	4.0	94.4
			Sprain		35	2.5	97.0
			Burn		17	1.2	98.2
			Sharp-cutting		15	1.1	99.3
			Dislocation		8	0.6	99.9
			Lethargy		2	0.1	100.0
Psychological symptoms (n = 5776) **			No		4044	70.0	70.0
			Yes		1732	30.0	100.0
Symptoms start with other chapter and change to chapter V of the ICD-10 until 20th expert record (n = 965)			No		768	79.6	79.6
			Yes		197	20.4	100.0
Symptoms start with chapter V of the ICD-10 and is kept until 20th expert record (n = 965)			No		740	76.7	76.7
			Yes		225	23.3	100.0
ICD chapter modified (n = 965)			No		332	45.0	45.0
			Yes		406	55.0	100.0

Refers to the worker's age at the first sick leave spell during the study period. * I—Certain infectious and parasitic diseases; II—Tumours (Neoplasms); III—Diseases of the blood and blood-forming organs and certain disorders involving the immune mechanism; IV—Endocrine, nutritional and metabolic diseases; V—Mental and behavioural disorders; VI-Diseases of the nervous system; VII—Diseases of the eye, adnexa. VIII—Diseases of the ear and mastoid process; IX—Diseases of the circulatory system; X—Diseases of the respiratory system; XI—Diseases of the digestive system; XII—Diseases of the skin and subcutaneous tissue; XIII—Diseases of the musculoskeletal system and connective tissue. XIV—Diseases of the genitourinary system; XV—Pregnancy, childbirth and the puerperium; XVI —Certain conditions originating in the perinatal period; XVII—Congenital malformations, deformations and chromosomal abnormalities; XVIII—Symptoms, signs and abnormal clinical and laboratory findings, not elsewhere classified; XIX—Injury, poisoning and certain other consequences of external causes; XX—External causes of morbidity and mortality; XXI—Factors influencing health status and contact with health services. ** Referred to by the doctor-expert in the record (based on complaints) of the consultation and extracted from the text.

More than one third (35%) of all sick leaves had, as primary (or main) cause, diseases classified as mental or behavioural disorders, according to the ICD-10 [29]. These were followed at a distance by diseases of the musculoskeletal system and of the connective tissue (17.8%). According to the medical evaluations, 20% of all cases affected the trunk; there was pain in up to 80% of the episodes; and there was psychological symptomatology in 30% of all cases.

Regarding the main cause according to the ICD-10, considering up to the 20th episode of sick leave (91.5% of cases), the cause of the first episode was modified in subsequent events in 45% of the cases, and it may have or not returned to the cause of the first episode. The main cause was subsequently modified to a diagnosis included in the chapter 'Mental and behavioural disorders' from the ICD-10 in 20% of the sick leaves that did not have a mental disorder as the main cause in the first episode. And, in about 23% of the cases, mental disorders were the main cause from the beginning until the end of the follow-up.

Table 2 shows that 26% (239) of the 965 workers who took a sick leave had to be readapted to work, with an average waiting period of 344 days. Of these, 77.7% (195) were readapted with some degree of activities' limitation when returning to work.

Table 3 presents the 51 most frequent causes of sick leave among the 150 diseases that were registered as the main cause in the period studied and that represent 90.1% of the total causes. Among the mental and behavioural disorders (Chapter V of the ICD-10), we see depressive disorders and the use of psychoactive substances as those that were most frequently recorded. Meantime, among the osteomuscular diseases (Chapter XIII of the ICD-10), dorsalgias, arthropathies and shoulder diseases were the most frequent. The other 99 diseases corresponded to 9.9% of the events among the 5776 registered spells of sick leave.

Table 3. Main causes of 5776 sick leaves (ICD diagnosis code or range).

P. *	ICD Diagnosis Code or Range	n	%	C % **
1	Major depressive disorder, recurrent	1131	19.6	19.6
2	Major depressive disorder, single episode, moderate	635	11.0	30.6
3	Dorsalgia	547	9.5	40.0
4	Convalescence after surgery	411	7.1	47.2
5	Shoulder lesions	254	4.4	51.6
6	Disorder of conjunctiva	159	2.8	54.3
7	Malignant neoplasm	158	2.7	57.0
8	Alcohol dependence	132	2.3	59.3
9	Arthropathies	103	1.8	61.1
10	Injuries of the knee and leg	96	1.7	62.8
11	Personality and behavioural disorders	81	1.4	64.2
12	Diseases of the veins and vessels and lymph nodes	80	1.4	65.6
13	Injuries of the ankle and foot	79	1.4	66.9
14	Other joint disorders	72	1.2	68.2
15	Disorder of nerves, roots and nerve plexuses	61	1.1	69.2
16	Ischemic diseases of the heart	58	1.0	70.2
17	Superficial trauma of the wrist and hand	57	1.0	71.2
18	Acute infections of the upper respiratory tract	54	0.9	72.2
19	Benign neoplasm	53	0.9	73.1
20	Diabetes Mellitus	51	0.9	74.0
21	Calculus of kidney	49	0.8	74.8
22	Disorders of the gallbladder, biliary tract and pancreas	49	0.8	75.7
23	Influenza (flu) and pneumonia	48	0.8	76.5
24	Hypertensive diseases	45	0.8	77.3
25	Diseases of the inner ear	36	0.6	77.9
26	Other local skin and subcutaneous tissue infections	36	0.6	78.5
27	Chronic diseases of the lower respiratory tract	32	0.6	79.1
28	Episodic and paroxysmal disorders	32	0.6	79.6
29	Pain and other conditions related to the female genital organs and the menstrual cycle	32	0.6	80.2
30	Dermatitis and eczema	30	0.5	80.7
31	Person in contact with health services due to other circumstances	29	0.5	81.2
32	Inflammatory polyarthropathy	29	0.5	81.7
33	Diseases of the esophagus, stomach and duodenum	27	0.5	82.2
34	Symptoms and signs that involve the digestive system and abdomen	27	0.5	82.6
35	Diseases of the oral cavity of the salivary glands and jaws	26	0.5	83.1
36	Other diseases of the upper respiratory tract	26	0.5	83.5
37	Other diseases of the urinary system	26	0.5	84.0
38	Other diseases of the intestines	26	0.5	84.4
39	Symptoms and general signs	26	0.5	84.9
40	Cerebrovascular diseases	24	0.4	85.3
41	Other viral diseases	24	0.4	85.7
42	Other forms of heart disease	24	0.4	86.1
43	Hernia	23	0.4	86.5
44	Organic mental disorders, including symptomatic disorders	22	0.4	86.9
45	Injuries of the forearm and elbow	22	0.4	87.3
46	Injuries of the shoulder and arm	22	0.4	87.7
47	Schizophrenia, schizotypal disorders and delusional disorders	21	0.4	88.0
48	Other bacterial diseases	20	0.3	88.4
49	Viral fevers transmitted by arthropods and hemorrhagic viral fevers	19	0.3	88.7
50	Obesity and other types of hyperalimentation	18	0.3	89.0
51	Other external causes of accidental injuries and falls	17	0.3	89.3
	Other (99 categories)	617	10.7	100
	Total	5776	100	

* Position; ** Cumulative percentage.

4. Discussion

First of all, it should be highlighted that the databases accessed to obtain the information used in this research contained data only on the civil servants who took at least one spell of sick leave during the study's period. Therefore, our results and their interpretation are valid only to this particular group of individuals and cannot be generalised to university civil servants in general.

The present study allows us to describe sick leave causes in a group of great importance because of its number and that is not usually studied, such as public university workers. This is a group of workers seen by many as privileged in terms of psychosocial risk protection due to their special work regime (for the most part of them), their job stability [30] and/or their educational levels above the average [7]. We identified a high percentage of sick leaves related to mental disorders (35%), of which 30% are depressive disorders. Having data on the causes, frequency and duration of sick leaves makes it possible to propose preventive measures related to organisational factors and aimed at improving the management of health services at these public institutions.

It must be borne in mind that the results presented in this study refer only to a subgroup of civil servants, statutory workers. However, the fact that the results show that workers with a medium level of education are the ones who take more sick leaves seems to corroborate the statement of health protection for that kind of worker. At the same time, it should be considered that these workers occupy lower positions in the employment hierarchy and perform less flexible activities, while those with a higher level of education tend to occupy management positions. These positions are frequently more flexible, and may be able to make use of informal agreements. Thus, their sick leaves may be under-registered in the system.

When a civil servant (regulated by statute or specific regulation, contributor of a provisional regime that belongs to an administrative unit, whether federal, state or municipal) requests a sick leave, he/she undergoes a medical expert examination that aims at the social and financial equilibrium of the institutions [31]. This study was conducted at an institution where the medical evaluations of sick leave are made by physicians who depend on the same employer of the workers they examine. This could mean that their decisions may not correspond to the reality of the diseased workers, for example, anticipating times of return to work. Although the medical evaluations carried out by these professionals may induce doubts, it is evident that the centralisation of these evaluations at the institution's own occupational medical service leads not only to reductions of travels to undergo examinations, but also facilitate the standardisation of criteria [32].

The expected work time until a worker takes a sick leave should be in accordance with the life cycle, in other words, older workers should be more likely to take sick leaves. This statement is corroborated in the present study, in which we see that 76% of workers were over 46 years of age and the average time they had spent in the institution until the first sick leave was over 21 years. However, other international studies on sick leaves due to non-work directly related causes show that this proportion is less than 30% [33].

Another finding of this research is that almost two thirds of the workers who took a sick leave were women, while in other scenarios women were less than 50% [33]. Consideration should be given to sex discrimination, which could influence the distribution of medium and higher education positions and its relation to the frequency of sick leaves. Although when analysing only sick leave cases without having the denominator of exposed workers, we cannot affirm that the proportion in one of the two sexes is greater or not. Likewise, it is well known from previous studies that women must attend to family emergencies to a greater extent than men, and this generates a higher percentage of sick leaves because there is no other mechanism that allows an individual to take care of children or other family members when such events arise [34].

The university unit with the highest proportion of sick leaves was the Human Health one (77.5%), in equal percentage to the proportion of workers of the Faculty of Medicine, and the university hospital accounted for 73% of those who composed this study's sample. It should be highlighted that almost half of the sick leaves were taken by health care workers, a fact that corroborates that, due to risks ranging from biological to organisational type [35–37], they are a population of workers quite vulnerable to temporary incapacities for work.

Making a reflection on the two previous considerations, the higher prevalence of workers from the Human Health unit can also determine the higher incidence of sick leaves among women, since the majority of the workers in the health sector are females, as stated by international and Brazilian literature [38–40].

The average duration of sick leaves for each worker probably varies in function of age, the type of work carried out and seriousness of the disease, associations that were not analysed since this is a descriptive study. However, it is necessary to highlight the multiplicity of events that the same worker can have, since 77% of the workers had more than one episode of sick leave in the study period and, of these, 45% had repeated episodes, maintaining the main cause from the first to the last episode. That is to say, it is very possible to infer tendencies of chronification of the diseases that originated the sick leaves, although they can also be explained, in part, by the greater age of the studied workers. However, to corroborate these hypotheses, no studies were found that had investigated predictors of the multiplicity of sick leaves.

Analysing chronic diseases, if we assume that longer sick leaves are a good example, we observe that these occurred to a greater extent among mental and behavioural diseases. This is consistent with the natural history of these diseases given that this type of pathologies produces acute symptoms to a lesser extent, except in some cases such as depressive disorders. However, if we analyse the records of the medical evaluations in less than a third of the registered sick leaves, psychological symptoms were identified as a complaint.

On the other hand, the same medical evaluation reports (when based on the initial complaints) that initially did not corroborate the diagnoses of the causes of temporary incapacity for work, now revealed that pain was present in 80% of all events. Thus, it is a widely found symptom in the majority of the acute causes that originated temporary incapacities for work, although they can also become chronic.

The finding that more than a third of the sick leaves had as their main cause mental and behavioural diseases is an important warning, especially because it does not agree with other populational studies [28]. In these, they are the fourth cause (and very close to the fifth), with a percentage close to 9% of the total. This was not either in accordance with other European studies where this group of diseases is the fifth cause and accounts for less than 8% of the sick leave total, behind musculoskeletal, respiratory, infectious diseases or those grouped in chapters XIX and XX of the ICD-10, generically described as external causes [32,33].

Depressive disorders were the most prevalent among all registered illnesses and one fifth of the workers had a main diagnosis related to mental health throughout their sick leave history. These results are congruent with previous studies [41] and can be explained by several reasons, which may also interact. We see how the mental health of civil servants is worse than that of the workers of the private sector. This leads us to believe that the recent changes in management mechanisms and work organisation that the civil sector has been through have led to work organisation models typical of the private initiative, based on productivity, which may impact more significantly on civil servants than in other sectors.

Another possible explanation is that the presence of psychiatrists among the physicians that work in the institution's own occupational medical service could lead to a better diagnosis or overdiagnosis of mental and behavioural diseases. It has been described, in previous publications, that the presence of such specialists can increase the diagnoses of mental illnesses and that such inadequate diagnoses and treatments can increase the risk for the said persons to develop physical disorders such as diabetes, cardiac disorders, weight gain, and other potentially serious health conditions [42].

In any case, due to overdiagnosis or not, addictions as a consequence of mental and behavioural disorders imply a large number of sick leaves to require medical treatment, in addition to great personal, institutional, economic and social losses, such as those derived from absenteeism, reduction of work ability and loss of productivity [15,22,26]. Substance addiction is also associated with jobs with high psychological demands and low work control [43,44], and the high prevalence obtained in this study can indicate that the work environment in the university presents such negative characteristics to workers' mental health.

There is consensus on the high cost of mental illness attributed to the loss of productivity and measured as absenteeism or lost work days. Thus, it is advisable to open lines of research that allow us to better understand the incidence, extent and recurrence of this type of diseases in this workers' population [45].

A large number of workers needed a readaptation of their previous work activity and, for many of them, with limitations. This aspect is important because we know from bibliography that the longer the duration of the sick leave the more it is related to the degree of disability and the lower the probability of returning to their original job [46].

Strength and Limitations

There are some limitations in this study. First, sick-leaves are multi-factorial and influenced not only by the health status of the individuals, but also by their work environment, social and psychological factors [47], attitudes and commitment to work as well as social insurance system. Thus, since the medical reports mainly contained health related information, we cannot make inferences about other possible sick leave causes related, for example, to psychosocial and workplace factors.

Second, it is a common problem for many registry-based studies of sick leaves that they only have access to one diagnosis, while we know that workers often struggle with several complaints and illnesses. Unfortunately, this was also the case of the databases that we had access to. They did not contain all the information we consider relevant, such as all the diagnoses related to each sick leave spell. In the system, only the main diagnosis of each sick leave spell is recorded. To identify all the workers with multiple complaints and their diagnoses, access to the medical records of each worker would be needed. However, we did not have access to these documents.

Third, we did not have access to the total number of workers at the units, forbidding the possibility to establish a denominator for the amount of sick leaves. This is a clear limitation, as it precludes us to know e.g. the overall prevalence and/or incidence of sick leaves in the units or to what extent the distributions of the various sociodemographic and work characteristics mirror that of the working population as a whole. The total number of workers at the units was not known, since it was fluctuating (due to hiring, layoffs, transfers and retirements), both during the entire study period and yearly. This made it difficult, if not almost impossible, to establish a precise estimation of the workers' population (needed denominator for prevalence and incidence calculation), and the decision to run an overall analysis of the entire six-year period made it even harder. A possible solution would be to use the number of workers recorded in the middle of 2012 (2364). However, this would bring even more inaccuracies and lead to the stratification of the analysis year by year, what would end up determining an annual analysis. Fourth, our results may be conditioned by the fact that the medical evaluations of sick leaves are made by physicians that work in the same university institution, being able to speed the return to work. However, a strength related to this centralisation of the evaluations, by the institution's own occupational medical service, is the standardisation of criteria.

The main difficulty to perform this study was that both databases were not integrated or built under the same computational architecture. This fact forced us to build the database used in the study manually, which was time-consuming and required extensive effort to collect information. These databases also presented most of the five methodological problems regarding the analysis of sickness absence described by Hensing et al. [48]. Solving these problems would facilitate the use of this useful source of information, not only for research purposes but also for the follow-up of sick leaves by the occupational medical service in the future.

5. Conclusions

Around 90% of all spells of sick leave were due to mental illness and musculoskeletal disorders. We would highlight that, when compared with other groups of sick workers, they have a higher number of sick leave spells due to mental illnesses, mostly depressive disorders. This fact has a negative effect on the workers involved and higher costs for the university. This is because they are a type of sick leave associated with higher levels of disability, fewer possibilities of return to work and that needs a process of readaptation to the previous job position. From a practical perspective, these results are of great relevance for those involved with workers' health management: they allow an overview of the diseases that are related to sick leaves in university workers, their burden, and also the widening of Occupational Health and Safety (OSH) managers' understanding about workers' sociodemographic data relation with sick leaves and return to work. Furthermore, the results might guide the construction of a workplace's preventive and protective measures and of health promotion interventions to reduce the burden on workers' health.

Using both record databases (Integrated Occupational Management Software and Health Medical System) to acquire the data used in this paper has allowed us to identify some points that must be improved in order to achieve the full potential of these tools, such as the absence of important data, the use of different computational architecture for both databases and the need of linkage between them. But this is not all, they have allowed us to demonstrate the usefulness of these databases for better sick leaves management by OSH managers and workers.

The analysis of data on sickness absences stored in computerised databases can lead to the detection of failures in the management system, the identification of groups, pathologies and organisational measures where action is needed. An example is the greater vulnerability found in the "Human health" unit that can be explained by being composed mostly by females and health personnel, two of the variables that in previous studies have been associated with a greater number of sick leave spells.

Finally, the effort to extract the data from both databases and reconstruct it under a unified database will contribute for OSH researchers and workers in concomitant and/or subsequent studies. With these, we intend to investigate some hypotheses that were generated during this study regarding predictors of multiple spells of sick leaves. For example, the ageing of the workforce due to not replacing retired workers and the effects of the economic crisis.

To conclude, the studied sick leaves taken by the university workers differ from those presented in previous publications, since more than a third of the sick leaves had as their main cause mental and behavioural diseases, also because women comprised almost two-thirds of the workers who took a sick leave and due to the fact that 76% of the workers who took a sick leave were over 46 years old, as previously stated in the discussion. Furthermore, the long duration of the sick leaves found in this study is remarkable and it may be related to the fact that multiple repetition of events occurred in several cases.

We would also like to highlight the important contingent of workers that were readapted to their previous work activity and the high percentage of those who were readapted to work with limitations. This is important since it is well known that the longer the sick leave is, the higher the disability levels and the lower the chances of return to work.

Author Contributions: Conceptualisation, A.D., J.M.B., M.M.F., C.R.-F. and J.G.-S.; Data curation, A.D., J.M.B., M.M.F., C.R.-F. and J.G.-S.; Formal analysis, A.D., J.M.B., M.M.F., C.R.-F. and J.G.-S.; Funding acquisition, A.D.; Investigation, A.D.; Methodology, A.D., J.M.B., M.M.F., C.R.-F. and J.G.-S.; Project administration, A.D.; Resources, A.D., J.M.B., M.M.F., C.R.-F. and J.G.-S.; Software, A.D., J.M.B., M.M.F., C.R.-F. and J.G.-S.; Supervision, A.D.; Validation, A.D. and J.M.B.; Visualisation, M.M.F., C.R.-F. and J.G.-S.; Writing—original draft, A.D., J.M.B., M.M.F., C.R.-F. and J.G.-S.

Funding: The São Paulo Research Foundation—FAPESP, process 2016-23096-1.

Acknowledgments: Botucatu Medical School/Research Unit of Public Health, Sandro Augusto Servilha Coquemala, Pedro Casagrande.

Conflicts of Interest: The authors declare no conflict of interests.

References

1. Whitaker, S. The management of sickness absence. *Occup. Environ. Med.* **2001**, *58*, 420–424. [CrossRef] [PubMed]
2. Marmot, M.G.; Rose, G.; Shipley, M.; Hamilton, P.J. Employment grade and coronary heart disease in British civil servants. *J. Epidemiol. Community Health* **1978**, *32*, 244–249. [CrossRef]

3. Johnson, W.; Bell, J.A.; Robson, E.; Norris, T.; Kivimäki, M.; Hamer, M. Do worse baseline risk factors explain the association of healthy, obesity with increased mortality risk? Whitehall II Study. *Int. J. Obes.* **2018**. [CrossRef]
4. Di Pietro, M.S.Z. *Direito Administrativo*, 29a ed.; GEN-Forense: São Paulo, Brazil, 2016.
5. Organization for Economic Cooperation and Development. *Government at a Glance*; Organization for Economic Cooperation and Development: Paris, France, 2015.
6. Ribeiro, C.V.S.; Mancebo, D. O servidor público no mundo do trabalho do século XXI. *Psicol. Ciênc. Prof.* **2013**, *33*, 192–207. [CrossRef]
7. Firpo, S. Emprego público protege quem não precisa. Folha de São Paulo. 2017. Available online: http://www1.folha.uol.com.br/mercado/2017/06/1893308-emprego-publico-protege-quem-nao-precisa.shtml (accessed on 25 October 2017).
8. Lacerda, J.A. *Capacitação e o perfil dos servidores públicos: UM estudo descritivo de uma Universidade Federal mineira*; UFL: Lavras, Brazil, 2013.
9. Carinhato, P.H. Neoliberalismo. reforma do estado e políticas sociais nas últimas décadas do século XX no Brasil. *Aurora* **2008**, *2*, 37–46.
10. Franco, T.; Druck, G.; Seligmann-Silva, E. As novas relações de trabalho. o desgaste mental do trabalhador e os transtornos mentais no trabalho precarizado. *Rev. Bras. Saude Ocup.* **2010**, *35*, 229–248. [CrossRef]
11. Silva, I.P. Neoliberalismo e as mudanças na estrutura do Estado: Ineficiência. cultura organizacional e hibridismo entre modelos de gestão. *Rev. Ciênc. Tecnol. Humanid. do IFPE* **2011**, *3*, 12–24.
12. Chiavegato Filho, L.G.; Navarro, V.L. A organização do trabalho em saúde em um contexto de precarização e avanço da ideologia gerencialista. In *O Avesso do Trabalho III*; Lourenço, E.A.S., Navarro, V.L., Eds.; Outras Expressões: São Paulo, Brazil, 2013; pp. 91–106.
13. Motta, P.R.M. O estado da arte da gestão pública. *Rev. Adm. Emp.* **2013**, *53*, 82–90. [CrossRef]
14. Metzger, J.L. Mudança Permanente: Fonte de penosidade no trabalho? *Rev. Bras. Saude Ocup.* **2011**, *36*, 12–24. [CrossRef]
15. Tonetto, E.S.; Prieb, S.A.M.; Tonetto, T.S. Os efeitos da reforma administrativa do estado sobre os servidores técnicos-administrativos da UFSM. *Rev. Univ. Soc.* **2011**, *21*, 54–61.
16. European Agency for Safety and Health at Work. *Management of Psychosocial Risks at Work: An Analysis of the Findings of the European Survey of Enterprises on New and Emerging Risks (ESENER)*; Observatory, E.R., Ed.; Publications Office of the European Union: Luxembourg, 2012; p. 64.
17. Ravalier, J.M.; McVicar, A.; Munn-Giddings, C. Public service stress and burnout over 12 months. *Occ. Med.* **2014**, *64*, 521–523. [CrossRef] [PubMed]
18. Briner, R.B. ABC of work related disorders. Absence from work. *BMJ* **1996**, *313*, 874–877. [CrossRef] [PubMed]
19. Porta, M.; Greenland, S.; Hernán, M.; Silva, I.S. *A Dictionary of Epidemiology*, 6th ed.; Oxford University Press: Oxford, UK, 2014; 377p.
20. Kivimaki, M.; Head, J.; Ferrie, J.E.; Shipley, M.J.; Vahtera, J.; Marmot, M.G. Sickness absence as a global measure of health: Evidence from mortality in the Whitehall II prospective cohort study. *Br. Med. J.* **2003**, *327*, 364–368. [CrossRef] [PubMed]
21. Permanent Commission and International Association on Occupational Health. Sub-committee on absenteeism: Draft recommendations. *Br. J. Ind. Med.* **1973**, *30*, 402–403.
22. Cruz, C.R.B.; Shirassu, M.M.; Barbosa, P.L.Q.; Santana, A.M.R. Transtornos mentais como causa de absenteísmo entre servidores públicos em São Paulo. *Rev. Psiq. Clin.* **2011**, *38*, 265–266. [CrossRef]
23. Fantazia, M.M. *Perfil do adoecimento dos trabalhadores de câmpus universitário do interior paulista: Análise dos dados de absenteísmo por motivo de doença*; Universidade Estadual Paulista: Botucatu, Brazil, 2015.
24. Costa, F.M.; Vieira, M.A.; Sena, R.R. Absenteísmo relacionado a doenças entre membros da equipe de enfermagem de um hospital escola. *Rev. Bras. Enferm.* **2009**, *69*, 38–44. [CrossRef]
25. Andrade, T.B.; Souza, M.G.C.; Simões, M.P.C.; Andrade, F.B. Prevalência de absenteísmo entre trabalhadores do serviço público. *Sci. Med.* **2008**, *18*, 166–171.
26. Braga, L.C.; Carvalho, L.R.; Binder, M.C.P. Condições de trabalho e transtornos mentais comuns em trabalhadores da rede básica de saúde de Botucatu (SP). *Ciênc. Saude Colet.* **2010**, *15*, 1585–1596. [CrossRef]

27. Braga, L.C.; Vendrameto, M.T. *Perfil de afastamento do trabalho por motivo de doença entre profissionais de enfermagem de uma instituição de ensino superior no interior paulista*; I Congresso Paulista de Medicina Legal e Perícias Médicas de São Paulo, APM: São Paulo, Brazil, 2012.
28. Brasil; Ministério da Fazenda; Secretaria de Previdência; Instituto Nacional do Seguro Social. *Empresa de Tecnologia e Informações da Previdência*; Anuário Estatístico da Previdência Social: Brasilia FD, Brazil, 2015; p. 918.
29. Organização Mundial da Saúde. *CID-10 Classificação Estatística Internacional de Doenças e Problemas Relacionados à Saúde*, 10a ed.; USP: São Paulo, Brazil, 1997.
30. *Constituição da República Federativa do Brasil. Art. 41*; IPSM: Brasilia FD, Brazil, 1988.
31. Nakano, S.M.S.; Rodrigues Filho, S.; Santos, I.C. Perícia Médica. In *Nakano SMS*; Braga, B.E., Ed.; Perícia Médica; CRM-GO: Goiânia, Brazil, 2007; pp. 31–46.
32. Cabanillas-Moruno, J.L.; Miner, M.G.; Gracia, J.M.L.; Doncel, J.D.V. *Tiempo óptimo personalizado de incapacidad temporal por diagnóstico*; Consejería de Salud y Bienestar Social de la Junta de Andalucía: Sevilla, Spain, 2012.
33. Torá-Rocamora, I.; Martínez, J.M.; Gimeno, D.; Alberti, C.; Jardí, J.; Manzanera, R.; Benavides, F.G.; Delclos, G. Assessment of the magnitude of geographical variations in the duration of non-work-related sickness absence by individual and contextual factors. *Gac. Sanit.* **2015**, *29*, 164–171. [CrossRef]
34. Blank, N.; Diderichsen, F. Short-term and long-term sick-leave in Sweden: Relationships with social circumstances. working conditions and gender. *Scand. J. Soc. Med.* **1995**, *23*, 265–272. [CrossRef]
35. Gianino, M.M.; Politano, G.; Scarmozzino, A.; Charrier, L.; Testa, M.; Giacomelli, S.; Benso, A.; Zotti, C.M. Estimation of sickness absenteeism among Italian healthcare workers during seasonal influenza epidemics. *PLoS ONE* **2017**, *12*. [CrossRef] [PubMed]
36. Andersen, L.N.; Juul-Kristensen, B.; Roessler, K.K.; Herborg, L.G.; Sorensen, T.L.; Sogaard, K. Efficacy of 'Tailored Physical Activity' in reducing sickness absence among health care workers: Design of a randomised controlled trial. *BMC Public Health* **2013**, *13*, 917. [CrossRef] [PubMed]
37. Moll, S.E. The web of silence: A qualitative case study of early intervention and support for healthcare workers with mental ill-health. *BMC Public Health* **2014**, *14*, 138. [CrossRef]
38. World Health Organization. *Gender and Health Workforce Statistics*; World Health Organization: Geneva, Switzerland, 2008.
39. McDonagh, K.J.; Bobrowski, P.; Hoss, M.A.K.; Paris, N.M.; Schulte, M. The leadership gap: Ensuring effective healthcare leadership requires inclusion of women at the top. *Open J. Leadersh.* **2014**, *3*, 20–29. [CrossRef]
40. Wermelinger, M.; Machado, M.H.; Tavares, M.D.F.L.; Oliveira, E.S.; Moysés, N.M.N. A força de trabalho do setor de saúde no Brasil: Focalizando a feminização. *Divulg. Saude Debate* **2010**, *45*, 55–71.
41. Dias, A.; Gómez-Salgado, J.; Bernardes, J.M.; Ruiz-Frutos, C. Factors Affecting Sick Leave Duration for Non-Work-Related Temporary Disabilities in Brazilian University Public Servants. *Int. J. Environ. Res. Public Health* **2018**, *15*, 2127. [CrossRef] [PubMed]
42. Caplan, P.J. *They Say You're Crazy: How the World's Most Powerful Psychiatrists Decide Who's Normal*; Perseus Books Group: New York, NY, USA, 1995; 358p.
43. Barbosa-Branco, A.; Bultmann, U.; Steenstra, I. Sickness benefit claims due to mental disorders in Brazil: Associations in a population-based study. *Cad. Saude Publica* **2012**, *28*, 1854–1866. [CrossRef] [PubMed]
44. Barbosa-Branco, A.; Souza, W.R.; Steenstra, I.A. Incidence of work and non-work-related disability claims in Brazil. *Am. J. Ind. Med.* **2011**, *54*, 858–871. [CrossRef] [PubMed]
45. Dewa, C.S.; Loong, D.; Bonato, S. Work outcomes of sickness absence related to mental disorders: A systematic literature review. *BMJ Open* **2014**, *4*, e005533. [CrossRef]
46. Vieira, E.R.; Albuquerque-Oliveira, P.R.; Barbosa-Branco, A. Work disability benefits due to musculoskeletal disorders among Brazilian private sector workers. *BMJ Open* **2011**, *1*, e000003. [CrossRef]

47. Lu, C.Y.; Tsai, M.C.; Muo, C.H.; Kuo, Y.H.; Sung, F.C.; Wu, C.C. Personal, Psychosocial and Environmental Factors Related to Sick Building Syndrome in Official Employees of Taiwan. *Int. J. Environ. Res. Public Health* **2018**, *15*, 7. [CrossRef] [PubMed]
48. Hensing, G.; Alexanderson, K.; Allebeck, P.; Bjurulf, P. How to measure sickness absence? Literature review and suggestion of five basic measures. *Scand. J. Soc. Med.* **1998**, *26*, 133–144. [CrossRef] [PubMed]

International Journal of
Environmental Research and Public Health

MDPI

Article

A Profile of Knee Injuries Suffered by Australian Army Reserve Soldiers

Ben Schram [1,*], Robin Orr [1] and Rodney Pope [1,2]

1 Tactical Research Unit, Bond University, Robina 4226, QLD, Australia; rorr@bond.edu.au (R.O.); rpope@csu.edu.au (R.P.)
2 School of Community Health, Charles Sturt University, Albury 2640, NSW, Australia
* Correspondence: bschram@bond.edu.au; Tel.: +61-5-595-5828

Received: 23 November 2018; Accepted: 18 December 2018; Published: 20 December 2018

Abstract: Despite having to perform the same occupational tasks as full-time soldiers, part-time soldiers may have lower levels of physical conditioning and report higher rates of injury per unit exposure to active service. The purpose of this study was to profile the leading body site of injury occurring in part-time soldiers to inform injury prevention strategies. Injury data from the Australian Army Reserve (ARES) spanning a two-year period were obtained from the Department of Defence Workplace Health, Safety, Compensation and Reporting database pertaining to locations, nature, mechanisms, and the activity being performed at the time of injury. Among the 1434 injuries reported by ARES personnel, the knee was the most common injury site (n = 228, 16%). Soft tissue injury due to trauma or unknown causes was the most common nature of knee injury (n = 177, 78%). Combat training was the most common activity being performed when soft tissue injuries occurred at the knee (n = 73, 42%), with physical training the second most common (n = 51, 30%), due to muscular stress (n = 36, 71%) and falls (n = 8, 16%). Targeted intrinsic and extrinsic approaches to injury minimization strategies for soft tissue knee injuries during combat and physical training should be designed.

Keywords: reserves; part-time; military; health and safety; defence; injury

1. Introduction

An effective military force is required to be agile, capable, efficient, and potent. Injuries to military personnel interrupt active duty service and detract from overall army capability [1]. Emphasis is on ensuring injury prevention strategies are put in place to minimise injuries sustained during military service [2–4]. To be effective however, these intervention strategies need to be informed by research investigating key types and sources of injuries, so that risk mitigation strategies are directed towards the most prevalent or serious types and sources of injury [2–4].

The Australian Defence Force is comprised of both part-time and full-time personnel [5]. Even though part-time personnel are not employed on a full time basis, these members are important contributors to the Army's capabilities [6]. With part-time members having similar training requirements, fitness standards, and occupational tasks as full-time personnel; injuries pose similar concerns for this population. Injuries may be of even greater concern for part-time soldiers, as previous research has shown part-time personnel report a substantially higher rate of injuries per unit exposure to active duty when compared to their full-time counterparts, with some showing up to double the rates in part-time compared to full-time personnel [7,8].

One possible reason for a heighted risk of injury in part-time personnel may be lower levels of aerobic fitness in part-time personnel [9–11]. Part-time personnel may have a lower fitness level when compared to full time personnel, possibly due to the necessity to balance both civilian life and military life [9]. It is well known that lower aerobic fitness is a risk factor for injuries in military personnel [10,12].

The lower limb has been shown to be the most commonly injured body site in military personnel [13]. However, further detail regarding the particular sites in the lower limb that are most frequently injured and the activities and mechanisms that give rise to injuries affecting those sites is lacking for part-time personnel [13]. This detail is needed to inform injury prevention efforts for part-time personnel and so enhance the readiness of this important element of Army capability. A detailed investigation of the nature and cause of injuries affecting specific lower limb sites will valuably inform selection and implementation of interventions designed to minimise both the incidence and severity of injuries suffered by the part-time army population. This approach is supported by previous research in the army context, which has provided positive evidence for injury rate reduction through targeted interventions, once high risk activities and locations have been identified [2,14–16]. The aim of this study was to profile the most common injury occurring in part-time soldiers with respect to the predominate location, nature, activity, and mechanism, with a view to informing injury prevention strategies for these part-time personnel.

2. Materials and Methods

The study employed a cross-sectional design, using Australian Department of Defence population data and records of injuries reported by Australian Army Reserve (ARES) personnel over a two-year period. The mean annual population size for the ARES across the period (n = 15,034) was ascertained from published Department of Defence Records [17,18]. The injury records for ARES personnel were sourced in a non-identifiable form from the Workplace Health, Safety, Compensation and Reporting (WHSCAR) database of the Australian Department of Defence, which constitutes the official record of incidents and injuries sustained by Army personnel [19]. The WHSCAR records provided to the researchers included, for each injury to an ARES soldier: details of the Service (Army) and service type (part-time), the type of occurrence the record reported (serious injury or minor injury), the injury date, the body site, the nature of the injury, the activity being undertaken at the time of the injury, the mechanism of injury, the soldier's duty status at the time of injury (on duty or off duty), age and rank, and a narrative description of the injury incident.

The injury records extracted from the WHSCAR database were included in the study if they related to: (1) ARES personnel; and (2) a minor or serious injury that occurred while the soldier was 'on duty'. The definitions of injury, whether for minor personal injury (MPI) or serious personal injury (SPI), were those provided by the Australian Department of Defence [19]. An SPI required immediate treatment as an in-patient in a hospital, whereas an MPI was defined as any minor injury which did not result in a fatality, SPI, illness, or dangerous incident. Records were excluded if they: (1) related to personnel from military services other than the Australian Army; (2) related to full-time Army personnel; (3) related to personnel from a foreign defence force, on secondment with the Australian Defence Force; or (4) contained missing or incomplete data pertinent to this study (for example, site of injury).

The WHSCAR data were manually cleaned following receipt to ensure that only eligible records were retained. Each record was reviewed, and duplicate and ineligible records were removed; the latter with reference to the inclusion and exclusion criteria listed above. Each datum record was further verified, corrected, or made more precise by manually comparing the allocated Type of Occurrence Classification System (TOOCS) classifications with the free text narrative data from the same record. When discrepancies were identified, precedence was given to the free text narratives and the TOOCS classification was adjusted accordingly, as narratives provided by incident reporters are considered more detailed and accurate than data entered by a third party using a finite coding system [20]. The adjusted dataset was employed in the data analysis. To increase data accuracy, brevity, and sensitivity, some TOOCS fields were aggregated, notably the 'nature of injury' and 'activity' fields. In the TOOCS 'nature of injury' classifications, 'soft tissue injuries due to trauma or unknown mechanism' subsumed 'trauma to muscle' (a soft tissue) and 'trauma to tendons' (another soft tissue). In addition, 'trauma to joints and ligaments' subsumed 'trauma to joints and ligaments, not elsewhere classified' and 'trauma to joints and ligaments unspecified'. In the TOOCS 'activity' classifications, all sports were merged into an aggregated classification, 'sport'. 'Running' was subsumed by 'physical training', and 'patrolling' and all weapon handling activities were subsumed by 'combat training'.

Data Analysis

Following this data cleaning process, descriptive analyses were employed to examine and describe the data to address the study aim. Injury incidence rates were first calculated as follows: the counts of minor injuries and serious injuries reported by ARES personnel across the two-year study period were each divided by the number of full-time-equivalent years of active service provided by ARES personnel across these two years and the result was then multiplied by 100 to derive the number of injuries reported by ARES personnel per 100 years of active service. In these calculations, one full-time-equivalent year of active service by ARES personnel was defined as 232 days of active service, based on the following:

Total days of active service in one full-time year = 365 days in a full year − 104 days of weekends (or equivalent days 'in lieu') − 20 days of annual leave − 9 days of public holidays = 232 days.

The proportion of reported occupational injuries in ARES personnel which occurred at each of the reported body locations was next calculated and these proportions were tabulated to enable identification of the most common body site of injuries in ARES personnel. Subsequently calculated were the proportions of knee injuries reported by ARES personnel which were associated with personnel in specific age brackets (less than 20 years, 20–29 years, 30–39 years, 40–50 years and greater than 50 years) or at specific rank levels, or which involved specific: (1) natures of injury; (2) activities being performed at the times injuries occurred; and (3) injury mechanisms. The latter proportions were used to identify the key natures, causes, and mechanisms of knee injuries reported by ARES personnel.

The Australian Defence Human Research Ethics Committee (ADHREC, LERP14-024) and the Bond University Human Research Ethics Committee (BUHREC, RO-1907) granted ethics approval for this study. As this data were retrospective and non-identifiable, it met the pre-requisites for a waiver of participant consent as there were no means through which the participants could be identified, and consent gained. Departmental authorisation for the project was obtained in parallel to the process for obtaining ADHREC approval. Authorization to publish this study was obtained from Joint Health Command.

3. Results

A total of 1434 injuries were reported by the ARES population of 15,034 personnel within the 2-year study period, representing a reported injury incidence rate of 30.5 injuries per 100 person-years of active service. Minor personal injuries (MPIs) accounted for 95.4% of these reported injuries (n = 1368), with the remaining 4.6% (n = 66) being classified as serious personal injuries (SPIs). The body sites of all lower limb MPI and SPI reported by ARES personnel in the two-year study period are listed in Table 1.

The knee was the most commonly reported specific body site of injury, accounting for 15.9% (n = 228) of all injuries reported by ARES personnel (Table 1) and therefore will be the focus for the rest of this investigation. Of the total 228 knee injuries reported by ARES personnel, 98% (n = 224) were MPIs and 2% (n = 4) were SPIs (Table 1). The SPIs which occurred at the knee were due to dislocation, one during parade and one while jogging.

The nature of soft tissue injuries suffered by part-time personnel can be found in Table 2 below. The most common nature of knee injuries reported by the ARES personnel was soft tissue injury due to trauma or unknown mechanisms, which was responsible for 81% of the injuries in this bodily location. This was followed by trauma to the joint and ligaments.

Table 1. Body sites of SPIs and MPIs reported by ARES personnel. Reported as number of injuries (percentage of overall injuries).

Location	MPI	SPI	MPI and SPI
Knee	224 (16.4%)	4 (6.1%)	228 (15.9%)
Ankle	139 (10.2%)	2 (3.0%)	141 (9.8%)
Foot	55 (4.0%)	2 (3.0%)	57 (4.0%)
Thigh	46 (3.4%)	0	46 (3.2%)
Lower limb general	35 (2.6%)	2 (3.0%)	37 (2.6%)
Gastroc-soleus complex	25 (1.8%)	0	25 (1.7%)
Hip	18 (1.3%)	1 (1.5%)	19 (1.3%)
Shins	15 (1.1%)	0	15 (1.1%)
Lower limb multiple	13 (1.1%)	0	13 (0.9%)
Pelvis	1 (0.1%)	0	1 (0.1%)

Data expressed as number of injuries (% of injuries). MPI = minor personal injury, SPI = serious personal injury.

Table 2. Nature of injuries of knee injuries in Australian Army Reserve (ARES) personnel.

Nature of Injury	MPI	SPI
Soft tissue injuries (trauma or unknown mechanisms)	181 (80.8%)	0
Trauma to joints and ligaments	16 (7.1%)	0
Contusion/bruising and superficial crushing	8 (3.6%)	0
Dislocation	6 (2.7%)	2 (50%)
Laceration	5 (2.2%)	0
Superficial injury	5 (2.2%)	0
Infectious and parasitic diseases	1 (0.4%)	0
Fracture	0	0
Multiple injuries	1 (0.4%)	0
Other diseases of skin and subcutaneous tissue	1 (0.4%)	0
Bursitis	0	1 (25%)
Other soft tissue diseases	0	1 (25%)
Total	224	4

Data expressed as number of injuries (% of injuries). MPI = minor personal injury, SPI = serious personal injury.

The activity being performed while soft tissue injuries were suffered at the knee can be found in Table 3 below. Combat training was the leading activity in which injuries occurred at the knee with 43% of injuries, while physical training was the second most common. Combining both combat training and physical training led to a total of 72% of soft tissue knee injuries and will therefore be explored further.

The most common mechanisms of injury reported by ARES personnel for soft tissue injuries at the knee joint that occurred while they undertook combat training were falls and muscular stress with no object being handled ($n = 27$, 37.0% and $n = 21$, 28.8%, respectively; Table 4). Similarly, ARES personnel reported muscular stress with no objects being handled and falls as the most prevalent mechanisms causing soft tissue injuries at the knee joint during physical training, accounting for 70.6% ($n = 36$) of the soft tissue injuries reported during physical training (Table 5).

Table 3. The activity in which soft tissue injuries occurred at the knee in part-time personnel.

Activity	MPI
Combat training	77 (42.2%)
Physical training	53 (29.5%)
Marching	14 (8.7%)
Walking	13 (6.9%)
Boarding/alighting a vehicle	5 (2.9%)
Manual/materials handling	4 (2.3%)

Table 3. *Cont.*

Activity	MPI
Sitting/standing	3 (1.7%)
Admin activities	2 (1.2%)
Driving	2 (1.2%)
Sport	3 (1.7%)
Construction/engineering	1 (0.6%)
Diving/immersion training	1 (0.6%)
Maintenance	1 (0.6%)
Sleeping	1 (0.6%)
Adventure training	1 (0.6%)
Total	181

Data expressed as number of injuries (% of injuries). MPI = minor personal injury.

Table 4. Knee injuries suffered during combat training. Number of injuries (% of injuries).

Mechanism	MPI
Falls	28 (36.4%)
Muscular stress with no object being handled	24 (31.2%)
Muscular stress while lifting carrying or putting	5 (6.5%)
Contact with moving or stationary object	13 (16.9%)
Other and multiple mechanisms	5 (6.5%)
Contact with or exposure to biological factors of non-human origin	1 (1.3%)
Stepping kneeling or sitting on objects	1 (1.3%)
Total	77

Data expressed as number of injuries (% of injuries). MPI = minor personal injury.

Table 5. Knee injuries suffered during physical training. Number of injuries (% of injuries).

Mechanism	MPI
Muscular stress with no object being handled	38 (71.7%)
Falls	8 (15.1%)
Muscular stress while lifting carrying or putting	1 (1.9%)
Contact with moving or stationary object	4 (7.5%)
Other and multiple mechanisms	2 (3.8%)
Total	53

Data expressed as number of injuries (% of injuries). MPI = minor personal injury.

Profiles of the Part-Time Soldiers Who Reported Knee Injuries

The mean age of the ARES personnel who reported knee injuries was 33.7 ± 11.1 years, ranging from 18 to 63 years of age, and the age and military rank distributions for the ARES personnel who reported these knee injuries are provided in Tables 6 and 7. The results presented in Table 6 indicate that while 43% of knee injuries reported by ARES personnel were reported by personnel in the 20–29-year age bracket, 54% of the reported knee injuries were reported by ARES personnel over the age of 30 years. Non-officers reported 183 of the knee injuries reported by ARES personnel (80.3%) while officers (including officer cadets) reported 45 of the knee injuries (19.7%; Table 7). Also, of note, 25% of the knee injuries reported by ARES personnel were reported by recruits, trainees and officer cadets and would therefore appear to have occurred during ARES initial training courses (Table 7).

Table 6. Ages of ARES personnel who reported knee injuries (n = number of injuries).

Age (years)	n	%
<20	7	3.1%
20–29	99	43.4%
30–39	45	19.7%
40–49	53	23.3%
≥50	24	10.5%
Total	228	100.0%

Table 7. Military ranks of ARES personnel who reported knee injuries (n = number of injuries).

Rank	n	%
Recruit	25	11.0%
Officer cadet	26	11.4%
Private trainee	6	2.6%
Private	44	19.3%
Private proficient	51	22.4%
Lance corporal	10	4.4%
Corporal	26	11.4%
Sergeant	11	4.8%
Warrant officer class 2	7	3.1%
Warrant officer class 1	3	1.3%
Lieutenant	4	1.8%
Captain	7	3.1%
Major	5	2.2%
Lieutenant colonel	2	0.9%
Colonel	1	0.4%
Total	228	100.0%

4. Discussion

The aim of this study was to identify the leading predominate locations, natures, activities, and mechanism of injuries occurring in part-time army personnel with a view to informing injury prevention strategies. This is the first known study to provide a detailed analysis of the leading body sites, natures, and causes of injuries reported by part-time army personnel. A key finding of this study was that the knee was the most commonly reported body site of injury in ARES personnel, accounting for 16% of all injuries reported by these part-time army personnel. Part-time personnel (30.5 injuries per 100 years of active service) appear to be injured more than their full-time colleagues with previous reports of full-time personnel injury rates of 16.72 injuries per 100 years of active service [7]).

This finding is in agreement with previous studies in military personnel, with injuries occurring at or below the knee most common [2,10,11,21]. Kaufman's review [2] included seven studies in which knee injuries comprised 10.2–34.3% of all reported injuries in a variety of military recruits including marines, army and naval special warfare candidates. Knapik found the knee to be the location of 21% of injuries for males and 19% for females in an army population, a similar finding to this current study [10]. In Knapik's study, the ankle and foot (20%) were commonly injured, in line with the findings of this study in which the ankle was the third most common site of injuries, accounting for 9.83% of all reported injuries (Table 1). Jennings found 18% of injuries in army soldiers were to the knee [21], while previous research on Australian military recruits has found that 24% of injuries occurred at the knee [11]. Across the Australian Army as a whole, aggregated injury data showed that knee injuries accounted for the highest proportion of lower limb injuries (35%) associated with a single body site and the highest proportion of working days lost (40%) [8].

Soft tissue injuries were the most common nature of injuries in the part-time, ARES population that was the subject of the current study, and these soft tissue injuries were most commonly due to either trauma or unknown mechanisms. It should be acknowledged however that the categorization of the nature of injury soft tissue injuries (trauma or unknown mechanisms) may be broad in nature and therefore may be over-represented because of this. Soft tissue injuries at the knee have previously been found to be the predominant type of injury amongst active duty military personnel, most commonly involve damage to structures such as the patella, meniscus, and ligaments [22]. The risk factors for soft tissue injuries affecting the knee amongst military personnel may include a history of prior injury to the affected knee, prior deployments, infantry service, and prior hip injury [22]. Hill et al. [22] also identified age greater than 30 years and increasing length of service to be risk factors for knee injuries. While this study similarly found that personnel over the age of 30 years featured heavily among those reporting knee injuries in this part-time, ARES population (53.51% of knee injuries), higher military ranks (and potentially lengths of service) did not appear to be strongly associated with higher injury rates.

In this study of part-time army personnel from the ARES, military combat training and physical training were the most common activities being performed when soft-tissue injuries occurred to the knee. Combat training is inherently more difficult for part-time personnel to prepare for. Unlike physical training which they can perform in their own time, combat training requires access to other personnel, restricted equipment, and preferably military styled tasks [23]. An example would be combat load carriage, which would preferably involve carrying their actual military loads and equipment [24]. This requirement is of importance given that military personnel are required to carry heavy combat loads, which can be in excess of 45 kg [25], and carrying these loads is a known cause of serious knee injuries. In a study of military soldiers conducting a 20-km march with a 46-kg load, Knapik et al. [26] observed an injury frequency of one per cent (two of 335). These two knee injuries equated to 14 days of limited duties. A subsequent study by Knapik et al. [27] found that, of six soldiers who could not complete a series of load carriage trials (six 20-km marches with loads ranging from 34 to 61 kg and utilising two difference pack designs), three were diagnosed with a knee strain, with the remaining three suffering injuries across three other body sites. To maintain specific fitness for combat load carriage, it is recommended that a load carriage training session using combat loads is conducted every seven to 14 days [28,29]. Considering this, it is noteworthy that part-time army personnel like those in the ARES may struggle to maintain this level of specific load carriage training, since having ARES personnel carrying military style equipment through urban areas in order to maintain their load carriage conditioning is likely to generate serious concerns among the general public, given current security threats.

Noting the importance of physical fitness for military personnel, it is of concern that physical training is a common source of injuries in both the general military population [8] and in this study. Injuries in physical training are often associated with sudden increases in training volume or intensity [30]. As such, while part-time personnel may be able to maintain some personal fitness, they may be at greater risk of injuries during unit physical training than full-time personnel due to undertaking lower volumes of military physical training than their full-time colleagues. Opportunities to increase military physical training are therefore needed for part-time personnel, potentially utilizing novel approaches like community-based training groups, where ARES personnel can be motivated to train in small groups, connected by close proximity or virtually, in order to maintain a suitable minimum level of fitness [23].

The most common mechanisms of injury during combat training and physical training were falls and muscular stress with no objects being handled. Injuries due to both microtrauma and macrotrauma appeared to occur during combat training in these part-time army personnel, whereas soft tissue injuries with no external stresses, such as overuse injuries, were more prevalent in physical training. Other studies within a military context have found injuries due to running and falls to be common [21], along with a high prevalence of overuse injuries due to repetitive activities [2], with some authors finding overuse mechanisms to be the cause of 75% of injuries in males recruits and 78% in females recruits [10].

Knee injuries in sport are known to occur more frequently in the latter stages of competition under conditions of fatigue, thought to be due to decreased neuromuscular control. Proprioceptive training for the lower limb with embedded cognitive challenges may therefore have a role in the minimization of ankle and knee injuries in those who have been identified with poor proprioception or a previous injury. Programs consisting of wobble boards and jump landing training have shown success in improving both ankle and knee proprioception [31], with wobble boards showing an optimization of ankle joint stability in landing tasks [32]. Poor landing mechanics have been linked to acute ankle and knee sprains [33] Generally increasing levels of fitness and endurance will enable soldiers to operate under less fatigue at the same relative work load, which may also play a role in injury reduction.

Investigating prevention strategies for overuse injuries in military personnel, a meta-analysis by Kollock et al. [34] has found a possible link between lower hip and thigh strength and overuse injuries of the knee. Despite focusing mainly on patello-femoral pain, the study found decreased hip external rotator, knee extensor, and knee flexor strength in symptomatic personnel, when compared to asymptomatic personnel. While acknowledging that physical training itself may be a cause of injury, it is possible that dedicated and specific strength and conditioning of the hip and knee of military personnel may be useful in minimizing these strength deficits in military personnel, as demonstrated in sporting populations [35]. For the lower limb in general, other injury prevention measures that may be useful in reducing lower limb loading during physical training include altering running surfaces [36], changing training loads [4], bracing ankles for certain activities [3], and use of shock-absorbing innersoles [2].

Not all injury prevention strategies are effective however. There is some evidence suggesting that pre-exercise static stretching, may be ineffective at reducing injury rates in military populations [11]. Likewise, the addition of balance and agility programs on top of physical training has been shown to increase injury rates when implemented in military recruits [37]. It is thought this may be due to this training being offered in addition to normal physical training within an already compact training schedule, leading to extra fatigue and a subsequent increase in injury risk [37]. This study adds to the current body of literature regarding ARES personnel and highlights the top site in which injuries occur among this service type. Differences in injuries between service type may be explained by less chronic conditioning, fewer opportunities to expose personnel to combat training, and time constraints to training in ARES personnel when compared to ARA personnel. Targeted approaches to injury prevention, such as specific physical training, load reduction, avoiding repetitive tasks, and use of ankle bracing may be of use in preventing these injuries. The findings of this study can be used to inform injury prevention efforts and future research for part-time army populations such as the ARES.

A limitation of this study was that data were extracted from a system in which injury information was collected by use of a formal injury report. This may have led to minor, or less severe injuries not being reported and therefore captured in this reporting system. A recent study has suggested that only 11–19% of injuries are captured with the WHSCAR system [7]. Under this system, the casualty is required to report to a system retrospectively and therefore the numbers of injuries reported in this study may underrepresent the absolute number of injuries in this population. It does remain likely that the proportional distributions of body sites, natures, and causes of injuries reported by ARES personnel are still representative of this part-time army population. There have been recommendations for a 'point of care' system of reporting to be utilized, in which health care personnel create a report at the time an injured soldier presents for health care, rather than relying on the casualty to report to a system retrospectively [7].

5. Conclusions

Soft tissue injuries affecting the knee were found to be the most common nature and site of injury amongst the part-time, ARES personnel. These injuries occurred most commonly during military combat training and physical training, due to falls, soft tissue injuries with no object being handled.

Author Contributions: Conceptualization, B.S., R.O., and R.P.; methodology, B.S., R.O., and R.P.; formal analysis, R.P.; writing—original draft preparation, B.S.; writing—review and editing, B.S., R.O., and R.P.

Funding: This study was supported by a Defence Health Foundation Grant.

Conflicts of Interest: The authors declare no conflict of interest.

References

1. Department of Defence. *Defence White Paper*; Australian Government Department of Defence: Canberra, Australia, 2016.
2. Kaufman, K.R.; Brodine, S.; Shaffer, R. Military training-related injuries: Surveillance, research, and prevention. *Am. J. Prev. Med.* **2000**, *18*, 54–63. [CrossRef]
3. Amoroso, P.J.; Ryan, J.B.; Bickley, B.; Leitschuh, P.; Taylor, D.C.; Jones, B.H. Braced for impact: Reducing military paratroopers' ankle sprains using outside-the-boot braces. *J. Trauma* **1998**, *45*, 575–580. [CrossRef] [PubMed]
4. Almeida, S.A.; Maxwell Williams, K.; Shaffer, R.A.; Luz, J.T.; Badong, K.E.; Brodine, S.K. *A Physical Training Program to Reduce Musculoskeletal Injuries in U.S. Marine Corps Recruits*; Naval Health Research Center, Technical Report; National Technical Information Service, U.S. Department of Commerce: Washington, DC, USA, 1997.
5. Australian Department of Defence. *Defence White Paper*; Australian Government Department of Defence: Canberra, Australia, 2013.
6. Smith, H.; Jans, N. Use them or lose them? Australia's defence force reserves. *Armed. Forces Soc.* **2011**, *37*, 301–320. [CrossRef]
7. Pope, R.; Orr, R. Incidence rates for work health and safety incidents and injuries in Australian army reserve vs. full time soldiers, and a comparison of reporting systems. *J. Mil. Veteran's Health* **2017**, *25*, 16–25.
8. Department of Defence. *Australian Defence Force Health Status Report*; Department of Defence: Canberra, Australia, 2000. Available online: http://www.Defence.Gov.Au/media/2000/health/01.Pdf. (accessed on 15 November 2016).
9. Warr, B.J.; Heumann, K.J.; Keating, C.J.; Swa, P.D.; Alvar, B.A.; Dodd, D.J.; Mitros, M.R. How do they compare? An assessment of predeployment fitness in the arizona national guard. *J. Strength Cond. Res.* **2011**, *25*, 2955–2962. [CrossRef] [PubMed]
10. Knapik, J.J.; Sharp, M.A.; Canham-Chervak, M.; Hauret, K.; Patton, J.F.; Jones, B.H. Risk factors for training-related injuries among men and women in basic combat training. *Med. Sci. Sports Exerc.* **2001**, *33*, 946. [CrossRef] [PubMed]
11. Pope, R.P.; Herbert, R.D.; Kirwan, J.D.; Graham, B.J. A randomized trial of preexercise stretching for prevention of lower- limb injury. *Med. Sci. Sports Exerc.* **2000**, *32*, 271–277. [CrossRef] [PubMed]
12. Pope, R. Prediction and Prevention of Lower Limb Injuries and Attrition in Army Recruits. PhD. Thesis, Charles Sturt University, Sydney, Australia, 2002.
13. McDonald, D.; Orr, R.M.; Pope, R. A comparison of work health and safety incidents and injuries in part-time and full-time Australian army personnel. *J. Athl. Train.* **2016**, *51*, 880–886. [CrossRef] [PubMed]
14. Pope, R.P. Injury surveillance and systematic investigation identify a rubber matting hazard for anterior cruciate ligament rupture on an obstacle course. *Mil. Med.* **2002**, *167*, 359–362. [CrossRef]
15. Pope, R.P. Rubber matting on an obstacle course causes anterior cruciate ligament ruptures and its removal eliminates them. *Mil. Med.* **2002**, *167*, 355–358. [CrossRef]
16. Pope, R.P. Prevention of pelvic stress fractures in female army recruits. *Mil. Med.* **1999**, *164*, 370–373. [CrossRef] [PubMed]
17. Department of Defence. *Agency Resources and Planned Performance*; Defence Housing Authority; Defence Material Organisation: Hague, The Netherlands, 2014.
18. Department of Defence. *Agency Resources and Planned Performance*; Defence Housing Authority; Defence Material Organisation: Hague, The Netherlands, 2013.
19. Department of Defence. *Incident Capture*; Department of Defence: Canberra, Australia, 2011.
20. Australian Safety and Compensation Council. *Type of Occurrence Classification System*; Australian Safety and Compensation Council: Canberra, Australia, 2008.
21. Jennings, B.M.; Yoder, L.H.; Heiner, S.L.; Loan, L.A.; Bingham, M.O. Soldiers with musculoskeletal injuries. *J. Nurs Scholarsh.* **2008**, *40*, 268–274. [CrossRef] [PubMed]

22. Hill, O.T.; Bulathsinhala, L.; Scofield, D.E.; Haley, T.F.; Bernasek, T.L. Risk factors for soft tissue knee injuries in active duty U. S. Army soldiers, 2000–2005. *Mil. Med.* **2013**, *178*, 676. [CrossRef] [PubMed]
23. Orr, R.; Knapik, J.J.; Pope, R. A physical training framework for reserve personnel: A rationalisation and recommendations. *Strength Cond. J.* **2016**, *28*, 36–41. [CrossRef]
24. Orr, R.M.; Pope, R.R. Load carriage: An integrated risk management approach. *J. Strength Cond. Res.* **2015**, *29* (Suppl. 11), S119. [CrossRef]
25. Orr, R.; Pope, R.; Johnston, V.; Coyle, J. Operational loads carried by Australian soldiers on military operations. *J. Health Saf. Environ.* **2015**, *31*, 451–457.
26. Knapik, J.; Reynolds, K.; Staab, J.; Vogel, J.A.; Jones, B. Injuries associated with strenuous road marching. *Mil. Med.* **1992**, *157*, 64. [CrossRef] [PubMed]
27. Knapik, J.J.; Johnson, R.F.; Ang, P.; Meiselman, H.; Bensel, C.K.; Johnson, W. Road march performance of special operations soldiers carrying various loads and load distributions. T14-93. In *Military Performance Division*; U.S. Army Research Institute of Environmental Medicine: Natick, MA, USA, 1993; p. 136.
28. Orr, R.; Pope, R.; Johnston, V.; Coyle, J. Load carriage: Minimising soldier injuries through physical conditioning-a narrative review. *J. Mil. Veteran's Health* **2010**, *18*, 31–38.
29. Knapik, J.J.; Harman, E.A.; Steelman, R.A.; Graham, B.S. A systematic review of the effects of physical training on load carriage performance. *J. Strength Cond. Res.* **2012**, *26*, 585–597. [CrossRef] [PubMed]
30. Prigg, S.K.; Jones, D.D.; Kolonel, L.N.; Warfe, P.; Colgrave, N. Developing injury prevention strategies for the Australian defence force. *J. Mil. Veteran's Health* **2000**, *19*.
31. Waddington, G.; Seward, H.; Wrigley, T.; Lacey, N.; Adams, R. Comparing wobble board and jump-landing training effects on knee and ankle movement discrimination. *J. Sci. Med. Sport* **2000**, *3*, 449–459. [CrossRef]
32. Silva, P.B.; Oliveira, A.S.; Mrachacz-Kersting, N.; Kersting, U.G. Effects of wobble board training on single-leg landing neuromechanics. *Scand. J. Med. Sci. Sports* **2018**, *28*, 972–982. [CrossRef] [PubMed]
33. McKay, G.D.; Goldie, P.A.; Payne, W.R.; Oakes, B.W. Ankle injuries in basketball: Injury rate and risk factors. *BJSM* **2001**, *35*, 103. [CrossRef] [PubMed]
34. Kollock, R.O.; Andrews, C.; Johnston, A.; Elliott, T.; Wilson, A.E.; Games, K.E.; Sefton, J.M. A meta-analysis to determine if lower extremity muscle strengthening should be included in military knee-overuse injury-prevention programs. *J. Athl.Train.* **2016**. [CrossRef] [PubMed]
35. Ferber, R.; Bolgla, L.; Earl-Boehm, J.E.; Emery, C.; Hamstra-Wright, K. Strengthening of the hip and core versus knee muscles for the treatment of patellofemoral pain: A multicenter randomized controlled trial. *J. Athl. Train.* **2015**, *50*, 366. [CrossRef] [PubMed]
36. Ross, J. A review of lower limb overuse injuries during basic military training. Part 1: Types of overuse injuries. *Mil. Med.* **1993**, *158*, 410–415. [CrossRef] [PubMed]
37. Goodall, R.L.; Pope, R.P.; Coyle, J.A.; Neumayer, R. Balance and agility training does not always decrease lower limb injury risks: A cluster-randomised controlled trial. *Int. J. Inj. Contr. Saf. Promot.* **2013**, *20*, 271–281. [CrossRef]

International Journal of
Environmental Research and Public Health

MDPI

Article

Occupational Diseases among Workers in Lower and Higher Socioeconomic Positions

Henk F. van der Molen *, Sanne de Vries and Judith K. Sluiter †

Amsterdam UMC, Coronel Institute of Occupational Health, Netherlands Center for Occupational Diseases, Amsterdam Public Health research institute, PO Box 22660, 1100 DD Amsterdam, The Netherlands; s.de.vries@scp.nl (S.d.V.); coronel@amc.nl (J.K.S.)

* Correspondence: h.f.vandermolen@amc.nl, Tel.: +312-0566-7857

† Dr. Judith K. Sluiter passed away last year.

Received: 13 November 2018; Accepted: 12 December 2018; Published: 13 December 2018

Abstract: *Background:* To determine differences between workers in lower and higher socioeconomic positions (SEP) in incidences of occupational disease (OD) and incapacity for work due to ODs. *Methods:* From a Dutch dynamic prospective cohort of occupational physicians (OPs), ODs assessed by OPs were retrieved for lower and higher SEP groups. *Results:* Among the lower SEP, musculoskeletal disorders, and noise-induced hearing loss (NIHL) comprised two-thirds of the OD diagnoses. Among the higher SEP, stress/burnout comprised 60% of the OD diagnoses. Temporary and permanent incapacity for work due to work-related lower back disorders and repetitive strain injuries differed significantly between workers in lower compared to higher SEP. *Conclusions:* Occupational diseases occur at a 2.7 higher incidence rate for workers in lower SEP compared with higher SEP. Incapacity for work varies between the type of OD and the level of SEP.

Keywords: occupational disease; socioeconomic position; incapacity for work

1. Introduction

Maintaining the health of workers in lower socioeconomic positions (SEP) is an increasing cause for concern [1,2]. In higher SEP jobs, however, task demands can also exceed individual capacities, as shown in a recent European overview regarding the effect of work on mental health [3]. Due to demographic changes, the age of workers is increasing, resulting in more frequent morbidity or, comorbidity, sickness absence [4], lower physical capacities, and higher cumulative work exposures. These changes increase the risk of work-related diseases [5,6].

Socioeconomic status as a determinant of health has been recognized widely and analysed as a composition of various underlying aspects such as education, income and social position [7]. Occupation is one dimension of socioeconomic status, and the weighing of occupations on education and income by job title [8] could reflect SEP. Job complexity could also be an indicator of SEP, with managerial and intellectually complex jobs at the higher end of SEP, and manual, less complex jobs at the lower end of SEP [9]. Ultimately, lower and higher SEP will reflect the distinction between blue and white-collar workers, with different task demands and working circumstances.

Registries of occupational diseases (ODs) can provide insight into job title, work-related diseases and incapacity for work. ODs are relevant outcomes, because they are clinically established diseases mainly caused by work [10,11]. In the Netherlands, OPs are obliged to report ODs to the Netherlands Center for Occupational Diseases (NCOD). In contrast to most other countries, there is no financial compensation system for diagnosed ODs in the Netherlands [12]. An OD is defined as a disease for which the work-related fraction is >50%. Each worker diagnosed with an OD is anonymously reported to the NCOD, with the following information recorded in its database: disease or pathology with clinical diagnosis, demographic characteristics, exposure, job title, economic sector, and incapacity for work [12].

It is hypothesized that workers in lower and higher SEP still differ in health disparities from an occupational perspective, with a higher burden of work-related diseases for lower SEP. The objective of this study is to determine differences between workers in lower and higher SEP occupational groups in (i) incidence and type of occupational disease and (ii) incapacity for work as a consequence of an occupational disease.

2. Methods

From a dynamic prospective cohort of occupational physicians (OPs), all ODs diagnosed by the OPs and reported to the Netherlands Centre for Occupational Diseases (NCOD) over a seven-year period (2010–2016) were retrieved for workers with lower and higher SEP. Elementary occupations and machine operating and assembly jobs (ISCO-08 groups 81–83, 91–96) were defined as lower SEP. Managerial and professional intellectual jobs (ISCO-08 groups 11–14, 21–26) were defined as higher SEP. The population size for the higher and lower SEP was retrieved from the database of Eurostat [13], consisting of 1,090,700 workers for the lower SEP and 2,642,00 workers for the higher SEP in 2016. During the period of 2010–2016, the annual populations varied between 1,002,400 and 1,207,000 workers for the lower SEP and between 2,478,800 and 2,642,000 workers for the higher SEP group.

An OD was defined as a clinically diagnosed disease (ICD-10 classification) that was predominantly caused by work-related factors [12]. Incidences were determined for all ODs and seven frequently occurring groups of ICD diagnosis, which were the following: noise-induced hearing loss (NIHL): H833, H919; non-specific low back pain: M545; repetitive strain injuries of the upper extremity: G560, G589, I730, M189, M199 (partly), M531, M700, M709 (partly), M770, M771; arthrosis of the knee and hip: M169, and M179; burnout/stress: Z730, F432; contact dermatitis: L239, L249, and L259; asthma/COPD: J439, J449, J450, J451, J458, J459, and J689.

Incidence of OD with incapacity for work was determined for the seven frequently occurring ODs. Trends in incidence were estimated using a multilevel negative binomial regression model. Annual incidence was determined by dividing the number of reported ODs in 2016 by the total working population. Differences in incapacity for work between lower and higher SEP were determined through chi-squared tests (IBM SPSS 24, IBM, Armonk, NY, USA). Trends in incidence rates were analysed with multilevel binomial regression analysis [14]. Case counts were analysed using a negative binomial regression model with 2010 as the reference year. Population estimates, as natural logarithms of the annual number of workers, were included in the regression model as an "offset". No report of a specific OD diagnosis was assumed to indicate a report of zero cases for that year. Trend analyses were performed with Stata 15.1 (StataCorp LLC, Texas, TX, USA).

3. Results

In total, 1233 OPs reported 13,917 ODs for workers in lower and higher SEP during the period of 2010–2016 (see Table 1). Lower SEP consisted of 8145 workers (82% male), of which 82% were aged over 40 years. Higher SEP consisted of 5772 workers (59% male), of which 71% were aged over 40 years.

Among the lower SEP, musculoskeletal disorders (37%) and NIHL (32%) comprised two-thirds of the OD diagnoses, with decreasing trends for non-specific low back pain (−12%; 95% CI: −18% to −6%) and NIHL (−7%; 95% CI: −11% to −3%). Among the higher SEP, stress/burnout comprised 60% of the OD diagnoses, with an increasing trend (6%; 95% CI: 3%–8%).

Incapacity for work varied between OD and SEP. It was rarely reported for NIHL (2%–3%), with no significant differences ($p = 0.177$) between SEP. Highest (temporary) incapacity for work was reported for stress/burnout (94%), with no significant differences ($p = 0.382$) between SEP. Occupational contact dermatitis, COPD and asthma, and knee and hip arthrosis showed the highest risks for permanent incapacity for work, varying from 13% to 32%, but no significant differences between SEP ($p > 0.50$). Incapacity for work due to work-related lower back disorders (69% vs. 9%) and repetitive strain injuries (89% vs. 47%) differed significantly ($p = 0.000$) between lower and higher SEP.

In 2016, 54 per 100,000 workers in Dutch elementary occupations, machine operating and assembly jobs, and managerial and professional jobs had an OD diagnosed, of which 98 per 100,000 workers were from lower SEP and 36 per 100,000 workers were from higher SEP.

Table 1. Occupational diseases and incapacity for work among workers in lower and higher socioeconomic positions (SEP).

International Classification of Diseases—10	N 2010–2016	Incidence per 100,000 2016	2010–2016		Incapacity for Work 2010–2016	
	Occupational Diseases		IRR *	95% CI	Temporary%	Permanent %
Total						
Lower SEP	8145	98	0.95	0.94–0.97		
Higher SEP	5772	36	1.03	1.01–1.05		
Noise Induced Hearing Loss						
Lower SEP	2599	23	**0.93**	**0.89–0.97**	0.8%	2%
Higher SEP	830	3	0.99	0.93–1.05	0.2%	2%
Non-specific Low Back Pain						
Lower SEP	635	6	**0.88**	**0.82–0.94**	**64%**	5%
Higher SEP	131	0.5	0.92	0.80–1.04	**7%**	**2%**
Arthrosis Knee/Hip						
Lower SEP	157	2	0.97	0.88–1.07	40%	27%
Higher SEP	19	0.1	0.97	0.71–1.22	32%	21%
Repetitive Strain Injury						
Lower SEP	2192	31	1.00	0.97–1.03	**83%**	6%
Higher SEP	339	2	0.95	0.89–1.02	**45%**	2%
Stress/Burnout						
Lower SEP	463	8	1.00	0.95–1.06	91%	3%
Higher SEP	3439	25	**1.06**	**1.03–1.08**	92%	2%
Contact Dermatitis						
Lower SEP	193	2	1.01	0.94–1.09	46%	13%
Higher SEP	28	0.1	1.09	0.88–1.29	36%	18%
COPD/Asthma						
Lower SEP	54	0.5	0.93	0.79–1.07	44%	32%
Higher SEP	20	-	0.84	0.60–1.07	40%	30%

* IRR = Incidence Rate Ratio (reference year 2010). Bold means $p < 0.05$.

4. Discussion

Occupational diseases occurred at a 2.7 higher incidence rate for workers in lower SEP compared with higher SEP in 2016. Among the workers in a lower SEP, musculoskeletal disorders and noise-induced hearing loss were the most frequently occurring ODs, with trends decreasing over a seven-year period. Among the workers in a higher SEP, stress/burnout was the most frequently occurring OD, with an increasing trend over a seven-year period. The highest temporary incapacity for work was reported for work-related stress/burnout, with no differences between SEP. Work-related knee and hip arthrosis, as well as dermal and lung diseases showed the highest risks for permanent incapacity for work, both in lower and higher SEP. Temporary and permanent incapacity for work due to work-related musculoskeletal disorders were higher in lower SEP workers compared with higher SEP workers.

Misclassification, selection bias, and uncertainty about missing values are methodological limitations in this study. Misclassification in SEP due to job title by ISCO-08 codes is possible, but considered to be non-differential. Selection bias may have been introduced due to differences in entrance to OPs; however, most employed workers visit their OPs when incapacity for work occurs or as a result of worker health monitoring, irrespective of SEP. Furthermore, the reporting of ODs may differ between SEP, e.g., OPs are more familiar with work-related musculoskeletal disorders, which may cause selection bias. Since many ODs emerge after cumulative exposures over time, the incidence of OD may depend on age; however, in our study no large differences in age between lower and higher SEP were found at the time of the assessed ODs. Uncertainty about missing values in regression analyses may have a large impact on the estimates of trends in OD incidence. To counteract this, we modified our methods to input zero reports only when an OP demonstrated being active in a specific year, thus assuming true zero reports [15]. The data in this paper were collected from the Dutch national registry. In future research, OD incidence and incapacity for work between lower and higher SEP could be enriched if SEP at an individual level also encompasses educational and income level.

Occupational diseases occur in both higher and lower SEP, although they differ in incidence, type of OD, and consequences for work capacity. Our results suggest that among lower SEP, hazardous workplaces and adverse work practices are still present, with known biomechanical, physical, and chemical risks factors still to be eliminated. In higher SEP requiring managerial and intellectual tasks, psychosocial demands seem to present the largest risk factors for mental disorders, accompanied by a temporary incapacity for work. Temporary and permanent incapacity for work due to work-related musculoskeletal disorders are higher for lower SEP compared with higher SEP, suggesting fewer opportunities to modify work tasks and working circumstances for lower SEP jobs. These findings are in line with evidence that work indeed explains socioeconomic inequalities in self-rated health among workers besides lifestyle factors [16], while differences in incidences of the specific ODs reflect the prevalence of risk factors in the lower SEP (e.g., noise levels [17] and biomechanical risk factors [18] and higher SEP (psychosocial risk factors [19]).

The understanding of whether SEP influences the possibility to stay in work with an OD is of considerable interest. Although adverse health conditions due to work hamper sustainable work ability, especially in lower SEP [20], higher SEP is at risk for especially work-related stress disorders. The frequently reported ODs among the Dutch working population revealed population attributable fractions varying between 3% and 25%, leaving considerable potential for taking preventive actions on work-related exposure in terms of the occurrence of ODs and their medical and productivity cost [21].

5. Conclusions

Occupational diseases occur at a 2.7 higher incidence rate for workers in lower SEP compared with higher SEP. Occupational diseases differ in incidence, type, and resulting incapacity for work between workers in higher and lower SEP. Among the workers in a lower SEP, musculoskeletal disorders and noise-induced hearing loss were the most frequently occurring ODs, with trends decreasing over a seven-year period. Among the workers in a higher SEP, stress/burnout was the most frequently occurring OD, with an increasing trend over a seven-year period. This provides further insight into disparities between workers in different socioeconomic positions in terms of their capacity to counteract negative consequences due to work.

Author Contributions: Conceptualization, H.F.v.d.M.; Data curation, S.d.V.; Formal analysis, H.F.v.d.M.; Writing—original draft, H.F.v.d.M.; Writing—review and editing, S.d.V. and J.K.S.

Patient Consent: Not applicable for this report/study.

Funding: This work was supported by the Dutch Ministry of Social Affairs and Employment (grant project number 21082).

Conflicts of Interest: The authors declare that they have no competing interests.

References

1. Schuring, M.; Robroek, S.J.W.; Otten, F.W.J.; Arts, C.H.; Burdorf, A. The effect of ill health and socioeconomic status on labor force exit and re-employment: A prospective study with ten years follow-up in the Netherlands. *Scand. J. Work Environ. Health* **2013**, *39*, 134–143. [CrossRef] [PubMed]
2. Schaap, R.; de Wind, A.; Coenen, P.; Proper, K.; Boot, C. The effects of exit from work on health across different socioeconomic groups: A systematic literature review. *Soc. Sci. Med.* **2017**, *198*, 36–45. [CrossRef] [PubMed]
3. Lastovkova, A.; Cardner, M.; Rasmussen, H.M.; Sjoberg, L.; de Groene, G.J.; Sauni, R.; Vevoda, J.; Vevodova, S.; Lasfargues, G.; Svartengren, M.; et al. Industrial Health Burnout syndrome as an occupational disease in the European Union: An exploratory study. *Ind. Health* **2017**. [CrossRef]
4. De Vroome, E.M.M.; Uegaki, K.; Ploeg, C.P.B. Burden of Sickness Absence Due to Chronic Disease in the Dutch Workforce from 2007 to 2011. *J. Occup. Rehabil.* **2015**, *25*, 675–684. [CrossRef] [PubMed]
5. Verbeek, J.; Mischke, C.; Robinson, R.; Ijaz, S.; Kuijer, P.; Kievit, A.; Ojajärvi, A.; Neuvonen, K. Occupational Exposure to Knee Loading and the Risk of Osteoarthritis of the Knee: A Systematic Review and a Dose-Response Meta-Analysis. *Saf. Health Work* **2017**, *8*, 130–142. [CrossRef] [PubMed]
6. Blanc, P.D.; Torén, K. COPD and occupation: Resetting the agenda. *Occup. Environ. Med.* **2016**, *73*, 357–358. [CrossRef]
7. American Psychological Association, Task Force on Socioeconomic Status. *Report of the APA Task Force on Socioeconomic Status*; American Psychological Association: Washington, DC, USA, 2007.
8. Maden, M.; Cunliffe, A.; McMahon, N. Use of programme theory to understand the differential effects of interventions across socio-economic groups in systematic reviews-a systematic methodology review. *Syst. Rev.* **2017**, *6*, 266. [CrossRef] [PubMed]
9. Fujishiro, K. Job Complexity, Race, and Socioeconomic Status: Examining Health Disparities from an Occupational Perspective. Available online: https://blogs.cdc.gov/niosh-science-blog/2017/10/05/job-complexity/ (accessed on 29 January 2018).
10. Bakusic, J.; Lenderink, A.; Lambreghts, C.; Vandenbroeck, S.; Verbeek, J.; Curti, S.; Mattioli, S.; Godderis, L. Methodologies to Identify Work-Related Diseases: Review of Sentinel and Alert Approaches. European Risk Observatory: Literature Review. Available online: https://limo.libis.be/primo-explore/fulldisplay?docid=LIRIAS1781378&context=L&vid=Lirias&search_scope=Lirias&tab=default_tab&lang=en_US&fromSitemap=1 (accessed on 29 January 2018).
11. Carder, M.; Hussey, L.; Money, A. The Health and Occupation Research Network: An Evolving Surveillance System. *Saf. Health Work* **2017**, *8*, 231–236. [CrossRef] [PubMed]
12. Van der Molen, H.F.; Kuijer, P.P.F.M.; Smits, P.B.A.; Schop, A.; Moeijes, F.; Spreeuwers, D.; Frings-Dresen, M.H.W. Annual incidence of occupational diseases in economic sectors in the Netherlands. *Occup. Environ. Med.* **2012**, *69*, 519–521. [CrossRef] [PubMed]
13. Eurostat. Available online: http://appsso.eurostat.ec.europa.eu/nui/show.do? (accessed on 29 January 2018).
14. Stocks, S.J.; McNamee, R.; van der Molen, H.F.; Paris, C.; Urban, P.; Campo, G.; Sauni, R.; Jarreta, B.M.; Valenty, M.; Godderis, L.; et al. Trends in incidence of occupational asthma, contact dermatitis, noise-induced hearing loss, carpal tunnel syndrome and upper limb musculoskeletal disorders in European countries from 2000 to 2012. *Occup. Environ. Med.* **2015**, *72*, 294–303. [CrossRef] [PubMed]
15. Van der Molen, H.F.; de Vries, S.C.; Stocks, S.J.; Warning, J.; Frings-Dresen, M.H.W. Incidence rates of occupational diseases in the Dutch construction sector, 2010–2014. *Occup. Environ. Med.* **2016**, *73*, 350–352. [CrossRef] [PubMed]
16. Dieker, A.C.M.; IJzelenberg, W.; Proper, K.I.; Burdorf, A.; Ket, J.C.F.; van der Beek, A.J.; Hulsegge, G. The contribution of work and lifestyle factors to socioeconomic inequalities in self-rated health—A systematic review. *Scand. J. Work Environ. Health* **2018**. [CrossRef] [PubMed]
17. Sayler, S.K.; Roberts, B.J.; Manning, M.A.; Sun, K.; Neitzel, R.L. Patterns and trends in OSHA occupational noise exposure measurements from 1979 to 2013. *Occup. Environ. Med.* **2018**. [CrossRef] [PubMed]
18. Driscoll, T.; Jacklyn, G.; Orchard, J.; Passmore, E.; Vos, T.; Freedman, G.; Lim, S.; Punnett, L. The global burden of occupationally related low back pain: Estimates from the Global Burden of Disease 2010 study. *Ann. Rheum. Dis.* **2014**, *73*, 975–981. [CrossRef] [PubMed]

19. Müller, G.; Brendel, B.; Freude, G.; Potter, G.; Rose, U.; Burr, H.; Falkenstein, M.; Martus, P. Work-Related determinants of burnout in a nationally representative sample of German employees. Results from the study on mental health at work. *JOEM* **2018**, *60*, 584–588. [PubMed]
20. Knowledge Agenda Prevention. *Dutch National Research Route Healthcare Research, Prevention and Treatment*; Nederlandse Federatie van Universitair Medische Centra (NFU) en ZonMw: Utrecht, The Netherlands, 2018.
21. Van der Molen, H.F.; Hulshof, C.T.J.; Kuijer, P.P.F.M. How to improve the assessment of the impact of occupational diseases at a national level? The Netherlands as an example. *Occup. Environ. Med.* **2018**. [CrossRef] [PubMed]

International Journal of
Environmental Research and Public Health

MDPI

Article

Executive Stress Management: Physiological Load of Stress and Recovery in Executives on Workdays

Beatriz Crespo-Ruiz [1,2,*], Shai Rivas-Galan [2], Cristina Fernandez-Vega [2], Carmen Crespo-Ruiz [2] and Luis Maicas-Perez [1]

1. Physical Activity and Sport Education Department, Faculty of Sport Sciences of Toledo at University of Castilla-La Mancha, 45002 Toledo, Spain; info@luismaicas.com
2. Freedom & Flow SL, 28050 Madrid, Spain; shai.rivas@freedomandflowcompany.com (S.R.-G.); Cristina.fernandez@freedomandflowcompany.com (C.F.-V.); carmen.crespo@freedomandflowcompany.com (C.C.-R.)

* Correspondence: beatriz.crespo@uclm.es; Tel.: +34-617-415-113

Received: 8 October 2018; Accepted: 2 December 2018; Published: 13 December 2018

Abstract: *Objective*: The use of high-performance sports technology to describe the physiological load of stress and the quality of recovery in a population of executives during the workday. *Methodology*: Heart rate variability values were recorded during 48 h from which the relationship between stress/recovery quality (stress balance) was obtained for three differentiated time slots: work, after work, and night in a workday. *Results*: We observed a negative stress balance during the 24 h of measurement in the course of a workday, being negative at work and after work, and positive at night. The stress generated or maintained outside working hours correlates significantly with a lower quality of recovery during the 24 h workday. *Conclusions*: It is necessary to prioritize strategies that help improve stress management in executives through the improvement of tools and strategies that mainly promote greater relaxation outside working hours.

Keywords: stress; stress management; human resources; executives; physiology; health; technology; business

---

1. Introduction

Stress is defined as the physical and mental responses of the body and adaptations to real and perceived changes and challenges in life. Stress is, for many, considered as the silent disease of the 21st century. However, it was not officially classified as a disorder or alteration to take into account differently to anxiety until the 5th edition of the Diagnostic and Statistical Manual of Mental Disorders (DSM) by the American Psychiatric Association published on 1 October 2016.

Nowadays society faces the great challenge of adapting to a continuous rate of change, connected to a large number of internal and external stimuli that, poorly managed, can become important daily stress triggers, with the physical and mental consequences that all of this involves in and out of working time. To this effect, there are several challenges that companies and governments must face when it comes to promoting health and well-being. Actually the increase of pathologies, such as stress, anxiety, and/or depression, have led to financial losses up to €136 million in companies reaching percentages of more than 75% of workers in the European Union who suffer daily stress being already more than 20% the working age population that suffer serious health problems, such as the chronic stress syndrome known as burnout [1].

In this sense, and due to the multifactorial nature of stress, other factors such as poor rest, physical inactivity, overweight, and obesity are increasingly present in today's companies, aggravating and increasing the risk of suffering cardiovascular diseases, immunological, as well as chronic diseases susceptible to reduce the quality of life of the individual [2–4], which affects not only at an individual level, but also at social and professional levels [5]. In this regard, and according to data from the European Heart Network, Spain is in the top ten European countries with a more sedentary lifestyle among adults; 42% of those over 18 say they do not do any physical activity during the week, against 6% in Sweden or 7% in Finland. In addition, data from the European Foundation for improving living and working conditions confirm that Spaniards spend an average of 1720 h a year at work [6].

Among the factors that currently have the greatest potential to become stressors, understood as stress triggering situations, could be any direct or indirect, external or internal stimulus (physical, chemical, acoustic or somatic, or sociocultural), that favors a disruption in the dynamic equilibrium of the organism (homeostasis) we can find environmental factors (work, family, work meetings, corporate culture, climate, environment, etc.) as those related to lifestyle (level of practice of physical activity, eating habits, and emotional management, among others) [7].

On a psychological level, a recent study detected through univariate and multivariate statistical analysis of the risk prediction score of cardiovascular disease (CVD), and of the general welfare of WHO, that a combination of general risk factors and organizational factors contribute to increase the risk and well-being of CVD, with a direct and inversely proportional relationship between work stress and the welfare index [8]. In addition, a study carried out with a sample of 2991 German and Chinese students where a lifestyle for positive mental health (PMH) and mental health problems (MHP) was analyzed through the Positive Mental Health Scale and a version of 21 items on the scale of anxiety, depression, and stress, obtained as results the importance of following a healthy lifestyle to improve psychological well-being and develop fewer mental health problems. Factors such as BMI, frequency of physical and mental activities, frequency of alcohol consumption, smoking, vegetarian diet and the irregularity of social rhythm were considered in this study to consider the lifestyle of the subjects [9].

Physiologically, the exposure to one or several stressors' stimuli triggers the response of the sympathetic nervous system (SNS), activating the hypothalamic pituitary adrenal axis in charge of releasing the hormone corticotropin (ACTH) that acts directly on the pituitary gland to secrete adrenocorticotropin, thereby increasing the levels of cortisol, cortisone, epinephrine, and norepinephrine into the blood. This chain reaction provoked by a stressor stimulus is responsible for increasing the levels of brain and blood glucose, heart rate (HR), and blood pressure, among others (Figure 1) [9].

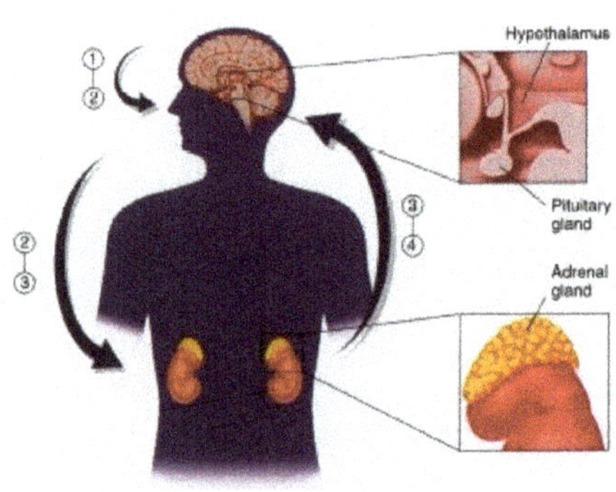

Figure 1. Neuroscience applied to stress control.

It is important to comprehend the physiological process that triggers stress to better understand the type of strategies that will be necessary to be implemented in stress management. Additionally, the response of our body to various stressors corresponds to a "mechanism of escape" whose magnitude of enrollment; both neuroendocrine and physiological depend on the duration and specific needs of the body. Its implementation not only involves a high energy expenditure, but also the release of hormones and substances that generate an over-excitation of the nervous system, which, maintained over time, can lead to an intensification in cellular aging, oxidative stress, inflammation of tissues, and cardiometabolic problems, among others [10].

To know the levels of stress in the body from a physiological point of view there are two non-invasive methodologies: the measurement of cortisol levels through saliva [11] and the recording of heart rate variability (HRV) understood as the variation between two consecutive beats: the greater the variation, the greater the parasympathetic activity [12] through devices recording the HR.

Studying the heart by HRV (Figure 2) provides us with a vast amount of information about our body. From beat to beat, heart rate is constantly changing to meet the needs of life. HRV means the variation in time between consecutive heartbeats. It is universally accepted as a non-invasive marker of autonomic nervous system (ANS) activity. A variety of physiological phenomena affect HRV, including:

- Inhalation and exhalation, control of breathing
- ANS adjustments
- Hormonal reactions
- Metabolic processes and energy expenditure
- Physical activity, exercise, and recovery from physical activity
- Movements and changes in posture
- Cognitive processes and mental load
- Stress reactions, relaxation, and emotional reactions

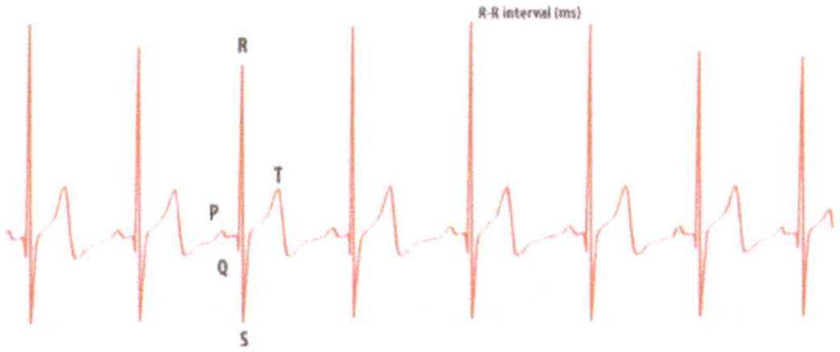

Figure 2. HRV means the variation in time between consecutive heartbeats.

Heart rate variability increases during relaxing and recovering activities and decreases during stress. Accordingly, HRV is typically higher when the heart is beating slowly and decreases as the heart beats more quickly. In other words, heart rate and HRV have a generally inverse relationship. Also, HRV changes from day to day based on activity levels and amount of work-related stress. In addition to these external stress factors, internal stress factors cause variation daily HRV levels. Internal stress factors include poor nutrition, alcohol use, illness, etc.

The principle of the method is to utilize HRV and HR reactions as a tool for analyzing autonomic nervous system activity in order to build a digital model of human physiology for recognizing different bodily states.

The human nervous system consists of central nervous system and peripheral nervous system. The latter has two major divisions, the voluntary and the autonomic systems. The voluntary nervous system is concerned mainly with movement and sensation. The ANS mainly controls functions over which we have less conscious control. These include for example the cardiovascular system, whose regulation is fast and involuntary.

The ANS is divided into sympathetic and parasympathetic nervous systems (Figure 3). Sympathetic and parasympathetic nerve cords start from the central nervous system and lead to different target organs all around the human body. Sympathetic and parasympathetic divisions typically function simultaneously in opposition to each other. The parasympathetic division is primarily involved in relaxation, helping the body to rest and recover. The sympathetic division prepares the body to fight by accelerating bodily functions, and is also associated with stress.

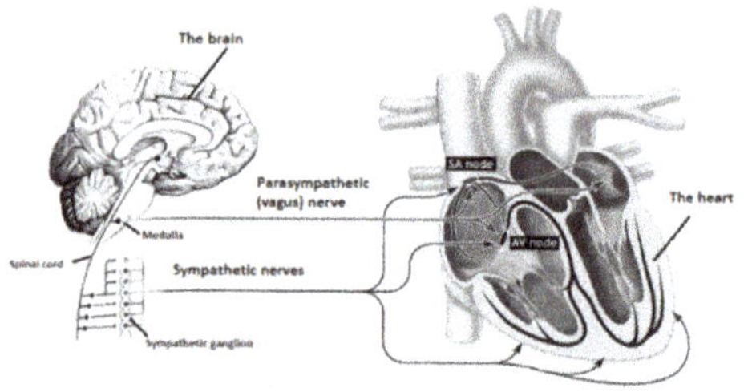

Figure 3. Autonomic nervous system controls different target organs via parasympathetic and sympathetic nerve cords. The parasympathetic nerve controlling the hearts is called the vagus nerve.

With stress reactions, the human body tries to cope with the demands of the surrounding environment. Positive stress gives energy "to get the job done". Negative stress causes negative emotions and reactions. Physiologically, the response to positive and negative stress is similar. As a result of the stress reaction, the ANS is activated and stress hormone production starts along with an increased rate and force of contraction of the heart [13]. The magnitude of the neuro-endocrine response reflects the metabolic and physiological demands required for the behavioral activity [14].

Therefore, although there is an ongoing debate of the exact definition of stress in the scientific literature, stress can be physiologically characterized by reduced recovery of the neuroendocrine reaction [14] and sympathetic dominance of the ANS function, whereas recovery is characterized as parasympathetic dominance.

In this study we will focus on HRV as an objective indicator to know the reactions to stress during the workday, as well as the quality of recovery of the nervous system (NS) during work, outside of work and at night. Its validity has been proven in several studies, both in the sports field with a focus on the study of high-performance training and in the workplace that concerns us [15–19]. In addition, a recent review of the literature on physiological biomarkers related to the study of stress in the workplace, concluded that the correlation between cortisol and work stress are less clear than those found with HRV [20].

In particular, the number of studies in which HRV has been used has been increasing in recent years. The most relevant findings show how acute stress correlates with a decrease in HRV during sleep [21] and during the day [22], finding a strong relationship between the decrease in HRV and work stress [5,12,18,23,24].

In order that the measurements made are accurate in a different environment to sports or medicine, much more accustomed to monitoring, it is necessary to take into account the technology to be implemented according to the characteristics of the population to be studied. Currently, there are several easy-to-use, mobile heart rate monitors that keep data of the intervals between beats (RR intervals) during the workday. Scientists to analyze HRV in sports science, medicine, and other fields of research have used commercial devices, such as heart rate monitors and activity clocks [25]. Recent studies have validated the HR recording devices in relation to different electrocardiogram systems with results that offer high reliability in the registration of RR interval series for the analysis of HRV similar to those offered by electrocardiography (ECG) equipment [26].

Among the new technologies applied in the workplace for HRV monitoring, we find the Body Guard 2 device of the Firstbeat® philanthropy as one of the best options at the scientific level [15–20], since it also provides information about the quality of recovery of the records obtained.

In this sense, the quality of recovery is one of the key variables to take into account in stress management and not only the level of daily reaction to it. It should also be noted that the quality of recovery in the executive sector not only gives the duration and quality of sleep. The characteristics of the executive profile make it necessary to acquire personalized strategies that can help them to combat stress during the workday, outside the working day, and during the night, independently of the areas and activities that they have assigned and the variability of them. To this effect, studies indicate that

HRV has been used to monitor the effort and recovery in sports such as judo or basketball [27,28], as well as after performing submaximal exercise [29]. However, there are few studies that analyze our target population specifically during the night to assess the quality of recovery; although there are studies carried out with Finnish workers (n = 16.275) that correlate a practice of high physical activity with lower percentages of stress during workdays and during one's work, as well as a balance of stress. Also positively related to a lower BMI with better recovery during sleep [30], the correct design of healthy strategies within the workplace, sustainable over time, could help the quality of recovery of workers within and out of work.

For everything described above, the aim of this study has been to describe the physiological burden of stress and the quality of recovery in a population of senior managers during the workday analyzed during three different time zones: work, after work, and night.

As a secondary objective, we mark the relocation of the use of high-performance technology for the objectification of parameters related to health management and stress in executive positions of high responsibility in a business environment.

Our hypothesis is that the physiological load derived from a low-quality recovery during the 24 h working day negatively influences the increase in the physiological load that results from stress in the manager in the medium-long term.

2. Materials and Methods

2.1. Participants

The study was carried out with a total of 48 subjects (n = 48). Of this total, 28 were men and 20 were women. All of them are senior managers of multinational companies based in Spain with high categories of responsibility during the working day. The sample had an age of 45.92 ± 6.97 years, height of 1.72 ± 0.09 m, weight of 76.04 ± 13.57 kg, and BMI of 25.54 ± 3.39.

The sample analyzed was of Caucasian race with a medium-high socioeconomic status and payroll above the Spanish average (1636 €/month). In addition, during the period of analysis, the sample did not express situations of stress beyond normal to the researcher group, so that the records were made in situations of habitual stress to them, performing their daily tasks during the HRV registry.

All subjects were healthy subjects who had not suffered any type of cardiovascular or nervous system disease/disorder. The exclusion criteria for participation in the RR interval recordings included severe heart disease, very high blood pressure (≥180/100 mmHg), type 1 or 2 diabetes with autonomic neuropathy, severe neurological disease, fever or other acute illnesses, and a BMI > 40 kg/m^2. These exclusion criteria represented by the manufacturer of the analysis software are presented in detail [31]. In all cases, acceptance and voluntary and informed signing of participation in the study was indispensable.

We certify that during the course of our investigation all the regulations marked on the ethical use of human volunteers marked in the Declaration of Helsinki were followed. In addition, the personnel in charge of collecting the data of the subjects included in the study did not include in the study data that could accurately identify the worker in accordance with the requirements of the General Data Protection Regulations (RGPD) (UE) 2016/679.

2.2. Material

The non-invasive device Firstbeat Bodyguard (Firstbeat Technologies Ltd., Jyväskylä, Finland) (Figure 4) was used to register the HRV. The data was recorded using Firstbeat Analysis Server software (version 6.3, Firstbeat Technologies Ltd.), which includes the artifact detection and correction function for irregular ectopic beats and signal noise. Its subsequent use was carried out with the exportation of the same to the software excel (version 15—year 2013) for the analysis of the individualized form of the relationship between stress and recovery (stress balance) in the different studied ranges: work, after work, and night, as well as the treatment of the different variables analyzed. All statistical analysis was performed with SPSS V.23. (SPSS Inc., Chicago, IL, USA) for Windows.

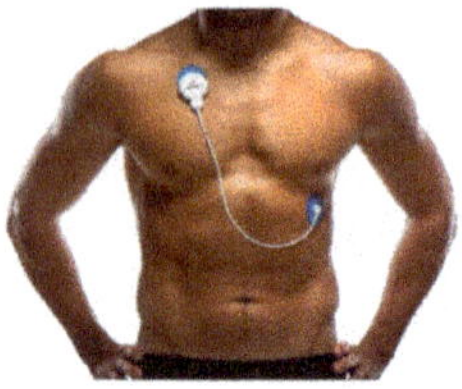

Figure 4. Firsbeat Bodyguard 2. Firstbeat Technologies Ltd.

The device is used through two disposable electrodes. The hydrogel electrodes that were used during the data collection in our sample were the model Kendall 530 foam (Meditrace). All participants were given the device and six additional electrodes so that they could exchange them when showering, since the device cannot get wet.

2.3. Protocol

The measurement data was interpreted following the Healthy Box® methodology for specialized research in companies (Freedom and Flow Company, Madrid, Spain). For the analysis of the data we took into account data such as sex, age, height, and weight for the interpretation of the results obtained through FirstBeat®. Ambulatory beat-to-beat R-R intervals were used to determine the amount and intensity of blood pressure (BP), stress, and recovery. The software calculates the HRV indices second by second using the short-time Fourier transform method and calculates the variables derived from HR and HRV of the respiration rate, oxygen consumption, on/off kinetics (increase or decrease of HR), and parameters describing the excess post-exercise oxygen consumption using neural networks. Subsequently, the software divides the measurement data into coherent data segments and categorizes these segments into different physiological states, such as physical activities (PA) of different intensities, stress, and recovery [32,33], taking into account the individual characteristics, levels, and scales of HR and HRV, and the individual relationships between HRV and autonomic control [34]. More information of this method of analysis is available in a document from Firstbeat Technologies Ltd [35].

All the participants received the device in hand in their respective offices, the protocol to be followed was explained to them during the next 48 h and they were given access to a diary where they indicated all the activities they would perform during the registration time, including working hours and sleeping time. All the participants had placed the device during 48 working hours with the objective of analyzing 24 full hours of registration, regardless of their lifestyle and working hours. This methodological decision was taken to try to homogenize to the maximum the different working hours that we can find in this studio population, where in some cases, the change of continental time between the different headquarters of the analyzed multinationals had to be taken into account.

2.4. Variables

To calculate the physiological load of stress and recovery we monitor through the Firstbeat® Bodyguard 2 device we measure the HR in beats per minute (PPM), the VFC measured in seconds (seconds), and the analysis of Root Mean Square of the Successive Differences (RMSSD) as is measured in milliseconds (ms) during a workday. From these parameters, the variables analyzed were [33]:

RMSSD: one of the few time domain tools used to evaluate the variability of heart rate. RMSSD searches for the successive difference between the R-R intervals in order to calculate the square of the middle root of the junction of the adjacent R-R intervals and provide an indicator of the vagal cardiac control (parasympathetic tone). Therefore, we can say that it is a parameter that informs us of those variations that occur in a short period between the R-R intervals, obtaining information on how the parasympathetic nervous system (SNP) affects the cardiovascular system. Thanks to the RMSSD we know with little time of measurement if there have been changes, the greater the RMSSD being the greater the parasympathetic activity.

Heart rate increases and, thus, the time between successive RR-intervals gets shorter during inhalation (inspiration) and longer during exhalation (expiration). This fluctuation in the time between the successive RR-intervals is called HRV. Image extracted by Stress and Recovery Analysis Methods based on 24 h heart rate variability, Firstbeat Technologies Ltd. (Figure 5).

- Time stress in 24 h (minutes): time in minutes of an average of 24 h reacting to stress.
- Stress percentage (%) (% Stress): percentage of reaction to stress in an average of 24 h.
- Recovery time in 24 h (minutes): total time, measured in minutes, in which the body is recovering.
- Percentage recovery (%) (% Recovery): percentage of total recovery time in 24 h.

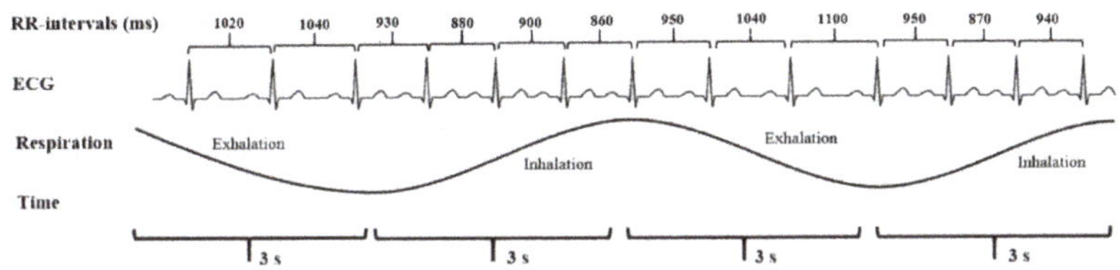

Figure 5. Electrocardiogram (ECG) exhibiting respiratory sinus arrhythmia.

The studies say that in 24 h, an adequate management of stress that impacts healthily in the professional and personal environment would entail between 40–60% of the time spent in activities that suppose a positive stress in the organism, indispensable for the high work performance, complemented with more than 30% of regenerative activities/recovery, which would be equivalent to 432 min of the 1440 min that day. We could summarize it (Figure 6):

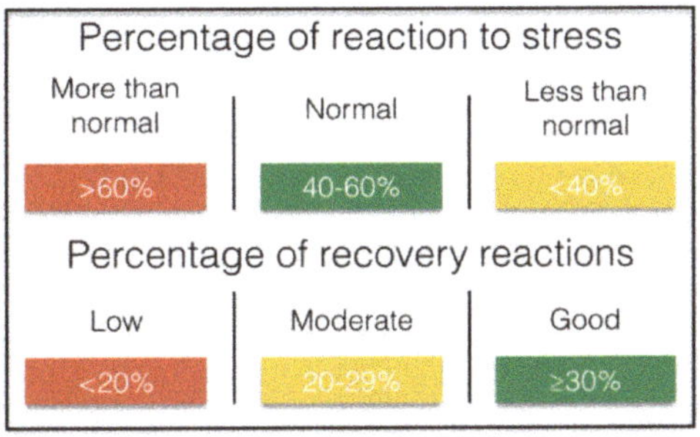

Figure 6. Values expressed in percentage of the impact of stress and recovery on performance.

It is important to note that stress is not always harmful. Stress can be positive or negative. The presence of stress may indicate that the person is experiencing something exciting or joyful. However, high stress indicators over a long period of time negatively impact personal well-being and health. Moderate stress levels during a normal working day are associated with high productivity at work.

Stress Balance: The 24 h stress balance features identify areas of stress in an executive's routine. This variable evaluates the balance between stress and recovery during the day or time slots analyzed, identifying if the body tendency reacts predominantly towards stress or relaxation.

Regular recovery is necessary for physiological systems to overcome the effects of stress. Recovery means reduced activation levels in the body in the absence of internal and external stress factors. During recovery, parasympathetic (vagal) activations dominate the ANS and psychophysiological resources are restored.

The connection between HRV and stress-recovery is commonly recognized. Strong indicators of recovery include individually low HR and high HRV. Night-time recovery rates are a key factor in stress balance.

The Firstbeat software gives us the stress balance value automatically for all the monitored record, this value being between 1 and -1 (values closer to 1 will indicate a correct recovery, while values close to -1 indicate a poor recovery) (Table 1).

Table 1. Stress balance areas.

High Tendency to Stress	Moderate Tendency to Stress	Moderate Tendency to Relaxation	High Tendency to Relaxation
From -1 to -0.5	From -0.49 to 0	From 0.1 to 0.49	From 0.5 to 1

Following the Healthy Box® methodologyy for specialized research in companies (Freedom and Flow Company, Spain) and in order to homogenize the recorded data as much as possible, we decided to divide the day into three strips and analyze the variables in a segmented manner for each of them, protocolizing the analysis and data processing:

- Work: in those cases in which the subject did not indicate an atypical variation of his work schedule, we applied the protocol of the type schedule (09:00 a.m. to 6:00 p.m.), as well as in the subjects who specified us schedule, and we filtered all the minutes worked throughout the 24 h of analysis, even if it was a split day.
- After Work: we consider here all the hours in which you are not working or sleeping, being the standardized hours from 6:00 pm to 11:00 pm, always respecting the specifics of the sample indicated by each subject.
- Night: For the evaluation of the recovery index, the results are highly individualized, since the method is to use a 4 h window that starts 30 min after going to bed, in order to compare the intensity of recovery with the highest measurement of registry.

For the calculation of stress balance, all the moments in which there is no signal or identification by the device, were broken. In this way, we were able to calculate the stress balance in each time slot through the following formula:

$$\text{Stress Balance} = \frac{(\text{Relaxion} + \text{Recovery from exercise}) - \text{“non} - \text{identificable”}}{(\text{Relaxion} + \text{Recovery from exercise}) + \text{“non} - \text{identificable”}}$$

The last of the analyzed data was training effect (TE), which represents the degree of alteration of the homeostasis resulting from a physical activity session (in our case of the 24 h measurement). The effect of training is based mainly on the values of COPD during the exercise, which is extended depending on the physical state or level of activity of the people. The higher the value of TE, the greater the expected increase in maximum performance after the exercise will also be. COPD (and TE) increases when the intensity or duration of exercise increases.

- Training effect describes the effect of the exercise on a scale of 0–1: 0.0–0.9 = no effect; 1.0–1.9 = minor effect; 2.0–2.9 = maintenance effect; 3.0–3.9 = improvement effect; 4.0–4.9 = highly improving effect; 5.0 = temporary overreach effect.

2.5. Statistics Analysis

The data processing was carried out in two general lines:

- Descriptive study of the physiological burden of stress and recovery during a workday in a sample of $n = 48$ executives. All values are shown as mean ± standard deviation (Med ± DS).
- Descriptive study comparative of the physiological load of stress and recovery during a workday between men ($n = 28$) and women ($n = 20$).

All statistical analyses were performed with SPSS® V.23. (SPSS Inc., Chicago, IL, USA) for Windows. All values are shown as mean ± standard deviation (Med ± DS). Due to the size of the sample, less than 50 subjects, the U-Mann Whitney test was carried out to verify the normality of the sample distribution. The level of significance was set at $p < 0.05$. Those variables that followed a normal distribution were applied the Student's T test for independent samples with two-tailed analysis, making the comparison with a confidence interval of 0.95 percent. In case of finding differences, and in order to avoid the type I errors that are made when making multiple comparisons, the Bonferroni post hoc test was performed. For those variables that needed their corresponding analysis of non-parametric type, Friedman's nonparametric test was used. To determine between which intervals differences were obtained, we used the nonparametric test of two Wilcoxon-related samples. The level of significance is set at $p < 0.05$. For the correlation tests, the Pearson or Spearman test was used according to parametric or nonparametric variables.

3. Results

In the descriptive study of the physiological burden of stress and recovery during a workday in a sample of $n = 48$ executives. All values are shown as mean ± standard deviation (Med ± DS).

The general aspects to consider are the reaction time to stress in minutes and percentage with respect to the total of the day. In this sense the reaction to stress can be positive or negative. An optimal average for work performance and health would be to find the percentage of reaction to stress between 40–60% of total hours of the day (9.6 h–14.4 h out of a total of 24 h). On the other hand, the relaxation time corresponds to the periods of time in which the body is recovering/regenerating. Important recovery periods include sleep and rest times during the day. As a reference, we should rest at least 30% (7.2 h) in a 24 h period. The result of the average percentage of time directly related to physiological reactions to stress during a 24 h workday in the group analyzed is 40.96 ± 18.91%, placing them within the values rated as habitual and optimal for performance. On the other hand, the average relaxation time in a 24 h period expressed as a percentage is 24.38 ± 11.45%, being lower than the recommended values (<30%). Significant differences have been found between stress time and relaxation time during the workday, a which mean that in a 24 h workday, stress is more present in the body than relaxation ($p < 0.05$). Below are the results analyzed for each time slot (Table 2).

Table 2. Descriptive analysis of the physiological load and recovery (Med ± SD).

	Relax Time (min)	%Relax Total	Stress Time (min)	%Stress Total	Stress Balance
Work	51.38 ± 89.14	3.57 ± 6.19%	310.11 ± 157.84 *	21.54 ± 10.96%	−0.59 ± 0.48 *
After Work	38.41 ± 45.67	2.67 ± 3.17%	212.89 ± 93.08 *	14.78 ± 6.46%	−0.52 ± 0.48 *
Night	276.13 ± 94.88 *	19.18 ± 6.59% *	85.78 ± 88.11 *	5.96 ± 6.12%	0.57 ± 0.43 *
Total	351.75 ± 164.86	24.38 ± 11.45%	589.88 ± 272.37	40.96 ± 18.91%	−0.31 ± 0.37

Min = minutes. * $p < 0.01$

As we can see in Table 2, the highest stress time is given in the time slot corresponding to the working hours, decreasing significantly in the after work range ($p < 0.00$) and during the night ($p < 0.00$). With respect to the relaxation time, we did not find significant differences in the time of relaxation inside and outside of work, although there we did between after work and night ($p < 0.00$), with other types of activities being able to exist outside the working hours that the device does not identify as stressors, and with it their corresponding impact on the SN, but that also do not allow the body to relax.

In the analysis of the impact of stress generated during working hours can generate in the rest of the variables, we found that there is a low positive correlation between the time of stress at work and stress time outside working hours (r = 0.30) ($p < 0.05$), being significantly different among them ($p < 0.00$), which indicates that the more stress at work, the more stress tends to be outside of working hours. We also found a low positive correlation between work stress and stress time present during the night time (r = 0.38) ($p > 0.05$), being significantly different, so, in this sense, having higher work stress is also relates to a greater tendency to suffer greater nighttime stress ($p < 0.00$). However, we did not find in the results any kind of correlation between the stress time shown during working hours and the nighttime relaxation time, which shows that the stress time generated during working hours does not have to involve lower values of relaxation during the night, although it does imply a significant decrease in the values of SB nocturne (r = −0.37) ($p < 0.05$).

On the other hand, when we analyze the impact of stress that is generated and/or remains outside of working hours after working hours, we find a moderate negative correlation between the stress time generated outside of working hours and the nighttime relaxation time, which indicates that the greater the hours of stress outside of work, the shorter the relaxation time during the night (r = −0.48) ($p < 0.01$) and the lower values of the SB at night (r = −0.35) ($p < 0.05$).

If we analyze separately the tendency of the organism to be in a state of stress or recovery during the full working day (24 h), the average found is identified with "moderate tendency to stress" (−0.31 ± 0.37), maintaining a high tendency to stress both within (−0.59 ± 0.48) and outside working hours (−0.52 ± 0.48), compensated with moderate recovery values only during the night (0.57 ± 0.43) (Figure 7).

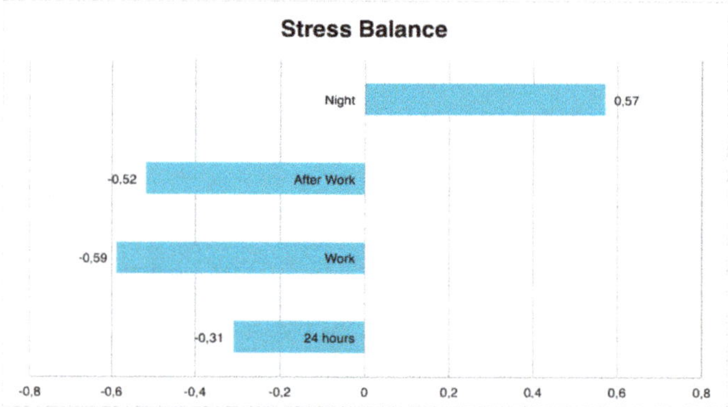

Figure 7. Stress balance for different time slots.

In the descriptive study of the physiological load of stress and recovery during a workday, segmented by gender (men, $n = 28$ and women, $n = 20$), we only found significant differences between gender in the time of reaction to stress by the night, being significantly lower in men (62.37 ± 73.0 min) than in women (119.0 ± 98.5 min) (Table 3).

In the descriptive study of the effect of training during a working day, we found that the analyzed sample obtained a TE of 1.69 ± 0.67, which means that it has a low level of physical activity (less training effect).

Table 3. Descriptive analysis of the physiological load and recovery segmented by sex (Med ± SD).

		Relax Time (min)	% Relax Total	Stress Time (min)	% Stress Total	Stress Balance
Work	Men	60.78 ± 104.02	4.22%	313.56 ± 175.72	21.78%	−0.63 ± 0.48
	Women	38.70 ± 64.33	2.69%	305.45 ± 134.25	21.21%	−0.55 ± 0.50
After work	Men	42.37 ± 45.84	2.94%	194.48 ± 90.32	13.50%	−0.46 ± 0.53
	Women	32.79 ± 46.07	2.28%	239.05 ± 92.98	16.60%	−0.61 ± 0.38
Night	Men	292.3 ± 90.79	20.30%	62.37 ± 73.05 *	4.33%	0.65 ± 0.43
	Women	253.16 ± 98.23	17.58%	119.05 ± 98.53 *	8.27%	0.47 ± 0.41
Total	Men	381.32 ± 182.87	26.48%	550.04 ± 294.57	38.20%	−0.23 ± 0.41
	Women	310.35 ± 128.91	21.55%	645.65 ± 233.66	44.84%	−0.41 ± 0.26

* $p > 0.05$.

4. Discussion

After analyzing the results, we explained that the main objective of this study was fulfilled, which was to describe the physiological burden of stress and the quality of recovery in a population of senior managers during the workday analyzed during three differentiated time slots: work, after work, and night. The marked secondary objective has also been met, through which it was sought to transfer the use of high-performance technology for the objectification of parameters related to health management and stress in executive positions of high responsibility to the business environment.

The hypothesis of research generated at the beginning of the study was fulfilled in which we established that the physiological load derived from a low quality of recovery during the 24 h workday, negatively influences the increase in the physiological load that stress entails in the manager in the medium-long term.

As we can see, the stress generated in the time interval between the work output and the time of going to bed is the one that significantly seems to influence more strongly in a low quality of recovery during the night since it does seem to influence the nighttime relaxation time with a negative correlation of $r = -0.48$. While the stress time generated during working hours does not correlate with it. In this case, whether in a general way or segmented by sex, the organism's longest period of relaxation occurs significantly at night, finding in this range the only positive SB values, related to a better quality of recovery.

To this effect, the data show a low positive and significant correlation between stress time at work and stress time outside working hours, which a priori indicates that the more stress at work, the more stress tends to exist outside working hours, thus influencing a worse quality of night recovery. However, if the stress is significantly lower after working hours but does not find significant differences in the relaxation time inside and outside of work, it may lead us to think that there may be other types of activities outside of work hours that, although not being identified by the body as stressors and are not directly related to work, nor allow the body to relax.

In line with this hypothesis, the device used identifies physical activity as an element different from stress/relaxation, which is why we include in the analysis of variables the effect of training derived from the time that the device collects as a practice of physical activity. In the analyzed population, the effect of the training is 1.69 ± 0.67 out of a maximum of 5.0, which means that they hardly did any physical activity during the day they wore the device, so we can rule out the practice of physical activity outside the working hours as a physical stressor responsible for the values recorded with respect to the time of stress and its relationship with relaxation time outside working hours, leaving the hypothesis open to the cause of stress outside working hours corresponds to other types of activities personal and/or professional.

In this regard, the study by Föhr et al., (2016) correlated in a sample of 16,275 lower Finnish workers percentages of stress during the days of work and during the work itself in those who had a practice of high daily physical activity, impacting also in its quality of recovery [28], In the upper management segment, the practice of physical activity is, thus, defined as a great compensatory tool for the stress generated during the day, deficient in the sample analyzed, which would serve to improve not only their levels of strength and aerobic capacity, but also improve the effects of training in general health and the management of physiological stress in particular.

On the other hand, our results confirm previous studies showing a strong relationship between the decrease in HRV and stress in the body [20,23,24], however most of these studies describe stress as "work-related stress". Analyzed in a general way, nevertheless, by segmenting the working day in three time zones—work, after work, and night—our results show how the stress generated during working hours is not directly responsible for the decrease in HRV sustained in time, and may not be in this case and for this sample, the problem to "manage" if the period included outside work hours (after work) until the time of going to bed.

Acute stress correlates with a decrease in HRV during sleep [21] and during the day [22], which may mean that the acute stress peaks that significantly decrease the quality of recovery during the night in our group are not given during work hours, but outside of work.

In this sense, the management of stress produced outside of work is decisive to achieve a quality of positive recovery and enough to compensate the reactions to stress the rest of the workday, if the stress generated outside of work is not caused for the practice of physical activity (positive stress), there are other personal or professional causes that strongly condition the quality of recovery in the upper management segment. In relation to this line of hypotheses, the team of Zoupanou et al. (2013) concluded in its study that employees strongly influenced by work are the ones with the highest negative stress, however, this result cannot be confirmed with our study, being necessary to continue expanding the sample with the aim of knowing which activities are those that cause an increase or maintenance of stress levels outside working hours, and cannot be directly attributed solely to the workload generated during the same.

5. Conclusions

The stress generated or maintained outside working hours correlates significantly with a lower quality of recovery during the 24 h workday.

It is necessary to prioritize strategies that help improve stress management in executives through the improvement of tools and strategies that promote greater relaxation outside working hours mainly.

The sample analyzes presents values of physical activity practice lower than those recommended by the World Health Organization.

6. Limitations

Variables, such as the IQ or socioeconomic status throughout the working life of the sample, were not analyzed in this study, with possible covariates that would improve the analysis.

The comparison of the stress obtained through HRV with self-perceived stress questionnaires could be very useful to obtain the physiological and mental relationship of stress both at a specific time of the day and a total balance throughout the same.

There is some limitation in the exact control of the work and after work bands in terms of the completion of the work moment and the start of after work, which can be a factor of confusion for the reader. The rest of the strips selected in the sample are very clear and precise. When developing the sample we analyzed its functions in a fixed physical place, and we could assess the possibility that these strips were inside the workplace and outside the workplace, as long as there was no mobility on the part of the subject.

Author Contributions: B.C.-R.: Director of the paper, managing all the processes of preparation of the study, data collection, analysis and supervision of the preparation of the manuscript. S.R.-G. and C.F.-V.: Data collection and organization of the database for statistical analysis. C.C.-R.: Coordinator of data collection and security in the protection thereof. L.M.-P.: Development and coordination of the study together with the management, coordination of data collection, statistical analysis and drafting of the manuscript with the supervision of the director.

Funding: This research received no external funding.

Conflicts of Interest: The authors declare no conflict of interest.

References

1. European Agency for Safety and Health at Work. May 2015. Available online: https://osha.europa.eu/en/tools-and-publications/blog (accessed on 10 June 2018).
2. Backe, E.M.; Seidler, A.; Latza, U.; Rossnagel, K.; Schumann, B. The role of psychosocial stress at work for the development of cardiovascular diseases: A systematic review. *Int. Arch. Occup. Environ. Health* **2012**, *85*, 67–79. [CrossRef] [PubMed]
3. Segerström, S.C.; Miller, G.E. Psychological Stress and the Human Immune System: A Meta-Analytic Study of 30 Years of Inquiry. *Psychol. Bull.* **2004**, *130*. [CrossRef] [PubMed]
4. Schneiderman, N.; Ironson, G.; Siegel, S.D. Stress and Health: Psychological, Behavioral, and Biological Determinants. *Annu. Rev. Clin. Psychol.* **2005**, *1*, 607–628. [CrossRef] [PubMed]
5. World Health Organization. *The European Health Report 2012—Charting the Way to Well-Being*; World Health Organization: Geneva, Switzerland, 2012.
6. EuroHeart II. June 2013. Available online: http://www.ehnheart.org/projects/euroheart-ii/euroheart-ii-publications.html (accessed on 10 June 2018).
7. Crespo-Ruiz, B.; León, M.; García-Unanue, J.; Gallardo, L.; Maicas-Pérez, L. *Estudio de Caso de Éxito: Implementación de Tecnología Para la Gestión del Estrés en el Entorno Laboral*; Leisure and Tourism Review; PODIUM Sport: Belfast, UK, 2017.
8. Lecca, L.I.; Campagna, M.; Portoghese, I.; Galletta, M.; Mucci, N.; Meloni, M.; Cocco, P. Work Related Stress, Well-Being and Cardiovascular Risk among Flight Logistic Workers: An Observational Study. *Int. J. Environ. Res. Public Health* **2018**, *15*, 1952. [CrossRef] [PubMed]
9. Velten, J.; Bieda, A.; Scholten, S.; Wannemüller, A.; Margraf, J. Lifestyle choices and mental health: A longitudinal survey with German and Chinese students. *BMC Public Health* **2018**, *18*, 632. [CrossRef] [PubMed]
10. Wolf, E.J.; Schnurr, P.P. PTSD-related cardiovascular disease and accelerated cellular aging. *Psychiatr. Ann.* **2016**, *46*, 527–532. [CrossRef] [PubMed]
11. An, K.; Salver, J.; Brown, R.E.; Kao, H.F.; Starkweather, A.; Shim, I. Salivary Biomarkers of Chronic Psychosocial Stress and CVD Risks: A Systematic Review. *Biol. Res. Nurs.* **2015**, *18*, 241–263. [CrossRef] [PubMed]
12. Van Amelsvoort, L.G.; Schouten, E.G.; Maan, A.C.; Swenne, C.A.; Kok, F.J. Occupational determinants of heart rate variability. *Int. Arch. Occup. Environ. Health* **2000**, *73*, 255–262. [CrossRef]
13. Chrousos, G.P.; Gold, P.W. The Concepts of Stress and Stress System Disorders—Overview of Physical and Behavioral Homeostasis. *J. Am. Med. Assoc.* **1992**, *267*, 1244–1252. [CrossRef]
14. Koolhaas, J.M. Stress revisited: A critical evaluation of the stress concept. *Neurosci. Biobehav. Rev.* **2011**, *35*, 1291–1301. [CrossRef]
15. Hanson, E.K.; Godaert, G.L.; Maas, C.J.; Meijman, T.F. Vagal cardiac control throughout the day: The relative importance of effort-reward imbalance and within-day measurements of mood, demand and satisfaction. *Biol. Psychol.* **2001**, *56*, 23–44. [CrossRef]
16. Hintsanen, M.; Elovainio, M.; Puttonen, S.; Kivimaki, M.; Koskinen, T.; Raitakari, O.T.; Keltikangas-Jarvinen, L. Effort-reward imbalance, heart rate, and heart rate variability: The Cardiovascular Risk in Young Finns Study. *Int. J. Behav. Med.* **2007**, *14*, 202–212. [CrossRef] [PubMed]
17. Riese, H.; Van Doornen, L.J.; Houtman, I.L.; De Geus, E.J. Job strain in relation to ambulatory blood pressure, heart rate, and heart rate variability among female nurses. *Scand. J. Work Environ. Health* **2004**, *30*, 477–485. [CrossRef] [PubMed]
18. Vrijkotte, T.G.; van Doornen, L.J.; de Geus, E.J. Effects of work stress on ambulatory blood pressure, heart rate, and heart rate variability. *Hypertension* **2000**, *35*, 880–886. [CrossRef] [PubMed]
19. Zanstra, Y.J.; Schellekens, J.M.; Schaap, C.; Kooistra, L. Vagal and sympathetic activity in burnouts during a mentally demanding workday. *Psychosom. Med.* **2006**, *68*, 583–590. [CrossRef] [PubMed]
20. Chandola, T.; Heraclides, A.; Kumari, M. Psychophysiological biomarkers of workplace stressors. *Neurosci. Biobehav. Rev.* **2010**, *35* (Suppl. S1), 51–57. [CrossRef] [PubMed]

21. Hall, M.; Vasko, R.; Buysse, D.; Ombao, H.; Chen, Q.; Cashmere, J.D.; Kupfer, D.; Thayer, J.F. Acute stress affects heart rate variability during sleep. *Psychosom. Med.* **2004**, *66*, 56–62. [CrossRef]
22. Dishman, R.K.; Nakamura, Y.; Garcia, M.E.; Thompson, R.W.; Dunn, A.L.; Blair, S.N. Heart rate variability, trait anxiety, and perceived stress among physically fit men and women. *Int. J. Psychophysiol.* **2000**, *37*, 121–133. [CrossRef]
23. Clays, E.; De Bacquer, D.; Crasset, V.; Kittel, F.; de Smet, P.; Kornitzer, M.; Karasek, R.; De Backe, G. The perception of work stressors is related to reduced parasympathetic activity. *Int. Arch. Occup. Environ. Health* **2011**, *84*, 185–191. [CrossRef]
24. Collins, S.M.; Karasek, R.A.; Costas, K. Job strain and autonomic indices of cardiovascular disease risk. *Am. J. Ind. Med.* **2005**, *48*, 182–193. [CrossRef]
25. Kaber, D.; Perry, C.; Segall, N.; Sheik-Nainar, M. Workload state classification with automation during simulated air traffic control. *Int. J. Aviat. Psychol.* **2007**, *17*, 371–390. [CrossRef]
26. Hernando, D.; Garatachea, N.; Almeida, R.; Casajús, J.A.; Bailón, R. Validation of Heart Rate Monitor Polar RS800 for Heart Rate Variability Analysis During Exercise. *J. Strength Cond. Res.* **2018**, *32*, 716–725. [CrossRef] [PubMed]
27. Morales, J.; Álamo, J.M.; García-Manso, X.; Buscà, B.; Lopez, J.L.; Serra-Añó, P.; González, L.M. Use of heart rate variability in monitoring stress and recovery in judo athletes. *J. Strength Cond. Res.* **2014**, *28*, 1896–1905. [CrossRef] [PubMed]
28. Dong, J.-G. The role of heart rate variability in sports physiology. *Exp. Ther. Med.* **2016**, *11*, 1531–1536. [CrossRef] [PubMed]
29. Danieli, A.; Lusa, L.; Potočnik, N.; Meglič, B.; Grad, A.; Bajrović, F.F. Resting heart rate variability and heart rate recovery after submaximal exercise. *Clin. Auton. Res.* **2014**, *24*, 53–61. [CrossRef] [PubMed]
30. Föhr, T.; Pietilä, J.; Helander, E.; Myllymäki, T.; Lindholm, H.; Rusko, H.; Kujala, U.M. Physical activity, body mass index and heart rate variability-based stress and recovery in 16 275 Finnish employees: A cross-sectional study. *BMC Public Health* **2016**, *16*, 701. [CrossRef] [PubMed]
31. Mutikainen, S.; Helander, E.; Pietilä, J.; Korhonen, I.; Kujala, U.M. Objectively measured physical activity in Finnish employees: A cross-sectional study. *BMJ Open* **2014**, *4*, e005927. [CrossRef]
32. Saalasti, S. *Neural Networks for Heart Rate Time Series Analysis;* University of Jyväskylä: Jyväskylä, Finland, 2003.
33. Kettunen, J.; Saalasti, S. Procedure for Deriving Reliable Information on Respiratory Activity from Heart Period Measurement. U.S. Patent 7,460,901, 2 December 2012.
34. Martinmäki, K.; Rusko, H.; Kooistra, L.; Kettunen, J.; Saalasti, S. Intraindividual validation of heart rate variability indexes to measure vagal effects on hearts. *Am. J. Physiol. Heart Circ. Physiol.* **2006**, *290*, 640–647. [CrossRef]
35. Firstbeat Technologies Ltd. *Stress and Recovery Analysis Method Based on 24-h Heart Rate Variability;* Firstbeat Technologies Ltd.: Jyväskylä, Finland, 2014.

International Journal of
Environmental Research and Public Health

MDPI

Article

Does Instruction of Oral Health Behavior for Workers Improve Work Performance? —Quasi-Randomized Trial

Naoki Toyama [1], Ayano Taniguchi-Tabata [2,*], Nanami Sawada [1], Yoshio Sugiura [1], Daiki Fukuhara [1], Yoko Uchida [1], Hisataka Miyai [1], Aya Yokoi [1], Shinsuke Mizutani [3,4], Daisuke Ekuni [1] and Manabu Morita [1]

1 Department of Preventive Dentistry, Okayama University Graduate School of Medicine, Dentistry and Pharmaceutical Sciences, Okayama University, Okayama 700-8558, Japan; pu171qxi@s.okayama-u.ac.jp (N.T.); de422027@s.okayama-u.ac.jp (N.S.); de421022@s.okayama-u.ac.jp (Y.S.); de20041@s.okayama-u.ac.jp (D.F.); de20006@s.okayama-u.ac.jp (Y.U.); pqpp0n70@s.okayama-u.ac.jp (H.M.); yokoi-a1@cc.okayama-u.ac.jp (A.Y.); dekuni7@md.okayama-u.ac.jp (D.E.); mmorita@md.okayama-u.ac.jp (M.M.)
2 Department of Preventive Dentistry, Okayama University Hospital, Okayama 700-8558, Japan
3 Section of Geriatric Dentistry and Perioperative Medicine in Dentistry, Division of Maxillofacial Diagnostic and Surgical Sciences, Faculty of Dental Science, Kyushu University, Fukuoka 812-8582, Japan; mizutani@dent.kyushu-u.ac.jp
4 OBT Research Center, Faculty of Dental Science, Kyushu University, Fukuoka 812-8582, Japan
* Correspondence: de19026@s.okayama-u.ac.jp; Tel.: +81-86-235-6712

Received: 31 October 2018; Accepted: 22 November 2018; Published: 24 November 2018

Abstract: Oral disease can cause economic loss due to impaired work performance. Therefore, improvement of oral health status and prevention of oral disease is essential among workers. The purpose of this study was to investigate whether oral health-related behavioral modification intervention influences work performance or improves oral health behavior and oral health status among Japanese workers. We quasi-randomly separated participants into the intervention group or the control group at baseline. The intervention group received intensive oral health instruction at baseline and a self-assessment every three months. Both groups received oral examinations and answered the self-questionnaire at baseline and at one-year follow-up. At follow-up, the prevalence of subjects who use fluoride toothpastes and interdental brushes/dental floss were significantly higher in the intervention group than in the control group. Three variables (tooth brushing in workplace, using fluoride toothpaste, and experience of receiving tooth brushing instruction in a dental clinic) showed significant improvement only in the intervention group. On the other hand, work performance and oral status did not significantly change in either group. Our intensive oral health-related behavioral modification intervention improved oral health behavior, but neither work performance nor oral status, among Japanese workers.

Keywords: work performance; oral health; intervention study; behavioral modification

1. Introduction

Health impairment influences work performance due to pain, absence for treatment and physical disability [1–4]. The World Health Organization states that protecting workers' health is important to household income, productivity, and economic development, and work-related health problems result in an economic loss of 4–6% of gross domestic product (GDP) for most countries [5].

Several chronic diseases, including oral diseases, were reported to cause economic loss due to impaired work performance [6]. In Japan, 34.8% of workers had problems with work due to oral diseases and impaired work performance [7]. Another study reported that oral diseases indirectly impose an economic burden, costing US$144 billion in terms of productivity losses due to absenteeism from work [8]. Thus, prevention and control of oral diseases is important for workers to avoid impaired work performance and subsequent economic loss.

Improving individual oral health behavior is effective for preventing oral diseases. Dentists or dental hygienists perform behavioral modification for improvement of patient oral health behavior [9–11]. Adopting methods for behavioral modification, such as "prompt self-monitoring of behavior", "prompt intention formation", "prompt specific goal setting", "provide feedback on performance", and "prompt review of behavioral goals", are effective [12,13]. However, there have been few studies investigating the effects of intervention for behavioral modification on work performance.

We hypothesize that oral health-related behavioral modification intervention will improve work performance by improving oral health behavior and oral health status. This study aims to investigate whether oral health-related behavioral modification intervention influences work performance or improves oral health behavior and oral health status among Japanese workers.

2. Materials and Methods

2.1. Study Population

We estimated the sample size using G*Power and calculated minimum sample sizes for a chi-squared test. We set the effect size at 0.3, alpha at 0.05, and power $(1 - \beta)$ at 0.80 [14]. The minimum sample size was 108 (chi-squared test). Assuming an attrition rate of 30% [15,16], the planned sample size was therefore a minimum of 308 participants (154 in each group).

Among central or branch offices in Okayama in Japan, we recruited companies that have never received oral examination in work places and agreed to participate in the study. A total of 14 companies in Okayama, Hiroshima, Osaka, and Kyoto cities in Japan agreed to participate in this study. Inclusion criteria for participant recruitment were to complete oral examinations and questionnaires, while exclusion criteria were participants who did not agree to participate. We enrolled 611 workers from April to December 2015 and performed re-examination from April to December 2016.

This study was an assessor-blinded, quasi-randomized trial (alternate allocation). All participants first received an oral examination and answered self-administered questionnaires, and were then divided into two groups in the order in which they came at baseline (2015). After alternate allocation (ratio; 1:1), participants were assigned to the intervention group or the control group. After oral examination, the intervention group received instructions for oral health-related behavioral modification. They were involved in further intervention by the mailing method, which was performed every three months. The control group received only oral examinations. After one year (follow-up) (2016), the two groups received re-examination and answered self-questionnaires.

All study protocols were approved by the Ethics Committees of Okayama University Graduate School of Medicine, Dentistry and Pharmaceutical Sciences and Okayama University Hospital (no. 1507-001). Written informed consent was obtained from all targeted participants. Moreover, this study was registered at the University Hospital Medical Information Network (no. 000023011) before commencing.

2.2. Oral Examination

At baseline and follow-up, six dentists (M.M., T.I., H.M., A.T.-T., A.Y., D.F.) who did not know the allocation performed oral examinations (single blind). The dentists assessed oral health status based on community periodontal index (CPI) [17], debris index-simplified (DI-S) [18] and bleeding on probing (BOP) using a CPI probe (YDM, Tokyo, Japan). CPI, DI-S, and BOP were measured for 10 representative teeth (maxilla: right first and second molar, right central incisor, left first and second molar; mandible: right first and second molar, left central incisor, left first and second molar). CPI scores were binarized; 0–2 vs. 3, 4. DI-S was evaluated in 4 grades (0–3). BOP was expressed as percentage (%BOP). In addition, the number of present teeth, decayed teeth, and filling teeth were recorded [17]. For assessment, all dentists received training and calibration. Data of CPI score (≤2/>2) were analyzed using a non-parametric kappa test. The kappa coefficients for intra- and inter-examiner reliability were 1.0 and 0.83, respectively.

2.3. Self-Questionnaire

Before oral examination, participants answered self-questionnaires on sex, age, job category [19], work pattern (daytime/daytime and nighttime/flextime), and 10 questions about oral health [20], as presented below:

(1) Do you have a family dental doctor? (Yes/No)
(2) Does your work disturb you going to dental clinic? (Yes/No)
(3) Do you brush your teeth in your workplace? (Always/Sometimes/No)
(4) Do you eat snack food between meals? (Always/Sometimes/No)
(5) Do you smoke tobacco? (Current smoking/Past smoking/Never)
(6) Do you brush your teeth before going to bed? (Always/Sometimes/No)
(7) Do you use fluoride toothpaste? (Yes/No/I don't know)
(8) Do you use interdental brushes/dental floss? (Always/Sometimes/No)
(9) Have you received tooth brushing instruction at a dental clinic? (Yes/No)
(10) Have you received oral examination in the past year at a dental clinic? (Yes/No)

Furthermore, to assess whether oral status influences work performance, we asked "Have you had any problems with work performance because of oral diseases?" [7]. The answer was given in a "yes/no" format. If the answer was "yes", work performance was assessed as impaired.

2.4. Intervention

The intervention group received individualized instruction for five minutes. During the study briefing, the participants set three goals for oral health behavioral modification to improve individual oral status and received advice on achieving the goals using a leaflet and a dental model. The instructors were dental hygienists or dentists who did not perform oral examinations. Moreover, we performed self-assessment questionnaires three times per year by mail (mailing method). In the mailing method, the intervention group evaluated the level of achievement of the goals, which were suggested at baseline intervention and reconsidered the direction. If the goals were achieved, new goals were established by participants.

2.5. Statistical Analysis

SPSS version 20 software (IBM, Tokyo, Japan) was used for statistical analyses. Values of $p < 0.05$ were considered to indicate significant associations. Chi-squared tests or non-paired t-tests were used to assess whether there were significant differences between the intervention group and the control group at both baseline and follow-up. McNemar test, McNemar-Bowker tests or paired t-tests were used to assess whether there were significant changes between baseline and follow-up.

3. Results

Figure 1 shows the flow chart for study participants. All participants agreed to participate in this study. As the participants who did not undergo re-examination or provided incomplete data were excluded, 371 workers out of 611 workers were included in the analysis (final follow-up rate; 60.7%).

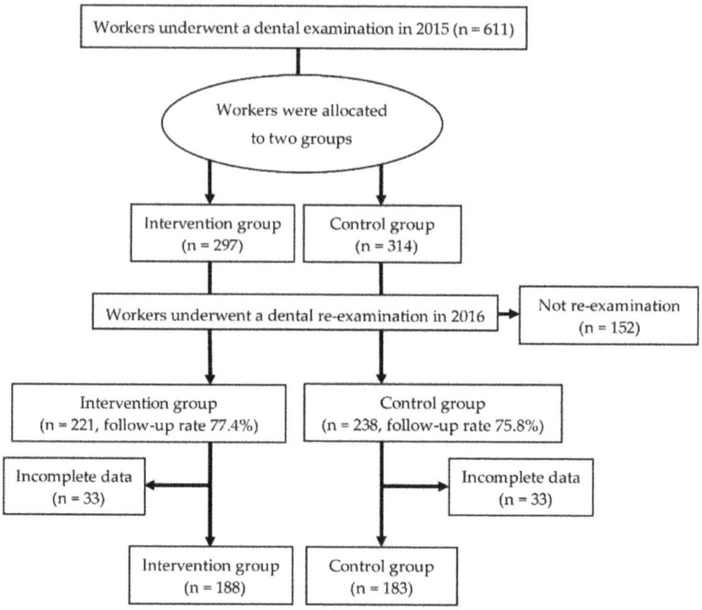

Figure 1. Flow chart showing the protocols for selecting analyzed workers from among those who agreed to participate in this study.

Table 1 shows the distribution of participants' characteristics at baseline. Data were not significantly different between the two groups at baseline ($p \geq 0.05$, chi-squared tests, data not shown). The most common job category was professional and technical workers (36.9%). Daytime workers accounted for 85.4% of participants.

Table 1. Characteristics of participants at baseline.

Variables	Intervention (*n* = 188)	Control (*n* = 183)
Sex		
Male	149 (79.3) [1]	148 (80.9)
Female	39 (20.7)	35 (19.1)
Age (y)	40.7 ± 11.9 [2]	41.4 ± 11.9
Job category		
Administrative and managerial workers	16 (8.5)	25 (13.7)
Professional and technical workers	67 (35.6)	70 (38.3)
Clerical workers	38 (20.2)	23 (12.6)
Sales workers	20 (10.6)	15 (8.2)
Service workers	3 (1.6)	4 (2.2)
Security workers	9 (4.8)	7 (3.8)
Manufacturing process workers	28 (14.9)	36 (19.7)
Transport and machine operation workers	7 (3.7)	3 (1.6)
Work schedule		
Daytime work	160 (85.1)	157 (85.8)
Daytime and nighttime work	8 (4.3)	6 (3.3)
Flextime work	20 (10.6)	20 (10.9)

[1] *n* (%); [2] Mean ± standard deviation.

In Table 2, we show a comparison of clinical variables between the two groups at baseline and at follow-up. All variables related to oral health status did not significantly differ between the two groups at baseline and follow-up ($p \geq 0.05$, non-paired t-tests or chi-squared tests, data not shown).

Table 2. Comparison of clinical variables between the intervention group and the control group at follow-up.

Variables		Baseline (2015)		Follow-up (2016)		p-Value
		Intervention (n = 188)	Control (n = 183)	Intervention (n = 188)	Control (n = 183)	
DI-S [1]		0.36 ± 0.34 [4]	0.38 ± 0.33	0.35 ± 0.36	0.34 ± 0.37	0.784 [6]
%BOP [2]		39.0 ± 30.5	40.5 ± 28.4	36.3 ± 27.3	37.4 ± 26.3	0.674
Present teeth		28.3 ± 2.4	28.5 ± 1.8	28.3 ± 2.4	28.6 ± 1.9	0.246
Decayed teeth		0.69 ± 1.58	0.77 ± 2.06	0.64 ± 1.60	0.60 ± 1.56	0.796
Filling teeth		8.67 ± 6.08	9.06 ± 5.73	8.66 ± 6.13	9.20 ± 5.64	0.376
CPI [3]	≤2	113 (60.1) [5]	110 (60.1)	121 (64.4)	116 (63.4)	0.845 [7]

[1] Debris index-simplified; [2] Percentage of bleeding on probing; [3] Community periodontal index; [4] Mean ± standard deviation; [5] n (%); [6] Non-paired t-test at follow-up; [7] Chi-squared test at follow-up.

The distribution of self-questionnaire answers between the intervention group and the control group is shown in Table 3. At baseline, there were no significant differences between the two groups ($p \geq 0.05$, chi-squared tests, data not shown). After intervention, the frequency of fluoride toothpaste and interdental brushes/dental floss use was higher in the intervention group than in the control group ($p < 0.05$). There were no significant differences in work performance.

Table 3. Comparison of qualitative variables between the intervention group and the control group at follow-up.

Vriables	Baseline (2015)		Follow-up (2016)		p-Value [1]
	Intervention (n = 188)	Control (n = 183)	Intervention (n = 188)	Control (n = 183)	
Have you had any problems with work performance because of oral diseases?					
Yes	9 (4.8) [2]	12 (6.6)	7 (3.7)	7 (3.8)	0.959
No	179 (95.2)	171 (93.4)	181 (96.3)	176 (96.2)	
Do you have a family dental doctor?					
Yes	118 (62.8)	116 (63.4)	126 (67.0)	122 (66.7)	0.942
No	70 (37.2)	67 (36.6)	62 (33.0)	61 (33.3)	
Does your work disturb you going to dental clinic?					
Yes	91 (48.4)	76 (41.5)	83 (44.1)	71 (38.8)	0.296
No	97 (51.6)	107 (58.5)	105 (55.9)	112 (61.2)	
Do you brush your teeth in your workplace?					
Always	56 (29.8)	46 (25.1)	51 (27.1)	50 (27.3)	0.07
Sometimes	38 (20.2)	43 (23.5)	62 (33.0)	42 (23.0)	
No	94 (50.0)	94 (51.4)	75 (39.9)	91 (49.7)	
Do you eat snack food between meals?					
Always	43 (22.9)	45 (24.6)	43 (22.9)	52 (28.4)	0.344
Sometimes	115 (61.2)	111 (60.7)	114 (60.6)	108 (59.0)	
No	30 (16.0)	27 (14.8)	31 (16.5)	23 (12.6)	

Table 3. *Cont.*

Vriables	Baseline (2015)		Follow-up (2016)		p-Value [1]
	Intervention (n = 188)	Control (n = 183)	Intervention (n = 188)	Control (n = 183)	
Do you smoke tobacco?					
Current smoking	43 (22.9)	44 (24.0)	45 (23.9)	43 (23.5)	0.994
Past smoking	33 (17.6)	29 (15.8)	31 (16.5)	30 (16.4)	
Never	112 (59.6)	110 (60.1)	112 (59.6)	110 (60.1)	
Do you brush your teeth before going to bed?					
Always	152 (80.9)	137 (74.9)	160 (85.1)	140 (76.5)	0.075
Sometimes	25 (13.3)	28 (15.3)	21 (11.2)	28 (15.3)	
No	11 (5.9)	18 (9.8)	7 (3.7)	15 (8.2)	
Do you use fluoride toothpaste?					
Yes	95 (50.5)	82 (44.8)	124 (66.0)	96 (52.5)	0.029
No	36 (19.1)	46 (25.1)	34 (18.1)	44 (24.0)	
I don't know	57 (30.3)	55 (30.1)	30 (16.0)	43 (23.5)	
Do you use interdental brushes/dental floss?					
Always	26 (13.8)	28 (15.3)	43 (22.9)	32 (17.5)	0.021
Sometimes	74 (39.4)	70 (38.3)	88 (46.8)	70 (38.3)	
No	88 (46.8)	85 (46.4)	57 (30.3)	81 (44.3)	
Have you received tooth brushing instruction at a dental clinic?					
Yes	129 (68.6)	129 (70.5)	146 (77.7)	135 (73.8)	0.382
No	59 (31.4)	54 (29.5)	42 (22.3)	48 (26.2)	
Have you received an oral examination in the past year at a dental clinic?					
Yes	72 (38.3)	65 (35.5)	89 (47.3)	87 (47.5)	0.969
No	116 (61.7)	118 (64.5)	99 (52.7)	96 (52.5)	

[1] Chi-squared test on differences between intervention and control groups at follow-up; [2] n (%).

Changes in measured variables from baseline to follow-up in each group were also compared (Table 4). Use of interdental brushes/dental floss and dental examinations in the past year improved significantly in both groups. On the other hand, three variables (tooth brushing in workplace, using fluoride toothpastes, and experience of receiving tooth brushing instruction) showed significant improvement only in the intervention group. Work performance and oral status did not change significantly.

Table 4. Changes in variables in intervention and control groups.

Variables	Intervention (n = 188)			Control (n = 183)		
	Baseline	Follow-up	p-Value [6]	Baseline	Follow-up	p-Value [6]
Continuous variables						
DI-S [1]	0.35 ± 0.36 [4]	0.36 ± 0.34	0.913	0.38 ± 0.33	0.34 ± 0.37	0.165
%BOP [2]	39.0 ± 30.5	36.3 ± 27.3	0.290	40.5 ± 28.4	37.4 ± 26.3	0.179
Present teeth	28.3 ± 2.36	28.3 ± 2.37	0.381	28.5 ± 1.78	28.6 ± 1.90	0.414
Decayed teeth	0.69 ± 1.58	0.64 ± 1.60	0.515	0.77 ± 2.06	0.60 ± 1.56	0.062
Filling teeth	8.67 ± 6.08	8.66 ± 6.14	0.969	9.06 ± 5.73	9.21 ± 5.64	0.337

Table 4. *Cont.*

Variables	Intervention (n = 188)			Control (n = 183)		
	Improved	Worsened	p-Value [7]	Improved	Worsened	p-Value [7]
Categorical variables						
CPI [3]	33 (17.6) [5]	25 (13.3)	0.358	32 (17.5)	26 (14.2)	0.512
Have you had any problems with work performance because of oral diseases?						
	9 (4.8)	7 (3.7)	0.804	10 (5.5)	5 (2.7)	0.302
Do you have a family dental doctor?						
	13 (6.9)	5 (2.7)	0.096	18 (9.8)	12 (6.6)	0.362
Does your work disturb you going to dental clinic?						
	26 (13.8)	18 (9.6)	0.291	25 (13.7)	20 (10.9)	0.551
Do you brush your teeth in your workplace?						
	30 (16.0)	16 (8.5)	0.003	22 (12.1)	19 (10.4)	0.256
Do you eat snack food between meals?						
	27 (14.4)	26 (13.8)	0.997	18 (9.8)	28 (15.3)	0.403
Do you smoke tobacco?						
	4 (2.1)	7 (3.7)	0.392	8 (4.3)	7 (3.8)	0.978
Do you brush your teeth before going to bed?						
	13 (6.9)	4 (2.1)	0.132	13 (7.1)	10 (5.4)	0.733
Do you use fluoride toothpaste?						
	53 (28.2)	7 (8.0)	<0.001	35 (19.1)	22 (12.0)	0.076
Do you use interdental brushes/dental floss?						
	50 (26.6)	7 (3.7)	<0.001	26 (14.2)	15 (8.2)	0.049
Have you received tooth brushing instruction at a dental clinic?						
	24 (12.8)	7 (3.7)	0.003	16 (8.7)	10 (5.5)	0.327
Have you received an oral examination in the past year at a dental clinic?						
	28 (14.9)	11 (5.9)	0.009	32 (17.5)	10 (5.5)	0.001

[1] Debris index-simplified; [2] Percentage of bleeding on probing; [3] Community periodontal index; [4] Mean ± standard deviation; [5] n (%); [6] Paired t-test; [7] McNemar test or McNemar-Bowker test.

Oral health behavioral interventions are not invasive. Therefore, there were no study-related serious adverse events in this study. Furthermore, outcomes did not change after the trial commenced.

4. Discussion

To the best of our knowledge, this was the first study to assess changes in work performance after oral health-related behavioral modification intervention. The study design was reliable as examinations were performed blinded, participants were quasi-randomly (alternate allocation) separated into either an intervention group or a control group, and the sample size was sufficiently large. Unfortunately, this intervention did not improve work performance, and there are several reasons for this. In a previous study [21], it was reported that work performance is mainly influenced by pain from oral diseases. In this study, there was a significant association between work performance and oral pain (baseline, $p = 0.002$; follow-up, $p = 0.019$; chi-squared tests; data not shown). However, there was no significant difference in the decrease in oral pain between the intervention and control groups ($p \geq 0.05$). A previous study showed that a combination of professional oral hygiene treatment and oral hygiene instructions contributed to a decrease in gingival-related pain [22]. Thus, in the future, we should investigate whether a combination of professional oral hygiene treatment and oral health instruction improves work performance.

Oral health-related behavioral modification intervention improved oral health behavior but not oral health status. A systematic review showed that oral hygiene instruction had short-term and long-term effects [10]. The short-term effects were improving knowledge, attitudes, self-efficacy, oral health behavior, and theory constructs. The long-term effects included improving the number of decayed teeth, plaque score, BOP, and gingival condition [10]. The results of this study may be included in the short-term effects. Menegaz et al. suggested that a follow-up time of less than one year led to a lack of efficacy for educational intervention [23]. In addition, Oshikohji et al. reported that workers who had more participation time for oral examination and oral health instruction had better periodontal condition than those with less time [24]. If the duration of this study and/or the frequency of instruction was increased, oral health status might improve.

The intervention in this study was advantageous as it included some of the known factors that lead to behavioral modification. We explained why the workers should change their behavior (prompt intention formation), let the workers set goals independently (prompt specific goal setting), and checked their improvement and prompted them to reconsider their goals (prompt self-monitoring of behavior and prompt review of behavioral goals) [12,13]. Goals to improve oral status were also set based on individual situations in this study. These concepts were supported by a previous study [25]. Finally, the intervention time was short (5 min), a factor which may be effective in workplaces to improve oral health behavior.

There were 17 participants who had problems with work because of tooth or gum disease (4.6% of participants) at baseline. These conditions agree with the prevalence of poor work performance caused by oral pain in previous studies, which ranged between 1.0–7.6% [25–28]. The percentage in this study was within this range. However, the job sector of participants in this study was skewed. The percentage of workers who belonged to the tertiary industry sector was high (83%), and there were no workers from the primary industry sector. Therefore, we should exercise caution when applying our results more generally.

There were some limitations with regard to the interpretation of these results. First, although most of the participants visited a dental clinic during the study period, the type of dental health instruction they received was not confirmed. The intensity of instruction may have affected the results. Second, the follow up rate was not high (approximately 60.7%). As >20% loss would pose a serious threat [29], the high percentage of loss to follow-up may have affected our results. In the intervention group, the ratios of work performance, oral status, and oral health behavior were not significantly different between the analyzed and non-analyzed workers (188 vs. 85 workers, chi-squared test and non-paired t-test, $p > 0.05$). However, in the control group, the percentage of those using interdental brushes/dental floss was significantly different (183 vs. 90 workers, chi-squared test, $p = 0.034$). In the control group, use of interdental brushes or dental floss might have been improved because more workers who did not use these were not analyzed. Other limitations include the short-term scale of the study period and the fact that this was not a randomized trial.

5. Conclusions

In conclusion, oral health-related behavioral modification intervention improved oral health behavior, but not work performance in Japanese workers.

Author Contributions: Conceptualization, A.T.-T., S.M., D.E. and M.M.; investigation, A.T.-T., N.S., Y.S., D.F., Y.U., H.M. and A.Y.; data curation, A.T.-T. and N.T.; writing—original draft preparation, N.T.; writing—review and editing, all authors; project administration, M.M.; funding acquisition, M.M.

Funding: The research was funded by the "Research Fund of Clinical Study for Industrial Accident and Disease" (14020101–01) from the Japanese Ministry of Health, Labour and Welfare.

Acknowledgments: The authors are grateful to Junko Emi (Animal Development and Reproductive Biotechnology, Okayama University Graduate School of Environmental and Life Science Okayama, Japan) for data entry and collection, Hirofumi Mizuno (Sasaki dental clinic, Aichi, Japan) for oral examination, and Yuko Kimura (International Dental Hygienist College, Okayama, Japan) for collaboration with regard to oral health behavioral modification intervention.

Conflicts of Interest: The authors declare no conflicts of interest.

References

1. Pronk, N.P.; Martinson, B.; Kessler, R.C.; Beck, A.L.; Simon, G.E.; Wang, P. The Association Between Work Performance and Physical Activity, Cardiorespiratory Fitness, and Obesity. *J. Occup. Environ. Med.* **2004**, *46*, 19–25. [CrossRef] [PubMed]
2. Suvinen, T.I.; Ahlberg, J.; Rantala, M.; Nissinen, M.; Lindholm, H.; Könönen, M.; Savolainen, A. Perceived stress, pain and work performance among non-patient working personnel with clinical signs of temporomandibular or neck pain. *J. Oral Rehabil.* **2004**, *31*, 733–737. [CrossRef] [PubMed]
3. Khubchandani, J.; Price, J.H. Association of Job Insecurity with Health Risk Factors and Poorer Health in American Workers. *J. Community Health* **2017**, *42*, 242–251. [CrossRef] [PubMed]
4. Sigurdardottir, V.; Drivelegka, P.; Svärd, A.; Jacobsson, L.T.H.; Dehlin, M. Work disability in gout: A population-based case—Control study. *Ann. Rheum. Dis.* **2018**, *77*, 399–404. [CrossRef] [PubMed]
5. Protecting Workers' Health. Available online: http://www.who.int/news-room/fact-sheets/detail/protecting-workers\T1\textquoteright-health (accessed on 26 October 2018).
6. Fouad, A.M.; Waheed, A.; Gamal, A.; Amer, S.A.; Abdellah, R.F.; Shebl, F.M. Effect of Chronic Diseases on Work Productivity: A Propensity Score Analysis. *J. Occup. Environ. Med.* **2017**, *59*, 480–485. [CrossRef] [PubMed]
7. Ichihashi, T.; Mutou, T.; Shibuya, K. Influence of Dental Diseaseon Workers in Terms of Hours Lost from Work or Daily Life Activities. *Jpn. Soc. Dent. Health* **2002**, *52*, 141–149. [CrossRef]
8. Listl, S.; Galloway, J.; Mossey, P.A.; Marcenes, W. Global Economic Impact of Dental Diseases. *J. Dent. Res.* **2015**, *94*, 1355–1361. [CrossRef] [PubMed]
9. Kay, E.; Vascott, D.; Hocking, A.; Nield, H.; Dorr, C.; Barrett, H. A review of approaches for dental practice teams for promoting oral health. *Community Dent. Oral Epidemiol.* **2016**, *44*, 313–330. [CrossRef] [PubMed]
10. Ghaffari, M.; Rakhshanderou, S.; Ramezankhani, A.; Buunk-Werkhoven, Y.; Noroozi, M.; Armoon, B. Are educating and promoting interventions effective in oral health?: A systematic review. *Int. J. Dent. Hyg.* **2018**, *16*, 48–58. [CrossRef] [PubMed]
11. Haresaku, S.; Tsutsui, A.; Sakai, K.; Ryu, C.; Kanesaki, N.; Hanioka, T.; Kashiwagi, S.; Mishima, K.; Chinju, N.; Ogawa, K. Relationships of Dental Factors for Behavior Change with the Effects of an Intervention Program in the Workplace and Consciousness of the Oral Health of Workers. *Jpn. Soc. Dent. Health* **2004**, *54*, 122–131. [CrossRef]
12. Michie, S.; Abraham, C.; Whittington, C.; McAteer, J.; Gupta, S. Effective techniques in healthy eating and physical activity interventions: A meta-regression. *Health Psychol.* **2009**, *28*, 690–701. [CrossRef] [PubMed]
13. Ishikawa, Y. Recent Global Trends in Standardized Reporting of Behavior Change Technique. *Jpn. J. Behav. Med.* **2014**, *20*, 41–46. [CrossRef]
14. Cohen, J. A power primer. *Psychol. Bull.* **1992**, *112*, 155–159. [CrossRef] [PubMed]
15. Davis, K.D.; Lawson, K.M.; Almeida, D.M.; Kelly, E.L.; King, R.B.; Hammer, L.; Casper, L.M.; Okechukwu, C.A.; Hanson, G.; McHale, S.M. Parents' Daily Time With Their Children: A Workplace Intervention. *Pediatrics* **2015**, *135*, 875–882. [CrossRef] [PubMed]
16. Yoshihara, A.; Yagi, M.; Sawamura, E.; Kanako, N.; Miyazaki, H. Evaluation of Personalized Oral Health Program with Mailing Pamphlets for Women. *Jpn. Soc. Dent. Health* **1999**, *49*, 809–815. [CrossRef]
17. World Health Organization. *Oral Health Surveys: Basic Methods*; World Health Organization: Geneva, Switzerland, 1997.
18. Greene, J.G.; Vermillion, J.R. The Simplified Oral Hygiene Index. *J. Am. Dent. Assoc.* **1964**, *68*, 7–13. [CrossRef] [PubMed]
19. Ministry of Internal Affairs and Communications. Japan Standard Industrial Classification 2013. Available online: http://www.soumu.go.jp/english/dgpp_ss/seido/sangyo/san13-3.htm (accessed on 23 November 2018).
20. Japan Dental Association. Lifelong Teeth Support Program. Available online: http://www.jda.or.jp/dentist/program/ (accessed on 23 November 2018).
21. Lawal, F.B.; Taiwo, J.O.; Oke, G.A. Impact of Oral Health on The Quality of Life of Elementary School Teachers. *Ethiop. J. Health Sci.* **2015**, *25*, 217–224. [CrossRef] [PubMed]

22. Arduino, P.G.; Lopetuso, E.; Carcieri, P.; Giacometti, S.; Carbone, M.; Tanteri, C.; Broccoletti, R. Professional oral hygiene treatment and detailed oral hygiene instructions in patients affected by mucous membrane pemphigoid with specific gingival localization: a pilot study in 12 patients. *Int. J. Dent. Hyg.* **2012**, *10*, 138–141. [CrossRef] [PubMed]
23. Menegaz, A.M.; Silva, A.E.R.; Cascaes, A.M. Educational interventions in health services and oral health: Systematic review. *Rev. Saúde Pública* **2018**, *52*. [CrossRef] [PubMed]
24. Oshikohji, T.; Shimazaki, Y.; Shinagawa, T.; Fukui, N.; Akifusa, S.; Yamashita, Y. Relationship between Receiving a Workplace Oral Health Examination Including Oral Health Instruction and Oral Health Status in the Japanese Adult Population. *J. Occup. Health* **2011**, *53*, 222–229. [CrossRef] [PubMed]
25. Abegg, C.; Fontanive, V.N.; Tsakos, G.; Davoglio, R.S.; de Oliveira, M.M.C. Adapting and testing the oral impacts on daily performances among adults and elderly in Brazil. *Gerodontology* **2015**, *32*, 46–52. [CrossRef] [PubMed]
26. Nagarajappa, R.; Batra, M.; Sanadhya, S.; Daryani, H.; Ramesh, G. Oral impacts on daily performance: Validity, reliability and prevalence estimates among Indian adolescents. *Int. J. Dent. Hyg.* **2018**, *16*, 279–285. [CrossRef] [PubMed]
27. Gülcan, F.; Nasir, E.; Ekbäck, G.; Ordell, S.; Åstrøm, A.N. Change in Oral Impacts on Daily Performances (OIDP) with increasing age: testing the evaluative properties of the OIDP frequency inventory using prospective data from Norway and Sweden. *BMC Oral Health* **2014**, *14*, 59. [CrossRef] [PubMed]
28. Peker, I.; Alkurt, M.T. Oral impacts on daily performance in Turkish adults attending a dental school. *J. Contemp. Dent. Pract.* **2014**, *15*, 92–98. [CrossRef] [PubMed]
29. Dettori, J.R. Loss to follow-up. *Evid.-Based Spine-Care J.* **2011**, *2*, 7–10. [CrossRef] [PubMed]

International Journal of
Environmental Research and Public Health

MDPI

Article

Multidisciplinary Intervention and Acceptance and Commitment Therapy for Return-to-Work and Increased Employability among Patients with Mental Illness and/or Chronic Pain: A Randomized Controlled Trial

Erik Berglund [1,*], Ingrid Anderzén [1], Åsa Andersén [1], Lars Carlsson [1,2], Catharina Gustavsson [1,2], Thorne Wallman [1,3] and Per Lytsy [1,4]

1. Department of Public Health and Caring Sciences, Uppsala University, Box 564, SE-75122 Uppsala, Sweden; Ingrid.Anderzen@pubcare.uu.se (I.A.); Asa.Andersen@pubcare.uu.se (Å.A.); Lars.Carlsson@ltdalarna.se (L.C.); Catharina.Gustavsson@ltdalarna.se (C.G.); Thorne.Wallman@dll.se (T.W.); Per.Lytsy@pubcare.uu.se (P.L.)
2. Centre for Clinical Research Dalarna, Uppsala University, SE-79182 Falun, Sweden
3. Centre for Clinical Research Sörmland, Uppsala University, SE-63188 Eskilstuna, Sweden
4. Department of Clinical Neuroscience, Division of Insurance Medicine, Karolinska Institute, SE-17177 Stockholm, Sweden

* Correspondence: erik.berglund@pubcare.uu.se; Tel.: +46-184716553; Fax: +46-184716675

Received: 10 September 2018; Accepted: 27 October 2018; Published: 31 October 2018

Abstract: Background: People on long-term sick leave often have a long-lasting process back to work, where the individuals may be in multiple and recurrent states; i.e., receiving different social security benefits or working, and over time they may shift between these states. The purpose of this study was to evaluate the effects of two vocational rehabilitation programs, compared to a control, on return-to-work (RTW) or increased employability in patients on long-term sick leave due to mental illness and/or chronic pain. Methods: In this randomized controlled study, 427 women and men were allocated to either (1) multidisciplinary team management, i.e., multidisciplinary assessments and individual rehabilitation management, (2) acceptance and commitment therapy (ACT), or (3) control. A positive outcome was defined as RTW or increased employability. The outcome was considered negative if the (part-time) wage was reduced or ceased, or if there was an indication of decreased employability. The outcome was measured one year after entry in the project and analyzed using binary and multinomial logistic regressions. Results: Participants in the multidisciplinary team group reported having RTW odds ratio (OR) 3.31 (95% CI 1.39–7.87) compared to the control group in adjusted models. Participants in the ACT group reported having increased employability OR 3.22 (95% CI 1.13–9.15) compared to the control group in adjusted models. Conclusions: This study of vocational rehabilitation in mainly female patients on long-term sick leave due to mental illness and/or chronic pain suggests that multidisciplinary team assessments and individually adapted rehabilitation interventions increased RTW and employability. Solely receiving the ACT intervention also increased employability.

Keywords: return-to-work; vocational rehabilitation; multidisciplinary rehabilitation; chronic pain; mental illness; sick leave

1. Introduction

Common mental illness and chronic pain are the two most frequent reasons for long-term sick leave in many countries, including Sweden [1,2]. In addition to the individual suffering related to mental illness and chronic pain, there is a major public/societal burden related to productivity losses [3]. In 2008/2009, the social insurance system in Sweden was reformed and maximum time sick-leave reimbursements were introduced; people on sick leave were transferred to the Swedish Public Employment Service (SPES) to have their work ability assessed [4]. During 2010–2012, about 40,000 people reached the maximum time for sick-leave compensation, and were among the first to have their work ability assessed by SPES, and thus be available for work in the labor market.

People on long-term sick leave often have a long-lasting process back to work [5], where the individuals may be in multiple and recurrent states; i.e., receiving different social security benefits or working, and over time they may shift between these states. This includes shifts between different social security benefits, programs, and part-time and full-time work [5]. Even if individuals do not necessarily move directly to return-to-work (RTW), they might come closer to, or further apart from, the labor market. Longer periods of sick leave are also known as a risk factor for not RTW [6,7]. Other factors that are associated with less RTW are female gender, age, pain, disability, depression, high work demands, previous sick leave, unemployment, and activity limitations [8].

Several strategies have been proposed to prevent work absence and facilitate RTW, and these interventions can be broadly classified as unimodal (for example individual psychotherapy), multimodal programs (team-based assessments and synchronized treatment by several health professionals), and interventions that target a structural level [9]. A recent systematic review of workplace interventions for RTW for musculoskeletal, pain-related, and mental health conditions concluded that there is strong evidence that multimodal intervention encompassing at least two of the three domains shortens duration away from work [10]. The current intervention project, which was carried out between 2010–2012, targeted people on long-term sick leave and at risk of losing their reimbursement from social insurance. Previous studies have foremost targeted people having short-term or medium-term sickness absence [10]. It is still not fully explored how people on very long-term sick leave RTW after experiencing mental illness or chronic pain. The aim of the study was to investigate the effects on RTW or changes in employability for people on long-term sick leave. The objective was to analyze the effects of two vocational rehabilitation interventions: a multidisciplinary team assessment and individualized treatment and/or unimodal psychotherapy with ACT intervention in patients on sick leave due to common mental disorders or chronic pain. To study an empirically relevant intervention outcome that reflects a stepwise rehabilitation perspective, individuals shifting between sources of income was used as an indicator of increased or decreased employability and RTW.

2. Materials and Methods

This study was conducted as a randomized controlled trial (RCT) and was implemented in two phases. In the first phase, only female participants were allocated to the multidisciplinary treatment (MDT) intervention group, the acceptance and commitment therapy (ACT) intervention group, or to the control group. In the second phase, both women and men participants were allocated either to the MDT group or the control group. The study sample from phase 1 has being used in previous studies [11,12]. The present study evaluates pooled data from both phases.

2.1. Subsection

Participants eligible for the study were women and men (men only in phase 2) on long-term sick leave or a temporary disability pension due to a mental illness and/or pain-related diagnosis in Uppsala County, Sweden. Mental illnesses included F-diagnoses (with the exceptions of the exclusion criteria diagnosis), and pain diagnoses included M-diagnoses and R-diagnoses defined in the International Statistical Classification of Diseases and Related Health Problems 10th revision (ICD-10). The office of the Swedish Social Insurance Agency (SSIA) identified 1331 individuals on sick leave, with these problems expected to reach their maximum time of sick leave between 2010–2012. After first inclusion, the individuals' sickness certificates were screened by a physician and an occupational therapist or psychologist to determine fulfilment of the inclusion criteria, and to ensure that they did not fulfil the exclusion criteria. The inclusion criteria were: (1) on sick leave for mental illness and/or chronic pain; (2) aged between 20–64 years. The exclusion criteria were: (1) at high risk for suicide; (2) ongoing alcohol/substance abuse; (3) major mental illness (schizophrenia, bipolar disorder type I, severe social dysfunction/personality disorder); (4) participation in psychotherapy or another vocational rehabilitation program. The SSIA initially identified 1331 people as eligible for the project; after screening, 418 were excluded from the project due to not meeting the inclusion criteria or meeting the exclusion criteria. The remaining 913 individuals were then contacted by mail with information about the project and invited to participate. Out of these, 473 did not respond or declined to participate. A further 13 people were excluded from the research part of the study (but received care in accordance with their allocation) due to being contacted before the formal approval by the ethics committee. The remaining 427 gave their consent to participate, and were randomized by the SSIA into the multidisciplinary team group (n = 178), ACT group (n = 102), or control group (n = 147). Out of these, 282 participants answered the outcome measure (see Figure 1). The inclusion, randomization, and allocation were performed consecutively during the project, about three to four months ahead of the date to match when participants were expected to transition to the SPES. Initially, the participants had an equal chance of being allocated into either the MDT, ACT, or control groups. In phase 2 of the study, two-thirds were randomized to the MDT group and one-third was allocated to the control group. The second phase also included men; the reason for also including men was an increased need among men for this type of intervention.

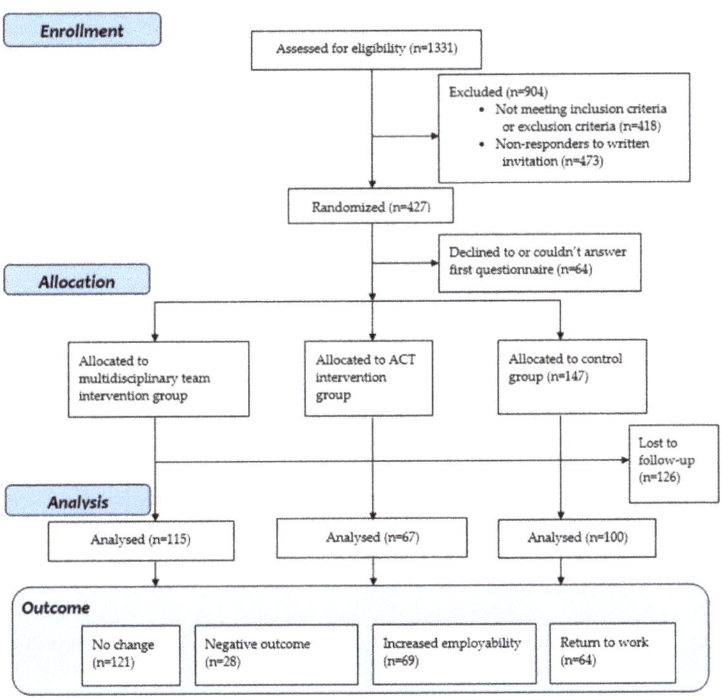

Figure 1. Flow chart of inclusion and follow-up procedure.

2.2. Interventions

The interventions started one to three months ahead of each participant's expected transfer to the SPES. Patients randomized to the MDT group met individually with professionals from a multidisciplinary team, including a psychologist (PS), a physician (MD), an occupational therapist (OT), and a social worker (SW). The health professional assessed the participant's strengths and limitations for RTW from each perspective. The team then met without the participant to establish an individualized rehabilitation plan, which was later brought back to the participant by one of the team members. The participants had the choice of accepting all, none, or parts of the rehabilitation plan's suggestions and interventions. The plan could involve further examinations, assessments, meetings, or psychotherapy (which then was delivered by the PS) for up to a period of one year. The team met weekly during the project period to evaluate the situation and synchronize the planned or ongoing activities for each participant. Participants allocated to the ACT group received solely ACT treatment. ACT is psychological therapy that uses cognitive behavioral therapy (CBT) and acceptance and mindfulness strategies, together with behavioral strategies, to increase function and quality of life rather than decreasing symptoms to increase psychological flexibility, which has shown to be of value for a number of long-lasting conditions [13]. Most psychotherapy sessions and meetings, for both the multidisciplinary team and ACT group, took place at the clinic, but there was also a possibility of conducting meetings at the participant's home, work, or elsewhere. Sessions were typically about an hour long.

In the second phase of the project, the possibility of being randomized to sole ACT treatment (ACT group) was omitted. The reason was that during phase 1, it turned out that some participants randomized to the ACT group were not interested in receiving ACT, but were interested in receiving other types of treatments. Participants randomized to the MDT group (in both phases) had the option of receiving ACT if suggested by the psychologist after assessment. In addition to the treatments, all of the participants also had scheduled collaboration meetings with their administrator at the SPES, the SSIA, and their contact person within the project. These meetings aimed to ascertain the rehabilitation plan and its goal for the individual as well as for the participating organizations.

The control group did not receive any intervention organized within the intervention project, but was free to receive the usual assistance and care provided by their regular contact with the SSIA, SPES, and potential contacts with healthcare providers. The control group responded to the same follow-up questionnaires as the intervention groups.

2.3. Questionnaires and Outcome Measures

Data collected before the intervention included demographics, such as the respondent's gender, age, and educational level (categorized as compulsory school, secondary school or equivalent, or university). Factors related to mental health were assessed using the Hospital Anxiety and Depression Scale (HADS) [14]. The HADS is a 14-item scale; seven of the items relate to anxiety, and seven relate to depression. The General Self-Efficacy scale (GSE) was used to measure the participants' perceived self-efficacy [15]. The GSE consists of 10 statements and is answered on a four-point Likert scale ranging from 1 = "Not at all true" to 4 = "Completely true". The items were summed to give a total score of 10 to 40. A mean value was calculated as the sum of all of the answers divided by the number of statements, as long as no more than three statements were missing [16]. The current version of the GSE has been translated into Swedish and has been validated [17]. There is no definite cut-off score for the self-efficacy scale. In this study, the mean value (2.3) of self-efficacy was used to categorize participants with lower (<2.3) versus higher ($\geq$2.3) self-efficacy. The work-related predictor variables that were used in this study included employment contract status (unemployed or employed), extent of sick leave (full-time or part-time), and years with income replacement, which were collected through SSIA registry data.

To measure intervention outcomes, the participants responded to a mailed follow-up questionnaire 12 months from randomization (see Figure 1).

This study's primary outcome uses self-reported sources of income at baseline and follow-up at 12 months to create an outcome variable with four exclusive categories that were believed to capture both changes in RTW as well as changes in employability. Outcome was measured by using the following question: "How do you provide for yourself?" Participants indicated answers in percentages of income from various sources currently and a year earlier. Income sources included: wages (through employment or own business); sickness compensation from the SSIA; and compensation through the SPES. The answers were then compared. If a person reported having increased their proportion of wage due to more work as source of income at 12 months, then they were categorized as "RTW" (having returned-to-work in full or to some degree). A person was categorized as having an "increased employability" if the compensation change indicated increased availability for work, such as increased compensation from the SPES instead of sick leave compensation from the SSIA, as an indication that the person was (more) eligible for work in the labor market. Outcome was considered "negative" if the (part-time) wage was reduced or stopped, or if there was an indication of decreased employability (increased compensation from the SSIA without increased wage). An unchanged outcome was defined as having no changes in wage, employability, or sickness benefits. The outcome variable was further dichotomized for the binary logistic regression analysis into those having a positive (having RTW or increased employability) or negative (having negative or unchanged outcome) outcome.

2.4. Analyses

Differences in outcome between the two intervention groups and the control group were investigated using Chi-square tests. The intervention's effects were analyzed using binary and multinomial logistic regression models. In randomized controlled trials, confounders are believed to be equally distributed between compared groups. However, it might be of interest to investigate the associations among different factors to the outcome. It might be of further interest to adjust for confounders that are potentially associated with the attrition. To adjust for potential predictors and confounders and other variables that may be associated with the outcome, a stepwise approach was performed using sets of variables. In model 1, the intervention group was adjusted for age and education level. In model 2, additional adjustments were made for HADS, self-efficacy, employment contract, extent of sick leave, and years with income replacement.

Multinomial logistic regressions were used comparing a negative outcome, increased employability, and RTW to those with no changes as a reference category. Multinomial logistic regressions were also performed and adjusted for potential confounders. A complete case analysis was performed in which respondents answered the outcome measure; also, due to a large number of missing values in the outcome variable (34.0%), a sensitivity analysis was performed, in which missing participants were assumed to have made no change in outcome (reference category). All of the tests were two-sided, and a level of $p < 0.05$ was considered statistically significant. The statistical analyses were performed using SPSS statistics (IBM Corp, Armonk, NY, USA), version 22.0.

2.5. Ethical Considerations and Trial Registration

All of the participants provided written informed consent for the study. The first phase of the study was approved by the Regional Ethical Review Board of Uppsala in 2010 (Reg. no. 2010/088) and the extension (second phase) of the project was approved in 2011 (Reg. no. 2010/088/1). In the reporting of the results of this trial, we have tried to follow the Consolidated Standards of Reporting Trials (CONSORT) checklist as far as possible. The study was registered at the Clinicaltrials.gov Register Platform (ID NCT03343457) on 15 November 2017 (retrospectively registered).

3. Results

The average age of the study group was 48.9 years (SD 8.3). The study group consisted of 94.7% women and 5.3% men. Secondary school was the most common completed education level. Most of the participants (68.1%) had an employer, and the average time on sick leave was 7.7 years (SD 3.2). About half of the participants were on full-time sick leave, and half were on part-time sick leave.

One-third of the participants were on sick leave for psychiatric disorders, about one-third were on sick leave for pain-related conditions, and about one-third were on sick leave for a combination of psychiatric and pain-related disorders. Common pain-related problems were fibromyalgia and pain in the back, neck, or joints. Common mental disorders were depression (current and recurrent) and stress-related and anxiety disorders.

Participants in the multidisciplinary team group attended on average 4.4 (SD 5.4) sessions delivered by the MD, OT, PT and SW, and 4.7 (SD 6.4) sessions with a psychologist who provided ACT, for a total average of 9.1 (SD 8.4) sessions. Participants in the ACT group attended on average 8.0 (SD 6.0) sessions with a psychologist providing ACT, as shown in Table 1. Of the complete cases in this study, 66% of the participants in the MDT group received at least one meeting with a psychologist providing ACT as one part of their individual plan.

Table 1. Characteristics of study participants.

Variable	Group/Measure	MDT Group	ACT Group	Control Group	Total
Sex	Female	90.4	100.0	93.9	93.9
	Male	9.6	0.0	6.1	6.1
Age, years	Mean (SD)	49.9 (8.5)	47.8 (7.8)	48.0 (8.3)	48.7 (8.3)
Education	Compulsory school	22.2	14.7	21.1	20.1
	Secondary school or equal	48.9	44.0	46.5	46.9
	University	28.9	41.3	32.5	33.0
HADS [a]	Anxiety, mean (SD)	10.9 (5.0)	10.1 (4.9)	11.1 (5.3)	10.8 (5.1)
	Depression, mean (SD)	9.5 (4.7)	8.5 (4.2)	9.1 (5.1)	9.1 (4.7)
SE [b]	SE, mean	2.3 (0.7)	2.4 (0.7)	2.3 (0.7)	2.3 (0.7)
Employment contract	Employed	66.3	57.8	61.9	62.8
	Not employed	33.7	42.2	38.1	37.2
Extent of sick leave	Full-time	55.7	53.9	55.2	55.1
	Part-time	44.3	46.1	44.8	44.9
Years with income replacement	Mean (SD)	8.1 (3.3)	7.6 (3.1)	7.5 (3.2)	7.8 (3.2)
Dosage of intervention	Sessions with psychologist, mean (SD)	4.7 (6.4)	8.0 (6.0)	0.0 (0.0)	3.9 (5.9)
	Sessions with MD [c]. OT [d]. PT [e] and SW [f], mean (SD)	4.4 (5.4)	0.0 (0.0)	0.0 (0.0)	1.8 (4.1)
	Total sessions in the project, mean (SD)	9.1 (8.4)	8.0 (6.0)	0.0 (0.0)	5.7 (7.4)

Figures as percentages if not stated otherwise. [a] Hospital Anxiety and Depression Scale, [b] Self-efficacy, [c] Physician, [d] Occupational therapist, [e] Physical therapist, [f] Social worker. ACT: acceptance and commitment therapy.

3.1. Return-to-Work, Increased Employability, Negative Outcome, or No Change

At the 12-month follow-up, 64 participants (22.7%) had RTW, 69 participants (24.5%) had increased employability, 28 participants (9.9%) had a negative outcome, and 121 participants (42.9%) had not changed in any direction. Among participants in the multidisciplinary team, 31.1% had RTW, 27.0% had increased employability, and 4.3% had a negative outcome. Among participants in the ACT group, 17.9% had RTW, 35.8% had increased employability, and 9.0% had a negative outcome, as shown in Table 2.

Table 2. Return to work, increased employability, negative, or unchanged outcome according to different groups.

Outcome	MDT Group	ACT Group	Control Group	Overall
RTW (%)	31.3 **	17.9 **	16.0 **	22.7
Increased employability (%)	27.0 **	35.8 **	14.0 **	24.5
Negative outcome (%)	4.3 **	9.0 **	17.0 **	9.9
No change (%)	37.4 **	37.3 **	53.0 **	42.9

Pearson Chi-Square test was used for proportions. ** $p \leq 0.01$. RTW: return-to-work.

3.2. Logistic Regression Models

The adjusted binary logistic regression analysis showed that the MDT group had an OR of 4.62 (95% CI 2.27–9.41) for RTW or increased employability. The corresponding number for the ACT group was OR 2.35 (95% CI 1.07–5.19), as shown in Table 3.

Table 3. Binary logistic regressions presenting odds ratios (OR) of reporting return to work or increased employability vs. negative or unchanged outcomes.

Variable	Group/Measure	Crude OR (95% CI)	Model 1 OR (95% CI)	Model 2 OR (95% CI)
Intervention group	Group			
	Control (ref.)	1	1	1
	MDT[a] group	3.26 ** (1.85–5.74)	4.22 ** (2.18–8.15)	4.62 ** (2.27–9.41)
	ACT[b] group	2.71 ** (1.42–5.16)	2.42 * (1.17–4.97)	2.35 * (1.07–5.19)
Demographic	Age	0.96 * (0.94–0.99)	0.96 * (0.92 - 0.99)	0.96 * (0.93–1.00)
	Education level			
	Compulsory school	1	1	1
	Secondary school-equal	1.87 (0.91–3.82)	1.60 (0.74–3.46)	1.98 (0.85–4.58)
	University	1.24 (0.58–2.66)	1.23 (0.55–2.77)	1.28 (0.53–3.11)
Health and work related factors	HADS[c], Anxiety	0.99 (0.94–1.04)		1.05 (0.96–1.14)
	HADS[c] Depression	0.97 (0.92–1.02)		0.97 (0.89–1.06)
	Self-efficacy (<2.30)	1		1
	Self-efficacy (≥2.30)	1.76 * (1.07–2.89)		2.75 ** (1.33–5.72)
	Employment contract			
	Not employed	1		1
	Employed	0.70 (0.42–1.15)		0.78 (0.38–1.61)
	Extent of sick leave			
	Full time	1		1
	Part time	0.67 (0.42–1.07)		0.56 (0.29–1.10)
	Years with income replacement	0.97 (0.90–1.05)		0.97 (0.88- 1.06)
Nagelkerke r^2			14.0%	24.1%

Odds ratio (OR), 95% CI: 95% confidence interval. * $p < 0.05$, ** $p < 0.01$. [a]Multidisciplinary treatment. [b]Acceptance and Commitment Therapy. [c]Hospital Anxiety and Depression Scale, ranging from 0 to 21. Model 1 = Intervention group + age + education level, Model 2 = Model 1 + HADS + Self-efficacy + Employment contract + Extent of sick leave + Years with income replacement.

3.3. Multinomial Regression Models

The adjusted multinomial logistic regression analysis showed that the multidisciplinary team group had an odds ratio (OR) of 3.31 (95% CI 1.39–7.87) for RTW, an OR of 4.24 (95% CI 1.60–11.26) for increased employability, and an OR of 0.19 (95% CI 0.05–0.72) on negative outcome. The adjusted multinomial logistic regression analysis showed that the ACT intervention group had an OR of 3.22 (95% CI 1.13–9.15) on increased employability, but no significant effect on RTW. See Table 4.

Due to a large number of internal missing values in the outcome measure (34.0%), a multinomial logistic regression analysis was also performed, in which non-responding participants were assumed to have made no change (reference category) in outcome. Similar results, despite somewhat lowered effects, showed that the multidisciplinary team group had an adjusted OR of 2.57 (95% CI 1.19–5.58) on RTW; an adjusted OR of 2.80 (95% CI 1.20–6.52) on increased employability; and an adjusted OR of 0.18 (95% CI 0.05–0.62) on negative outcome. The ACT intervention group had an adjusted OR of 2.79 (95% CI 1.12–6.97) on increased employability.

Table 4. Results of multinomial logistic regression of intervention group's effect on negative outcome, return to work, or increased employability.

Variable		Return to Work or Change in System Position					
		Negative Outcome		Increased Employability		Return to Work	
		Crude OR (95% CI)	Adjusted OR (95% CI)	Crude OR (95% CI)	Adjusted OR (95% CI)	Crude OR (95% CI)	Adjusted OR (95% CI)
Intervention group	Group						
	Control (ref.)	1	1	1	1	1	1
	MDT[a] group	0.36 (0.12–1.06)	0.19 * (0.05–0.72)	2.73 ** (1.29–5.77)	4.24 ** (1.60–11.26)	2.77 ** (1.36–5.66)	3.31 ** (1.39–7.87)
	ACT[b] group	0.75 (0.26–2.13)	0.36 (0.10–1.35)	3.63 ** (1.61–8.19)	3.22 * (1.13–9.15)	1.56 (0.66–3.86)	1.36 (0.48–3.86)
Demographic	Age	0.99 (0.94–1.04)	0.94 (0.88–1.01)	0.95 ** (0.92–0.99)	0.94 * (0.90–0.99)	0.97 (0.93–1.01)	0.96 (0.92–1.01)
	Education level						
	Compulsory school	1	1	1	1	1	1
	Secondary school or equal	1.41 (0.40–4.91)	0.76 (0.16–3.57)	3.78 * (1.31–10.92)	4.52 * (1.29–15.87)	1.16 (0.49–2.77)	1.08 (0.40–2.89)
	University	1.44 (0.40–5.22)	0.61 (0.13–2.98)	1.79 (0.57–5.64)	2.24 (0.58–8.71)	1.10 (0.45–2.74)	0.85 (0.30–2.39)
Health and work-related factors	HADS[c], Anxiety	0.93 (0.85–1.01)	0.92 (0.80–1.06)	0.99 (0.93–1.06)	1.02 (0.92–1.14)	0.96 (0.90–1.02)	1.05 (0.94–1.16)
	HADS[c], Depression	0.93 (0.85–1.02)	1.14 (0.96–1.35)	0.96 (0.90–1.02)	0.98 (0.87–1.10)	0.96 (0.89–1.02)	1.01 (0.90–1.13)
	Self-efficacy (<2.30)	1	1	1	1	1	1
	Self-efficacy (≥2.30)	1.99 (0.84–4.73)	1.81 (0.52–6.34)	1.74 (0.93–3.25)	2.71* (1.07–6.91)	2.35 * (1.22–4.50)	3.31 ** (1.34–8.15)
	Employment contract						
	Not employed	1	1	1	1	1	1
	Have work	3.96 * (1.13–13.93)	1.66 (0.32–8.70)	0.52 * (0.28–0.95)	0.64 (0.27–1.54)	1.55 (0.78–3.11)	1.09 (0.44–2.71)
	Extent of sick leave						
	Full time	1	1	1	1	1	1
	Part time	15.65 ** (3.55–68.94)	34.57 ** (3.84–311.31)	0.56 (0.30–1.05)	0.44 (0.17–1.02)	1.65 (0.89–3.05)	1.42 (0.62–3.21)
	Years, with income replacement	1.07 (0.94–1.22)	1.07 (0.89–1.29)	0.99 (0.90–1.09)	0.99 (0.89–1.12)	0.98 (0.89–1.07)	0.96 (0.85–1.07)

Reference outcome category: No change. For the adjusted model, Nagelkerke r^2 = 37.8%. * $p < 0.05$, ** $p < 0.01$. [a]Multidisciplinary treatment. [b]Acceptance and Commitment Therapy. [c]Hospital Anxiety and Depression Scale, ranging from 0 to 21. Odds ratio (OR), significant level and confidence interval (CI) for having made RTW or (positive) system position change or negative change.

4. Discussion

This study aimed to investigate the effects on RTW and increased employability of two vocational rehabilitation interventions in patients on long-term sick leave due to mental illness and/or chronic pain. In this study, a non-dichotomous outcome was used to capture not only RTW, but also changes in increased or decreased employability. The results indicate that multidisciplinary interventions and individualized treatments may increase RTW and employability in patients on long-term sick leave due to common mental illness and/or chronic pain. The results in this study are similar to results presented in other studies regarding RTW [18–23]. Also, in review studies, this type of multi-domain intervention seems to be the most effective intervention for RTW outcome when managing musculoskeletal and pain-related conditions [10]. The results also suggest that multidisciplinary team and ACT interventions may increase employability, i.e., transferring individuals in the insurance system to increased availability for employment and work.

One reason for removing the separate ACT group in the second phase of the project was that the intervention providers discovered that some people who were randomized to ACT were not keen on receiving psychological therapy [24]; this might also explain the somewhat weaker outcome of the ACT group.

At the time when the study was conducted, the participants were about to lose their sickness insurance benefits due to a major change in the social insurance system. These circumstances may have led to the inclusion of participants who would not otherwise have been motivated to participate in vocational rehabilitation, thus creating a study population with relatively low motivation and belief in their own ability to RTW. Since longer periods of sick leave and absence from the labor market are known risk factors for RTW failure [6,7], this project was believed to target a difficult group. Taking all of the factors into account, including the interventions, the multinomial regression explained 37.8% (r^2) of the outcome, which leaves a 62.2% unexplained variance that is dependent on factors that were not assessed in the model. This indicates that there are other factors outside the intervention program that affect the outcomes. For instance, this study did not include any work-directed modifications or interventions, which is seen as a factor to increase the chances of RTW goals [25]. The causal chain between sick leave, mental illness, and chronic pain is not fully explored. Sick leave is warranted by an inability to work, but sick leave may in itself also contribute to depression, unhealthy living, and stress [26]. Previous research has identified several important factors for RTW [8]. Current demands in the labor market are important for re-entry to the workforce, including factors on a systemic/organizational level [27]. Many of these factors are not affected by health and rehabilitation interventions such as this project. Instead, several of these factors are found "upstream" in the analogy of a "river", which is used to describe how previous social, financial, environmental, and historic factors ultimately go on to profoundly influence present outcomes [28]. In the present study, this implies that even if a participant in the project reduces their ill health and increases employability, these results might not be captured in a sole RTW outcome; thus, RTW is (also) dependent on upstream factors that are determined outside the reach of the project. Especially when considering the long-term sick leave period among the project participants (on average 7.7 years), it is reasonable to assume that the labor market has changed in several aspects during their absence, such as work content and demands etc. Therefore, an outcome measure was constructed that also captures changes in different transition stages made by program participants, such as increased employability. This does not apply to all of the participants; several had part-time jobs.

In Sweden, as well as in many other countries, concern and efforts provided by society for people on sick leave are regulated by different laws and principals and divided among different authorities. There have been doubts about whether a multi-actor model is optimal, and limitations have been found in the system. This project included several authorities and professions with one collaborative goal: to support the participants in their vocational rehabilitation and increase their likelihood for RTW. This project was also a collaborative challenge, as different professions in the MDT worked closely with one goal. It should be noted that the MDT and ACT groups received about the same total number of sessions in the project. The ACT group only received sessions with an ACT psychologist; the MDT group received on average about half of the sessions from an ACT psychologist and half from the other professions.

The major findings in this study imply that a multidisciplinary team-based intervention directed at people on long-term sick leave, including ACT counseling, seems to help people, even those on long-term sick leave, to RTW. The findings add to the evidence that multidisciplinary interventions such as vocational rehabilitation may increase RTW among patients with mental illness and/or chronic pain [29].

There is a need to further investigate multidisciplinary RTW interventions, determine their core components, and consider combining them with workplace collaboration, including the employer and interventions in the work environment.

Strengths and Limitations

The strengths of this study include the randomized prospective controlled design and the experimental design, which suggest that the effects on RTW are in fact effects of the interventions.

This study also has some limitations. Reliable evidence for RTW should be assessed using information on validated employment and work activity. In this study, the outcome was based on self-reported data and actual RTW was not measured; instead, a changed proportion of income source was used as an indicator for changes in working status and employability. However, similar studies often use proxy variables for measuring RTW [23]. Since the data—both exposures and outcomes—are self-reported, there is a risk of recall bias. Another limitation of this study is that education level, HADS, and self-efficacy were measured after randomization, so the scores could have already been influenced by the knowledge of intervention group affiliation. The results were not adjusted by type of disease (mental illness or chronic pain).

Many participants did not show up, dropped out, or did not answer the follow-up questionnaires, which weakens the assessment of the outcomes. There could be different reasons for the high attrition: perhaps the participants did not actually want to be part of the project, were too sick to participate, or felt they had a problem that would not benefit from the project.

Since participants in the treatment groups received individual treatment as well as organizational collaboration, this raises the question of which of these interventions mediated the effect, if either. The reason to include organizational collaboration was to set and mutually agree on each individual's RTW goal. Another potential problem with this study is that the two types of multidisciplinary team interventions that were combined were not identical, but they were similar.

5. Conclusions and Practice Implications

This study of vocational rehabilitation in men and women on long-term sick leave due to mental illness and/or chronic pain showed that multidisciplinary team assessments and individually adapted rehabilitation interventions increased RTW and employability. Sole ACT intervention increased employability.

The study implies that it is possible to increase RTW among people on long-term sick leave due to mental illness and/or chronic pain with a multidisciplinary rehabilitation intervention. Multidisciplinary team rehabilitation and sole ACT also seem to be useful for increasing employability and gradually moving people in a stepwise positive direction, through the welfare system, and eventually toward RTW.

Author Contributions: E.B. designed the study, undertook the statistical modeling and led the writing. I.A., Å.A. and P.L. designed the study, contributed to data interpretation, handling of data and drafting of the manuscript. L.C., C.G., and T.W. contributed to data interpretation and drafting of the manuscript. All authors approved the final version of the manuscript.

Funding: This work was supported by REHSAM, under Grant RS2011/010, a research program financed by the Swedish Ministry of Health and Social Affairs, the Social Insurance Agency. We are also grateful to all of the respondents who took the time to answer the questionnaires.

Conflicts of Interest: The authors declare no conflict of interest.

References

1. Henderson, M.; Harvey, S.B.; Overland, S.; Mykletun, A.; Hotopf, M. Work and common psychiatric disorders. *J. R. Soc. Med.* **2011**, *104*, 198–207. [CrossRef] [PubMed]
2. Linder, J.; Ekholm, K.S.; Jansen, G.B.; Lundh, G.; Ekholm, J. Long-term sick leavers with difficulty in resuming work: Comparisons between psychiatric-somatic comorbidity and monodiagnosis. *Int. J. Rehabil. Res.* **2009**, *32*, 20–35. [CrossRef] [PubMed]
3. Dewa, C.S.; Loong, D.; Bonato, S.; Joosen, M.C.W. The effectiveness of return-to-work interventions that incorporate work-focused problem-solving skills for workers with sickness absences related to mental disorders: A systematic literature review. *BMJ Open* **2015**, *5*, e007122. [CrossRef] [PubMed]
4. Government Offices of Sweden. Regeringens Proposition 2007/08:136. En Reformerad Sjukskrivningsprocess för ökad Återgång i Arbete. [Government Proposition 2007/08: 136. A Reformed Sick Leave Process to Increase Return to Work]. Available online: https://www.riksdagen.se/sv/dokument-lagar/dokument/proposition/en-reformerad-sjukskrivningsprocess-for-okad_GV03136/html (accessed on 29 May 2018).
5. Oyeflaten, I.; Lie, S.A.; Ihlebaek, C.M.; Eriksen, H.R. Multiple transitions in sick leave, disability benefits, and return to work—A 4-year follow-up of patients participating in a work-related rehabilitation program. *BMC Public Health* **2012**, *12*, 748. [CrossRef] [PubMed]
6. Marnetoft, S.U.; Selander, J. Long-term effects of early versus delayed vocational rehabilitation—A four-year follow-up. *Disabil. Rehabil.* **2002**, *24*, 741–745. [CrossRef] [PubMed]

7. Roelen, C.A.; Norder, G.; Koopmans, P.C.; van Rhenen, W.; van der Klink, J.J.; Bultmann, U. Employees sick-listed with mental disorders: Who returns to work and when? *J. Occup. Rehabil.* **2012**, *22*, 409–417. [CrossRef] [PubMed]
8. Cancelliere, C.; Donovan, J.; Stochkendahl, M.J.; Biscardi, M.; Ammendolia, C.; Myburgh, C.; Cassidy, J.D. Factors affecting return to work after injury or illness: Best evidence synthesis of systematic reviews. *Chiropr. Man. Ther.* **2016**, *24*, 32. [CrossRef] [PubMed]
9. Van der Klink, J.J.; Blonk, R.W.; Schene, A.H.; van Dijk, F.J. The benefits of interventions for work-related stress. *Am. J. Public Health* **2001**, *91*, 270–276. [PubMed]
10. Cullen, K.L.; Irvin, E.; Collie, A.; Clay, F.; Gensby, U.; Jennings, P.A.; Hogg-Johnson, S.; Kristman, V.; Laberge, M.; McKenzie, D.; et al. Effectiveness of workplace interventions in return-to-work for musculoskeletal, pain-related and mental health conditions: An update of the evidence and messages for practitioners. *J. Occup. Rehabil.* **2018**, *28*, 1–15. [CrossRef] [PubMed]
11. Lytsy, P.; Larsson, K.; Anderzen, I. Health in women on long-term sick leave because of pain or mental illness. *Int. J. Rehabil. Res.* **2015**, *38*, 27–33. [CrossRef] [PubMed]
12. Lytsy, P.; Carlsson, L.; Anderzen, I. Effectiveness of two vocational rehabilitation programmes in women with long-term sick leave due to pain syndrome or mental illness: 1-Year follow-up of a randomized controlled trial. *J. Rehabil. Med.* **2017**, *49*, 170–177. [CrossRef] [PubMed]
13. Hacker, T.; Stone, P.; MacBeth, A. Acceptance and commitment therapy—Do we know enough? Cumulative and sequential meta-analyses of randomized controlled trials. *J. Affect. Disord.* **2016**, *190*, 551–565. [CrossRef] [PubMed]
14. Zigmond, A.S.; Snaith, R.P. The hospital anxiety and depression scale. *Acta Psychiatr. Scand.* **1983**, *67*, 361–370. [CrossRef] [PubMed]
15. Schwarzer, R.; Jerusalem, M. Self-efficacy measurement and generalized self-efficacy scale. In *Measures in Health Psychology: A User's Portfolio*; Johnston, M.W., John, S.C.W., Eds.; NFER-NELSON: Windsor, UK, 1995; pp. 33–39.
16. Schwarzer, R. Everything You Wanted to Know about the General Self-Efficacy Scale but Were Afraid to Ask. Available online: http://userpage.fu-berlin.de/~health/faq_gse.pdf (accessed on 6 July 2016).
17. Love, J.; Moore, C.D.; Hensing, G. Validation of the Swedish translation of the general self-efficacy scale. *Qual. Life Res.* **2012**, *21*, 1249–1253. [CrossRef] [PubMed]
18. Van der Klink, J.J.; Blonk, R.W.; Schene, A.H.; van Dijk, F.J. Reducing long term sickness absence by an activating intervention in adjustment disorders: A cluster randomised controlled design. *Occup. Environ. Med.* **2003**, *60*, 429–437. [CrossRef] [PubMed]
19. Franche, R.-L.; Cullen, K.; Clarke, J.; Irvin, E.; Sinclair, S.; Frank, J. Workplace-based return-to-work interventions: A systematic review of the quantitative literature. *J. Occup. Rehabil.* **2005**, *15*, 607–631. [CrossRef] [PubMed]
20. Brouwers, E.P.; Tiemens, B.G.; Terluin, B.; Verhaak, P.F. Effectiveness of an intervention to reduce sickness absence in patients with emotional distress or minor mental disorders: A randomized controlled effectiveness trial. *Gen. Hosp. Psychiatry* **2006**, *28*, 223–229. [CrossRef] [PubMed]
21. Van Rhenen, W.; Blonk, R.W.; Schaufeli, W.B.; van Dijk, F.J. Can sickness absence be reduced by stress reduction programs: On the effectiveness of two approaches. *Int. Arch. Occup. Environ. Health* **2007**, *80*, 505–515. [CrossRef] [PubMed]
22. Netterstrøm, B.; Friebel, L.; Ladegaard, Y. Effects of a multidisciplinary stress treatment programme on patient return to work rate and symptom reduction: Results from a randomised, wait-list controlled trial. *Psychother. Psychosom.* **2013**, *82*, 177–186. [CrossRef] [PubMed]
23. Momsen, A.H.; Stapelfeldt, C.M.; Nielsen, C.V.; Nielsen, M.B.; Aust, B.; Rugulies, R.; Jensen, C. Effects of a randomized controlled intervention trial on return to work and health care utilization after long-term sickness absence. *BMC Public Health* **2016**, *16*, 1149. [CrossRef] [PubMed]
24. Hayes, S.C.; Luoma, J.B.; Bond, F.W.; Masuda, A.; Lillis, J. Acceptance and commitment therapy: Model, processes and outcomes. *Behav. Res. Ther.* **2006**, *44*, 1–25. [CrossRef] [PubMed]
25. Nieuwenhuijsen, K.; Faber, B.; Verbeek, J.H.; Neumeyer-Gromen, A.; Hees, H.L.; Verhoeven, A.C.; van der Feltz-Cornelis, C.M.; Bultmann, U. Interventions to improve return to work in depressed people. *Cochrane Database Syst. Rev.* **2014**, *12*, CD006237. [CrossRef] [PubMed]

26. Vingard, E.; Alexanderson, K.; Norlund, A. Swedish council on technology assessment in health care (SBU). Chapter 9. Consequences of being on sick leave. *Scand. J. Public Health Suppl.* **2004**, *63*, 207–215. [CrossRef] [PubMed]
27. Soklaridis, S.; Ammendolia, C.; Cassidy, D. Looking upstream to understand low back pain and return to work: Psychosocial factors as the product of system issues. *Soc. Sci. Med.* **2010**, *71*, 1557–1566. [CrossRef] [PubMed]
28. Gehlert, S.; Sohmer, D.; Sacks, T.; Mininger, C.; McClintock, M.; Olopade, O. Targeting health disparities: A model linking upstream determinants to downstream interventions: Knowing about the interaction of societal factors and disease can enable targeted interventions to reduce health disparities. *Health Aff.* **2008**, *27*, 339–349. [CrossRef] [PubMed]
29. Salmi, P.; Svedberg, P.; Hagberg, J.; Lundh, G.; Linder, J.; Alexanderson, K. Outcome of multidisciplinary investigations of long-term sickness absentees. *Disabil. Rehabil.* **2009**, *31*, 131–137. [CrossRef] [PubMed]

International Journal of
Environmental Research and Public Health

MDPI

Article

Reduced Lung Function among Workers in Primary Coffee Processing Factories in Ethiopia: A Cross Sectional Study

Samson Wakuma Abaya [1,2,3,*], Magne Bråtveit [2], Wakgari Deressa [1], Abera Kumie [1] and Bente E. Moen [2,3]

1 Department of Preventive Medicine, School of Public Health, Addis Ababa University, P.O. Box 90861000 Addis Ababa, Ethiopia; deressaw@gmail.com (W.D.); aberakumie2@yahoo.com (A.K.)
2 Occupational and Environmental Medicine, Department of Global Public Health and Primary Care, University of Bergen, 5020 Bergen, Norway; Magne.Bratveit@uib.no (M.B.); Bente.Moen@uib.no (B.E.M.)
3 Centre for International Health, Department of Global Public Health and Primary Care, University of Bergen, 5009 Bergen, Norway
* Correspondence: samson_wakuma@yahoo.com; Tel.: +251-92-394-0998

Received: 13 October 2018; Accepted: 28 October 2018; Published: 31 October 2018

Abstract: Dust exposure is one of the major risk factors for respiratory health in many workplaces, including coffee factories. The aim of this study was to assess the prevalence of respiratory symptoms and lung function reduction among workers in Ethiopian primary coffee processing factories, compared to a control group of workers. A total of 115 coffee workers and 110 water bottling workers were involved in this study, from 12 coffee and 3 water bottling factories in Ethiopia, respectively. The chronic respiratory symptoms were assessed using a structured interview, using a standardized questionnaire adopted from the American Thoracic Society (ATS). The lung function tests were performed according to the ATS recommendation for spirometry. The coffee workers had a significantly higher prevalence of coughing, coughing with sputum, breathlessness, work-related shortness of breath, and wheezing compared with the controls. The prevalence ratio of work-related shortness of breath (PR = 3.7, 95% CI: 1.6–8.7) and wheezing (PR = 3.3, 95% CI: 1.3–8.4) was significantly higher for the coffee workers compared to the controls. The coffee workers in the age groups 28–39 years and ≥40 years, had a significantly lower forced vital capacity and forced expiratory volume in 1 s compared to the controls in the similar age groups. The findings indicated the need for longitudinal studies on the possible effect of coffee dust on respiratory health of coffee production workers.

Keywords: coffee workers; dust exposure; Ethiopia; lung function; respiratory symptoms

1. Introduction

Several studies have indicated an association between working in coffee factories and respiratory health problems. Allergies have been suggested to be related to the problems [1–7]. A few older studies conducted in primary coffee processing factories have indicated that exposure to coffee dust is likely to cause acute and chronic respiratory symptoms in these factories as well [8–11].

Recently, studies were conducted in primary coffee processing factories in Tanzania. These demonstrated a higher prevalence of chronic respiratory symptoms in coffee workers than among the controls [11,12]. The primary coffee processing factories are factories that perform mechanical cleaning of the debris from the coffee-making process, such as the hulling, grading, hand picking, and packing of green coffee beans. The lung function parameters were not different between the coffee workers and the controls [12]. The Robusta coffee workers had higher prevalence of asthma symptoms than Arabica coffee workers [12]. The findings related to lung function were not clear, and more studies are needed for conclusive information regarding the respiratory health of coffee workers. Ethiopia produces exclusively Arabica coffee. The respiratory health impact of working with these coffee beans has not yet been explored. In addition, the coffee pre-processing methods used on the farms in Ethiopia is different from the ones used in Tanzania. Moreover, a recent study conducted in the coffee factories of Ethiopia found much higher levels of personal dust exposure compared with the levels measured in the Tanzanian factories [13].

In Ethiopia, more than 50% of foreign income comes from coffee, with an estimated 15 million people relying on coffee production for their livelihood [14]. Understanding the level of respiratory problems in Ethiopian coffee processing factories can generate information that could aid policy makers and other relevant stakeholders to develop any necessary preventive and control methods.

Studying respiratory disease is difficult in these types of factories, as a healthy worker effect may occur. This means that workers developing an illness may stop working, and may therefore not be found at the work sites. Cohort studies are difficult to perform, as the methods for tracing persons over longer periods is challenging. Case-control studies are also difficult to perform in Ethiopia, as the population does not have easy access to hospitals, and are treated at a large number of small health units. Therefore, a comparative cross-sectional study design was chosen, where the coffee factory workers were compared to a control group.

The aim of this study was to assess the prevalence of respiratory symptoms and to study the lung function among workers in the primary coffee processing factories of Ethiopia, and to compare these findings with a control group of water bottling workers. The methodology can detect early signs of respiratory diseases and is therefore useful in a company setting of relatively healthy workers.

2. Materials and Methods

2.1. Study Site and Period

There are about 746 primary coffee processing factories in Ethiopia. Almost all are found in three regions, Oromia; Addis Ababa; and Southern Nations, Nationalities and Peoples' Region (SNNPR). We did a power calculation before beginning the study in order to estimate the required number of workers. Taking into consideration the available resources, we selected 12 primary coffee processing factories for inclusion in this study. The 12 primary coffee processing factories were divided equally among the three regions (i.e., four factories from each of the three regions), and the factories were selected randomly. The study was conducted from May to October 2016.

2.2. Control Group

The workers from three water bottling factories, one from each of the three study areas, were selected as the control group. Water bottling factories were chosen as their workers experience less dust exposure at work. Water bottling workers' tasks are loading bottled water to the trucks. There are about 38 water bottling factories in Ethiopia.

2.3. Dust Exposure Levels

The personal total dust was sampled in the workers' breathing zone using 25-mm three pieces, conductive cassettes with a cellulose acetate filter attached to a Side Kick Casella (SKC) pump with a flow rate of 2 l min^{-1} [15] Altogether, 360 full-shift exposure measurements were conducted on randomly chosen days of the week, and repeated sampling was conducted the next day. The sampling process is described in a previous paper [13]. A total of 60 full-shift personal exposure measurements were conducted in the water bottling factories. The arithmetic mean (range) of the personal total dust exposure was 17.36 mg/m^3 (1.12–81.61 mg/m^3) and 0.33 mg/m^3 (0.11–1.16 mg/m^3) for the coffee workers and controls, respectively. The personal total dust exposure levels among the coffee workers were significantly higher than among the control workers with geometric means (GM) of

12.30 and 0.30 mg/m^3, respectively. The dust samples were analyzed gravimetrically using a standard microbalance scale AT261 Mettler Toledo with a detection limit of 0.01 mg/m^3, in the accredited laboratory SINTEF MOLAB in Norway.

2.4. Study Population and Sample Size

The sample size for this study was calculated using a double population formula considering that the prevalence of wheezing among the primary coffee workers in Tanzania was 16% and 4.3% among the controls [12]. An 80% power was set to detect a difference in the wheezing between the two groups at significance level of 0.05. After considering 15% for non-response, a total of 240 participants (i.e., 120 from coffee factories and 120 from water bottling) were selected by systematic random sampling method, using the workers' registration list as a sampling frame. All of the participants were male. In the coffee factories, only workers directly related to coffee processing were involved in this study. Office workers and guards were not included in this study.

2.5. Data Collection

2.5.1. Chronic Respiratory Symptoms Interview

The chronic respiratory symptoms among participants were assessed with an interview, using a standardized questionnaire from the American Thoracic Society (ATS) [16]. This questionnaire was chosen because it has been used in previous occupational studies of respiratory health in East-Africa [12], making comparisons possible. The questionnaire was translated from English to Amharic and Afan Oromo languages, and translated back to English. A pre-test was conducted prior to the actual data collection for the validation of the data collection tool. Questions that were not easy for the participants to understand were rephrased to make them more easily understood. The interviews were conducted in an office located at their workplaces in absence of other people, in order to help the interviewee speak freely. The interviews lasted between 25 and 40 min per respondent.

The data were collected by the principal investigator together with an experienced research assistant. The questionnaire included socio-demographic data (age, height, weight, and Body Mass Index (BMI)), occupational history (years of work experience in the present and other dusty factories), past respiratory diseases (pneumonia, tuberculosis, bronchitis, asthma, and chest injury), and smoking habits (current smoker, ex-smoker, and never smoker). The questionnaire also included questions about the use of respiratory protective devices while working (yes/no), and the reason for not using respiratory protective devices (RPD). We asked the workers about this information to see how many of the workers use of RPD. The use of RPD during work might reduce respiratory health problems. The questionnaire also included questions about chronic respiratory symptoms—coughing, coughing with sputum, breathlessness, work related shortness of breath, wheezing, and chronic bronchitis.

2.5.2. Lung Function Test

Lung function tests were performed for a total of 225 participants (i.e., 115 coffee workers and 110 control workers), according to the ATS [17] recommendation for spirometry. A portable spirometer (SPIRARE 3 sensor model SPS 320) was used to measure the lung function. The standing height and weight of the participants was measured using standard weight and height measure. The test was performed during the day shift between 08:00 and 16:00, with the workers in a sitting position. Three acceptable maneuvers with consistent ("repeatable") results were retained and the best of all of these was recorded. Only the absolute values for the lung function are given in the results, as there are currently no reference equations for the Ethiopia population for obtaining predicted values. The lung function parameters included were FVC and FEV_1, as well as the percentage ratio of FEV_1/FVC. The participants with $FEV_1/FVC < 0.70$ were considered to have airflow limitations [18]. FEV1 is the maximal volume of air exhaled in the first second of a forced expiration from a position of full inspiration. FVC is the maximal volume of air exhaled with maximally forced effort from a maximal inspiration.

Eleven spirometer results among coffee workers and seven among the controls were excluded from the analysis because of unacceptable readings.

2.6. Operational Definition of Variables

Current smoker: participants who smoke currently or those who stopped smoking less than one year ago.

Ex-smoker: participants who had stopped smoking more than one year ago.

Never smoker: participants who had never smoked.

Cough: participants were considered to have coughed if they answered "yes" to at least one of the following four questions; cough first thing in the morning, cough during the day or night, cough as much as four to six times a day in a week, or cough for most days for as much as three consecutive months during the year.

Cough with sputum: participants were considered to have cough with sputum if they answered "yes" to at least one of the four questions: cough with sputum first thing in the morning, cough with sputum during the day or night, cough with sputum as much as four to six times a day in a week, or cough with sputum for most days for as much as three consecutive months during the year.

Breathlessness: participants were considered to have breathlessness if he/she was troubled by a shortness of breath when hurrying on level ground or walking up a slight hill, or get shortness of breath when walking at his/her own pace on the level ground.

Work-related shortness of breath participants were considered to have work-related shortness of breath if he/she usually experience chest tightness while at work or just after work.

Wheezing: participants were considered to have wheezing if his/her chest ever sounded wheezy (whistling sound).

2.7. Data Management and Analysis

The collected data were checked for completeness and consistencies by the principal investigator through a close follow up during the data collection period. The data were coded, and no names were included in the database. The code list as well as the data were kept confidential, and were accessed only by the research team.

Independent *t*-tests were used to compare mean values for the continuous variables. The Pearson chi-square test or Fisher's exact test, if the expected value was less than 5, were used to test the difference between the groups regarding the categorical variables. Poisson regression analysis with a robust variance was used to determine the prevalence ratio of the different respiratory symptoms between the coffee workers and controls, with a corresponding 95% confidence interval, and the statistical significance level was set to a p-value less than 0.05. As the prevalence of the chronic respiratory symptoms was high, we chose the prevalence ratio over the odds ratio, because the odds ratio overestimated the strength of association [19].

Analysis of covariance (ANCOVA) were used to compare the mean lung function parameters between the coffee workers and controls when adjusting for height and education level. We adjusted for education level, because there was a significant difference in the educational level between the coffee workers and the controls.

2.8. Ethical Approval

The Institutional Review Board of the College of Health Sciences of Addis Ababa University (Protocol number: 051/15/SPH) and the National Research Ethical Review Committee of the Federal Ministry of Science and Technology (NRERC-3/10/110/2016) approved the study. Permission to conduct the study was obtained from the factory managers. Written informed consent was obtained from each participant, and participation in the study was voluntary. Participants with lung function impairments were advised to consult the nearest health center.

3. Results

3.1. Characteristics of the Study Participants

All of the participants were men. A total of 115 coffee workers and 111 controls participated in the study, making the response rate 94%. The reasons for non-response were that five workers refused to participate, seven workers were in sick leave, and two had stopped working. The coffee workers were older and had a lower educational level than the controls (Table 1). No difference was found between the groups regarding weight, height, BMI, and past respiratory diseases (Table 1).

Table 1. Characteristics of the participants.

Variable	Coffee Workers (n = 115)	Control (n = 110)	*p*-Value
Age (years); AM (range)	35.1 (18.0–75.0)	30.9 (18.0–71.0)	0.008 $
Weight (Kg); AM (range)	59.8 (43.0–88.0)	60.0 (45.0–90.0)	0.9 $
Height (cm); AM (range)	169.3 (148.0–187.0)	169.9 (153.0–183.0)	0.5 $
BMI (Kg/m^2); AM (range)	20.8 (15.4–30.5)	20.7 (16.6–29.1)	0.8 $
Duration of employment at present work years AM (range)	6.5 (1.0–30.0)	3.4 (1.0–6.0)	0.001 $
Years worked in other dusty factories AM (range)	0.23 (0.0–12.0)	0.5 (0.0–12.0)	0.2 $
Education			
Illiterate; n (%)	14 (12.2)	3 (2.7)	0.007 †
Primary education & above; n (%)	101 (87.8)	107 (97.3)	0.007 †
Smoking habits			
Ex smoker; n (%)	4 (3.5)	1 (0.9)	0.37 ±
Current smoker; n (%)	3 (2.6)	4 (3.6)	0.71 ±
Cigarettes smoked per day for current smokers AM (range)	3 (2–4)	2 (1–3)	0.2 $
Cooking			
Cooking food at home; n (%)	103 (89.6)	97 (82.2)	0.74 †
Kitchen located inside the living room; n (%)	34 (33)	31 (32)	0.87 †
Use biomass for cooking; n (%)	96 (93.2)	86 (88.7)	0.26 †
Previous Respiratory Disease			
Pneumonia; n (%)	7 (6.1)	5 (4.5)	0.61 †
Bronchitis; n (%)	3 (2.6)	1 (0.9)	0.62 ±
Tuberculosis; n (%)	4 (3.5)	2 (1.8)	0.68 ±
Asthma; n (%)	8 (7)	4 (3.6)	0.27 ±
Participants who have had at least one of the respiratory diseases, n (%)	22 (19.1)	12 (10.9)	0.09 †

AM: arithmetic mean; $ Independent *t* test between control and coffee workers; † Pearson chi square test; ± Fisher's exact test. BMI—body mass index; "n": Number of study participants.

3.2. Use of Respiratory Protective Device (RPD)

The majority of the 112 (97.4%) coffee workers did not use any type of respiratory protective devices (RPD). Among the non-users of RPD, 109 (97.3%) of the coffee workers indicated that the reason for not using RPD was because it was not available or not provided at the work place. Others reported that the reasons for not using RPD were because it was not comfortable (one worker) (0.9%), and that the worker experienced that the RPD did not protect from the dust (one worker) (0.9%).

3.3. Chronic Respiratory Symptoms

The prevalence of chronic respiratory symptoms was in the range of 5.2–55% and 2.7–12.7% among the coffee workers and controls respectively (Table 2). Six of the coffee workers (5.2%), and none of the controls had chronic bronchitis. The prevalence ratio of all of the respiratory symptoms was significantly higher for the coffee workers compared to the controls after adjusting for age, education, years worked in other dusty factories, and previous respiratory disease (Table 2). As the number of current smokers were few, the analysis was also performed after excluding the smokers. This did not change the results substantially.

Table 2. Prevalence of chronic respiratory symptoms among coffee workers and controls.

Variable	Coffee Workers n = 115	Control n = 110	Prevalence Ratio, 95% CI	*p*-Value
Cough; n (%)	52 (46.4)	8 (7.5)	5.6 (2.9–11.7)	<0.001
Cough with sputum; n (%)	26 (23.2)	2 (1.9)	11.4 (2.7–47.8)	<0.001
Breathlessness; n (%)	40 (35.7)	12 (11.3)	2.9 (1.6–5.3)	<0.001
Work-related shortness of breath; n (%)	22 (19.6)	6 (5.5)	3.7 (1.6–8.7)	0.003
Wheezing; n (%)	20 (17.9)	5 (4.7)	3.3 (1.3–8.4)	0.01

CI, confidence interval while adjusting for age; education, years worked in other dusty factories and previous respiratory disease; *p*-value when comparing coffee workers vs. controls; "n": Number of study participants.

3.4. Lung Function

Table 3 shows the result of lung function stratified age among the coffee workers and controls. The coffee workers in the age group 28–39 years and ≥40 years, had significantly lower FVC and FEV_1 compared with the controls in the similar age category. The FEV_1/FVC-ratio was significantly lower among the coffee workers compared to the controls in the oldest age group (Table 3). The prevalence of airflow limitation ($FEV_1/FVC < 0.7$) was higher among the coffee workers compared to the controls in all of the age categories (Table 3). The analyses were also performed again without including education level in the model, and the results were quite similar (data not shown).

Table 3. Lung function among primary coffee processing factories and control groups stratified by age (three age groups).

Lung Function Parameters	Age Group	No of Participants		Absolute Value Mean (SD)		*p*-Value
		Coffee Workers n = 104	Controls n = 103	Coffee Workers	Controls	
FVC (l)	18–27	35	57	4.60 (0.43)	4.70 (0.49)	0.35
	28–39	35	23	4.08 (0.47)	4.43 (0.46)	<0.001
	≥40	34	23	3.38 (0.53)	3.67 (0.51)	0.05
	All age group	104	103	4.03 (0.69)	4.41 (0.63)	<0.001
FEV_1 (l)	18–27	35	57	3.74 (0.46)	3.87 (0.39)	0.15
	28–39	35	23	3.29 (0.58)	3.63 (0.47)	0.02
	≥40	34	23	2.60 (0.50)	3.05 (0.51)	<0.001
	All age group	104	103	3.22 (0.69)	3.63 (0.54)	<0.001
FEV_1/FVC	18–27	35	57	0.81 (0.08)	0.83 (0.05)	0.43
	28–39	35	23	0.80 (0.09)	0.82 (0.07)	0.48
	≥40	34	23	0.77 (0.09)	0.83 (0.06)	0.02
	All age group	104	103	0.80 (0.09)	0.83 (0.06)	0.01
$FEV_1/FVC < 0.7$; n (%)	18–27	35	57	3 (8.6)	0	-
	28–39	35	23	2 (5.7)	1 (4.3)	1 *
	≥40	34	23	9 (26.5)	0	-

Analysis of covariance between coffee worker and controls while adjusting for height and education level. * Fisher exact test between coffee workers and controls; *p*-value: significance level; "n": Number of study participants.

4. Discussion

This study found a significantly higher prevalence of respiratory symptoms and lower lung function among the coffee workers compared to controls. Our results are consistent with studies conducted in primary coffee processing factories in Papua New Guinea, Uganda, and Tanzania [8,9,11]. All of these studies show that coffee workers have high prevalence of respiratory health problems. However, our present study found a higher prevalence of some of the respiratory symptoms compared with the studies conducted among Arabica coffee workers in Tanzania, where the prevalence of breathlessness was 14%, wheezing 13%, and chronic bronchitis 3.1% [12]. One of the reasons for this difference could be the higher personal total dust exposure in Ethiopian coffee factories (GM = 12.3 mg/m^3) compared with the comparable job groups in Tanzanian primary coffee factories (GM = 2.1 mg/m^3) [20]. The different methods of coffee pre-processing could be another reason; the Arabica coffee is pre-processed only by a wet-method in the Tanzanian factories, whereas in Ethiopia, Arabica coffee is pre-processed either by dry or wet method, based on the individual farmers' interests. In addition, only 3% of the workers used RPD in Ethiopia, compared to 33% in the coffee workers in Tanzania. The lack of RPD use makes it more likely that the workers actually were exposed to the dust levels measured in the factories. There may have been other additional factors that were not identified in the present study that may also have influenced the respiratory health of the workers.

Similarly, the prevalence of a cough with sputum and wheezing in our study was higher than in the study in Uganda; where the prevalence was 5.2% and 13.5%, respectively [9]. This might be due to the different types of coffee species between the two countries; the Robusta and Arabic coffee were processed in Ugandian factories, whereas only Arabica coffee was processed in Ethiopia.

For a cough with sputum, we found a higher prevalence than reported in the study in Papua New Guinea (8.7%) [8]. This difference might be due to higher dust exposure in the present study compared with what was measured in Papua New Guinea (0.7–10 mg/m^3). In addition, the difference in working environments, coffee processing methods, and level of awareness among the coffee workers about the impact of dust exposure on their health might be the reason for the difference in the symptom prevalence. In addition, there may be differences between these countries regarding the presence of, for instance, lung infections or sequela after lung infections. Infections may cause respiratory symptoms and influence lung function. This possibility is not very likely, as the examined workers are performing hard physical work, but this factor needs to be considered, because of the high prevalence of tuberculosis as well as HIV in East-African countries [21]. However, it is not likely that this type of health problem is different among the workers in the two factory types included in our study.

The present study's results showed that in the two oldest age groups of coffee workers, the FVC and FEV_1 were lower than among the controls, while FEV_1/FVC was lower in the oldest age group of coffee workers than among the controls. In the Tanzanian study, there were no difference in the FVC and FEV_1 between coffee workers and controls [12]. The considerably higher dust exposure in the Ethiopian study (GM = 12.3 mg/m^3) [13] compared to the levels reported for the processing of Arabica coffee in Tanzania (GM = 2.1 mg/m^3) [20] may have contributed to the difference in findings related to lung function. Also, the study conducted in Papua New Guinea, where the dust levels were lower than in the present study, did not find significant differences in FVC and FEV_1/FVC between the coffee workers and controls.

Both FEV_1 and FVC were reduced among the coffee workers, indicating both obstructive and restrictive lung effects. However, in the oldest age group, the FEV_1/FVC ratio was less than 0.70 for about 27% of the coffee workers, which indicates the presence of an obstructive lung disease [18]. It is noteworthy that such a result was found, even though these workers were present at the workplaces in physically demanding work.

No statistically significant difference was observed in the incidence of past respiratory diseases between the coffee workers and controls; unfortunately, we have no information about when these past respiratory diseases occurred. For example, they could have been before starting work in coffee factories or after starting working in the factories. We only asked the participants if they had ever had any previous respiratory disease.

The control group in the present study was from another production factory, with very low dust levels. Another possibility would have been to choose a control group from the general population, but this would have introduced other types of bias in the study, related to socioeconomic differences between the factory workers and the population.

This is the first study to assess the prevalence respiratory symptoms and lung function among coffee workers in Ethiopia. However, as this study is a cross sectional study, the cause and effect association between dust exposure, and respiratory symptoms and lung function reduction cannot be drawn based on our findings. Our analyses were adjusted for other factors, including age, which may affect lung function. However, it is worth noting that there may be other variables present, which we have not identified. We would therefore recommend that a longitudinal study is undertaken in order to characterize the association between dust exposure and lung function reduction.

This study used a questionnaire-based interview to assess the respiratory symptoms that might result in recall and interviewer bias. However, similar questions were used to assess the respiratory symptoms in both the coffee workers and control groups. To minimize bias, a well-trained interviewer was involved in interviewing both groups. Also, the reported symptoms agreed with the objective measures from the spirometry. Symptoms such as coughing, wheezing, and breathlessness are often associated with obstructive lung disease [22].

This study included workers from all three coffee growing and processing regions of Ethiopia, and the factories are considered to be representative to all similar primary coffee processing factories in Ethiopia. Similar results might also be expected by any African coffee factory with a similar dust exposure level and similar production type of Arabica coffee beans.

As this study showed that the majority of the coffee workers did not use any type of respiratory protective devices, an immediate action to reduce respiratory health problems among coffee workers would be to provide proper facemasks.

5. Conclusions

Workers in primary coffee processing factories in Ethiopia had a higher prevalence of chronic respiratory symptoms and lower lung function than the controls. This might represent early signs of lung disease. A longitudinal study on the possible effects of coffee dust on respiratory health among coffee production workers is recommended.

Author Contributions: S.W.A. planned the study, collected and analyzed data, and drafted the manuscript in consultation with other authors. M.B., W.D., A.K., and B.E.M. participated in the design, collection and analysis of data, and provided scientific support throughout the project and commented on the manuscript. All of authors have read and approved the final manuscript.

Funding: This research was funded by the Norwegian Program for Capacity Building in Higher Education and Research for Development (NORHED).

Acknowledgments: We would like to thank the coffee factory management teams and workers for their permission to conduct the study and for participating in the study.

Conflicts of Interest: The authors declare that they have no competing interest.

References

1. Figley, K.D.; Rawling, F.F.A. Castor bean an industrial hazard as a contaminant of green coffee dust and used burlap bags. *J. Allergy* **1950**, *21*, 545–553. [CrossRef]
2. Karr, R.M.; Lehrer, S.B.; Butcher, B.T.; Salvaggio, J.E. Coffee worker's asthma: A clinical appraisal using the radioallergosorbent test. *J. Allergy Clin. Immunol.* **1978**, *62*, 143–148. [CrossRef]
3. Bruun, E. Allergy to coffee: An occupational diseases. *Acta Allergol.* **1957**, *11*, 150–154. [CrossRef] [PubMed]
4. Kaye, M.; Freedman, S. Allergy to Raw Coffee—An Occupational Disease. *Can. Med. Assoc. J.* **1961**, *84*, 469–471. [PubMed]
5. Larese, F.; Fiorito, A.; Casasola, F.; Molinari, S.; Peresson, M.; Barbina, P.; Negro, C. Sensitization to green coffee beans and work-related allergic symptoms in coffee workers. *Am. J. Ind. Med.* **1998**, *34*, 623–627. [CrossRef]
6. Osterman, K.; Zerterstrom, O.; Johansson, S.G.O. Coffee Worker's Allergy. *Allergy* **1982**, *37*, 313–322. [CrossRef] [PubMed]
7. Zuskin, E.; Vali, F.; Skuri, Z. Respiratory function in coffee workers. *Br. J. Ind. Med.* **1979**, *36*, 117–122. [CrossRef] [PubMed]

8. Smith, D.; Brott, K.; Kokisource, G. Respiratory Impairment in Coffee Factory Workers in the Asaro Valley of Papua New Guinea. *Br. J. Ind. Med.* **1985**, *42*, 495–498. [CrossRef] [PubMed]
9. Sekimpi, K.; Agaba, E.; Okot-Nwang, M.; Ogaram, D. Occupational coffee dust allergies in Uganda. *Afr. Newsl. Occup. Health Saf.* **1996**, *6*, 6–9.
10. Uragoda, C.G. Acute symptoms in coffee workers. *J. Trop. Med. Hyg.* **1988**, *91*, 169–172. [PubMed]
11. Sakwari, G.; Bråtveit, M.; Mamuya, S.H.D.; Moen, B.E. Dust exposure and chronic respiratory symptoms among coffee curing workers in Kilimanjaro: A cross sectional study. *BMC Pulm. Med.* **2011**, *11*, 54–61. [CrossRef] [PubMed]
12. Sakwari, G.; Mamuya, S.H.D.; Bråtveit, M.; Moen, B.E. Respiratory Symptoms, Exhaled Nitric Oxide, and Lung Function Among Workers in Tanzanian Coffee Factories. *JOEM* **2013**, *55*, 544–551. [CrossRef] [PubMed]
13. Abaya, W.S.; Bråtveit, M.; Deressa, W.; Kumie, A.; Moen, B.E. Personal dust exposure and its determinants among workers in primary coffee processing in Ethiopia. *Ann. Work Expo. Health* **2018**. [CrossRef] [PubMed]
14. United State AID. Ethiopian Coffee Industry Value Chain Analysis. 2010. Available online: https://agoa.info/images/documents/5157/Ethiopian_Coffee_Industry_Value_Chain_Analysis_2010.pdf (accessed on 22 May 2018).
15. Occupational Safety and Health Administration. OSHA Technical Manual: Section II, Chapter 1: Personal Sampling for Air Contaminants. Occupational Safety and Health Administration. 2014. Available online: https://www.osha.gov/dts/osta/otm/otm_ii/otm_ii_1.html#total_dust (accessed on 20 May 2018).
16. America Thoracic Society-Division of Lung Diseases. Recommended Respiratory Disease Questionnaires for Use with Adults and Children in Epidemiological Research. ATS. 1978. Available online: http://citeseerx.ist.psu.edu/viewdoc/download?doi=10.1.1.607.2516&rep=rep1&type=pdf (accessed on 22 May 2018).
17. America Thoracic Society. Standardization of Spirometry, 1994 Update. America Thoracic Society. *Am. J. Respir. Crit. Care Med.* **2005**, *152*, 1107–1136.
18. Pauwels, A.; Buist, S.; Calverley, A.; Jenkins, R.; Hurd, S. Globally Strategy for the diagnosis management and prevention of Chronic Obstructive Pulmonary Disease: NHLBI/WHO Global Initiative for Chronic Obstructive Lung Disease (GOLD) Workshop Summary. *Am. J. Respir. Crit. Care Med.* **2001**, *163*, 1256–1276. [CrossRef] [PubMed]
19. Tamhane, A.R.; Westfall, A.O.; Burkholder, G.A.; Cutter, G.R. Prevalence odds ratio versus prevalence ratio: Choice comes with consequences. *Stat. Med.* **2016**, *35*, 5730–5735. [CrossRef] [PubMed]
20. Sakwari, G.; Mamuya, S.H.D.; Bråtveit, M.; Larsson, L.; Pehrson, C.; Moen, B.E. Personal Exposure to Dust and Endotoxin in Robusta and Arabica Coffee Processing Factories in Tanzani. *Ann. Occup. Hyg.* **2012**, *57*, 173–183. [PubMed]
21. Belay, M.; Bjune, G.; Abebe, F. Prevalence of tuberculosis, HIV, and TB-HIV co-infection among pulmonary tuberculosis suspects in a predominantly pastoralist area, northeast Ethiopia. *Glob. Health Action* **2015**, *8*, 27949. [CrossRef] [PubMed]
22. Siafakas, N.M.; Vermeire, P.; Pride, N.A.; Paoletti, P.; Gibson, J.; Howard, P.; Yernault, J.C.; Decramer, M.; Higenbottam, T.; Postma, D.S. Optimal assessment and management of chronic obstractive pulmonary disease (COPD). *Eur. Respir. J.* **1995**, *8*, 1398–1420. [CrossRef] [PubMed]

International Journal of
Environmental Research and Public Health

MDPI

Article

The Epidemiology, Cost, and Occupational Context of Spinal Injuries Sustained While 'Working for Income' in NSW: A Record-Linkage Study

Lisa N. Sharwood [1,2,3,*], Holger Mueller [4], Rebecca Q. Ivers [4,5], Bharat Vaikuntam [1,2], Tim Driscoll [6] and James W. Middleton [1,2,7]

1 Sydney Medical School, University of Sydney, Camperdown, NSW 2050, Australia; bvai6198@uni.sydney.edu.au (B.V.); james.middleton@sydney.edu.au (J.W.M.)
2 John Walsh Centre for Rehabilitation Studies, Kolling Institute, St Leonards, NSW 2065, Australia
3 Department Epidemiology and Preventive Medicine, Monash University, Melbourne, VIC 3004, Australia
4 The George Institute for Global Health, Newtown, NSW 2042, Australia; hmoeller@georgeinstitute.org.au (H.M.); rivers@georgeinstitute.org.au (R.Q.I.)
5 School of Public Health, University of New South Wales, Kensington, NSW 2033, Australia
6 School of Public Health, University of Sydney, Camperdown, NSW 2050, Australia; tim.driscoll@sydney.edu.au
7 Agency for Clinical Innovation, Chatswood, NSW 2067, Australia
* Correspondence: lisa.sharwood@sydney.edu.au

Received: 8 September 2018; Accepted: 23 September 2018; Published: 27 September 2018

Abstract: This study aimed to describe the epidemiological characteristics, the occupational context, and the cost of hospitalised work-related traumatic spinal injuries, across New South Wales, Australia. A record-linkage study of hospitalised cases of work-related spinal injury (ICD10-AM code U73.0 or workers compensation) was conducted. Study period 2013–2016. Eight hundred and twenty-four individuals sustained work-related spinal injuries; 86.2% of whom were males and had a mean age of 46.6 years. Falls led to 50% of the injuries; predominantly falls from building/structures, ladders or between levels. Falls occurred predominantly in the construction industry (78%). Transport crashes caused 31% of injuries and 24% in heavy vehicles. Half of all the transport injuries occurred 'off road'. The external cause was coded as 'non-specific work activity' in 44.5% of cases; missing in 11.5%. Acute care bed days numbered at 13,302; total cost $19,500,000. High numbers of work-related spinal injuries occurred in the construction industry; particularly falling from a height. Off-road transport-related injuries were significant and likely unaddressed by 'on-road' prevention policies. Medical record documentation was insufficient in injury mechanism and context specificity. Workers in the construction industry or those using vehicles off-road were at high risk of spinal injury, suggesting inefficient systems approaches or ineffective prevention policies. Reducing the use of non-specific external cause codes in patients' medical records would improve the measurement of policy effectiveness.

Keywords: workplace injuries; spinal trauma; record-linkage data

1. Introduction

Traumatic spinal injuries (TSI) can comprise column fractures, spinal cord injury or both. They are among the most severe injuries with potential long-term, physical, psychological, and social consequences. The leading causes of TSIs are widely reported as falls and motor vehicle crashes [1–5]; some of these occur in occupational settings, placing a significant financial burden on both employer and employee, the compensation system, and the health care system. Safe Work Australia calculated the cost of work-related falls to be at $6,640,000, in 2012–2013 [6,7]. The economic cost of work-related injury and illness, more broadly, has been estimated at ranging from 1.8% to 6.5%, of a country's gross domestic product [8]. Safe Work Australia's current "Work Health and Safety Strategy" [9] has set one of its three national targets as a 30% reduction in serious workplace injury compensation claims, by 2022.

The global epidemiology of TSI has recently been estimated in a systematic review [10]. The modelled overall global incidence was 10.5 cases per 100,000 persons; meaning around 768,000 new cases across the world per year. These authors reviewed 102 studies, reporting the TSI from work-related falls to be more common in low-to-middle-income countries, than in high-income countries. Road traffic crashes and falls were the most common mechanisms of injury in all income strata, however, low-to-middle-income countries had a higher proportion of cord injuries, only, as part of the injury profile in TSI. While comprehensive, this review was unable to report, more specifically, the industry context of the work-related TSIs. Numerous studies describing TSI epidemiology have been single hospital or trauma centre-based only and have not apportioned attributable risk to work-related incidents [2,3,11]. The authors recognised the paucity of the literature, globally, in examining TSI in population-based studies [10], particularly relative to the preponderance of studies considering solely cord injuries. If we are to consider only injuries to the spinal cord, and which are attributable to work globally, this was estimated at between 10–25%, in 2001 [12]. More recently, the Australian Institute for Health and Welfare (AIHW) reported the incidence and prevalence of traumatic spinal cord injuries across Australia [13]; "working for an income" was the second most common specified activity type at the time of injury, over the five-year period; accounting for 13% of all spinal injuries. A notable limitation of the AIHW data is that it is compiled using only data provided by consenting patients from the participating spinal cord injury units (SCIUs), in Australia, therefore likely to be an underestimate, based on an analysis of state-wide record-linked data, in New South Wales (NSW) [14]. Further, a vital missing component of these reports is the examination of the activity, at the time of injury.

The primary aim of this study was to describe the population-based epidemiology and occupational context of hospitalised traumatic spinal column and cord injuries, that occurred while 'working for an income' in NSW, the most populous state in Australia. The study does not include work-related 'back' injuries, for example, only musculoskeletal injuries without any spinal column or cord injuries. Traumatic spinal cord and column injuries are severe, and highly unlikely to avoid a period of hospitalisation; hence, the capacity of this study to accurately describe the health system burden of these injuries. A secondary aim was to describe the completeness of activity-coded data.

2. Methods

The study is set in the most populous Australian state—NSW, with approximately 7.5 million inhabitants, spread over 800,000 km^2 in suburban, rural, and very remote areas [15]. The study time period covered from 1 June 2013–30 June 2016.

Study inclusion criteria were: patients aged $\geq$16 years, who had a recorded TSI as the reason for their index admission and an indication that this injury was related to work. Work-relatedness was defined by the International Classification of Diseases and Related Health Problems, 10th Version, Australian Modification (ICD10-AM) [16] code U73.0, or at least some of the costs covered by funding from workers compensation, in either the index admission or any subsequent episode of care within the acute care continuous period of stay.

Study exclusion criteria were: patients aged <16 years, and those for whom the first admission with a record of spinal injury was for rehabilitation.

Spinal injuries included all traumatic spinal cord injuries or spinal column injuries, defined on the basis of specific ICD-10-AM [16] codes (Appendix A). Probabilistic data linkage was undertaken by the Centre for Health Record Linkage (CHeReL), linking all patients where a TSI code was either a principal or additional diagnosis, for any separation within the Admitted Patient Data Collection (APDC). The APDC contains records for all patients admitted to all public hospitals across the state of

NSW. Corresponding records were linked with the Emergency Department (ED) Data, NSW Mortality data, NSW Ambulance data collections, and the NSW District Network Return (DNR) activity-based funding data. The NSW APDC contains all inpatient records including patient demographics, comprehensive admission, transfer and discharge data, ICD-10-AM [16] diagnosis codes, Australian Refined-Diagnostic Related Group (AR-DRG) codes, procedure codes, separation mode (discharges, transfers and deaths), and financial information from all NSW public hospitals, private hospitals, and day procedure centres. The NSW DNR records the individual patient-level health service activity, enabling the estimation of the costs incurred by the health service providers, in a bottom-up approach. The first hospital episode for the patient, satisfying inclusion criteria conditions, as well as all other contiguous episodes of care, including nested/non-nested transfers, was recognised as the 'index event'. The Socio-Economic Indexes for Areas (SEIFA); developed by the Australian Bureau of Statistics, to rank areas in the country according to the relative socio-economic disadvantage or advantage, was derived from the patients' residential postcodes to describe the population relative to their education and occupation, within this index.

Activity and the place of injury were derived from the first record, or from subsequent records of the first continuous period of stay, if relevant information was missing in the first record. The sub-codes of the root U73.0 were used to identify the attributed industry (U73.00–U73.09). Type of TSI and body region affected was derived from any record within the first continuous period of stay. Length of stay was calculated for the first continuous period of stay. Costs were derived from the NSW DNR, which included the ED and the admitted costs.

Descriptive statistics were used to report the prevalence of various factors. Values were reported as the mean and the standard deviation (SD), in normally distributed continuous variables, or proportions; median and interquartile range (IQR) for non-normally distributed continuous variables. All statistical analyses were performed using Stata version 15.0 (Stata Corporation, College Station, TX, USA). Standardised reporting of the demographic and other variables, as recommended by De Vivo et al. [17], was followed where possible. The incidence of injury was based on the NSW Labour Force, aged 15 years and over [18],—note that the numerator data are based on persons 16 years and over—with 95% confidence intervals calculated, assuming a Poisson distribution [19].

This study was approved by the Cancer Institute NSW, Population and Health Services Research Ethics Committee: AU RED Reference: HREC/16/CIPHS/19, Cancer Institute NSW reference number: 2016/07/647.

3. Results

From this record-linked administrative dataset, 824 patients aged 16 years or over were identified as having sustained a TSI in NSW, while working for an income over the period June 2013–June 2016. Injury victims were predominantly male (86.2%), with a gender ratio of 6.22. Almost half of these injuries occurred as a result of a fall (49.2%), and more than half of these (55.1%) were falls from building structures, scaffolding or ladders (Table 1). Of the 254 (31%) transport-related spinal injuries, 50% occurred in an off-road setting. Fewer workplace injuries occurred in summer (20%), compared with other seasons, but the variation between seasons was not substantial (note that the proportion of 'winter injuries' includes one more month—June 2013—than the other seasons). Workplace-related spinal injuries represented almost 5% of all acute TSI, identified in this dataset.

Table 2 shows that the most common injury was a fracture and/or dislocation to the lumbosacral region (58%). Comorbid head, chest or abdominal injury was also sustained in 21% of incidents. Table 2 also quantifies the measure of resource required caring for these injuries. The mean length of the acute-care stay was more than two weeks (16.1 days). The total number of acute-care bed days, used by the 824 injured persons, was 13,302 at a total cost of $ 19,500,000 (95%CI $16 M–$23 M). The mean (SD) per patient cost for acute admission was $23,681.00 ($62,304.00); median (IQR) per patient cost was $7436.50 ($3381.50–$20,393.00).

Table 1. Characteristics of the patient population and context of injury occurrence (n = 824).

Characteristics	n (%)
Sex	
- male	710 (86.2)
- female	114 (13.8)
Age category years	
- 16–29	145 (17.6)
- 30–44	233 (28.3)
- 45–59	280 (33.9)
- 60–74	144 (17.5)
- 75+	22 (2.7)
Season of injury	
- Summer	165 (20.0)
- Autumn	205 (24.9)
- Winter	230 (27.9)
- Spring	224 (27.2)
Mechanism of injury (more detail Table 3)	
- Falls (W00–W19)	405 (49.2)
- Transport (V01–V99)	254 (30.8)
o Traffic	127 (50.0)
o Non-traffic (off-road)	127 (50.0)
- Mechanical forces (W20–W64)	135 (16.4)
- Other and unspecified (X58–X59)	30 (3.6)
Place of injury occurrence	
- Industrial and construction area	161 (19.5)
- Street and highway	124 (15.0)
- Farm	84 (10.2)
- Trade and service area	57 (6.9)
- Home	37 (4.5)
- Sports and athletics area	27 (3.3)
- Other specified	49 (5.9)
- Unspecified	285 (34.6)
Industry (external cause—within activity code)	
- Construction	163 (19.8)
- Agriculture, forestry, and fishing	104 (12.6)
- Transport and storage	82 (9.9)
- Manufacturing	13 (1.6)
- Other specified work for income	183 (22.2)
- Unspecified	184 (22.3)
- Missing	95 (11.5)
SEIFA Index (Education/Occupation: quintiles) *	
- First quintile #	138 (17.3)
- Second quintile	193 (24.1)
- Third quintile	202 (25.3)
- Fourth quintile	151 (18.9)
- Fifth quintile ##	116 (14.5)
- Missing	24 (2.9)

* derived from patient's residential postcode # lowest education and occupation status ## highest education and occupation status.

For the 47 patients who had inpatient rehabilitation (130 hospital separations), the mean (SD) length of stay in rehabilitation was 40 days (44).

Table 2. Injury detail and consequent hospitalisation.

Injuries Sustained	Number	%
Spinal cord injury	62	7.5
Cervical level fracture/dislocation	183	22.2
Thoracic level fracture/dislocation	295	35.8
Lumbosacral level fracture/dislocation	480	58.3
Co-morbid traumatic brain injury	65	7.9
Co-morbid severe chest injury	93	11.3
Co-morbid severe abdominal injury	33	4
Subsequent rehabilitation admission = yes	47	5.7
Length of stay acute care days (mean (SD))	16.1	(39.7)
Length of stay acute care days (median (IQR))	4.9	(1.7–11.5)
Length of stay rehabilitation days (mean (SD))	40	44
Length of stay rehabilitation days (median (IQR))	24.3	(13.9–45.9)

Table 3 further investigates the activity within each broad mechanism of injury category, permitting a greater understanding of the circumstances of injury, within certain activities. The most common type of fall injury was related to falling from a building or structure (24.4%), while the most common transport injury was sustained as an occupant of a heavy vehicle (23.6%). Over half the workplace TSIs caused by a mechanical force resulted from being struck by a projected or falling object (54.1%).

Table 3. A detailed description of injury in the context of activity.

Specific Activity Leading to Injury	*n* (%)
Falls	
- From building/structure	99 (24.4)
- On and from ladder	91 (22.5)
- Other from one level to another	77 (19.0)
- On and from scaffolding	33 (8.1)
- On and from stairs	27 (6.7)
- Same level	24 (5.9)
- Other same level	22 (5.4)
- Other & unspecified	21 (5.2)
- From tree	11 (2.7)
Total falls	405 (100)
Transport accidents	
- Occupant of heavy transport vehicle (V60–V69)	60 (23.6)
- Car occupant (V40–49)	48 (18.9)
- Animal-rider (V80)	37 (14.6)
- Motorcycle (V20–V29)	21 (8.3)
- Occupant of special all-terrain vehicle (V86)	21 (8.3)
- Pedestrian (V01–V09)	12 (4.7)
- Occupant of pick-up truck (V50–V59)	11 (4.3)
- Other and unspecified (V98–V99)	11 (4.3)
- Occupant-vehicle mainly used in agriculture (V84)	9 (3.5)
- Other	9 (3.5)
- Pedal cycle (V10–V19)	8 (3.1)
- Occupant-vehicle used on industrial premises (V83)	7 (2.8)
Total transport accidents	254 (100)
Mechanical forces	
- Struck by thrown, projected or falling object (W20)	73 (54.1)
- Bitten or struck by other mammals (W55)	21 (15.6)
- Contact with other and unspecified machinery (W31)	17 (12.6)
- Striking against or struck by other objects (W22)	13 (9.6)
- Other specified	11 (8.1)
Total mechanical forces	135 (100)

The external cause activity was coded as 'other or unspecified' in 44.5% of cases, and 'missing' in another 11.5% of cases (Table 1). Of the remaining cases where codes were specified to an industry, 78.8% of all falls occurred to persons in the construction industry, as did 48.3% of all mechanical force injuries. Transport-related injuries occurred predominantly in the transport and storage industry (51%) or agriculture/forestry industry (41.5%), and rarely in the construction industry (4%).

The annual rate of workplace-related spinal injuries was 7.2 (95% CI 6.8–7.7) per 100,000 persons, with the rate per 100,000 persons for males (11.6, 95% CI 10.7–12.5) being six times that of females (2.2, 95% CI 1.8–2.6).

4. Discussion

This study identified 824 persons during a three-year period who sustained TSIs while working for income. Almost half of these injuries resulted from a fall (49.2%); often from building structures, scaffolding or ladders (55.1%). Given that only 18% of TSI occurred in the 16–29 years age group, developmental vulnerability, and inexperience do not seem to be major contributing factors. The SEIFA index classifying education and occupational status shows a slightly higher proportion in the lowest three quintiles (67%), than in the higher two. The only comparator to this study analysed NSW hospitalisation and workers compensation data almost 20 years ago and considered all injury types, and not TSI alone [20].

Almost half of all work-related spinal injuries in our study were due to falls. Fall risk in Australian workplaces has been the focus of national attention over recent years. A Working at Heights Association survey [21], in 2014, found concerning failure rates of unsafe equipment installation, where 94% of fixed ladders were identified as potentially fatal. Despite numerous publications of codes of practice promoting workplace health and safety (WHS), and strong WHS laws, our results suggest that increased local surveillance of safety systems and stricter enforcement of relevant legislation may be required to reduce risks and, therefore, fall-related injuries.

Heavy transport vehicle crashes were the leading cause of transport-related spinal injuries in this study. A heavy vehicle driving crash risk is known to be reduced by the consumption of caffeinated substances [22], however, increased with night shift driving, insufficient breaks, and lack of vehicle safety devices [23]. Industry safety for heavy vehicle drivers has a long chain of responsibility that involves general practitioners in driver licensing, logistics managers, employers of various sizes, loading managers, goods consigners, and many others. Where multiple parties may be responsible at different stages in risk profiles, it is clear that all parties must work seamlessly together to reduce overall risk.

The reliability of the external cause codes in ICD10-AM [16] has been previously proven to be questionable, with high levels of missing activity codes, and 'non-specific' coding to describe events surrounding injury cause [24,25]. Analysis of a nationally representative sample of injury admissions across Australia, in 2002, revealed an underestimation of around 32%, in hospital coding, of the true burden of occupational injury [26]. The sub-codes of the root U73.0, used to identify the attributed industry (U73.00–U73.09), within which the activity was being undertaken at the time of injury; was missing or coded as 'other' or unspecified, in more than half of all cases (56%). Lack of coding specificity clearly hampers the provision of information to injury prevention activities and policy and likely leads to underestimation of actual events. The importance of improving the quality of clinical documentation, and particularly the level of specificity surrounding the injury events has been previously highlighted by Soo et al. [25]. These authors suggested that this perhaps indicated a relatively lower perceived importance of activity information, compared to injury mechanism codes, which have been more completely coded [25].

A particular strength of this study is its comprehensive profile of work-related TSIs, drawn from a population-based record linkage; not previously offered in Australia. Despite the undoubted under-reporting due to medical coding issues, these data aptly inform the current policy targets from the Australian Work Health and Safety Strategy 2012–2022 [9], to achieve a "reduction in the incidence rate of claims resulting in one or more weeks off work of at least 30%" for workplace injuries. Baseline data for this policy included serious non-fatal workers' compensation claims, reportedly around 11.5 claims per 1000 employees, over the 2009–2010 to 2011–2012 period. The objective of 30% reduction is acknowledged as 'ambitious' but thought to be attainable, if 'concerted and sustainable effort is made to target the most common causes of injury in those industry sectors that experience both high numbers and high rates of injury' [27]. This study did not consider TSIs related to other workplace injuries, however, this injured population certainly would be included within a '30% reduction' target. A replicated follow-up record linkage, in 2022, would ideally quantify the measure of any reduction achieved.

Limitations of this study included the unavailability of various important variables about the injured worker, such as ethnicity, level of education and experience, the employment situation (e.g., whether permanent/part-time/casual), and specific occupation. Indigenous status was not identified within the APDC collection; the population of NSW has 2.9% of indigenous people. These variables may influence the risk profile within particular industries or worker groups. The source data coding issues have been discussed earlier. Finally, the APDC does not include hospitalisation data for patients who were admitted to private hospitals across NSW. The degree of under-representation that this presents is uncertain, however, such severe injuries are much more likely to be treated within the public hospital system.

5. Conclusions

Work-related traumatic spinal injuries create a significant burden of cost and disability for the Australian workforce but are preventable, and also fall under a current focus of the Safe Work Australia policy to reduce serious injury compensation claims, by 30%, by 2022. This study demonstrates that the construction industry is still experiencing a high burden of work-related spinal trauma, particularly related to falling from heights, with a need for more effective policies, risk management strategies, and countermeasures for prevention. Transport injury prevention efforts equally need to address heavy vehicle occupant risk. Further research is required to better understand the factors contributing to traumatic spinal injuries in the workplace, including worker risk profiles, job design, work environment, culture, and leadership. Finally, the design and tailoring of industry-specific injury prevention strategies would be greatly assisted by improving the quality of medical record documentation, including, specifically, a reduction in the use of non-specific external cause codes. A more accurate identification of the activities and sectors which give rise to workplace spinal trauma, has policy relevance, as injury circumstances inform public health initiatives to target injury prevention.

Author Contributions: Conceptualisation, L.N.S. and T.D.; Methodology, L.N.S., H.M. and B.V.; Software, H.M. and L.N.S.; Formal Analysis, L.N.S, H.M. and B.V.; Data Curation, L.N.S., H.M. and B.V., Writing-Original Draft Preparation, L.N.S.; Writing-Review & Editing, J.W.M., R.I., H.M. and T.D.; Supervision, J.W.M.; Project Administration, L.N.S.; Funding Acquisition, L.N.S.

Funding: This research was funded by icare™; the article processing charge was funded by icare™.

Acknowledgments: The authors would like to thank the Meteor coding assistant team at the Australian Institute of Health and Welfare, for their strategic advice in the clarification of search and usage of activity codes.

Conflicts of Interest: The authors declare no conflict of interest. The founding sponsors had no role in the design of the study; in the collection, analyses, or interpretation of data; in the writing of the manuscript, and in the decision to publish the results.

Appendix A

ICD10-AM Codes provided to the Centre for Health Record Linkage, in order to identify persons aged 16 years or over, at admission, who were admitted after sustaining a traumatic spinal injury: S12, S12.0, S12.1, S12.2, S12.21, S12.22, S12.23, S12.24, S12.25, S12.7, S12.8, S12.9, S13.1, S13.10, S13.11, S13.12, S13.13, S13.14, S13.15, S13.16, S13.17, S13.18, S13.2, S13.3, S14.0, S14.10, S14.11, S14.12, S14.13, S14.70, S14.71, S14.72, S14.73, S14.74, S14.75, S14.76, S14.77, S14.78, S22.0, S22.00, S22.01, S22.02, S22.03,

S22.04, S22.05, S22.06, S22.1, S24.0, S24.1, S24.10, S24.11, S24.12, S24.7, S24.70, S24.71, S24.72, S24.73, S24.74, S24.75, S24.76, S24.77, S32, S32.0, S32.00, S32.01, S32.02, S32.03, S32.04, S32.05, S34.0, S34.1, S34.3, S34.70, S34.71, S34.72, S34.73, S34.74, S34.75, S34.76, T06.0, T06.1, T09.3.

References

1. Lenehan, B.; Street, J.; Kwon, B.; Noonan, V.; Zhang, H.; Fisher, C.G.; Dvorak, M.F. The epidemiology of traumatic spinal cord injury in British Columbia, Canada. *Spine* **2012**, *37*, 321–329. [CrossRef] [PubMed]
2. Leucht, P.; Fischer, K.; Muhr, G.; Mueller, E. Epidemiology of traumatic spine fractures. *Injury* **2009**, *40*, 166–172. [CrossRef] [PubMed]
3. Oliver, M.; Inaba, K.; Branco, B.; Barmparas, G.; Scnhuriger, B.; Lustenberger, T.; Tang, A.; Demetriades, D. The changing epidemiology of spinal trauma: A 13-year review from a Level I trauma centre. *Injury* **2012**, *43*, 1296–1300. [CrossRef] [PubMed]
4. Passias, P.G.; Poorman, G.W.; Segreto, F.A.; Jalai, C.M.; Horn, S.R.; Bortz, C.A.; Vasquez-Montes, D.; Diebo, B.G.; Vira, S.; Bono, O.J.; et al. Traumatic Fractures of the Cervical Spine: Analysis of Changes in Incidence, Cause, Concurrent Injuries, and Complications Among 488,262 Patients from 2005 to 2013. *World Neurosurg.* **2018**, *110*, e427–e437. [CrossRef] [PubMed]
5. Price, C.; Makintubee, S.; Hemdon, W.; Istre, GR. Epidemiology of traumatic spinal cord injury and acute hospitalization and rehabilitation charges for spinal cord injuries in Oklahoma, 1988–1990. *Am. J. Epidemiol.* **1994**, *139*, 37–47. [CrossRef] [PubMed]
6. Safe Work Australia. *The Cost of Work-Related Injury and Illness for Australian Employers, Workers and the Community: 2012–2013*; Safe Work Australia: Canberra, Australia, 2015.
7. Van den Berg, M.E.; Castellote, J.M.; Mahillo-Fernandez, I.; de Pedro-Cuesta, J. Incidence of spinal cord injury worldwide: A systematic review. *Neuroepidemiology* **2010**, *34*, 184–192. [CrossRef] [PubMed]
8. Takala, J.; Jamalainen, P.; Saarela, K.; Yun, L.; Manickam, K.; Jin, T.; Heng, P.; Tjong, C.; Kheng, L.; Lim, S.; et al. Global Estimates of the Burden of Injury and Illness at Work in 2012. *J. Occup. Environ. Hyg.* **2014**, *11*, 326–337. [CrossRef] [PubMed]
9. Safe Work Australia. *Australian Work Health and Safety Strategy 2012–2022*; Safe Work Australia: Canberra, Australia, 2012.
10. Kumar, R.; Lim, J.; Mekary, R.; Rattani, A.; Dewan, M.; Sharif, S.; Osorio-Fonseca, E.; Park, K.B. Traumatic Spinal Injury: Global Epidemiology and Worldwide Volume. *World Neurosurg.* **2018**, *113*, e345–e363. [CrossRef] [PubMed]
11. Tuma, M.; El-Menyar, A.; Al-Thani, H.; Al-Hassani, A.; Recicar, J.; Al Yazeedi, W.; Yazeedi, W.A.; Maull, K.I. Epidemiology of workplace-related fall from height and cost of trauma care in Qatar. *Int. J. Crit. Ill. Inj. Sci.* **2013**, *3*, 3–7.
12. Sekhon, L.; Fehlings, M. Epidemiology, demographics, and pathophysiology of acute spinal cord injury. *Spine* **2001**, *26*, S2–S12. [CrossRef] [PubMed]
13. AIH, W.; Harrison, J. *Spinal Cord Injury, Australia: Summary 2008–2009 to 2012–2013*; Institute of Health and Welfare: Canberra, Australia, 2018.
14. Sharwood, L.; Boufous, S.; Muecke, S.; Middleton, J. Health Service Pathways Analysis as Evidence Base for Trauma Policy Change: A Retrospective Study of Patients with Traumatic Spinal Cord Injury. *Emerg. Med.* **2017**, *7*. [CrossRef]
15. Australian Bureau of Statistics. *Australian Demographic Statistics*; Australian Bureau of Statistics: Canberra, Australia, 2017.
16. National Centre for Classification in Health. *ICD-10-AM/ACHI/ACS TENTH EDITION*; Australian Consortium for Classification Development: Sydney, Australia, 2017.
17. DeVivo, M.; Biering-Sorensen, F.; New, P.; Chen, Y. Standardization of data analysis and reporting of results from the International Spinal Cord Injury Core Data Set. *Spinal Cord* **2011**, *49*, 596–599. [CrossRef] [PubMed]
18. Australian Bureau of Statistics. *Labour Force, Australia*; Australian Government: Canberra, Australia, 2018.
19. Pezzullo, J. Exact Binomial and Poisson Confidence Intervals 2009. Available online: http://statpages.info/confint.html (accessed on 18 September 2018).
20. Boufous, S.; Williamson, A. Work-related injury in NSW hospitalisation and workers' compensation datasets: A comparative analysis. *Aust. N. Z. J. Public Health* **2003**, *27*, 352–357. [CrossRef] [PubMed]

21. Working for Heights Association. 2018. Available online: https://www.waha.org.au/?home (accessed on 2 August 2018).
22. Sharwood, L.; Elkington, J.; Meuleners, L.; Ivers, R.; Boufous, S.; Stevenson, M. Use of caffeinated substances and risk of crashes in long distance drivers of commercial vehicles: Case-control study. *BMJ* **2013**, *346*. [CrossRef] [PubMed]
23. Stevenson, M.; Elkington, J.; Sharwood, L.; Meuleners, L.; Ivers, R.; Boufous, S.; Williamson, A.; Haworth, N.; Quinlan, M.; Grunstein, R.; et al. The role of sleepiness, sleep disorders, and the work environment on heavy-vehicle crashes in 2 Australian states. *Am. J. Epidemiol.* **2014**, *179*, 594–601. [CrossRef] [PubMed]
24. Hayen, A.; Mitchell, R. *NSW Injury Profile: A Review of Injury Hospitalisations during 1989–1990 to 2003–2004*; Centre NIRMR, University of New South Wales: Sydney, Australia, 2006.
25. Soo, I.; Lam, M.; Rust, J.; Madden, R. Do we have enough information? How ICD-10-AM Activity codes measure up. *Health Inf. Manag. J.* **2009**, *38*, 22–34. [CrossRef]
26. McKenzie, K.; Mitchell, R.; Scott, D.; Harrison, J.; McClure, R. The reliability of information on work-related injuries available from hospitalisation data in Australia. *Aust. N. Z. J. Public Health* **2009**, *33*, 332–338. [CrossRef] [PubMed]
27. Safe Work Australia. *Measuring Progress towards Targets: Reducing the Incidence of Work-Related Death, Injury and Illness*; Safe Work Australia: Canberra, Australia, 2012.

International Journal of
Environmental Research and Public Health

MDPI

Article

Data-Driven Approach to Improving the Risk Assessment Process of Medical Failures

Shih-Heng Yu [1], Emily Chia-Yu Su [2,3] and Yi-Tui Chen [1,*]

1 Department of Health Care Management, College of Health Technology, National Taipei University of Nursing and Health Sciences, Taipei 10845, Taiwan; shihhengyu@gmail.com
2 Graduate Institute of Biomedical Informatics, College of Medical Science and Technology, Taipei Medical University, Taipei 11031, Taiwan; emilysu@tmu.edu.tw
3 Clinical Big Data Research Center, Taipei Medical University Hospital, Taipei 11031, Taiwan
* Correspondence: yitui@ntunhs.edu.tw; Tel.: +886-2-2388-5111

Received: 13 August 2018; Accepted: 18 September 2018; Published: 20 September 2018

Abstract: In recent decades, many researchers have focused on the issue of medical failures in the healthcare industry. A variety of techniques have been employed to assess the risk of medical failure and to generate strategies to reduce the frequency of medical failures. Considering the limitations of the traditional method—failure mode and effects analysis (FMEA)—for risk assessment and quality improvement, this paper presents two models developed using data envelopment analysis (DEA). One is called the slacks-based measure DEA (SBM-DEA) model, and the other is a novel data-driven approach (NDA) that combines FMEA and DEA. The relative advantages of the three models are compared. In this paper, an infant security case consisting of 16 failure modes at Western Wake Medical Center in Raleigh, North Carolina, U.S., was employed. The results indicate that both SBM-DEA and NDA may improve the discrimination and accuracy of detection compared to the traditional method of FMEA. However, NDA was found to have a relative advantage over SBM-DEA due to its risk assessment capability and precise detection of medical failures.

Keywords: failure mode and effects analysis; medical failure; novel data-driven approach; data envelopment analysis; healthcare

---

1. Introduction

In recent decades, medical failures, which are referred to as errors or adverse events in a medical service, have attracted much attention in the healthcare industry due to the increasing concern for patient safety [1]. The occurrence of medical failures may result in additional costs and a reduction in medical quality [2]. The U.S. Institute of Medicine reported that preventable medical failures result in 1,000,000 injuries and 44,000–98,000 deaths in hospitalized patients [3] and incur a loss of $17,000,000 [4] each year in America. In Taiwan, approximately 500 medical conflicts each year await legal mediation or trial [5]. Researchers suggest that reducing medical failures is critical for improving patient safety in healthcare systems. The prevention of medical failures may consist of two stages: risk assessment and quality improvement to monitor medical failures that may occur in a system. In general, risk assessment is processed by categorizing medical errors and predicting the probability of their occurrence [6]. The Joint Commission on Accreditation of Healthcare Organizations (JCAHO) requires all accredited hospitals or other healthcare organizations to complete at least one proactive risk assessment annually to assess the risk of errors and to continuously improve quality [7].

The techniques of risk assessment and quality improvement involve a variety of methods to prevent medical failures, including Six Sigma, hazard analysis and critical control points (HACCP), failure mode and effect analysis (FMEA) or healthcare failure mode and effect analysis (HFMEA), the Toyota production system (TPS), hazard and operability studies (HAZOP), total quality management/continuous quality improvement (TQM/CQI), root cause analysis (RCA), and probabilistic risk assessment (PRA) [8]. Among these methods, FMEA is widely accepted and employed to assess the risk of medical failures [9–11] and thus serves as a basis for generating preventive actions [12]. The validity of FMEA is commonly noted for the assessment of medical risk by the JCAHO. In FMEA, three indexes, including severity (S), occurrence (O) and detection (D), are applied to assess risk, where S denotes the seriousness of the effect of failure, O is the probability or frequency of the failure, and D represents the probability that the failure will be detected before the impact of the effect is realized. However, weaknesses in the process of assessing risk in FMEA have been reported [13,14]. Based on a review of previous studies, the limitations of FMEA include the following: (1) FMEA may not provide sufficient information regarding S, O, and D because it assumes that the relative importance of S, O and D is equal [13]; (2) due to insufficient discriminative power, the prioritization for the failure mode with different combinations of S, O, and D may yield the same value for the risk priority number (RPN), resulting in difficulty in ranking priorities [15]; and (3) FMEA provides limited corrective information on S, O and D for each failure mode.

Inspired by the technique of data envelopment analysis (DEA), this paper proposes two methods to overcome the weaknesses of FMEA. One is called the slacks-based measure DEA (SBM-DEA) model, and the other is a novel data-driven approach (NDA) that combines FMEA and DEA. The proposed modified DEA models are applied to risk index datasets of S, O and D. The realistic solutions, including complete prioritization and effective mitigation strategy, are generated to provide risk managers in healthcare organizations with insights into the degree of risk of medical errors for each medical service. Furthermore, the proposed models are also helpful for carrying out further process redesign for risk mitigation.

The subsequent sections of this paper are organized as follows. The methodology is presented in Section 2, in which the basic DEA model is briefly presented and three risk assessment approaches are described. In Section 3, the numerical results of FMEA, SBM-DEA and NDA are presented. Section 4 presents a comparison of the three approaches. Section 5 concludes with a summary of findings.

2. Methodology

FMEA was first developed to solve reliability and safety problems in the aerospace industry in the late 1950s. Because FMEA emphasizes the proactive prevention of medical failures rather than solutions, it can assist managers in identifying failures and causes/effects and in eliminating failures by instituting corrective actions in the risk assessment process [16]. In FMEA, a documented method is employed, asking the manager to provide structural and formalized information for the risk control and assessment of potential failures in terms of what might go wrong, what might cause it to go wrong, and what effects it would have [17]. The prioritization of failure modes is determined by the RPN, which is calculated by multiplying the scales of S, O and D. Higher values of RPN imply that corrective action is more urgently needed. The calculation of the RPN is expressed as follows:

$$\text{RPN} = \text{S} \times \text{O} \times \text{D} \tag{1}$$

DEA is a non-parametric analysis technique used to measure the relative efficiencies of decision-making units (DMUs). By using mathematical programming, DEA yields a composite efficiency score between zero and one for each DMU having multiple inputs and outputs. A DMU is said to be efficient if and only if it has an efficiency score of one. In DEA, an assumption of the weights for all of the productive indicators is not required. A set of weights is objectively generated via a programming process in which favorable weights for all DMUs under evaluation are determined by maximizing their efficiency scores. The result obtained from DEA may help decision-makers to identify the inefficient units and to consequently establish improvement strategies.

To overcome the weakness of FMEA, a numerous studies suggest that DEA may be an effective option for enhancing the assessment capability of FMEA [18–20]. DEA is a well-known data-driven approach for measuring the relative efficiencies among DMUs [21]. According to the efficiency perspective, DEA aggregates all productive indicators and yields a composite score to reveal the distance between a DMU's position and efficiency frontier. The frontier is formed by efficient DMUs, also called best -practices, representing the boundary condition for the whole system, which all DMUs can benchmark at their current production technology [22].

In this paper, a slacks-based measure (SBM) was used to assess the risk of failure modes in the healthcare industry. Suppose that there are n DMUs, each DMU_j ($j = 1, \ldots, n$) uses m inputs x_{ij} ($I = 1, \ldots, m$) to produce s outputs y_{rj} ($r = 1, \ldots, s$). Let DMU_o be the DMU under evaluation, and its ith input and rth output are denoted by x_{io} and y_{ro}, respectively. The SBM score of DMU_o, calculated using the input orientation, is expressed by the following programming model:

$$\text{Minimize} \quad \theta_o^{SBM} = 1 - \frac{1}{m}\sum_{i=1}^{m} s_i^- / x_{io}$$

s.t.

$$\begin{array}{ll} x_{io} = \sum_{j=1}^{n} \lambda_j x_{ij} + s_i^- & i = 1, \ldots, m \\ y_{ro} \leq \sum_{j=1}^{n} \lambda_j y_{rj} & r = 1, \ldots, s \\ \lambda_j \geq 0, s_i^- \geq 0 & j = 1, \ldots, n \end{array} \tag{2}$$

Model (2) is commonly referred to as the envelopment form and is the dual problem of the multiplier form. In model (2), $s^- \in R^m$ is the slack vector for the input, and $\lambda_j \in R^n$ is the non-negative vector connecting all inputs and outputs to form an efficiency frontier. s_i^- denotes the excess amounts in the input that can be decreased non-radially comparing with efficient DMUs. The θ_o^{SBM*} is the SBM efficiency of DMU_o. If $s_i^{-*} > 0$, DMU_o is identified as an inefficient unit, i.e., $\theta_o^{SBM*} < 1$; otherwise, it is an efficient unit. Compared with a traditional radial DEA model, SBM provides a clearer view for determining the specific input variable that causes the inefficiency. Through the optimal slack amount, s_i^{-*}, the direction for improving inefficient DMUs can also be easily obtained.

Figure 1 depicts the process of risk assessment, including four steps:

Step 1: Collect the risk index report of failure modes.

Step 2: Generate a dataset of risk indexes (severity, occurrence, and detection).

Step 3: Assess the risk of failure modes using modified DEA, including SBM-DEA and NDA, as discussed in this paper, and generate the risk rankings for all failure modes.

Step 4: Provide improvement strategies by mitigating risk for the prevention of medical failures.

Because the S, O, and D dataset in FMEA has the property of "the lower, the better", which is similar to inputs, this paper considers the risk indexes of S, O, and D as inputs. Thus, by applying SBM, as depicted in Equation (2), the FMEA model yields the following:

$$\text{Minimize} \quad \theta_o^{RPN} = 1 - \left(s^{s-}/S_o + s^{O-}/O_o + s^{D-}/D_o\right)/3$$

s.t.

$$\begin{array}{ll} S_o = \sum_{j=1}^{n} \lambda_j S_j + s^{S-} & \text{for severity} \\ O_o = \sum_{j=1}^{n} \lambda_j O_j + s^{O-} & \text{for occurrence} \\ D_o = \sum_{j=1}^{n} \lambda_j D_j + s^{D-} & \text{for detection} \\ 1 = \sum_{j=1}^{n} \lambda_j & j = 1, \ldots, n \\ \lambda_j, s^{S-}, s^{O-}, s^{D-} \geq 0 & \end{array} \tag{3}$$

where s^{S-}, s^{O-} and s^{D-} denote the slack for S, O, and D, respectively. The θ_o^{RPN*} represents a composed RPN index for each failure mode and is further employed as the basis for prioritizing n failure modes. A failure mode with $\theta_o^{RPN*} = 1$ and $s^{S-*} = 0$, $s^{O-*} = 0$, $s^{D-*} = 0$ represents a safer mode, whereas failure modes with $\theta_o^{RPN*} < 1$ represent riskier modes. For risky failure modes, the improving targets $\left(S_o - s^{S-*}, O_o - s^{O-*}, D_o - s^{D-*}\right)$ may be generated automatically by using the optimal slacks (s^{S-*}, s^{O-*}, s^{D-*}). In this paper, Equation (3) is referred to as the SBM-DEA model.

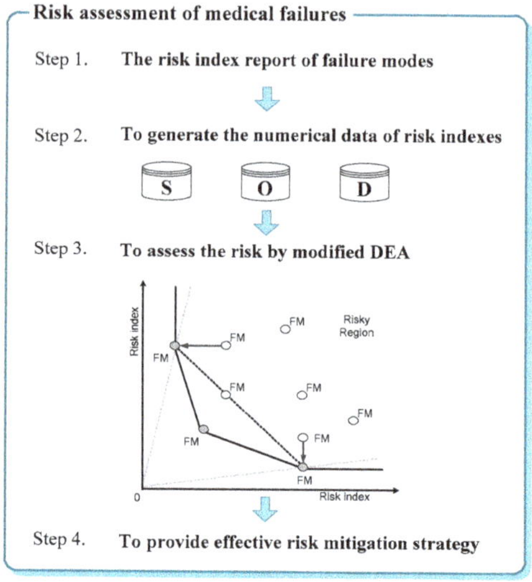

Figure 1. The process of risk assessment. DEA: data envelopment analysis.

SBM-DEA may successfully improve the discriminatory problem of traditional RPN, i.e., some failure modes have the same RPN composed of different combinations of S, O and D, providing an alternative adjustment as quantitative information for each risky failure mode. However, SBM-DEA may present two chief shortcomings: (1) for safer failure modes, it is unable to generate the complete prioritization, as they all have a unity score $\theta_o^{RPN*} = 1$; and (2) for risky failure modes, the improving targets waste of risk mitigation resources.

To overcome the problem arising from SBM-DEA, this paper presents the NDA, expressed in Equations (4) and (5). All failure modes are classified into two sets: safe failure modes and risky failure modes. We then apply the Super SBM model developed by Tone [23] and a minimum distance model developed by Aparicio et al. [24] to evaluate the RPN indexes of safe failure modes and risk failure modes, respectively.

For safer failure modes:

Assume that there are n safe failure modes with $\theta_o^{RPN*} = 1$. To differentiate them, the RPN for each safe failure mode is defined as the optimal value δ_o^{RPN*} in the following model.

$$\text{Minimize } \delta_o^{RPN} = 1 + \left(s^{S+}/S_o + s^{O+}/O_o + s^{D+}/D_o\right)/3$$

s.t.

$$\begin{array}{ll} S_o \geq \sum_{j=1, j\neq o}^{n-1} \lambda_j S_j - s^{S+} & \text{for severity} \\ O_o \geq \sum_{j=1, j\neq o}^{n-1} \lambda_j O_j - s^{O+} & \text{for occurrence} \\ D_o \geq \sum_{j=1, j\neq o}^{n-1} \lambda_j D_j - s^{D-} & \text{for detection} \\ 1 = \sum_{j=1, j\neq o}^{n-1} \lambda_j & j = 1, \ldots, n-1,\ j \neq o \\ \lambda_j, s^{S+}, s^{O+}, s^{D+} \geq 0 & \end{array} \quad (4)$$

For risky failure modes:

Let E be the set of safe failure modes with $\theta_o^{RPN} = 1$ and $\lambda_j = 1$. Thus, the RPN index for each risky failure mode can be solved by the following model.

$$\text{Maximize } \theta_o^{RPN} = 1 - \left(s^{s-}/S_o + s^{O-}/O_o + s^{D-}/D_o\right)/3$$

s.t.

$$\begin{array}{ll} S_o = \sum_{j=1,\ j\in E}^{n} \lambda_j S_j + s^{S-} & \text{for severity} \\ O_o = \sum_{j=1,\ j\in E}^{n} \lambda_j O_j + s^{O-} & \text{for occurrence} \\ D_o = \sum_{j=1,\ j\in E}^{n} \lambda_j D_j + s^{D-} & \text{for detection} \\ 1 = \sum_{j=1,\ j\in E}^{n} \lambda_j & j \in E \\ -(v^S S_j + v^O O_j + v^D D_j) + u = -d_j & \\ v^S, v^O, v^D,\ u \geq 1 & \\ 0 \leq d_j \leq M b_j & \\ 0 \leq \lambda_j \leq M(1 - b_j) & \\ b_j \in \{0,1\} & \\ s^{S-}, s^{O-}, s^{D-} \geq 0 & \end{array} \quad (5)$$

where M is a large positive variable, and b_j is the binary variable. The v^S, v^O and v^D are the weights for severity, occurrence and detection, respectively, which comply with the corresponding constraint to the multiplier form.

Compared to SBM-DEA, in the NDA model, the safe failure modes to be evaluated are removed from the safe frontier (λ_j, $j \neq 0$). In addition, all of the slacks (s^{S-}, s^{O-} and s^{D-}) in the constraints and objective function are modified from positive to negative. Thus, the RPN for each safe failure mode can be obtained as $\delta_o^{RPN*} \geq 1$.

Data Collection in the Healthcare Industry

In this section, we reuse a case from Western Wake Medical Center in Raleigh, North Carolina, which was first introduced by applying FMEA to mitigate the risk of preventing infant abduction in Reichert [25]. The dataset is tabulated in Table 1 and consists of 16 failure modes, which were identified by a managerial team in the medical service process.

Table 1. Risk indexes (S, O, D) in failure mode and effects analysis (FMEA) for preventing infant abduction.

No.	Failure Modes	Severity	Occurrence	Detection
FM1	Child not banded	10	7	5
FM 2	Insufficient IS info provided to mom	5	4	8
FM 3	Mom not paying attention	5	8	8
FM 4	Info not understood	5	2	8
FM 5	Baby may not be HUGS banded prior to washing	10	9	3
FM6	Info not entered into computer system, including name/room	10	8	5
FM7	Delay in entering info into computer system	10	4	5
FM8	"Unfounded" Alarms	10	3	10
FM9	Alarm ringing—doors not locking	10	2	10
FM10	HUGS band not applied until reaching post-partum (sometimes)	10	5	2
FM11	Bands loosening	8	9	6
FM12	Bands not checked and/or tightened properly	8	3	8
FM13	Not checked against census	7	8	7
FM14	Transferred rooms, not updated	7	7	7
FM15	HUGS band may not be checked when moving to nursery, other, for blood draws, circ, etc	5	7	3
FM16	Leaving SCN other than for discharge w/o HUGS band (may include family room visiting)	8	5	8

Note: HUGS: Hugs infant security system SCN: special care nursery.

3. Results

This paper applies the failure mode data in Table 1 to the three models: FMEA, SBM-DEA and NDA. The results are demonstrated in Figure 2 regarding the prioritization of failure modes among the three different approaches. For each approach, the horizontal axis displays the ranked set of failure modes sorted from highest to lowest risk, whereas the risk index is shown on the vertical axis. Additionally, we divided all ranked FMs into four quartiles (designated Q1 to Q4), with Q1 representing the highest 25th percentile of risk for FMs requiring urgent action. In Figure 2, we use the reciprocal of optimal scores obtained by SBM-DEA and the NDA model for simple ranking. A risky FM with θ_o^{RPN*}, $\delta_o^{RPN*} < 1$ has the covered risk index $1/\theta_o^{RPN*}$, $1/\delta_o^{RPN*} > 1$, which serves as the basis for ranking.

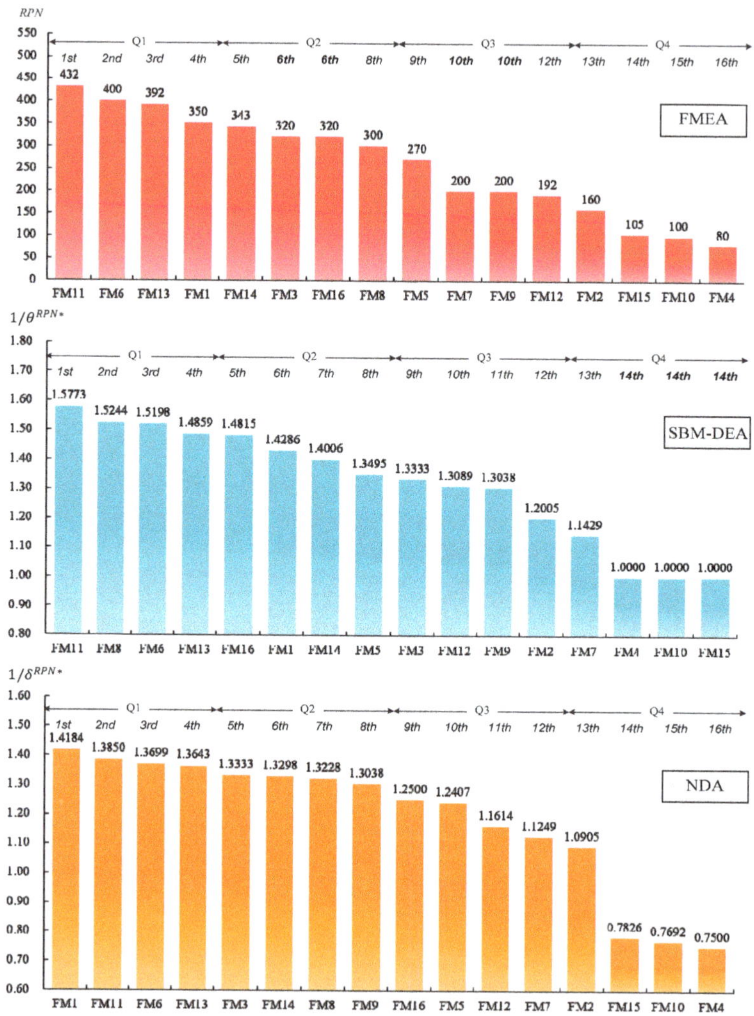

Figure 2. Prioritization of failure modes from risk priority number (RPN), slack-based measure (SBM) and our approach. FMEA: failure mode and effects analysis; SBM-DEA: slacks-based measure; NDA: data-driven approach.

In terms of FMEA, the subsets of the four quartiles included Q1 = {FM 11, FM 6, FM 13, FM 1}, Q2 = {FM 14, FM 3, FM 16, FM 8}, Q3 = {FM 5, FM 7, FM 9, FM 12} and Q4 = {FM 2, FM 15, FM 10, FM 4}. It became clear that the discrimination of FM 3 from FM 16 (an ordinal number of 6th) and FM 7 from FM9 (an ordinal number of 10th) was quite low due to their use of different combinations of S, O and D to compose the same RPN, i.e., FM 3 and FM 16 have RPN = 320; FM 7 and FM 9 have RPN = 200.

SBM-DEA may overcome such discriminatory problems, identifying the following risk priorities: FM 3 ($1/\theta_3^{RPN*} = 1.333$) $\prec$ FM 16 ($1/\theta_{16}^{RPN*} = 1.482$) and FM 7 ($1/\theta_7^{RPN*} = 1.143$) $\prec$ FM 9 ($1/\theta_9^{RPN*} =$

1.304). However, the ranking is still not sufficiently complete. The risk indexes for FM 4, FM 10 and FM 15 in Q4 imply that they are relative safe modes requiring no corrective action. However, advanced information on the priority of the modes is lacking because these three failure modes have the same unity score. Furthermore, the analytical results for the failure modes in Q1 = {FM 11, FM 8, FM 6, FM 13} and Q2 = {FM 16, FM 1, FM 14, FM 5} by SBM-DEA are not well matched to the results from FMEA. Only 75% of failures in Q1 and 50% in Q2 are in agreement with the FMEA results.

According to the results from the NDA model in Figure 2, all of the problems mentioned above were clearly solved. First, the weak discriminatory power of FMEA was improved upon. Risk rankings between FM 3 and FM 16 and between FM 7 and FM 9 were obtained using the NDA model. The risk index for FM 3 was ($1/\delta_3^{RPN*} = 1.333$) greater than that for FM 16 ($1/\delta_{16}^{RPN*} = 1.25$), and the risk index for FM 7 ($1/\delta_7^{RPN*} = 1.125$) was smaller than that for FM 9 ($1/\delta_9^{RPN*} = 1.304$). Second, three safe modes, including FM 4, FM 10 and FM 15, analyzed by SBM-DEA, showed the same unity score. Through the analysis depicted in Equation (4), the risk of these three failure modes was completely ranked using the NDA model. The priority ranking was determined as FM 15 $\succ$ FM 10 $\succ$ FM 4. Such a result helps risk managers to obtain full prioritization. Finally, the prioritization of Q1 = {FM 1, FM 11, FM 6, FM 13} and Q2 = {FM 3, FM 13, FM 8, FM 9} based on NDA is virtually a match, with the same results as FMEA, i.e., 100% in Q1 and 75% in Q2.

4. Discussion

The RPN value calculated using FMEA provides very limited information for establishing improvement strategies. Compared with the traditional FMEA, both SBM-DEA and the NDA model not only can generate a composite risk index from an efficiency perspective for each FM but also provide the risk control team with the quantitative information to set explicit targets for improving their strategies. This quantitative information can be determined from the difference between risky failure modes and their projection targets. However, these projection targets may differ between SBM-DEA and the NDA model because the former uses the maximum difference, while the latter concerns the minimum difference under programming.

Table 2 provides a detailed list of optimal scores, projection targets and difference rates for all failure modes calculated from SBM-DEA and the NDA model. Both the SBM-DEA model (left-hand side) and the NDA model (right-hand side) identify that FM 4, FM 10 and FM 15 are relatively safe modes. For each, the SBM-DEA model yields a score of one and projection target of S, O and D that are equivalent to the original data, such that the reduction rates are all zero. In contrast, the NDA model provides a score of more than one that can be used as the basis for further ranking. Moreover, the positive rates of S, O and D express additional information on risk-taking ability, i.e., FM 4 can increase 100% of O, FM 10 can increase 40% of O and 50% of D, and FM 15 can increase 83% of S.

Table 2. Comparative results of SBM-DEA and novel data-driven approach (NDA).

SBM-DEA					NDA				
Modes θ_o^{RPN*}	Index	Original	Projection	Rate	Modes δ_o^{RPN*}	Index	Original	Projection	Rate
FM1 0.700	S	10	5.0	−50.00%	**FM1** 0.705	S	10	7.5	−25.00%
	O	7	7.0	0.00%		O	7	3.5	−50.00%
	D	5	3.0	−40.00%		D	5	5.0	0.00%
FM2 0.833	S	5	5.0	0.00%	**FM2** 0.917	S	5	5.0	0.00%
	O	4	2.0	−50.00%		O	4	4.0	0.00%
	D	8	8.0	0.00%		D	8	6.0	−25.00%
FM3 0.750	S	5	5.0	0.00%	**FM3** 0.750	S	5	5.0	0.00%
	O	8	2.0	−75.00%		O	8	2.0	−75.00%
	D	8	8.0	0.00%		D	8	8.0	0.00%
FM4 1.000	S	5	5.0	0.00%	**FM4** 1.333	S	5	5.0	0.00%
	O	2	2.0	0.00%		O	2	4.0	100.00%
	D	8	8.0	0.00%		D	8	8.0	0.00%
FM5 0.741	S	10	10.0	0.00%	**FM5** 0.806	S	10	9.2	−8.33%
	O	9	5.0	−44.44%		O	9	4.5	−50.00%
	D	3	2.0	−33.33%		D	3	3.0	0.00%
FM6 0.658	S	10	5.0	−50.00%	**FM6** 0.730	S	10	7.5	−25.00%
	O	8	7.0	−12.50%		O	8	3.5	−56.25%
	D	5	3.0	−40.00%		D	5	5.0	0.00%
FM7 0.875	S	10	7.5	−25.00%	**FM7** 0.889	S	10	6.7	−33.33%
	O	4	3.5	−12.50%		O	4	4.0	0.00%
	D	5	5.0	0.00%		D	5	5.0	0.00%
FM8 0.656	S	10	5.0	−50.00%	**FM8** 0.756	S	10	6.7	−33.33%
	O	3	2.0	−33.33%		O	3	3.0	0.00%
	D	10	8.0	−20.00%		D	10	6.0	−40.00%
FM9 0.767	S	10	5.0	−50.00%	**FM9** 0.767	S	10	5.0	−50.00%
	O	2	2.0	0.00%		O	2	2.0	0.00%
	D	10	8.0	−20.00%		D	10	8.0	−20.00%
FM10 1.000	S	10	10.0	0.00%	**FM10** 1.300	S	10	10.0	0.00%
	O	5	5.0	0.00%		O	5	7.0	40.00%
	D	2	2.0	0.00%		D	2	3.0	50.00%
FM11 0.634	S	8	5.0	−37.50%	**FM11** 0.722	S	8	6.7	−16.67%
	O	9	7.0	−22.22%		O	9	3.0	−66.67%
	D	6	3.0	−50.00%		D	6	6.0	0.00%
FM12 0.764	S	8	5.0	−37.50%	**FM12** 0.861	S	8	6.7	−16.67%
	O	3	2.0	−33.33%		O	3	3.0	0.00%
	D	8	8.0	0.00%		D	8	6.0	−25.00%
FM13 0.673	S	7	5.0	−28.57%	**FM13** 0.733	S	7	7.0	0.00%
	O	8	7.0	−12.50%		O	8	3.2	−60.00%
	D	7	3.0	−57.14%		D	7	5.6	−20.00%
FM14 0.714	S	7	5.0	−28.57%	**FM14** 0.752	S	7	7.0	0.00%
	O	7	3.0	−57.14%		O	7	6.2	−11.43%
	D	7	7.0	0.00%		D	7	2.6	−62.86%
FM15 1.000	S	5	5.0	0.00%	**FM15** 1.278	S	5	9.2	83.33%
	O	7	7.0	0.00%		O	7	7.0	0.00%
	D	3	3.0	0.00%		D	3	3.0	0.00%
FM16 0.675	S	8	5.0	−37.50%	**FM16** 0.800	S	8	8.0	0.00%
	O	5	2.0	−60.00%		O	5	5.0	0.00%
	D	8	8.0	0.00%		D	8	3.2	−60.00%

Note: FM15 and 16 are taken as two examples to elaborate the calculations of SBM-DEA and NDA (See Appendix A). NDA: novel data-driven approach, SBM-DEA: slacks-based measure DEA (data envelopment analysis).

For risky failure modes with scores of less than one, the reduction rate with respect to the corresponding original data provides the scales for improving the effort of S, O and D (see the fifth and tenth columns of Table 2). By following these rates, the risky failure modes can be made safer, i.e., either to achieve the projection targets or to produce a score of $\theta_o^{RPN*} = 1$ for the SBM-DEA model and $\delta_o^{RPN*} \geq 1$ for the NDA model. Table 2 also shows large differences in optimal scores and reduction rates between the SBM-DEA model and the NDA model. On the basis of the optimal scores, the first three extreme cases include FM 16 ($\theta_{16}^{RPN*} = 0.675$ and $\delta_{16}^{RPN*} = 0.800$), FM 8 ($\theta_8^{RPN*} = 0.756$ and $\delta_8^{RPN*} = 0.656$) and FM 12 ($\theta_{12}^{RPN*} = 0.861$ and $\delta_8^{RPN*} = 0.764$). Regarding these failure modes, the SBM-DEA model suggests that reduction rates are S (−37.5%), O (−60%), and D (0%) for FM 16; S (−50%), O (−33.33%), and D (−20%) for FM 8; and S (−37.5%), O (−33.33%), and D (0%) for FM 12. These targets seem unattainable. In contrast, the NDA model obviously provides a more attainable (less effort) target for safety improvement with reduction rates of S (0%), O (0%), and D (−60%) for FM 16, S (−33.33%), O (0%), and D (−40%) for FM 8 and S (−16.67%), O (0%), and D (−25%) for FM 12. None of the reduction rates of S, O and D by the NDA model are ensured to be less than those obtained by SBM-DEA. For instance, the NDA model suggests that FM 5 may reach the safety frontier by reducing 8.33% of S and 50% of O, whereas the projection target provided by SBM-DEA asks FM 5 to reduce 44% of O and 33.33% of D. Figure 3 compares the average reduction rates between the SBM-DEA model and the NDA model. The reduction rate calculated by the difference between the projection target and the original data is 21.71% for the NDA model and 22.26% for the SBM-DEA model. The result demonstrates that the projection target of NDA is more closed to FEMA. And thus, on an average, safety improvement recommended by the NDA model are significantly more effective than those provided by the SBM-DEA model.

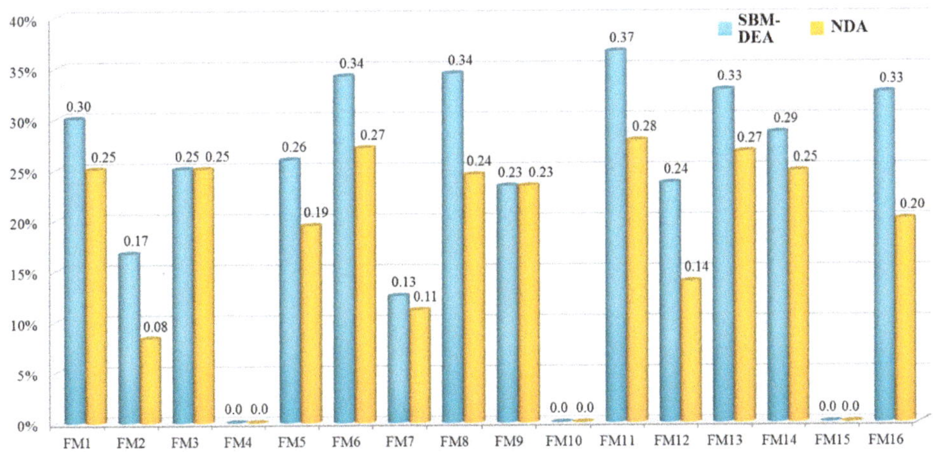

Figure 3. The average reduction rates between SBM and our approach.

In brief, SBM-DEA may yield biased measurements of risk and generate unrealistic solutions with two main shortcomings in comparison to the NDA model. First, SBM-DEA imperfectly generates a complete prioritization for all failure modes. Second, the improvement strategy generated by SBM-DEA for risk mitigation is feasible, but it results in a waste of resources.

5. Conclusions

Given the growing awareness of and pressure for healthcare quality and patient safety in today's healthcare environment, both academics and practitioners are increasingly concerned with risk management in medical services to avoid the effects of medical failures. FMEA is a well-known systematic procedure that is widely used to identify medical errors and to provide the necessary corrective actions. In this paper, we presented two models for improving the traditional FMEA method and compared the relative advantages among the three models. The analysis was based on an infant security case at Western Wake Medical Center in Raleigh, North Carolina, U.S.

Both the SBM-DEA model and the NDA model aim to solve the problem of discriminatory power arising from FMEA, which may result in the same RPN with different combinations of S, O and D for some failure modes. The results indicate that the SBM-DEA model and the NDA model, by integrating both two models and FMEA, may provide realistic solutions on optimal targets for safety improvement, whereas the risk mitigation strategies resulting from FMEA remain scarce. However, SBM-DEA might be imperfect, as the corrective direction generated from the optimizing process was unrealistic, resulting in a waste of resources. Additionally, SBM-DEA is incapable of providing complete prioritization for all failure modes.

The NDA model was found to successfully overcome the problems associated with the SBM-DEA model, as the NDA model can provide precise and complete prioritizations of failure modes in the healthcare industry. The NDA model attempts to find the minimum distance for each failure mode and then yields a strategy for improving medical failures. The corrective actions obtained from the NDA model are guaranteed to require less effort. As risk mitigation is a vital activity for reducing any further damages to safety once the risk assessment process is completed, risk mitigation plays a critical role in enhancing safety. The empirical results clarify the superiority of the NDA model. In light of the limited resources of healthcare organizations, the NDA model is a more effective and precise approach for risk management and costs less.

Author Contributions: S.-H.Y. conceived the study; Y.-T.C. and S.-H.Y. analyzed the data and wrote the draft; Y.-T.C. and E.C.-Y.S. edited the manuscript. All authors have approved the final manuscript.

Funding: The research was partly funded by Ministry of Science and Technology of Taiwan under grant No. MOST 106-2410-H-227-001 to Y.-T.C.

Acknowledgments: The authors would like to thank the editorial team of International Journal of Environmental Research and Public Health and anonymous reviewers who provided valuable comments and constructive suggestions for improving the quality of this paper.

Conflicts of Interest: The authors declare no conflict of interest.

Appendix A. Calculations of SBM-DEA and NDA for FM 15 and 16

SBM-DEA solves the following linear problems to obtain the optimal objective values of FM 15 θ_{15}^{RPN*} = 1.000 and FM 16 θ_{16}^{RPN*} = 0.675, respectively.

$$\text{Minimize} \quad \theta_{15}^{RPN} = 1 - \left(s^{s-}/5 + s^{O-}/7 + s^{D-}/3\right)/3$$

s.t.

$$\begin{aligned}
&5 = (10\lambda_1 + 5\lambda_2 + 5\lambda_3 + 5\lambda_4 + 10\lambda_5 + 10\lambda_6 + 10\lambda_7 + 10\lambda_8 + 10\lambda_9 + 10\lambda_{10} + 8\lambda_{11} + 8\lambda_{12} + 7\lambda_{13} + 7\lambda_{14} + 5\lambda_{15} + 8\lambda_{16}) + s^{S-}\\
&7 = (7\lambda_1 + 4\lambda_2 + 8\lambda_3 + 2\lambda_4 + 9\lambda_5 + 8\lambda_6 + 4\lambda_7 + 3\lambda_8 + 2\lambda_9 + 5\lambda_{10} + 9\lambda_{11} + 3\lambda_{12} + 8\lambda_{13} + 7\lambda_{14} + 7\lambda_{15} + 5\lambda_{16}) + s^{O-}\\
&3 = (5\lambda_1 + 8\lambda_2 + 8\lambda_3 + 8\lambda_4 + 3\lambda_5 + 5\lambda_6 + 5\lambda_7 + 10\lambda_8 + 10\lambda_9 + 2\lambda_{10} + 6\lambda_{11} + 8\lambda_{12} + 7\lambda_{13} + 7\lambda_{14} + 3\lambda_{15} + 8\lambda_{16}) + s^{D-}\\
&1 = (\lambda_1 + \lambda_2 + \lambda_3 + \lambda_4 + \lambda_5 + \lambda_6 + \lambda_7 + \lambda_8 + \lambda_9 + \lambda_{10} + \lambda_{11} + \lambda_{12} + \lambda_{13} + 7\lambda_{14} + \lambda_{15} + \lambda_{16})\\
&\lambda_{1:16}, s^{S-}, s^{O-}, s^{D-} \geq 0
\end{aligned}$$

$$\text{Minimize} \quad \theta_{16}^{RPN} = 1 - \left(s^{s-}/8 + s^{O-}/5 + s^{D-}/8\right)/3$$

s.t.

$$\begin{aligned}
&8 = (10\lambda_1 + 5\lambda_2 + 5\lambda_3 + 5\lambda_4 + 10\lambda_5 + 10\lambda_6 + 10\lambda_7 + 10\lambda_8 + 10\lambda_9 + 10\lambda_{10} + 8\lambda_{11} + 8\lambda_{12} + 7\lambda_{13} + 7\lambda_{14} + 5\lambda_{15} + 8\lambda_{16}) + s^{S-}\\
&5 = (7\lambda_1 + 4\lambda_2 + 8\lambda_3 + 2\lambda_4 + 9\lambda_5 + 8\lambda_6 + 4\lambda_7 + 3\lambda_8 + 2\lambda_9 + 5\lambda_{10} + 9\lambda_{11} + 3\lambda_{12} + 8\lambda_{13} + 7\lambda_{14} + 7\lambda_{15} + 5\lambda_{16}) + s^{O-}\\
&8 = (5\lambda_1 + 8\lambda_2 + 8\lambda_3 + 8\lambda_4 + 3\lambda_5 + 5\lambda_6 + 5\lambda_7 + 10\lambda_8 + 10\lambda_9 + 2\lambda_{10} + 6\lambda_{11} + 8\lambda_{12} + 7\lambda_{13} + 7\lambda_{14} + 3\lambda_{15} + 8\lambda_{16}) + s^{D-}\\
&1 = (\lambda_1 + \lambda_2 + \lambda_3 + \lambda_4 + \lambda_5 + \lambda_6 + \lambda_7 + \lambda_8 + \lambda_9 + \lambda_{10} + \lambda_{11} + \lambda_{12} + \lambda_{13} + 7\lambda_{14} + \lambda_{15} + \lambda_{16})\\
&\lambda_{1:16}, s^{S-}, s^{O-}, s^{D-} \geq 0
\end{aligned}$$

NDA solves the following linear problems to obtain the optimal objective values of FM 15 δ_{15}^{RPN*} = 1.278 and FM 16 δ_{16}^{RPN*} = 0.800, respectively.

$$\text{Minimize } \theta_{15}^{RPN} = 1 + \left(s^{s+}/5 + s^{O+}/7 + s^{D+}/3\right)/3$$

s.t.

$$\begin{array}{l}
5 \geq (10\lambda_1 + 5\lambda_2 + 5\lambda_3 + 5\lambda_4 + 10\lambda_5 + 10\lambda_6 + 10\lambda_7 + 10\lambda_8 + 10\lambda_9 + 10\lambda_{10} + 8\lambda_{11} + 8\lambda_{12} + 7\lambda_{13} + 7\lambda_{14} + 8\lambda_{16}) + s^{S+} \\
7 \geq (7\lambda_1 + 4\lambda_2 + 8\lambda_3 + 2\lambda_4 + 9\lambda_5 + 8\lambda_6 + 4\lambda_7 + 3\lambda_8 + 2\lambda_9 + 5\lambda_{10} + 9\lambda_{11} + 3\lambda_{12} + 8\lambda_{13} + 7\lambda_{14} + 5\lambda_{16}) + s^{O+} \\
3 \geq (5\lambda_1 + 8\lambda_2 + 8\lambda_3 + 8\lambda_4 + 3\lambda_5 + 5\lambda_6 + 5\lambda_7 + 10\lambda_8 + 10\lambda_9 + 2\lambda_{10} + 6\lambda_{11} + 8\lambda_{12} + 7\lambda_{13} + 7\lambda_{14} + 8\lambda_{16}) + s^{D+} \\
1 = (\lambda_1 + \lambda_2 + \lambda_3 + \lambda_4 + \lambda_5 + \lambda_6 + \lambda_7 + \lambda_8 + \lambda_9 + \lambda_{10} + \lambda_{11} + \lambda_{12} + \lambda_{13} + 7\lambda_{14} + \lambda_{16}) \\
\lambda_{1:16(\neq 15)}, s^{S+}, s^{O+}, s^{D+} \geq 0
\end{array}$$

$$\text{Maximize } \theta_{16}^{RPN} = 1 - \left(s^{s-}/8 + s^{O-}/5 + s^{D-}/8\right)/3$$

s.t.

$$\begin{array}{l}
8 = (5\lambda_4 + 10\lambda_{10} + 5\lambda_{15}) + s^{S-} \\
5 = (2\lambda_4 + 5\lambda_{10} + 7\lambda_{15}) + s^{O-} \\
8 = (8\lambda_4 + 2\lambda_{10} + 3\lambda_{15}) + s^{D-} \\
1 = (\lambda_4 + \lambda_{10} + \lambda_{15}) \\
-\left(v^S 5 + v^O 2 + v^D 8\right) + u = -d_4 \\
-\left(v^S 10 + v^O 5 + v^D 2\right) + u = -d_{10} \\
-\left(v^S 5 + v^O 7 + v^D 3\right) + u = -d_{15} \\
0 \leq d_4 \leq M b_4 \\
0 \leq d_{10} \leq M b_{10} \\
0 \leq d_{15} \leq M b_{15} \\
0 \leq \lambda_4 \leq M(1 - b_4) \\
0 \leq \lambda_{10} \leq M(1 - b_{10}) \\
0 \leq \lambda_{15} \leq M(1 - b_{15}) \\
v^S, v^O, v^D,\ u \geq 1 \\
s^{S-}, s^{O-}, s^{D-} \geq 0 \\
b_4, b_{10}, b_{15} \in \{0, 1\}
\end{array}$$

References

1. Giraldo, P.; Sato, L.; Sala, M.; Comas, M.; Dywer, K.; Castells, X. A retrospective review of medical errors adjudicated in court between 2002 and 2012 in Spain. *Int. J. Qual. Health Care* **2016**, *28*, 33–39. [CrossRef] [PubMed]
2. Valentini, R.P. Patient safety and quality improvement: What the pediatric trainee needs to know. *Prog. Pediatr. Cardiol.* **2017**, *44*, 47–53. [CrossRef]
3. Kohn, L.T.; Corrigan, J.M.; Donaldson, M.S. *To Err is Human: Building a Safer Health System*; A Report of the Committee on Quality of Health Care in America; National Academies Press: Washington, DC, USA, 2000.
4. Green, S.F. The cost of poor blood specimen quality and errors in preanalytical processes. *Clin. Biochem.* **2013**, *46*, 1175–1179. [CrossRef] [PubMed]
5. Ministry of Health and Welfare. MIHW News. Available online: https://www.mohw.gov.tw/np-16-1.html (accessed on 10 June 2018).
6. Classen, D.C.; Resar, R.; Griffin, F.; Federico, F.; Frankel, T.; Kimmel, N.; Whittington, J.C.; Frankel, A.; Seger, A.; James, B.C. Global trigger tool shows that adverse events in hospitals may be ten times greater than previously measured. *Health Affairs* **2011**, *30*, 581–589. [CrossRef] [PubMed]
7. Marx, D.A.; Slonim, A.D. Assessing patient safety risk before the injury occurs: An introduction to sociotechnical probabilistic risk modelling in health care. *Qual. Saf. Health Care* **2013**, *12*, 33–38. [CrossRef]
8. Aspden, P.; Corrigan, J.M.; Wolcott, J.; Erickson, S.M. Quality improvement and proactive hazard analysis models: Deciphering a new Tower of Babel. In *Patient Safety: Achieving a New Standard for Care*; National Academies Press: Washington, DC, USA, 2004.
9. Chiozza, M.L.; Ponzetti, C. FMEA: A model for reducing medical errors. *Clin. Chim. Acta* **2009**, *404*, 75–78. [CrossRef] [PubMed]

10. Fattahi, R.; Khalilzadeh, M. Risk evaluation using a novel hybrid method based on FMEA, extended MULTIMOORA, and AHP methods under fuzzy environment. *Saf. Sci.* **2018**, *102*, 290–300. [CrossRef]
11. Rezaee, M.J.; Yousefi, S.; Valipour, M.; Dehdar, M.M. Risk analysis of sequential processes in food industry integrating multi-stage fuzzy cognitive map and process failure mode and effects analysis. *Comput. Ind. Eng.* **2018**, *123*, 325–337. [CrossRef]
12. Vandenbrande, W.W. How to use FMEA to reduce the size of your quality toolbox. *Qual. Prog.* **1998**, *31*, 97–100.
13. Liu, H.C.; Liu, L.; Liu, N.; Mao, L.X. Risk evaluation in failure mode and effects analysis with extended VIKOR method under fuzzy environment. *Expert Syst. Appl.* **2012**, *39*, 12926–12934. [CrossRef]
14. Chang, D.S.; Chung, J.H.; Sun, K.L.; Yang, F.C. A novel approach for evaluating the risk of health care failure modes. *J. Med. Syst.* **2012**, *36*, 3967–3974. [CrossRef] [PubMed]
15. Chang, D.S.; Sun, K.L.P. Applying DEA to enhance assessment capability of FMEA. *Int. J. Qual. Reliab. Manag.* **2009**, *26*, 629–643. [CrossRef]
16. Kim, K.O.; Zuo, M.J. General model for the risk priority number in failure mode and effects analysis. *Reliab. Eng. Syst. Saf.* **2018**, *169*, 321–329. [CrossRef]
17. Sankar, N.R.; Prabhu, B.S. Modified approach for prioritization of failures in a system failure mode and effects analysis. *Int. J. Qual. Reliab. Manag.* **2001**, *18*, 324–336. [CrossRef]
18. Chin, K.S.; Wang, Y.M.; Poon, G.K.K.; Yang, J.B. Failure mode and effects analysis by data envelopment analysis. *Decis. Support Syst.* **2009**, *48*, 246–256. [CrossRef]
19. Parameshwaran, R.; Srinivasan, P.S.S.; Punniyamoorthy, M. An integrated approach for performance enhancement in automobile repair shops. *Int. J. Bus. Excel.* **2010**, *3*, 77–104. [CrossRef]
20. Rezaee, M.J.; Salimi, A.; Yousefi, S. Identifying and managing failures in stone processing industry using cost-based FMEA. *Int. J. Adv. Manuf. Technol.* **2017**, *88*, 3329–3342. [CrossRef]
21. Zhu, J. *Quantitative Models for Performance Evaluation and Benchmarking: DEA with Spreadsheets*; Springer Press: New York, NY, USA, 2014.
22. Ozcan, Y.A.; Tone, K. *Health Care Benchmarking and Performance Evaluation: An Assessment Using Data Envelopment Analysis (DEA)*; Springer Press: New York, NY, USA, 2014.
23. Tone, K. A slacks-based measure of super-efficiency in data envelopment analysis. *Eur. J. Oper. Res.* **2002**, *143*, 32–41. [CrossRef]
24. Aparicio, J.; Ruiz, J.L.; Sirvent, I. Closest targets and minimum distance to the Pareto-efficient frontier in DEA. *J. Prod. Anal.* **2007**, *28*, 209–218. [CrossRef]
25. Reichert, T.A. Applying failure modes and effects analysis (FMEA) in healthcare: Preventing infant abduction, a case study. In Proceedings of the 2004 Society for Health Systems Presentation, Raleigh, NC, USA, 20–21 February 2004.

International Journal of
Environmental Research and Public Health

MDPI

Article

Nurses' Occupational and Medical Risks Factors of Leaving the Profession in Nursing Homes

Carole Pélissier [1,2,*], Barbara Charbotel [3,4], Jean Baptiste Fassier [3,5], Emmanuel Fort [3] and Luc Fontana [1,2]

1 Unité Mixte de Recherche Épidémiologique et de Surveillance Transport Travail Environnement (UMRESTTE, UMR_T9405), Institut français des sciences et technologies des transports, de l'aménagement et des réseaux (IFSTTAR), Université de Lyon, Université Lyon 1, Université de St Etienne, 42055 Saint-Etienne, France; luc.fontana@chu-st-etienne.fr
2 Service de Santé au Travail et Pathologies Professionnelles, CHU de Saint-Etienne, 42055 Saint-Etienne, France
3 Unité Mixte de Recherche Épidémiologique et de Surveillance Transport Travail Environnement (UMRESTTE, UMR_T9405), Institut français des sciences et technologies des transports, de l'aménagement et des réseaux (IFSTTAR), Université de Lyon, Université Lyon 1, F-69373 Lyon, France; barbara.charbotel-coing-boyat@univ-lyon1.fr (B.C.); jean-baptiste.fassier@chu-lyon.fr (J.B.F.); emmanuel.fort@univ-lyon1.fr (E.F.)
4 Hospices Civils de Lyon, Centre Hospitalier Lyon Sud, Service de Pathologies Professionnelles, F-69495 Pierre Bénite, France
5 Hospices Civils de Lyon, Service de Médecine et Santé au Travail, 69002 Lyon, France
* Correspondence: Pelissier.carole.chu@gmail.com; Tel.: +33-(0)4-7782-8325; Fax: +33-(0)4-7782-8139

Received: 8 August 2018; Accepted: 23 August 2018; Published: 27 August 2018

Abstract: This study aimed to evaluate the association between intention to leave work, and working conditions and health status among female care-staff in nursing homes. A multicenter cross-sectional study included female care-staff in 105 nursing homes for the elderly. We used validated questionnaires to assess occupational, psychosocial and medical data in a multicenter transverse study. Univariate analysis on chi^2 test was performed with stratification according to job (nurse, nursing assistant), and variables found to be significant on each dimension were included on multivariate models. 1428 nursing assistants and 342 registered nurses were included. 391 nursing assistants and 85 registered nurses intended to leave their work with the elderly. The registered nurses' intention to leave was associated with deteriorated care-team or residents relations, and with perceived elevated hardship due to the proximity of residents' death. The nursing assistants' intention to leave was associated with deteriorated management relation, with job insecurity and elevated hardship due to the residents' intellectual deterioration. Impaired physical or psychological health status also correlated with this intention. Policy to reduce voluntary turnover of care-staff in nursing homes for the elderly could be based on multifactorial management, acting on work organization and reducing psychosocial stress.

Keywords: care workers' intention to leave; nursing homes for the elderly; psychosocial factors; musculoskeletal complaints; impaired well-being

1. Introduction

High rates of staff turnover in nursing homes are not a recent phenomenon, especially among those who work most closely with the residents: registered nurses and nursing assistants. Nursing homes for the elderly differ in functioning from hospitals in that they have lower level of medical presence. They are residential establishments caring for increasingly elderly, dependent persons with multiple comorbidities. Care is given by nursing assistants with various kinds of initial training and by registered nurses. Registered nurses usually ensure technical care and coordinate the work of the nursing assistants. As well as catering and accompaniment, nursing assistants are in charge of hygiene, comfort and preventive and curative care and are under the supervision of a nurse. About 17.5% of new nurses leave their first job within one year of starting their jobs [1]. The proportion of nurses considering or intending to leave the profession varied from 4% to 54% [2]. The cost of turnover from the organizational perspective includes replacement costs (including training), lost productivity, lost quality and lowered morale [3,4]. A previous study argued that these costs may well be reflected in the quality of care that residents receive [3,5]. Three broad categories of factors that influence turnover have been identified: general economic, work-related and personal factors [3]. Registered nurses and nursing assistants in nursing homes are subject to strong mental and physical demands (e.g., lifting and carrying, work schedule), and frequently describe their working environment as distressing [6]. The physical and mental deterioration of elderly patients and the proximity to death were more often perceived as a source of hardship by registered nurses and nursing assistants. Registered nurses and nursing assistants are more often confronted by aggressive patients than in hospitals or facilities for the disabled [7–9]. Registered nurses who had experienced burnout or stress were more likely to intend to leave the profession [2,10]. Fochsen et al. have focused on the relationship between musculoskeletal disorders and intent to leave the profession in staff of nursing-homes for the elderly [11]. Several studies underlined an association between impaired mental well-being in nursing home care workers and psychosocial factors in health caregivers, but there has been less research on the association between impaired mental well-being in nursing home care workers and health caregivers' intention to leave has hardly been studied [12–15]. Understanding why health care workers abandon their current employer and/or their job in the nursing profession is important in retention of health providers. The objective of the present study was to analyze occupational and medical factors associated with the intention to leave work with the elderly, comparing between nursing assistants and registered nurses, considering the differences in their tasks.

2. Materials and Methods

2.1. Design

The study was designed as a cross-sectional questionnaire survey design.

2.2. Participants

The target population of the survey was female employees working in with elderly patients in nursing homes in the Rhône-Alpes Region of France. The occupational physicians of the Region were asked to participate in the survey by the Regional Department of Businesses, Competition, Consumption, Work and Employment (DIRECCTE), a state business consultancy. Volunteer occupational physicians filled out a working conditions assessment questionnaire, and asked all employees meeting the inclusion criteria in the nursing homes which they oversaw to take part. Only employees who had been working with the elderly for at least 6 months on at least a half-time basis were included. The occupational physician handed over the self-administered questionnaire to subjects included in the study and collected data on working conditions and health status in nursing staff. The number of subjects who refused to participate was anonymously collected by the occupational physicians.

2.3. Data Collection

Between October 2009 and September 2010, data were collected by self-administered questionnaires during periodic follow-up medical examinations or during company visits. These self-administered questionnaires comprised personal characteristics (age, gender, family status, number of children), health characteristics and work-related characteristics and used four questionnaires measuring Job related hardship, musculoskeletal complaints, impaired mental well-being, and psychosocial demands [16–21].

2.4. Measures

Job related hardship: The questionnaire included visual analog hardship scales (1 = no hardship, to 10 = great hardship) related to: premises (disrepair, stairs, clutter), lifting and carrying the elderly, patients' mental and physical deterioration, and proximity of death [16–18]. The choice of these particular categories was based on the literature [21]. Hardship scores were categorized as slight ($\leq$3), moderate (4–7) or severe hardship ($\geq$8).

Musculoskeletal complaints: Musculoskeletal complaints were assessed on the Nordic Musculoskeletal Questionnaire, comprising multiple choice questions for each body part (such as upper limbs, lower limbs, neck and back): "During the last 12 months, have you had trouble (such as ache, pain, discomfort)?". The Nordic Musculoskeletal Questionnaire is a standardized questionnaire with reliability and validity moderate to high, which makes is a good instrument for epidemiological survey into musculoskeletal disorders and complaints [19].

Impaired mental well-being: Developed as a screening tool to detect the workers likely to have or to risk of developing psychiatry disorders, the General Health Questionnaire (GHQ) is a measure of the common mental health problems, domains of depression, anxiety, somatic symptoms and social withdrawal. It's the 12-item version (GHQ-12) was used. Respondents had to indicate how frequently they had recently experienced the various symptoms listed. Each item was rated on a 4-point scale, with weights from 0 to 3 according to Likert-like type scale (0 = less than usual, 1 = no more than usual, 2 = rather more than usual, and 3 = much more than usual) [20]. Scores higher than 12 were considered as indicating impaired mental wellbeing [22,23].

Psychosocial demands: Psychosocial demands at work were assessed on the effort-reward imbalance (ERI) model using the Siegrist questionnaire. In this model, chronic work-related stress is identified as non-reciprocity or imbalance between high efforts spent and low rewards received. Conversely, positive emotions evoked by appropriate social rewards promote well-being, health and survival [16]. This questionnaire has three scales: two measuring the extrinsic components of 'effort' (6 items) and 'reward' (11 items covering earnings, esteem and job security) and one measuring the intrinsic component of 'over-commitment' (six items) [16,17]. Effort was measured either by six items on the demanding aspect of the work environment (three measuring quantitative load, one qualitative load, one increase in total load over time, and one physical load), rated as 1 = does not apply, 2 = does apply but subject does not consider herself distressed, 3 = does apply and subject considers herself somewhat distressed, 4 = does apply and subject considers herself distressed, or 5 = does apply and subject considers herself very distressed. A sum score of these ratings was totalled, as documented in several studies [16,17]. According to the ERI model, extrinsic and intrinsic effort scores are directly proportional to effort, whereas the rewards score is inversely proportional to reward. ERI was measured by calculating the ratio between the extrinsic effort index (E) and the inverse reward index (R): $E/(R^*c)$, with c as a correction factor (c: 6/11); ERI >1 indicates a critical condition of high-cost/low-gain, or effort-reward imbalance [16,17]. To obtain a more precise view of which rewards were related to which indicators of employee health, three occupational rewards (earnings, esteem and job security) were assessed separately. All three reward scores were dichotomized separately, using the most adverse tercile to indicate low reward: the higher the reward score, the lower the reward [16–18,21,24,25].

2.5. Ethical Considerations

Approval by the French Ministry of Health Research (Comité Consultatif pour le Traitement de l'Information en Matière de Recherche dans le Domaine de la Santé, 09.320) was obtained before starting the study. The participants were given an information leaflet explaining the study objectives and participation was voluntary.

2.6. Data Analysis

The continuous quantitative variable of seniority in the establishment was transformed into an ordinal qualitative variable for statistical purposes.

A descriptive step characterized the employee population according to personal characteristics, working conditions, including occupational psychosocial factors, and mental health status. Distinguishing between registered nurses and nursing assistants, associations were sought between the intent to leave work with the elderly and personal factor, occupational factors, psychosocial factors and medical factors. Frequencies were compared on chi-squared tests, with chi-squared trend tests depending on the results of cross-analysis. Ratios of event probabilities per case of intent to leave were studied. As the prevalence of each event was high, odds ratios would not provide a good estimate of relative risk, and a log-linked binomial model was applied, using the PROC GENMOD procedure in the SAS statistical package (version 9.3) with the DIST = BINOMIAL and LINK = LOG options.

Univariate and multivariate analyses were performed stratified on job category (nurse/nursing assistant). The binary response of each case of intent to leave was modeled in two steps: Firstly, all independent variables underwent univariate analysis; secondly, multivariate analyses were performed for each dimension (sociodemographic, occupational, psychosocial, and personal health); variables with p-value ≤ 0.1 were included in a multivariate model on a descending procedure, and variables with p-value < 0.05 were kept in the model. The psychosocial and medical dimension models were adjusted on age. For the psychosocial dimension, the global ERI variable is classically used, but in the present study we sought to investigate the questionnaire sub-dimensions in greater detail, studying the four variables of extrinsic effort and the three types of reward (esteem, earnings, and job security) in the multivariate models. From these four multivariate models, multivariate regression was performed on a descending procedure, with a significance threshold of 5%. In case of non-convergence of PROC GENMOD because the maximum likelihood estimate (MLE) lay on the boundary of the parameter space, the SAS COPY macro was used, which provides a good approximation to the exact maximum likelihood estimates, as well as yielding good estimates of the true population parameters [26].

3. Results

3.1. Socio-Occupational and Medical Data

1770 women (19.6% registered nurses, 80.4% nursing assistants) working in direct contact with the elderly in 105 nursing homes were included. Twenty-nine registered nurses and nine nursing assistants refused to participate, leading to a global participation rate of 98%. Four hundred and seventy-six of the 1808 women (26.3%), wished to leave their work with the elderly: 391 nursing assistants (26.8%) and 85 registered nurses (24.2%).

3.2. Factors Associated with Intention to Leave Work on Univariate Analysis

Occupational factors: In both nursing assistants and registered nurses, severe hardship related to residents' physical deterioration, to proximity to death, or to lack of equipment was significantly associated with intention to leave. In nursing assistants, weak attachment to the elderly residents, understaffing, and severe hardship related to lifting and carrying residents, to premises, or to residents' intellectual deterioration, were significantly associated with intention to leave (Table 1). In both nursing assistants and registered nurses, work contract, seniority in work with elderly, working time, night work and type of working hours were not associated with intention to leave.

Table 1. Sociodemographic, occupational, psychosocial and medical factors associated with registered nurses' and nursing assistants' intention to leave work with the elderly, on univariate analysis.

		Nursing Assistants' Intention to Leave (n = 391)				Registered Nurses' Intention to Leave (N = 85)			
Sociodemographic Factors		N	%	PR	[95% CI]	N	%	PR	[95% CI]
Age	<30 years	118	33.9	1 ****	17	27.9	1 ▽		
	30–39 years	97	31.0	0.91	0.74–1.14	24	33.3	1.19	0.71–2.01
	40–49 years	110	24.5	0.72	0.58–0.90	24	25.8	0.93	0.54–1.57
	≥50 years	65	20.5	0.60	0.46–0.78	20	17.2	0.62	0.35–1.09
Marital status	Single	92	32.7	1 *	10	29.4	1		
	In couple	237	25.4	0.77	0.64–0.94	62	24.8	0.84	0.48–1.48
	Separated, divorced, widowed	58	28.6	0.87	0.66–1.15	13	22.8	0.77	0.38–1.57
Do you have children?	Yes	267	25.4	1 **	68	24.9	1		
	No	123	33.0	1.30	1.09–1.55	17	24.6	0.98	0.62–1.57
Occupational Factors		**N**	**%**	**PR**	**[95% CI]**	**N**	**%**	**PR**	**[95% CI]**
Hardship: lifting and carrying	Mild	36	16.4	1 ****	18	20.4	1		
	Moderate	108	22.6	1.37	0.97–1.93	34	25.0	1.22	0.74–2.02
	Severe	245	34.1	2.07	1.51–2.85	32	28.6	1.40	0.84–2.31
Hardship: premises	Mild	161	11.4	1 **	28	20.3	1		
	Moderate	133	30.7	1.31	1.08–1.59	27	26.0	1.28	0.80–2.03
	Severe	245	32.7	1.40	1.13–1.73	30	31.60	1.56	0.99–2.42
Hardship: equipment	Mild	139	21.3	1 ****	32	20.0	1 *		
	Moderate	143	30.7	1.44	1.18–1.76	27	25.5	1.27	0.81–1.99
	Severe	103	36.9	1.73	1.39–2.14	25	36.2	1.81	1.16–2.81
Hardship: residents' intellectual deterioration	Mild	54	16.8	1 ****	14	15.4	1		
	Moderate	115	25.1	1.44	1.18–1.76	28	21.1	1.57	0.88–2.80
	Severe	218	34.4	1.73	1.40–2.14	43	32.6	2.11	1.24–3.64
Hardship: residents' physical deterioration	Mild	46	17.1	1 ****		13	15.7	1 *	
	Moderate	112	24.7	1.45	1.06–1.96	30	23.3	1.48	0.82–2.68
	Severe	230	33.1	1.94	1.46–2.57	42	38.8	2.09	1.20–3.66
Hardship: proximity to death	Mild	90	22.4	1 **		24	19.7	1 *	
	Moderate	128	27.0	1.21	0.95–1.52	32	22.7	1.15	0.72–1.85
	Severe	172	31.7	1.41	1.13–1.76	29	37.7	1.91	1.21–3.03
Do you get attached to the residents ?	Very often	59	21.4	1 *		6	13.0	1 ▽	
	Often	235	27.5	1.29	1.00–1.65	52	24.9	1.91	0.87–4.17
	Seldom	78	31.8	1.49	1.11–1.99	24	34.3	2.63	1.16–5.93
	Rarely/never	19	39.6	1.85	1.22–2.81	3	20.00	1.53	0.44–5.39
Staffing levels adequate?	Yes	58	20.1	1 ***		10	15.6	1 ▽	
	No	331	29.4	1.46	1.14–1.87	75	27.4	1.75	0.96–3.19

Table 1. *Cont.*

		Nursing Assistants' Intention to Leave (n = 391)				Registered Nurses' Intention to Leave (N = 85)			
Psychosocial Factors		N	%	PR	[95% CI]	N	%	PR	[95% CI]
Victim of verbal aggression	No	51	17.6	1 ****		12	23.5	1	
	Yes	340	29.8	1.69	1.29–2.20	73	25.1	1.06	0.62–1.82
Victim of physical aggression	No	137	22.2	1 ****		41	23.7	1	
	Yes	254	31.3	1.41	1.18–1.69	44	26.0	1.09	0.76–1.59
Relations with team	Satisfactory/very satisfactory	308	26.5	1 $^{\nabla}$		60	21.1	1 ***	
	Moderately satisfactory/unsatisfactory	81	31.6	1.19	0.98–1.46	25	43.9	2.07	1.43–3.00
Relations with patients	Satisfactory/very satisfactory	339	26.0	1 ***		66	22.1	1 **	
	Moderately satisfactory/unsatisfactory	52	42.3	1.63	1.29–2.04	19	45.2	2.05	1.38–3.04
Relations with families	Satisfactory/very satisfactory	287	25.5	1 ****		58	24.1	1	
	Moderately satisfactory/unsatisfactory	76	40.6	1.59	1.30–1.95	27	28.4	1.18	0.79–1.74
Relations with management	Satisfactory/very satisfactory	231	22.4	1 ****		52	22.4	1	
	Moderately satisfactory/unsatisfactory	153	40.4	1.80	1.52–2.12	33	30.6	1.36	0.94–1.98
Effort/reward imbalance	No	317	25.0	1 ****		72	23.2	1 *	
	Yes	70	48.3	1.93	1.59–2.34	13	43.3	1.87	1.18–2.95
Overcommitment	No	268	25.2	1 **		48	21.0	1 *	
	Yes	123	33.7	1. 34	1.12–1.60	37	32.7	1.56	1.08–2.25
Extrinsic effort	No	243	22.6	1 ****		49	22.6	1	
	Yes	148	41.8	1.85	1.57–2.18	36	28.8	1.27	0.88–1.85
Reward	Yes	234	22.3	1 ****		60	22.2	1 *	
	No	157	41.6	1.87	1.59–2.20	25	34.7	1.56	1.06–2.30
Earnings	Yes	151	20.8	1 ****		45	20.9	1 *	
	No	226	35.8	1.72	1.44–2.05	37	33.0	1.57	1.09–2.28
Esteem	Yes	174	20.9	1 ****		41	20.3	1 **	
	No	202	37.6	1.80	1.51–2.13	43	35.6	1.65	1.15–2.39
Job security	Yes	128	19.1	1 ****		31	16.6	1 ****	
	No	258	35.9	1.89	1.57–2.26	54	35.8	2.15	1.46–3.17
Medical Factors		N	%	PR	[95% CI]	N	%	PR	[95% CI]
Psychological distress	No	200	37.8	1 ****		45	31.5	1 *	
	Yes	189	21.5	1.76	1.49–2.08	39	19.7	1.59	1.10–2.32
Spinal complaints	No	98	19.6	1 ***		22	17.9	1 *	
	Yes	293	31.7	1.62	1.32–1.98	61	28.2	1.58	1.02–2.44
Upper-limb complaints	No	303	26.2	1 *		63	22.9	1 $^{\nabla}$	
	Yes	85	33.5	1.28	1.05–1.56	21	33.3	1.45	0.96–2.19
Lower-limb complaints	No	311	25.8	1 ***		64	22.8	1 *	
	Yes	77	37.6	1.45	1.19–1.78	21	36.8	1.62	1.08–2.42

PR: Prevalence Ratio; CI: Confidence Interval. $^{\nabla}$ p-value < 0.1; * $p < 0.05$; ** $p < 0.01$; *** $p < 0.001$; **** $p \leq 10^{-4}$.

Psychosocial factors: In both nursing assistants and registered nurses, intention to leave was significantly associated with impaired relations with residents, poor reward in terms of earnings, job security, and esteem, over-commitment, and ERI.

In nursing assistants, intention to leave was significantly associated with physical, or verbal aggression, and impaired relations with management, or families.

In registered nurses, intention to leave was significantly associated with impaired relations with the care-team (Table 1).

Med Psychosocial factors: In both nursing assistants and registered nurses, intention to leave was significantly associated with impaired relations with residents, poor reward in terms of earnings, job security, and esteem, over-commitment, and ERI.

In nursing assistants, intention to leave was significantly associated with physical, or verbal aggression, and impaired relations with management, or families.

In registered nurses, intention to leave was significantly associated with impaired relations with the care-team (Table 1).

ical factors: For both nursing assistants and registered nurses, psychological distress and spinal, or lower-limb complaints were significant. Upper-limb musculoskeletal disorder was significantly associated with intention to leave in nursing assistants (Table 1).

3.3. Factors Associated with Intention to Leave Work on Multivariate Analysis

Occupational factors: Severe hardship related to proximity to death was associated with intention to leave in registered nurses, as was severe hardship related to residents' intellectual deterioration and weak attachment to residents in nursing assistants (Tables 2–4). In this global multivariate analysis, hardship related to inadequate equipment no longer featured as a significant factor (Table 4).

Psychosocial factors: Impaired relations with management in nursing assistants, impaired relations with residents or with care team in registered nurses, remained associated with intention to leave. In nursing assistants, high levels of effort and poor reward in terms of job security were associated with intention to leave. Poor esteem from colleagues no longer featured as a significant factor on global multivariate analysis (Tables 2 and 4).

Medical factors: Lower limb complaints and spinal complaints remained associated with intention to leave in nursing assistants but not registered nurses on global multivariate analysis (Table 4).

Table 2. Significant associations between nursing assistants' intention to leave work with the elderly and sociodemographic, occupational, psychosocial and medical factors on intermediate multivariate analysis.

Variables		PR	[95% CI]
Sociodemographic Factors			
Age	<30 years	1 ***	
	30–39 years	0.91	0.74–1.14
	40–49 years	0.72	0.58–0.90
	≥50 years	0.60	0.46–0.78
Occupational Factors			
Work contract	Permanent	1 *	
	Temporary	0.78	0.63–0.97
Hardship: equipment	Mild	1 **	
	Moderate	1.23	1.00–1.51
	Severe	1.45	1.17–1.79
Hardship: residents' intellectual deterioration	Mild	1 ****	
	Moderate	1.41	1.05–1.89
	Severe	1.94	1.48–2.55
Do you get attached to the residents?	Very often	1 **	
	Often	1.29	1.00–1.66
	Seldom	1.48	1.11–1.97
	Rarely/never	1.96	1.33–2.87

Table 2. *Cont.*

Variables		**PR**	**[95% CI]**
Psychosocial Factors			
Relations with management	Satisfactory/very satisfactory	1 *	
	Moderately satisfactory/unsatisfactory	1.26	1.04–1.55
Extrinsic effort	No	1 **	
	Yes	1.31	1.08–1.60
Esteem	Yes	1 *	
	No	1.26	1.01–1.57
Job security	Yes	1 ***	
	No	1.51	1.21–1.89
Medical Factors			
Psychological distress	No	1 ****	
	Yes	1.55	1.31–1.84
Spinal complaints	No	1 **	
	Yes	1.38	1.13–1.70
Lower-limb complaints	No	1 ***	
	Yes	1.39	1.15–1.69

PR: Prevalence Ratio; CI: Confidence Interval.* $p < 0.05$; ** $p < 0.01$; *** $p < 0.001$; **** $p \leq 10^{-4}$.

Table 3. Significant associations between registered nurses' intention to leave work with the elderly and sociodemographic, occupational, psychosocial and medical factors on intermediate multivariate analysis.

Variables		**PR**	**[95% CI]**
Sociodemographic Factors			
Age	<30 years	1 *	
	30–39 years	1.20	0.71–2.01
	40–49 years	0.93	0.54–1.57
	≥50 years	0.62	0.35–1.10
Occupational Factors			
Hardship: equipment	Mild	1 *	
	Moderate	1.25	0.80–1.95
	Severe	1.75	1.14–2.68
Hardship: proximity to death	Mild	1 ***	
	Moderate	1.17	0.73–1.89
	Severe	1.95	1.23–3.08
Psychosocial Factors			
Relations with team	Satisfactory/very satisfactory	1 **	
	Moderately satisfactory/unsatisfactory	1.98	1.32–2.98
Relations with patients	Satisfactory/very satisfactory	1 *	
	Moderately satisfactory/unsatisfactory	1.43	0.93–2.19
Medical Factors			
Psychological distress	No	1 **	
	Yes	1.66	1.14–2.39
Spinal complaints	No	1 *	
	Yes	1.65	1.07–2.53

PR: Prevalence Ratio; CI: Confidence Interval. * $p < 0.05$; ** $p < 0.01$; *** $p < 0.001$.

Table 4. Significant associations between registered nurses' and nursing assistants' intention to leave work with the elderly and sociodemographic, occupational, psychosocial and medical factors on global multivariate analysis.

Nursing Assistants				Registered Nurses			
Variables		**PR**	**[95% CI]**	**Variables**		**PR**	**[95% CI]**
Sociodemographic Factors					**Sociodemographic Factors**		
Age	<30 years	1 ***		Age	<30 years	1 *	
	30–40 years	0.92	0.75–1.12		30–40 years	0.97	0.60–1.57
	40–50 years	0.74	0.61–0.90		40–50 years	0.80	0.49–1.33
	>50 years	0.58	0.46–0.74		>50 years	0.53	0.30–0.92
Occupational Factors					**Occupational Factors**		
Hardship: residents' intellectual deterioration	Mild	1 ****		Hardship: proximity to death	Mild	1 *	
	Moderate	1.38	1.04–1.83		Moderate	1.23	0.79–1.93
	Severe	1.77	1.36–2.30		Severe	1.82	1.18–2.82
					Psychosocial Factors		
Do you get attached to the residents?	Very often	1 **		Relations with team	Satisfactory/very satisfactory	1 **	
	Often	1.28	1.01–1.63		Moderately satisfactory/unsatisfactory	1.71	1.15–2.56
	Seldom	1.33	1.02–1.73	Relations with patients	Satisfactory/very satisfactory	1 *	
	Rarely/never	1.96	1.63–2.82		Moderately satisfactory/unsatisfactory	1.52	1.02–2.26
Psychosocial Factors							
Relations with management	Satisfactory/very satisfactory	1 ***					
	Moderately satisfactory/unsatisfactory	1.34	1.14–1.58				
Extrinsic effort	No	1 *					
	Yes	1.22	1.02–1.45				
Job security	Yes	1 ***					
	No	1.42	1.17–1.72				
Medical Factors							
Spinal complaints	No	1 *					
	Yes	1.27	1.04–1.55				
Lower-limb complaints	No	1 **					
	Yes	1.34	1.13–1.59				

PR: Prevalence Ratio; CI: Confidence Interval. * $p < 0.05$; ** $p < 0.01$; *** $p < 0.001$; **** $p \leq 10^{-4}$.

4. Discussion

In the present study, care-workers' intention to leave was significantly related to certain psychosocial factors and impaired health status. This study of 1770 female registered nurses and nursing assistants in 105 nursing homes for the elderly in the Rhône-Alpes Region of France had a 98% response rate. This study has the advantage of having exploited for the administration of the questionnaires the periodic visits conducted by the occupational physicians. This method usually allows a high participation and minimizes the possibility that the answers are influenced by other workers, because the time in the waiting room is very limited [27].

Validated questionnaires assessed psychosocial demand, musculoskeletal complaints and psychological distress. The interest of the study lay in correlating intention to leave work with the elderly and working conditions (psychosocial and organizational demand) while taking into account the registered nurses' and nursing assistants' psychological and physical health status. This cross-sectional study does not allow us to know the temporal relation between the different phenomena that influence the intention to leave. However, previous studies have made it clear that the various factors, violence and stress, are cyclically related to each other [28–30].

Four hundred and seventy-six (26.3%) of respondents wished to leave their work with the elderly, and nursing assistants (26.8%) more frequently than registered nurses (24.2%). This finding agrees with Fochsen et al., who reported that "being an assistant nurse was associated with leaving nursing care" [11]. The NEXT-Study (Nurses' early exit study) was established to investigate the degree, reasons, circumstances, and consequences of premature departure from the nursing profession in Europe. The proportion of nurses (24.9%) who had frequently considered leaving their profession in nursing homes was higher in our study than in the French data of the longitudinal NEXT-Study (16.5%), in which nurses were working in residential care for the elderly, hospital structures or home-care [31]. The negative relation-ship between age and turnover intent has been widely reported in previous studies [13,32]. It has been argued that young nurses who belong to generation Y (born after 1980) hold different attitudes and values towards their work, which may influence their retention. According to Lavoie-Tremblay et al., the generation Y nurses reported that recognition was a key motivator. Their needs are stability, flexible work schedules and shifts, recognition, opportunities for professional development, and adequate supervision [33].

The study highlighted a significant association between hardship in relation to proximity to death and intention to leave work with the elderly. Previous study showed that nursing home staff who had had palliative care training were less liable to report severe hardship in relation to proximity to death, suggesting that palliative care training has positive impact on perceived hardship in relation to proximity to death [34]. Better training in the management of dementia patients and in palliative care might reduce the intention to leave work with the elderly.

A number of researchers have reported an association between workload, stress and turnover intention [35,36]. In this cross-sectional study, both workplace violence and bad relationships (which often fall into verbal violence) are significantly associated with the intention to leave work. The effect was higher in younger workers; this confirms what observed in previous Italian cohorts of nurse and nursing students [37]. Previous studies suggested that the psychologically strenuous and stressful nature of the work causes nurses to consider leaving the nursing profession [38–40]. In the present study, intention to leave was significantly related to certain psychosocial factors. First effort/reward imbalance was significantly related to intention to leave in nursing assistants. The ERI model was used to analyze intention to leave the nursing profession in nurses (n = 21,299) in seven European countries, in the NEXT-Study: ERI was associated with the frequency of considering leaving the nursing profession [31]. Secondly, overcommitment was not significantly associated with intention to leave in the present study, in agreement with previous findings [31,40]. According to Zeytinoglu et al., nurses with higher levels of career commitment showed statistically significantly lower levels of propensity to leave nursing [10]. Wang et al. found that a higher level of occupational commitment was related to stronger intention to stay [41]. Low affective commitment to the profession was associated with greater intention to leave the profession [2]. Moreover, Takase et al. found that nursing staff commitment was directly related to reduce intention to quit the profession [42]. The present study highlighted weak attachment to residents on the part of nurses and nursing assistants as associated with intention to leave. Then high levels of effort were an important work environment factor for intention to leave, consistent with previous findings [31–40]. Finally, for nursing assistants, poor reward in terms of job security, but in terms of not earnings, was significantly associated with intention to leave on multivariate analysis. Pay was found not a significant predictor for Jordanian nurses to leave their organization [43]. According to Lavoie-Tremblay et al., the reasons most often given for quitting the profession by nurses were difficult working conditions and a lack of job stability [34]. Improving the psychosocial work environment and specifically occupational rewards may be helpful in retaining caregivers.

Poor relations with management for nursing assistants and poor relations with the care-team and patients for nurses were significantly associated with intention to leave [44]. Nursing assistants seemed to exchange little with nurses according to an ergonomic study of geriatric care-staff [45]. In France, the working week was reduced to 35 h, which may have had the effect of reducing the time available for verbal exchanges within the team. Moreover, increasing administrative work for nurses and the increased work-load reported may have reduced the time available for verbal exchanges between patients and nurses, impairing the nurse-patient relationship. Cowden et al., in a systematic review of the literature, found a positive relationship between transformational leadership, supportive work environments and staff nurses intentions to stay [46]. Creating a supportive work environment, with supportive leadership gives nurses the confidence to stay [47,48]. Healthy and supportive work relationships have been shown to be related to greater intention to stay in work for nurses [49,50].

The present study revealed a significant association between intention to leave and impaired health status. First, lower-limb and spinal musculoskeletal complaints were significantly associated with intention to leave for nursing assistants. Fochsen and Sjögren showed that musculoskeletal problems of the neck/shoulder and knees were associated with leaving nursing care [11,51]. Secondly, psychological distress was significantly associated with intention to leave for both nursing assistants and nurses, in line with the longitudinal study of 6441 caregivers by Kivimaki et al. [52]. Bartram et al. found that emotional labor has an indirect effect on intention to leave via burnout nurses experience [53].

5. Conclusions

Care-staff in nursing homes for the elderly are exposed to elevated psychological and physical demands in caring for dependent elderly persons often with comorbidities. The present study found that some of the demands experienced by nurses and nursing assistants underlie an intention to leave work with the elderly. The results highlight the importance of perceived working conditions in this intention to leave. Policy to reduce voluntary turnover in nursing homes for the elderly could be based on a multifactorial approach involving work organization, reduced psychosocial demand and access to certain training modules such as in palliative care and the management of patients in dementia. Reorganization to reduce nurses' administrative workload by delegating tasks to administration workers should allow nurses more time for exchanges with both patients and nursing assistants. Having more time to devote to relational aspects would enhance verbal exchange between residents and caregivers, which in turn should improve job satisfaction and quality of care. Greater involvement in drawing up personalized care projects and reinforcing and developing caregiver autonomy in performing everyday care tasks should improve the caregivers' image of the job. Better recognition of the work accomplished could be achieved by increasing the time available for exchanges between colleagues and with management, and by improving job security.

Author Contributions: Conceptualization, B.C. and L.F.; Data curation, C.P., E.F. and B.C.; Formal analysis, C.P. and E.F.; Funding acquisition, B.C.; Investigation, C.P. and B.C.; Methodology, C.P., B.C., J.B.F., E.F. and L.F.; Project administration, B.C. and J.B.F.; Supervision, B.C. and L.F.; Validation, C.P., B.C., E.F., J.B.F. and L.F.; Visualization, C.P., J.B.F., E.F. and L.F.; Writing—original draft, C.P.

Funding: This research was funded by [Department of Businesses, Competition, Consumption, Work and Employment (DIRECCTE)].

Acknowledgments: The authors thank all of the occupational physicians who agreed to assist with this study.

Conflicts of Interest: The authors declare no conflict of interest.

References

1. Kovner, C.T.; Brewer, C.S.; Fatehi, F.; Jun, J. What does nurse turnover rate mean and what is the rate? *Policy Politics Nurs. Pract.* **2014**, *15*, 64–71. [CrossRef] [PubMed]
2. Flinkman, M.; Leino-Kilpi, H.; Salanterä, S. Nurses' intention to leave the profession: Integrative review. *J. Adv. Nurs.* **2010**, *66*, 1422–1434. [CrossRef] [PubMed]
3. Brannon, D.; Zinn, J.S.; Mor, V.; Davis, J. An Exploration of Job, Organizational, and Environmental Factors Associated with High and Low Nursing Assistant Turnover. *Gerontologist* **2002**, *42*, 159–168. [CrossRef] [PubMed]
4. Mukamel, D.B.; Spector, W.D.; Limcangco, R.; Wang, Y.; Feng, Z.; Mor, V. The costs of turnover in nursing homes. *Med. Care* **2009**, *47*, 1039. [CrossRef] [PubMed]
5. Cohen-Mansfield, J. Turnover among nursing home staff. A review. *Nurs. Manag.* **1997**, *28*, 59–62, 64. [CrossRef]
6. Pelissier, C.; Fontana, L.; Fort, E.; Agard, J.P.; Couprie, F.; Delaygue, B.; Glerant, V.; Perrier, C.; Sellier, B.; Vohito, M.; et al. Occupational risk factors for upper-limb and neck musculoskeletal disorder among health-care staff in nursing homes for the elderly in France. *Ind. Health* **2014**, *52*, 334–346. [CrossRef] [PubMed]
7. Moss, A.J.; Harris-Kojetin, L.D.; Sengupta, M.; Park-Lee, E.; Caffrey, C.; Rosenoff, E.; Wiener, J.M.; Greene, A.M. Design and Operation of the 2010 National Survey of Residential Care Facilities. *Vital Health Stat Ser. 1 Programs Collect Proced.* **2011**, *54*, 1–131.
8. Spidla, V. *Long Term Care in the European Union*; European Commission: Brussels, Belgium, 2008.
9. Pélissier, C.; Vohito, M.; Fort, E.; Sellier, B.; Agard, J.P.; Fontana, L.; Charbotel, B. Risk factors for work-related stress and subjective hardship in health-care staff in nursing homes for the elderly: A cross-sectional study. *J. Occup. Health* **2015**, *57*, 285–296. [CrossRef] [PubMed]
10. Zeytinoglu, I.U.; Denton, M.; Davies, S.; Baumann, A.; Blythe, J.; Boos, L. Retaining nurses in their employing hospitals and in the profession: Effects of job preference, unpaid overtime, importance of earnings and stress. *Health Policy* **2006**, *79*, 57–72. [CrossRef] [PubMed]
11. Fochsen, G.; Josephson, M.; Hagberg, M.; Toomingas, A.; Lagerström, M. Predictors of leaving nursing care: A longitudinal study among Swedish nursing personnel. *Occup. Environ. Med.* **2006**, *63*, 198–201. [CrossRef] [PubMed]
12. Pélissier, C.; Fontana, L.; Fort, E.; Vohito, M.; Sellier, B.; Perrier, C.; Glerant, V.; Couprie, F.; Agard, J.P.; Charbotel, B. Impaired mental well-being and psychosocial risk: A cross-sectional study in female nursing home direct staff. *BMJ Open* **2015**, *5*, e007190. [CrossRef] [PubMed]
13. Chiang, Y.-M.; Chang, Y. Stress, depression, and intention to leave among nurses in different medical units: Implications for healthcare management/nursing practice. *Health Policy* **2012**, *108*, 149–157. [CrossRef] [PubMed]
14. Jolivet, A.; Caroly, S.; Ehlinger, V.; Kelly-Irving, M.; Delpierre, C.; Balducci, F.; Sobaszek, A.; De Gaudemaris, R.; Lang, T. Linking hospital workers' organisational work environment to depressive symptoms: A mediating effect of effort-reward imbalance? The ORSOSA study. *Soc. Sci. Med.* **2010**, *71*, 534–540. [CrossRef] [PubMed]
15. Van Vegchel, N.; de Jonge, J.; Bosma, H.; Schaufeli, W. Reviewing the effort–reward imbalance model: Drawing up the balance of 45 empirical studies. *Soc. Sci. Med.* **2005**, *60*, 1117–1131. [CrossRef] [PubMed]
16. Siegrist, J.; Starke, D.; Chandola, T.; Godin, I.; Marmot, M.; Niedhammer, I.; Peter, R. The measurement of effort–reward imbalance at work: European comparisons. *Soc. Sci. Med.* **2004**, *58*, 1483–1499. [CrossRef]

17. Niedhammer, I.; Siegrist, J.; Landre, M.F.; Goldberg, M.; Leclerc, A. Psychometric properties of the French version of the Effort-Reward Imbalance model. *Revue d'Epidemiologie et de Sante Publique* **2000**, *48*, 419–437. [PubMed]
18. Niedhammer, I.; Siegrist, J. Psychosocial factors at work and cardiovascular diseases: Contribution of the Effort-Reward Imbalance model. *Revue d'Epidemiologie et de Sante Publique* **1998**, *46*, 398–410. [PubMed]
19. Kuorinka, I.; Jonsson, B.; Kilbom, A.; Vinterberg, H.; Biering-Sørensen, F.; Andersson, G.; Jørgensen, K. Standardised Nordic questionnaires for the analysis of musculoskeletal symptoms. *Appl. Ergon.* **1987**, *18*, 233–237. [CrossRef]
20. Lesage, F.-X. Validation of the *General Health Questionnaire* (GHQ-12) adapted to a work-related context. *Open J. Prev. Med.* **2011**, *1*, 44–48. [CrossRef]
21. Bouletreau, A.; Chouanière, D.; Wild, P.; Fontana, J. Concevoir, traduire et valider un quetsionnaire à propos d'un exemple EUROQUEST. *INRS* **2009**, *178*, 1–49. (In French)
22. Estryn-Behar, M.; Kaminski, M.; Peigne, E.; Bonnet, N.; Vaichere, E.; Gozlan, C.; Azoulay, S.; Giorgi, M. Stress at work and mental health status among female hospital workers. *Br. J. Ind. Med.* **1990**, *47*, 20–28. [CrossRef] [PubMed]
23. Charbotel, B.; Croidieu, S.; Vohito, M.; Guerin, A.C.; Renaud, L.; Jaussaud, J.; Bourboul, C.; Imbard, I.; Ardiet, D.; Bergeret, A. Working conditions in call-centers, the impact on employee health: A transversal study. Part II. *Int. Arch. Occup. Environ. Health* **2009**, *82*, 747–756. [CrossRef] [PubMed]
24. Niedhammer, I.; Chea, M. Psychosocial factors at work and self reported health: Comparative results of cross sectional and prospective analyses of the French GAZEL cohort. *Occup. Environ. Med.* **2003**, *60*, 509–515. [CrossRef] [PubMed]
25. Langevin, V.; François, M.; Boini, S.; Riou, A. Déséquilibre efforts/récompense. *Doc. Pour. Médecin. Trav.* **2011**, *125*, 111–115.
26. Deddens, J.; Petersen, M.; Lei, X. Estimation of prevalence ratos when PROC GENMOD does not converge. In Proceedings of the 28th Annual SAS Users Group International Conference, Washington, DC, USA, 30 March–2 April 2003; Seattle Wash SAS Institute: Cary, NC, USA, 2003.
27. Magnavita, N.; Garbarino, S. Social psychiatry in the waiting room. What a physician can learn about occupational stress from workers waiting to be examined. *Psychiatry J.* **2013**, *2013*, 701872. [CrossRef] [PubMed]
28. Magnavita, N. The exploding spark. Workplace violence in an infectious disease hospital—A longitudinal study. *BMRI BioMed Res. Int.* **2013**, *2013*, 316358. [CrossRef] [PubMed]
29. Magnavita, N. Workplace violence and occupational stress in health care workers: A chicken and egg situation—Results of a 6-year follow-up study. *J. Nurs. Scholarsh.* **2014**, *46*, 366–376. [CrossRef] [PubMed]
30. Halter, M.; Boiko, O.; Pelone, F.; Beighton, C.; Harris, R.; Gale, J.; Gourlay, S.; Drennan, V. The determinants and consequences of adult nursing staff turnover: A systematic review of systematic reviews. *BMC Health Serv. Res.* **2017**, *17*, 824. [CrossRef] [PubMed]
31. Hasselhorn, H.-M.; Tackenberg, P.; Peter, R. Effort–Reward Imbalance among Nurses in Stable Countries and in Countries in Transition. *Int. J. Occup. Environ. Health* **2004**, *10*, 401–408. [CrossRef] [PubMed]
32. Ramoo, V.; Abdullah, K.L.; Piaw, C.Y. The relationship between job satisfaction and intention to leave current employment among registered nurses in a teaching hospital. *J. Clin. Nurs.* **2013**, *22*, 3141–3152. [CrossRef] [PubMed]
33. Lavoie-Tremblay, M.; O'brien-Pallas, L.; Gélinas, C.; Desforges, N.; Marchionni, C. Addressing the turnover issue among new nurses from a generational viewpoint. *J. Nurs. Manag.* **2008**, *16*, 724–733. [CrossRef] [PubMed]
34. Pélissier, C.; Fontana, L.; Fort, E.; Charbotel, B. Pénibilité ressentie et accès aux formations chez le personnel féminin travaillant auprès des résidents dans les maisons de retraite médicalisées: Une enquête transversale. *Gériatrie Psychol. Neuropsychiatr. Vieil.* **2015**, *13*, 396–406.
35. Brannon, D.; Barry, T.; Kemper, P.; Schreiner, A.; Vasey, J. Job Perceptions and Intent to Leave Among Direct Care Workers: Evidence from the Better Jobs Better Care Demonstrations. *Gerontologist* **2007**, *47*, 820–829. [CrossRef] [PubMed]
36. Liu, Y.; Wu, L.-M.; Chou, P.-L.; Chen, M.-H.; Yang, L.-C.; Hsu, H.-T. The Influence of Work-Related Fatigue, Work Conditions, and Personal Characteristics on Intent to Leave Among New Nurses. *J. Nurs. Scholarsh.* **2016**, *48*, 66–73. [CrossRef] [PubMed]

37. Magnavita, N.; Heponiemi, T. Workplace violence against nursing students and nurses. An Italian experience. *J. Nurs. Scholarsh.* **2011**, *43*, 203–210. [CrossRef] [PubMed]
38. Cho, S.-H.; Park, M.; Jeon, S.H.; Chang, H.E.; Hong, H.-J. Average Hospital Length of Stay, Nurses' Work Demands, and Their Health and Job Outcomes. *J. Nurs. Scholarsh.* **2014**, *46*, 199–206. [CrossRef] [PubMed]
39. Li, J.; Fu, H.; Hu, Y.; Shang, L.; Wu, Y.; Kristensen, T.S.; Mueller, B.H.; Hasselhorn, H.M. Psychosocial work environment and intention to leave the nursing profession: Results from the longitudinal Chinese NEXT study. *Scand. J. Public Health* **2010**, *38* (Suppl. 3), 69–80. [CrossRef] [PubMed]
40. Tominaga, M.T.; Miki, A. Factors associated with the intention to leave among newly graduated nurses in advanced-treatment hospitals in Japan. *Jpn. J. Nurs. Sci.* **2011**, *8*, 33–46. [CrossRef] [PubMed]
41. Wang, L.; Tao, H.; Ellenbecker, C.H.; Liu, X. Job satisfaction, occupational commitment and intent to stay among Chinese nurses: A cross-sectional questionnaire survey. *J. Adv. Nurs.* **2012**, *68*, 539–549. [CrossRef] [PubMed]
42. Takase, M.; Yamashita, N.; Oba, K. Nurses' leaving intentions: Antecedents and mediating factors. *J. Adv. Nurs.* **2008**, *62*, 295–306. [CrossRef] [PubMed]
43. Al-Hussami, M.; Darawad, M.; Saleh, A.; Hayajneh, F.A. Predicting nurses' turnover intentions by demographic characteristics, perception of health, quality of work attitudes. *Int. J. Nurs. Pract.* **2014**, *20*, 79–88. [CrossRef] [PubMed]
44. Zeytinoglu, I.U.; Denton, M.; Plenderleith, J.M. Flexible employment and nurses' intention to leave the profession: The role of support at work. *Health Policy* **2011**, *99*, 149–157. [CrossRef] [PubMed]
45. Estryn-Behar, M.; Chaumon, E.; Garcia, F.; Milanini-Magny, G.; Fry, C.; Bitot, T.; Ravache, A.E.; Deslandes, H. la souffrance au travail en gériatrie comprendre et agir. *La Revue Francophone de Gériatrie et de Gérontologie* **2013**, *20*, 6–27.
46. Cowden, T.; Cummings, G.; Profetto-Mcgrath, J. Leadership practices and staff nurses' intent to stay: A systematic review. *J. Nurs. Manag.* **2011**, *19*, 461–477. [CrossRef] [PubMed]
47. Kaewboonchoo, O.; Yingyuad, B.; Rawiworrakul, T.; Jinayon, A. Job stress and intent to stay at work among registered female nurses working in Thai hospitals. *J. Occup. Health* **2014**, *56*, 93–99. [CrossRef] [PubMed]
48. Mrayyan, M.T. Differences of hospitals' organisational climates and nurses' intent to stay: Nurses' perspectives. *J. Res. Nurs.* **2009**, *14*, 465–477. [CrossRef]
49. Tourangeau, A.E.; Cranley, L.A. Nurse intention to remain employed: Understanding and strengthening determinants. *J. Adv. Nurs.* **2006**, *55*, 497–509. [CrossRef] [PubMed]
50. Tourangeau, A.E.; Cummings, G.; Cranley, L.A.; Ferron, E.M.; Harvey, S. Determinants of hospital nurse intention to remain employed: Broadening our understanding. *J. Adv. Nurs.* **2010**, *66*, 22–32. [CrossRef] [PubMed]
51. Sjögren, K.; Fochsen, G.; Josephson, M.; Lagerström, M. Reasons for leaving nursing care and improvements needed for considering a return: A study among Swedish nursing personnel. *Int. J. Nurs. Stud.* **2005**, *42*, 751–758. [CrossRef] [PubMed]
52. Kivimäki, M.; Vanhala, A.; Pentti, J.; Länsisalmi, H.; Virtanen, M.; Elovainio, M.; Vahtera, J. Team climate, intention to leave and turnover among hospital employees: Prospective cohort study. *BMC Health Serv. Res.* **2007**, *7*, 170. [CrossRef] [PubMed]
53. Bartram, T.; Casimir, G.; Djurkovic, N.; Leggat, S.G.; Stanton, P. Do perceived high performance work systems influence the relationship between emotional labour, burnout and intention to leave? A study of Australian nurses. *J. Adv. Nurs.* **2012**, *68*, 1567–1578. [CrossRef] [PubMed]

International Journal of
Environmental Research and Public Health

MDPI

Article

The Safe Use of Pesticides: A Risk Assessment Procedure for the Enhancement of Occupational Health and Safety (OHS) Management

Mario Fargnoli [1,2], Mara Lombardi [2], Daniele Puri [3], Laura Casorri [4], Eva Masciarelli [4], Stefan Mandić-Rajčević [5,*] and Claudio Colosio [5]

1 Department of Rural Development, Ministry of Agriculture, Food and Fishery, DISR I, via XX Settembre 20, 00187 Rome, Italy; mario.fargnoli@uniroma1.it
2 Department of Chemical Engineering Materials Environment (DICMA), Sapienza-University of Rome, via Eudossiana 18, 00184 Rome, Italy; mara.lombardi@uniroma1.it
3 Department of Technological Innovations and Safety of Plants, Products and Anthropic Settlements (DIT), National Institute for Insurance against Accidents at Work (INAIL), Via Fontana Candida 1, 00078 Monte Porzio Catone (RM), Italy; d.puri@inail.it
4 Department of Technological Innovations and Safety of Plants, Products and Anthropic Settlements (DIT), National Institute for Insurance against Accidents at Work (INAIL), Via R. Ferruzzi, 38/40, 00143 Rome, Italy; l.casorri@inail.it (L.C.); e.masciarelli@inail.it (E.M.)
5 Department of Health Sciences of the University of Milan, International Centre for Rural Health of the SS. Paolo and Carlo Hospital, Via San Vigilio 43, 20142 Milan, Italy; claudio.colosio@unimi.it
* Correspondence: stefan.mandic-rajcevic@unimi.it

Received: 16 December 2018; Accepted: 19 January 2019; Published: 23 January 2019

Abstract: The attention paid to the use of pesticides has increased notably in recent years as demonstrated by the issue of laws and regulations requiring their safe and environmentally-conscious use (e.g. Directive 2009/128/EC and Regulation (EC) no. 1272/2008). Despite the benefits that can be achieved by pursuing the targets of stricter legislative framework, the difficulties for farmers in complying with it are remarkable, especially for small-sized companies. In fact, in contrast to other occupational health and safety (OHS) contexts, in the case of pesticides even a preliminary analysis on the relationship between pesticide use and the consequent exposure risks for the workers is a complex task. In order to reduce the above-mentioned gap, the present study is focused on the development of an easy-to-use tool for carrying out occupational risk assessment of agricultural activities related to the use of pesticides. The procedure was developed by starting from the Agricultural Health Study (AHS) approach and its improvements, and continuing to the thorough development of a tool for preliminary risk assessment, providing a simplified model for its practical application by farmers. A case study concerning olive cultivation was used for its first verification. The results achieved should be considered as an initial step for the promotion of safer practices when using pesticides, providing a consistent base for their further validation.

Keywords: occupational health and safety; risk assessment; chemical risks; occupational exposure; pesticides; occupational risk management; olive orchards

1. Introduction

In recent years, matters concerning the safer and more sustainable use of chemical products in agriculture have risen in importance worldwide [1,2]. In the European Union this goal is represented by the implementation of the Integrated Pest Management (IPM) policy [3], which relies on a series of legislative interventions starting from the issue of Directive 2009/128/EC, establishing a framework for community action to achieve the sustainable use of pesticides [4]. This directive, together with the related acts affecting, among others, the safety requirements of the machinery for pesticide application [5], the placing of plant protection products on the market [6], the classification, labelling, and packaging of substances and mixtures [7], and the requirements for the registration, evaluation, authorization, and restriction of chemicals [8–10], have had a large impact on farmers and companies operating in the agricultural sector.

These new and stricter obligations concern the whole cycle of pesticide use, starting from their purchase up to the disposal of packaging and residues. As requested by Directive 2009/128/EC, the mandatory requirements that should be satisfied for the proper use of pesticides are defined by Member States through their National Action Plans (NAPs) [11]. From the farmers' perspective, this new approach towards a low pesticide-input in agriculture affects several aspects, ranging from the change of agronomic practices to the compliance with more rigorous specifications for both machinery maintenance as well as occupational health and safety (OHS) measures [12–14].

Besides the unquestionable benefits for the environment, human health, and social costs that can be achieved pursuing the targets proposed by this new legislative framework, the difficulties for farmers in complying with it are also remarkable [15,16].

The goal of the present study was to investigate the latter aspect, focusing on the assessment of the occupational risks related to the use of pesticides. Numerous studies addressing risk assessment from the epidemiological point of view can be found in the literature [17–21]. On the other hand, only few studies have dealt with the practical needs of the companies, in particular agricultural enterprises, of implementing risk assessment and management to guarantee the safe use of pesticides [8,22]. In particular, one of the major problems at the practical level, especially for small companies, is represented by the provision of a document where, as per Article 9 of Directive 89/391/EEC, "an assessment of the risks to safety and health at work, including those facing groups of workers exposed to particular risks" is reported. Hence, companies have to implement and document a risk assessment procedure that includes, among other aspects, the best practices, information, and training issues coming from the application of Directive 2009/128/EC, and information provided by the safety data sheet as defined by Regulation (EC) no. 1907/2006 in conjunction with Regulation (EC) no. 1272/2008. Contrary to pesticide exposure, in other types of exposure to particular occupational risks, such as vibrations, noise, or ultraviolet (UV) radiation, it is possible to provide a preliminary evaluation of the exposures and risks. Specifically, when dealing with vibrating tools and machines the exposure levels can be properly defined thanks to the availability of databases recognized from scientific bodies/authorities [23,24]. Based on this, a preliminary risk assessment can be performed considering the dose and the duration of exposure in a hands-on manner [25].

In the case of pesticides, the exposure depends on many factors and workers doing apparently the same job might be exposed to different levels of an active substance. There is a lack of clear evidence on how the dose levels or the repeated exposure might influence workers' health [18,26–28]. Moreover, the products put on the market are in continuous evolution [29], and, although some pesticide databases exist [30], their recognition by the OHS authorities is difficult. As a consequence, even a preliminary risk assessment, providing information on the relationships between the pesticides' use and the consequent exposure risks for the workers, is certainly a complex task [31], requiring additional efforts and resources particularly in the case of small-sized companies [32,33]. In such a context, in fact, safety knowledge, attitudes, and practices are still inadequate [34–36], even when dealing with a proper understanding of safety pictograms [37–40].

In order to reduce the above-mentioned gap, the present study is focused on the development of an easy-to-use tool for carrying out occupational risk assessment of agricultural activities related to the use of pesticides. Such a tool is aimed at supporting companies in verifying the compliance with mandatory requirements and providing OHS management indications to achieve and maintain safe working conditions when using pesticides.

In the next section, an analysis of the legislative framework that the risk assessment activities have to comply with is provided. Then, in Section 3 a background analysis on the scientific issues related to the solution of such a problem is reported. Section 4 presents the research approach/methodology, illustrating the proposed risk assessment procedure, while in Section 5 its practical application in a case study is reported. Section 6 discusses the achieved results and conclusive remarks are presented in Section 7.

2. Legislative Framework

Table 1 synthetizes the interwoven combination of legislative acts, considering their implementation in the Italian legislation and the main issues related to the safe use of pesticides.

Table 1. EU legislation, its implementation in the Italian legislation, the context, and the related main issues.

Main Legislative Source	Italian Legislation	Context	Main Issues
Directive 89/391/EEC	Decree 81/2008	Occupational health and safety (OHS) of professional workers	Specific risk assessment of working activities related to the use of chemical products; Specific information and training of the operators that use pesticides; Provision of safe working equipment and specific personal protective equipment (PPE).
Directive 2009/128/EC	Decree 150/2012 and National Action Plan (NAP)	Sustainable use of pesticides	Certified information and training of the users, distributors, and advisors; Certified inspection of pesticide application equipment in professional use; Documented regular calibrations and technical checks of the pesticide application equipment; Proper handling and storage of pesticides and treatment of their packaging and remnants; Implementation of practices and products allowing low pesticide-input pest management.
Directive 2006/42/EC	Decree 17/2010	Machinery safety	Specific essential health and safety requirements for the construction and maintenance of machinery for pesticide application.
Regulation (EC) no. 1272/2008		Classification, labelling, and packaging of substances and mixtures	New type of classification and labelling of hazardous substances.
Regulation (EC) no. 1907/2006		Registration, evaluation, authorization and restriction of chemicals	New requirements for safety data sheets (containing information concerning hazards, first-aid measures, handling and storage, personal protection, etc.)

Notes: (1) In the table, only the main legislative acts are mentioned, while their further updates/amendments were not cited: e.g. concerning Directive 2006/42/EC, Directive 2009/127/EC was not mentioned. Similarly, when citing Directive 89/391/EEC we intend its consolidated text, including for example Directive 2009/39/EC. (2) Regulation (EC) no. 1907/2006 and its amendments (the so-called "REACH") have not had a strong impact on pesticide users; it was included in the table due to the new rules on safety data sheets.

From the risk assessment point of view, the combination of the mandatory requisites provided by such legislative frameworks can be translated into the following requirements, which companies have to deal with:

- Provide a documented risk assessment report, demonstrating that the employer has taken into account all the risks derived from the use of pesticides;
- The risk assessment of the activities related with the use of pesticides should consider the worst situation of exposure for each activity;
- All the phases of the process should be considered, starting from handling, preparation of the mixture, setting of the application equipment, mixing, loading, and application, up to the final operations related to the equipment cleaning and maintenance, as well as dealing with the management of the cleaning water and the pesticide residues;
- The risk assessment has to take into account the hazardous properties of the pesticides, the information on health and safety provided by the safety sheet of each product, the level of exposure, and the duration of the exposure, as well as any occupational exposure limit values or biological limit values associated with each product;

- The preventive and protective measure applied, as well as the re-entry safety periods for each type of application have to be defined.

The practical implementation of these provisions requires a high level of expertise and, although a specific training for operators is mandatory to use pesticides, difficulties can arise in correctly understanding and putting them into practice [41]. Moreover, if we consider the Italian context, the companies operating in the agricultural sector are mainly small-sized or family-run enterprises [42–44], where the lack of human and financial resources often represents a drawback in properly implementing occupational health and safety duties [45].

To reduce these difficulties, which are similar for small and medium sized enterprises (SMEs) operating in different contexts [46–48], a specific easy-to-use risk assessment procedure was developed, which can allow companies to comply with the abovementioned requirements.

3. Background Analysis

The risk assessment activities are based on the estimation of the probability of occurrence of a certain event and the severity of its consequences. In the case of chemical risk, such a basic rule can be translated into the evaluation of the toxicity of the chemical product (e.g., based on the acceptable operator exposure level (AOEL) or the "lethal dose" criterion) and the level of exposure of the worker, intended as intensity of exposure per exposure time [49]. The assessment of the exposure to pesticides has been discussed by numerous studies [1,27,29,30,50,51] and different approaches have been proposed, which can be roughly distinguished into: (1) biomonitoring of exposure to pesticides, i.e., the measurement of a pesticide, its metabolite(s), or biotransformation products in biological fluids such as urine or blood [52]; (2) environmental monitoring, consisting in the measure of the exposure in the working environment [53].

Nevertheless, measuring the level of exposure is a difficult and complex task, due to the particularities that characterize the agricultural activities, the differences among the operators and working environments [54]. Accordingly, alternative methods for exposure and risk assessment have been developed, which vary from the use of expert opinion [55,56] and pre-marketing models [57,58] to the use of combination of data from the literature, measurements, and expert opinion [54,59]. In particular, premarketing models were introduced due to the mandatory need for evaluating the exposure of operators as well as for residents and bystanders [60], providing calculators based on databases, such as the BROWSE model [61], EUROPOEM [57], or TOXSWA [62]. Despite their ease of access, these models suffer from several drawbacks when applied in a practical context for occupational risk assessment [63,64]. Similarly, the so-called job exposure matrices (JEMs) [65] present with limited effectiveness when considering the agricultural activities [59,66], and for effective results in the determination of intensity of exposure they should be used in combination with algorithms that take into account other parameters such as the application rate, the type of equipment, and the characteristics of the crop [67].

The latter category includes the widespread Agricultural Health Study (AHS) model [68], developed for the estimation of the exposure to more than 50 individual pesticides, using questionnaire responses and pesticide information published in the literature. Such an approach is considered the most effective means for estimating the intensity level of the exposure to pesticides [69]. Without going into detail since a large literature can be found on the AHS augmentation (e.g., in [18,27,54,70–72]), the approach can be summarized in the following equation:

$$I = (MIX + APPL + REPAIR) \times PPE, \tag{1}$$

where

- I represents the intensity score level, i.e., the exposure level of the operator;
- MIX indicates the exposure during the mixing/preparation activities;

- APPL indicates the exposure during the pesticide application activity;
- REPAIR stands for the exposure during the repair/maintenance/regulation operations of the equipment for pesticide application; and
- PPE refers the personal protective equipment used (e.g., eye glasses, gloves, etc.).

As noted by Mandić-Rajčević [73], the weights of these factors are based on the monitoring data published in the scientific literature. Although both positive and negative examples of using the AHS algorithm exist in the literature, this system was constructed for epidemiological studies and not for the purposes of the mandatory issues of the OHS legislation. In order to provide a method for the risk assessment of activities related to the use of pesticides, Colosio et al. [54] provided an augmented algorithm based on the AHS approach, which allows a semi-quantitative estimation of the occupational exposure and risk level consequent to pesticide application. Such a study provided practical criteria for the assessment of the exposure factors, which are summarized in Table 2.

Table 2. Criteria used in the algorithm proposed by the Agricultural Health Study (AHS).

Factors	Criteria
MIX	Number of loadings; concentration of the active principle; type of formulation; duration of mixing and loading
APPL	Use rate; application pressure; treated area; interventions on machines during application; condition of the equipment; duration of the application
REPAIR	Maintenance of the equipment; duration of the maintenance

Also, modifying factors such as the type of tractor, the type of the PPE used, and the training/skill of the operator were considered. In order to evaluate the toxicity, the criterion used consisted in deriving the toxicity scores based on the risk phrases allocated to the compound of the pesticides used. The advantage of this approach is that it uses the data readily available on the label of the product and does not require any extra training in toxicological evaluation of active substances for the workers. In line with such a framework, other studies (e.g., [74,75]) also provided practical criteria for the estimation of the exposure during re-entry (especially for specific types of farming, such as cultivation in greenhouses), which are based on the density of the plants and the type of pesticide.

Even though the above mentioned studies provide effective guidelines for the assessment of operators' exposure to pesticides and the related risk levels, they were developed for the purposes of historical exposure assessment in epidemiological studies. Therefore, the models and their various extensions fail to provide a documented risk assessment needed for companies to comply with the health and safety legislation. One example is the option of non-use of proper PPE, which is a legitimate option in epidemiological studies, but is not allowed by the legislation (Directive 89/391/EEC). Additional examples include the specific training of operators as well as the maintenance/calibration of the equipment (Directive 2009/128/EC), which are also cogent requirements.

Additionally, the risk phrases and precautionary statements have been replaced by the "hazard statements" and the related codes due to the entry into force of Regulation (EC) 1272/2008, which would make the approach proposed by Colosio et al. (2012) obsolete [54].

Based on the above considerations, we tried to extend the above-mentioned approaches considering the perspective of an employer that has to draw-up a document where:

1. An assessment of the risks to safety and health at work is reported, including those facing the workers exposed to chemical risks;
2. The protective measures to be taken as well as the personal protective equipment to be used are defined; and
3. The specific training of operators and the related mandatory certificates are listed.

4. Materials and Methods

The proposed approach consists of three main phases (Figure 1). In the first phase, a preliminary check is carried out in order to verify if the company is compliant with general OHS requirements related to the use of pesticides. Then, the specific assessment in case of chemical risks is carried out, evaluating the exposure level of the operator related to the toxicity of the products used. Although the procedure we propose represents a simplified and preliminary assessment of chemical risk, in accordance with the national and EU OHS legislation, we use the locution "chemical risk assessment" for this phase. Finally, the improvement options are proposed for a proper risk management.

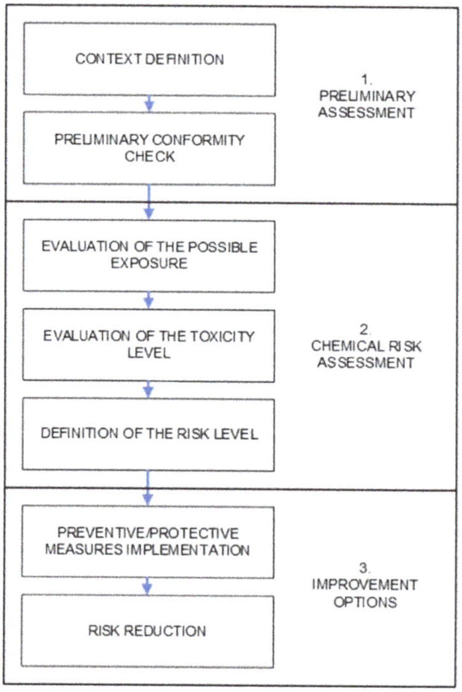

Figure 1. Scheme of the proposed approach.

4.1. Preliminary Assessment

In this phase, a preliminary analysis of the context has to be performed in order to understand the company's practical needs and the working tasks that should be performed. Accordingly, the employer has to verify the compliance with the general OHS requirements regarding the following topics:

1. Professional information and training of the operator and the related certification as the pesticides' professional user;
2. Machinery conformity (tractor and pesticide application equipment);
3. Selection of the proper pesticides depending on the company needs;
4. Functional calibration of the application equipment;
5. Definition of working procedures for the pesticides' application;
6. Selection of the proper PPE based on the type of pesticides and machinery used; and
7. Conformity with the health surveillance requisites.

The fulfilment of all these requirements is mandatory and to support their management a specific checklist was developed (Appendix A). The accomplishment of such requirements provides the necessary input to perform the specific evaluation of the so-called "chemical risks".

4.2. Chemical Risk Assessment

This analysis consists of a preliminary assessment (i.e., before the application of the pesticides is carried out) aimed at the definition of an exposure risk profile, and it is realized through a three-step approach. In the first step, the levels of exposure are estimated, considering all the possible exposure determinants present in the scenario under evaluation. Based on their conditions in this scenario, a numeric weight is assigned, and the obtained values are elaborated through a specific algorithm, to obtain and estimate of the possible level of exposure. Then, a value of toxicity is assigned considering the characteristics of the product that will be used. Finally, the estimation of the risk level is computed combining these values.

4.2.1. Evaluation of the Possible Exposure

To evaluate the possible exposure level (I_{exp}) of the operators, the algorithm proposed by Colosio et al. [54] and Mandić-Rajčevič [73] was improved as follows:

$$I_{exp} = [(MIX \times t_M + APPL \times t_A + REPAIR \times t_R + RE\text{-}ENTRY \times t_{RE}) \times SKILL \times PPE] \times FREQ \quad (2)$$

where the possible re-entry of the operator was included (RE-ENTRY), as well as a reducing factor considering the experience of the operator (SKILL), while PPE considers the status of the personal protective equipment and FREQ indicates how many times in a year the operator carries out activities involving the use of pesticides. With reference to the latter aspect, it has to be noted that, according to the current Italian OHS legislation, the employer has to update the risk assessment document at least yearly. As far as the time t is concerned, t_M, t_A, t_R, and t_{RE} represent the percentage of time dedicated to the MIX, APPL, REPAIR, and RE-ENTRY activities, respectively in a working day, taking into account that according to the Italian OHS legislation the duration of a working day is of 8 h. In other words, we assumed that the sum of these factors is not more than 100% of time of a regular working day, since the abovementioned activities cannot overlap each other as they are carried out sequentially by one operator only in a working day. Regarding the factor SKILL, the criteria used to introduce this aspect in Equation (2) are based on the information provided by the technical guideline provided by the International Social Security Association (ISSA) [76], where the skills of the operator are estimated considering its experience in carrying out a specific task.

As far as the RE-ENTRY working activities are concerned, they usually consist in any type of activity performed in a field where pesticides were previously used. From the legislative point of view, in line with the provisions of the Italian NAP, the re-entry in the field is allowed only 24 h after the pesticide's application. Then, during the following 24 h the operator can enter in the field only with the proper PPE; after that (i.e., after 48 h) the use of the pesticides' PPE is not mandatory. From an agronomic perspective, it has to be underlined that in some types of cultivations (e.g., maize or rice) the re-entry is not foreseen and thus it should not be computed. In our study, we included in this category the following situation: the operator needs to refill the atomizer's tank to complete the application and goes back and forward from the loading point to the application area. In case the cultivated field has more than one access, the latter activity is not computed if the operator can use other entry points avoiding the already sprayed areas. Although such criteria might appear quite simple, they are based on the experiences with farmers, which are often oriented towards practices that allow them to save time and resources.

The assessment criteria and the relative scores of the elements of Equation (2) are reported as follows: Table 3 (MIX), Table 4 (APPL), Table 5 (REPAIR), Table 6 (RE-ENTRY), and Table 7 (PPE, SKILL, and FREQ). The criteria used in the following tables are based on multiple sources: the starting point consisted in the findings and the related scientific review provided by [36,64,73]; as additional references for the weighting factors we have considered technical guidelines in the field of pesticide management [77] and from other fields such as mechanical hazards [76]. Moreover, the weighting factors were further discussed in a group of experts in order to verify their usability and effectiveness.

Table 3. Exposure factors during mixing and loading activities.

MIX = (LOAD × CONC) × COMP		
LOAD	Number of loads per day	Score
	1	0.5
	2–5	1
	>5	2
CONC	Concentration of the active principle	Score
	<50%	0.5
	50–90%	1
	>90%	2
COMP	Type of formulation/compound	Score
	Soluble bags	0.5
	Granules/liquid	1
	Powder	2

MIX: mixing; LOAD: loads; CONC: concentration; COMP: compound.

It has to be noted that CONC refers to the concentration of the active principle used in the product: expressed as a percentage: this information can be depicted from the product's Safety Data Sheet (SDS) and it is expressed as a weight/weight (w/w) percentage (as indicated in Regulation (EC) no. 1272/2008).

Table 4. Exposure factors during the application activities.

APPL = [(DOSE × SURF × BAR) ×TRACT] + INT + EQUIP		
DOSE	Quantity of pesticide used (kg/ha)	Score
	<0.1	1
	0.1–2.5	2
	>2.5	3
SURF	Application surface (ha)	Score
	<3	0.5
	3–10	1
	10–20	2
	>20	3
BAR	Application pressure/type of equipment (bar)	Score
	<3	1
	3–5	2
	5–10	3
	>10	4
TRACT	Type of tractor used to operate the pesticide application equipment	Score
	Without cabin	3
	With a non air-conditioned cabin	2
	With an air-conditioned cabin	1
	With an air-conditioned cabin equipped with activated carbon filters	0
INT	Number of in-field interventions to calibrate the equipment	Score
	0	0
	1–2	1
	>2	2

Table 4. *Cont.*

APPL = [(DOSE × SURF × BAR) ×TRACT] + INT + EQUIP		
EQUIP	Condition of the application equipment	Score
	Good	0
	Not good	8

APPL: application; DOSE: dose; SURF: surface; BAR: pressure; TRACT: tractor; INT: interventions; EQUIP: equipment.

It has to be noted that in Table 4, both INT and EQUIP were considered as additional weighting factors of the exposure risk during the application phase. This is because especially in small companies the attention paid to the condition of the application equipment is still limited [78–80].

Table 5. Exposure factors during in-field maintenance of the application equipment.

	Equipment Maintenance Operations	**Score**
REPAIR	Maintenance operations are carried out by a different person	0
	Maintenance operations are carried out by the operator	30

Table 6. Exposure factors during re-entry activities.

RE-ENTRY = (DOSE × H/D) × EARL		
H/D	Plants height/foliage density	score
	Low/Low	1
	Low/High	2
	High/Low	3
	High/High	4
EARL	Time before re-entering in the field after the pesticide application in order to carry out other activities	score
	>2 days	0
	1–2 days (24–48 h)	1.5

Table 7. Exposure factors related to the condition of PPE, the operator's experience, and the application frequency.

	Condition of PPE	**Score**
PPEs	Good	0.5
	Not good	1
	Experience/Skills of the Operator in Using Pesticides	**Score**
SKILL	>5 year	0.25
	1–5 years	0.5
	<1 year	1
	Number of Days Per Year Dedicated to the Use of Pesticides	**Score**
FREQ	<5	0.5
	5–10	1
	10–20	2
	>20	3

Based on the results obtained by means of equation (2), for each pesticide used it is possible to define an exposure level (I_{exp}), which can be classified as depicted in Table 8 following the criteria proposed in [42].

Table 8. Levels of possible exposure.

Exposure Level (I_{exp})	
Score	**Meaning**
≤5	Very low level of possible exposure
6–15	Low level of possible exposure
16–30	Medium level of possible exposure
31–50	High level of possible exposure
≥51	Very high level of possible exposure

4.2.2. Evaluation of the Toxicity Level

The creation of a grid for the evaluation of the toxicity exposure needs the synthesis of toxicity levels in ranked numeric values. As observed by Maroni et al. [31], despite its qualitative nature, the use of the information provided by the product labels for a preliminary risk assessment in an OHS context can be considered effective. Such an approach can answer to the needs of safety managers or entrepreneurs that can use the data provided by the pesticides' producers in compliance with the mandatory authorization's requirements [9], as practical information for a safe management of pesticides. For this reason, as a reference we used the list of substances provided by Regulation (EC) no. 1272/2008, although other types of lists proposed at the international level [81,82] can be found.

Based on this, we defined five levels of toxicity using as a surrogate of the potential toxicity the hazard statements (H) established for toxic substances by the Regulation (EC) no. 1272/2008. The grid is shown in Table 9, where a 1 to 5 toxicity index (I_{tox}) is considered (1 = very low; 5 = very high). The use of a Likert scale [83], ranging from 1 (not important) to 5 (extremely important) is quite common in qualitative assessment and its application in risk assessment is foreseen by the ISO/IEC 31010 standard [84].

Table 9. List of the toxicity levels based on Regulation (EC) no. 1272/2008.

Code	Hazard Statement	Toxicity Index (I_{tox})
H302	Harmful if swallowed	1
H319	Causes serious eye irritation	
H335	May cause respiratory irritation	
H315	Causes skin irritation	
EUH066	Repeated exposure may cause skin dryness or cracking	
H332	Harmful if inhaled	2
H312	Harmful in contact with skin	
H301	Toxic if swallowed	
H314	Causes severe skin burns and eye damage	
H318	Causes serious eye damage	
H331	Toxic if inhaled	3
H300	Toxic in contact with skin	
H317	May cause an allergic skin reaction	
H336	May cause drowsiness or dizziness	
H330	Fatal if inhaled	4
H310	Fatal in contact with skin	
H334	May cause allergy or asthma symptoms or breathing difficulties if inhaled	
H361f	Suspected of damaging fertility	
H360Fd	May damage fertility. May damage the unborn child	
H362	May cause harm to breast-fed children	
H304	May be fatal if swallowed and enters airways	
H371	May cause damage to organs	

Table 9. Cont.

Code	Hazard Statement	Toxicity Index (I_{tox})
H373	May cause damage to organs prolonged or repeated exposure	
H370	Causes damage to organs	
H351	Suspected of causing cancer	
H372	Causes damage to organs through prolonged or repeated exposure	5
H360F	May damage fertility	
H340	May cause genetic defects	
H360D	May damage the unborn child	

In the grid both hazard statements (H) and supplemental hazard statements relating to particular physical and health properties (EUH) were included: they were selected considering the pesticides most used in Italy. From the practical standpoint, it is worth noting that most of the products available on the market present more than one hazard statement. Hence, when carrying out the risk assessment, the value given to the product is established based on the highest score of the toxicity index.

4.2.3. Definition of the Risk Level

The estimation of the risk level (R_E) is performed combining the possible exposure level (I_{exp}) and the toxicity index (I_{tox}) by means of the following equation:

$$R_E = I_{exp} \times I_{tox} \quad (3)$$

The output of the second phase consists in the classification of the exposure risk level based on the criteria exposed in Table 10: the definition of the different levels' ranges are based on the suggestion provided by the ISO/IEC 31010 technical standard [84] for the implementation on the risk matrix.

Table 10. Levels of the exposure risk (R_E).

R_E	Level	Meaning
≤15	I	Acceptable level of exposure risk
16–60	II	Medium level of exposure risk
61–150	III	High level of exposure risk
≥151	IV	Unacceptable level of exposure risk

4.3. Improvement Options

Based on the results obtained in the second phase, and the levels of risk pointed out, the next phase of the evaluation consists in the definition of the need of risk management options addressed at reducing the risk to acceptable values. In Table 11 the main preventive interventions which can be done by the company are shown.

Table 11. Improvement measures depending on the exposure risk's level.

Exposure Risk Level (R_E)	Improvement Measures
Level I	No additional interventions are required.
Level II	Update information and training activities; verify the adequacy and the condition of PPE. Verify the adequacy of the pesticides used.
Level III	Update information and training activities; verify the adequacy and the condition of PPE. Verify the adequacy of the pesticides used and the possibility of selecting less hazardous products, providing specific biological/environmental monitoring. Verify the adequacy and the condition of the pesticide application equipment and its maintenance operations. Update the operative procedures and instructions and carry out a new risk assessment.
Level IV	The adequacy of the pesticides used needs to be verified and the use of less hazardous products should be considered. A specific biological/environmental monitoring, as well as the operators' health surveillance have to be implemented. Verify the selection of PPE and its condition as well as the adequacy of operative procedures and instructions. Verify the adequacy and the condition of the pesticide application equipment and its maintenance operations. Carry out a new risk assessment.

Once the preventive/protective measures are put into practice, the level of the exposure risk has to be assessed again in order to verify the levels of risk anticipated after the intervention. It is worth noting that the advantage of this approach is that the risk is assessed before the application, and the application is done only when it has been proved the absence of an unacceptable risk.

Following the provisions of the OHS legislation, this information has to be documented in a proper risk assessment file concerning each type of pesticide used by the company. If the company uses more than one pesticide, the whole procedure described in the previous sections has to be applied for each product. Hence, the proper preventive/protective interventions have to be defined considering all the information collected, i.e., the overall risk assessment activities described in this section.

5. Case Study

In order to validate the proposed approach, we carried out, in collaboration with an Italian company engaged in olive oil production, an "in-field study". In particular, we considered a field of about 2 hectares, where 210 olive trees are cultivated (Figure 2).

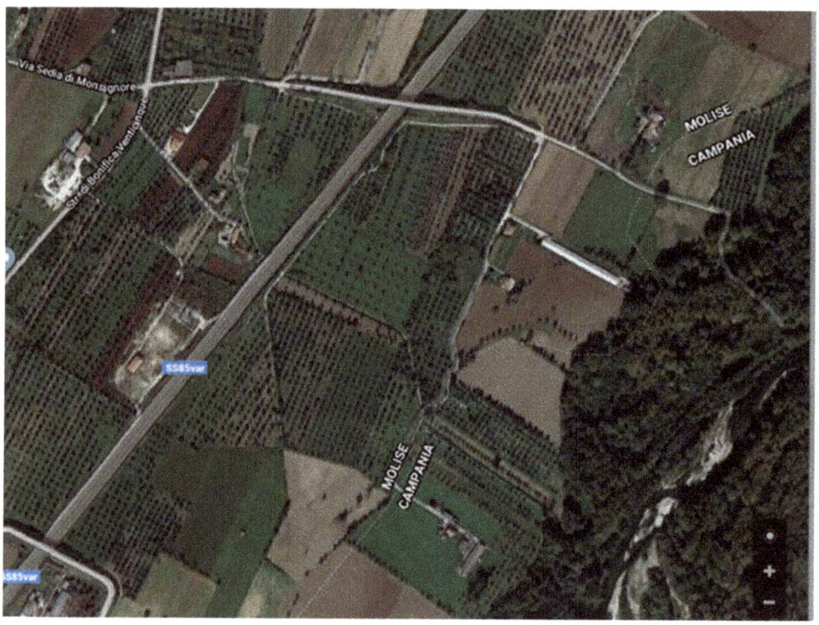

Figure 2. Aerial photo of the field.

5.1. Preliminary Assessment

The typical pathologies that can affect the olive trees and their fruits in the area where the company's fields are located (middle part of Italy) are the olive fly (*Bactrocera* or *Dacus oleae*) and the so-called "olive peacock spot" (*Spilocaea oleaginea*), which are quite common in olive cultivation [85]. More in detail, considering the number and the dimensions of the trees, as well as the characteristics of the field, the following products are used by the company:

- Product "A" against the "olive fly": a synthetic pyrethroid is used, whose active principle is based on the presence of deltamethrin (whose concentration derived from the SDS is 1.51 %). As far as the quantity of product is concerned, the use of 0.9 L of pesticide was estimated for 1000 L of water (i.e., the company uses 0.45 L of product A per hectare). The re-entry time is fixed in 3 days after the treatment.

- Product "B" against the "olive peacock spot": a copper compound is used, i.e., a tribasic copper sulfate (whose concentration derived from the SDS is 24%). The needed quantity was estimated in 3.0 L per 1000 L of water (i.e., the company uses 1.5 L of product B per hectare). The re-entry time is fixed in 20 days after the treatment.

The sprayer used for the application is a tractor-mounted mist blower for medium volume air treatment with a capacity of 500 L. Thus in both cases it has to be used twice. The tractor is equipped with a non air-conditioned cabin. As far as the treatments' schedule is concerned, both of them are applied in a 1 day working shift.

All the requisites of the conformity checklist (Appendix A) were verified positively: in particular, the three operators attended the specific training, holding the certificate of competence as professional pesticide users. One of them has 1 year of experience, while the other two have more than 5 years. Hence, in the assessment the case of the first one is considered. The PPE was considered adequate to the type of substances used and resulted in good condition.

5.2. Evaluation of the Possible Exposure Level

Two different assessments were done, for each of the two products used by the company. In particular, the evaluation of the possible exposure level related to both the product "A" and "B" are summarized in Table 12. In detail, for both products the scoring related to the considered surface (SURF) is equal to 0.5 (as per values indicated in Table 4), while for the estimation of DOSE we assumed that the specific weight of the formulation is roughly that of water (1 L = 1 kg). Then, following the criteria exposed in Table 4, in both cases the DOSE = 2.

Table 12. Scores related to the calculation of the possible exposure level.

	Code		Product "A"	Product "B"
1. MIX	1.1	LOAD	1	1
	1.2	CONC	0.5	0.5
	1.3	COMP	1	1
	1.4	t_M	0.042 (20 min)	0.042 (20 min)
2. APPL	2.1	DOSE	2	2
	2.2	SURF	0.5	0.5
	2.3	BAR	4	4
	2.4	TRACT	2	2
	2.5	INT	0	0
	2.6	EQUIP	0	0
	2.7	t_A	0.312 (2.5 h)	0.312 (2.5 h)
3. REPAIR	3.1	REPAIR	30	30
	3.2	t_R	0.125 (1 h)	0.125 (1 h)
4. REENTRY	2.1	DOSE	2	2
	4.1	H/D	3	3
	4.2	EARL	1.5	1.5
	4.3	t_{RE}	0.042 (20 min)	0.042 (20 min)
5. PPE			0.5	0.5
6. SKIL			0.5	0.5
7. FREQ			1	2
I_{exp}			2.036	4.073

Based on the criteria exposed in Table 8, both the potential exposure levels can be ascribed as belonging the level 1, i.e., "very low level of possible exposure". It has to be noted that in both cases the re-entry activities were considered only once, when the operator has to refill the sprayer's tank.

5.3. Evaluation of the Toxicity Level

The analysis of the toxicity level of the pesticides used by the company is carried out based on the information provided in their safety sheets (Table 13).

Table 13. Evaluation of the Toxicity Index of both products.

Code	Hazard Statement	Toxicity Index (I_{tox})
	Product "A"	
H302	Harmful if swallowed	1
H315	Causes skin irritation	1
H301	Toxic if swallowed	2
H318	Causes serious eye damage	2
H331	Toxic if inhaled	3
H317	May cause an allergic skin reaction	3
	Product "B"	
H302	Harmful if swallowed	1
H319	Causes serious eye irritation	1
H315	Causes skin irritation	1
H317	May cause an allergic skin reaction	3
H330	Fatal if inhaled	4
H372	Causes damage to organs through prolonged or repeated exposure	5

5.4. Evaluation of the Risk Level

Combining the possible exposure level and the toxicity level as per Equation (3), the exposure risk level (R_E) for both products was estimated (Table 14).

Table 14. Scores related to the calculation of the exposure risk.

	I_{exp}	I_{tox}	R_E	Level
Product "A"	2.0361	3	$R_E = 6.11$	I
Product "B"	4.073	5	$R_E = 20.36$	II

5.5. Improvement Options

While the risk level when using the product "A" resulted "acceptable" and no further interventions are required, in the case of "B" the risk level is higher mainly due to the limited experience of the younger operator. For this reason, additional training activities were foreseen, and the company decided to assign the application of "B" only to the two more experienced operators. Consequently, the risk index was reduced to $R_E = 10.18$, reaching the level of acceptability. A further improvement could be achieved providing a proper route in the orchard in order to avoid or reduce the exposure time during the re-entry when the refill of the sprayer is needed.

6. Discussion

The results achieved were considered positively by the company since our approach allowed them to perform a complete analysis, updating their risk assessment documents in a user-friendly manner. Moreover, the checklist for the preliminary assessment was considered a useful tool for monitoring the proper application of safety procedures.

From a more general perspective, the problem of providing tools that allow the estimation of the risk of the exposure to pesticides, contributing to the definition of exposure limits and to the prevention of the toxic effects on workers is widely discussed in the literature [1,67,81]. As a matter of facts, the risk assessment related to the exposure to pesticides presents numerous variables, making it a more complex task than when dealing with other types of hazards agricultural workers are exposed to [28]. In such a context, the definition of a tool aimed at supporting safety managers in the documented preliminary risk assessment of working activities related to the use of pesticides represents a narrow aspect of the problem, although the relevant impact it might have on the practical needs of companies. In such a research niche, the present study can be considered a first attempt of merging all the mandatory issues related to the use of pesticides in an easy-to-use procedure for the correct implementation of OHS risk assessment activities.

In particular, our study is based on the results achieved in the epidemiological literature, together with the provisions of technical guidelines and the experts' opinions, translating them in an OHS context. This result is in line with the research hints provided by Lichtenberg et al. [41] and Damalas and Koutroubas [29]. To the authors' knowledge this represents a novelty in context of the OHS literature.

The proposed algorithm constitutes a basis for a simplified risk assessment procedure for the pesticides' use and its implementation in a knowledge management system for risk assessment activities [86] is currently being considered, as well as its implementation in an OHS management system.

In addition, the current paper also aims at increasing the knowledge on the safe use pesticides. Such a result, in line with the practical needs highlighted by Rijal et al. [87], provides a general framework that integrates different disciplines and stakeholders.

Moreover, although the proposed approach is based on the requirements of the Italian legislation, its general framework could be extended to other national contexts easily. As a matter of fact, the preliminary characterization of exposure levels scenarios allows safety managers to better define the potential damage and the evolution of hazard's scenarios [88], supporting both the entrepreneur and the appointed physicians in effectively perform the workers' health surveillance (WHS) that is mandatory in an OHS context in the EU countries [89].

Thanks to its simplicity and its task-based approach, the proposed methodology can be used also as a reference framework to augment the operators' knowledge and awareness on a safe behavior, allowing the increase of all safety aspects within the company [90].

Beside these positive aspects, the study limitations have to be addressed as well. From a practical point of view, we have to consider that the selection of the types of toxicity listed in Table 9 cannot be considered exhaustive and a further analysis of possible toxicity typologies that can be found in the pesticides available on the market nowadays should be carried out. The whole approach of using hazard statements as a proxy of toxicity of substances needs validation, but any improvement in this aspect would easily be implemented in the proposed method. It has to be noted that in the present study the hazard statements related to the toxicity for the environment were not taken into account. For instance, for both product "A" and "B" the statement H400 (very toxic to aquatic life) was listed in the safety sheets. Since environmental concerns were not an objective of this study, an augmented approach considering also these issues could be beneficial for a more holistic risk assessment. In such a context, also the equipment's cleaning operations should be included.

Furthermore, we also need to underline that improved solutions such as the so-called mass trapping systems and bait sprays for the prevention of the olive fly were not considered in the study, since the proper use of such solutions to define the reduction of pesticide use quantitatively requires an expert's analysis, which was not available when the case study was carried out. Nevertheless, we are aware that the implementation and promotion of eco-friendlier solutions to replace the use of hazardous substances is an important issue that needs to be investigated largely, as stressed by Damalas and Koutroubas [91].

From a scientific perspective, the proposed approach needs validation, which should be carried out by the parallel use of the proposed approach and environmental or biological monitoring to verify the effectiveness of the proposed factors and weights. This can be beneficial for a more accurate definition of the different weights' ranges used for the computation of the various factors. Finally, the type of results achieved through a single case-study as a research tool can be considered exploratory and used to define new research questions and new understandings [92,93], but the findings' external validity is limited by the sample concerned [94]. Accordingly, the application to different case studies concerning other types of cultivations and hence of pesticides is necessary.

7. Conclusions

The paper illustrates a procedure for the risk assessment of activities related to the application of pesticides, addressing the needs of farmers in complying with the recent legislative issues. This approach is based on studies concerning the application of the AHS algorithm and the related literature review [54,64,73]; through the integration of their findings with the provisions of technical guidelines and experts' opinion, a preliminary risk assessment framework that can be used at a practical level to comply with the OHS legislation was defined.

The merit of this paper consists in the overall development of a tool for the preliminary risk assessment, providing a simplified approach for its practical application. Our algorithm aims at evaluating all the parameters that might influence the exposure to pesticides, providing a qualitative result thorough the evaluation of a realistic situation. This supports the findings of Acquavella et al. [95], highlighting the limitations of the risk assessment approaches based on passive dosimetry in evaluating individual exposure situations effectively.

This study is at an initial step of implementation and the validation of the proposed approach through biological monitoring is already planned. Thus, researchers and practitioners are also invited to contribute to its further development.

Author Contributions: Conceptualization, M.F., M.L., D.P., L.C., S.M-R., and C.C.; methodology, M.F., M.L., D.P., L.C., S.M-R., and C.C..; case study, M.F., M.L., D.P., L.C., E.M., S.M-R., and C.C.; writing—review and editing, M.F., M.L., D.P., S.M-R., and C.C.

Funding: This research received no external funding.

Acknowledgments: We wish to thank Marco Zeoli, Eng. MD for the support in the case study development.

Conflicts of Interest: The authors declare no conflicts of interest.

Appendix A

The appendix contains an excerpt of the preliminary conformity checklist.

Working Equipment (Tractor)		
Type of tractor		
Verify the following items:	(Y/N)	Type and status
ROPS		
PTO protection		
Cabin		
Is the tractor functionality safe and adequate for the working activities? (Yes/No)		

Working Equipment (Sprayer)		
Type of sprayer		
Verify the following items:	(Y/N)	Date
CE mark		
Periodical functional control		
Calibration		
Is the sprayer functionality safe and adequate for the working activities? (Yes/No)		

Personal Protective Equipment (PPE)					
Type	Aim	Applicable		Specify the type of PPE chosen (model, category, etc.)	Quantity needed
		YES	NO		
Protection of head	Helmet				
Protection of eyes	Safety spectacles, face-shields, etc.				
Protection of ears	Earplugs, earmuffs, etc.				
Protection of hands	Gloves				
Respiratory protective equipment	Filtering face-pieces, masks, etc.				
Protection of body	Boilersuits, chemical suits, etc.				
Protection of foots	Shoes				
Is the selected PPE adequate for the type of working activities? (Yes/No)					
Is the selected PPE properly assigned to the operator/s? (Yes/No)					

Is adequate information and training on the use and maintenance of PPE provided? (Yes/No)		
Training and Information of the Operators		
Training and information requirements	Name of the operator	Date of the certificate
Pesticides' use	1.	
	2.	
	3.	
Tractor's use	1.	
	2.	
	3.	
PPE use and maintenance	1.	
	2.	
	3.	
Is the training and information of the operators adequate for the working activities? (Yes/No)		
NOTE: *If all the requirements are not satisfied, the company needs to apply the necessary preventive and protective measures to comply with them before carrying out the working activities.*		

References

1. Machado, S.C.; Martins, I. Risk assessment of occupational pesticide exposure: Use of endpoints and surrogates. *Regul. Toxicol. Pharmacol.* **2018**, *98*, 276–283. [CrossRef] [PubMed]
2. Möhring, N.; Gaba, S.; Finger, R. Quantity based indicators fail to identify extreme pesticide risks. *Sci. Total Environ.* **2019**, *646*, 503–523. [CrossRef]
3. Lamichhane, J.R. Pesticide use and risk reduction in European farming systems with IPM: An introduction to the special issue. *Crop Prot.* **2017**, *97*, 1–6. [CrossRef]
4. Skevas, T.; Lansink, A.O.; Stefanou, S.E. Designing the emerging EU pesticide policy: A literature review. *NJAS-Wagening. J. Life Sci.* **2013**, *64*, 95–103. [CrossRef]
5. Directive 2009/127/EC of the European Parliament and of the Council of 21 October 2009 Amending Directive 2006/42/EC with Regard to Machinery for Pesticide Application. Available online: http://data.europa.eu/eli/dir/2009/127/oj (accessed on 7 November 2018).
6. Regulation (EC) No. 1107/2009 of the European Parliament and of the Council of 21 October 2009 Concerning the Placing of Plant Protection Products on the Market and Repealing Council Directives 79/117/EEC and 91/414/EEC. Available online: https://eur-lex.europa.eu/legal-content/EN/TXT/?uri=celex%3A32009R1107 (accessed on 7 November 2018).
7. Regulation (EC) No. 1272/2008 of the European Parliament and of the Council of 16 December 2008 on Classification, Labelling and Packaging of Substances and Mixtures, Amending and Repealing Directives 67/548/EEC and 1999/45/EC, and Amending Regulation (EC) No. 1907/2006. Available online: https://eur-lex.europa.eu/eli/reg/2008/1272/oj (accessed on 7 November 2018).
8. Briggs, D.J. A framework for integrated environmental health impact assessment of systemic risks. *Environ. Health* **2008**, *7*, 61. [CrossRef]

9. Handford, C.E.; Elliott, C.T.; Campbell, K.A. Review of the global pesticide legislation and the scale of challenge in reaching the global harmonization of food safety standards. *Integr. Environ. Assess. Manag.* **2015**, *11*, 525–536. [CrossRef]
10. Dugger-Webster, A.; LePrevost, C.E. Following pesticide labels: A continued journey toward user comprehension and safe use. *Curr. Opin. Environ. Sci. Health* **2018**, *4*, 19–26. [CrossRef]
11. PANE (Pesticide Action Network Europe). NAP Best Practice—Sustainable use of pesticides: Implementing a National Action Plan. 2010. Available online: https://www.pan-europe.info/old/Resources/Reports/NAP_best_practice.pdf (accessed on 7 November 2018).
12. Cunha, J.P.; Chueca, P.; Garcerá, C.; Moltó, E. Risk assessment of pesticide spray drift from citrus applications with air-blast sprayers in Spain. *Crop Prot.* **2012**, *42*, 116–123. [CrossRef]
13. Biocca, M.; Pochi, D.; Fanigliulo, R.; Gallo, P.; Pulcini, P.; Marcovecchio, F.; Perrino, C. Evaluating a filtering and recirculating system to reduce dust drift in simulated sowing of dressed seed and abraded dust particle characteristics. *Pest Manag. Sci.* **2017**, *73*, 1134–1142. [CrossRef] [PubMed]
14. Alix, A.; Capri, E. Modern Agriculture in Europe and the Role of Pesticides. *Adv. Chem. Pollut. Environ. Manag. Prot.* **2018**, *2*, 1–22. [CrossRef]
15. Lechenet, M.; Makowski, D.; Py, G.; Munier-Jolain, N. Profiling farming management strategies with contrasting pesticide use in France. *Agric. Syst.* **2016**, *149*, 40–53. [CrossRef]
16. Hillocks, R.J. Farming with fewer pesticides: EU pesticide review and resulting challenges for UK agriculture. *Crop Prot.* **2012**, *31*, 85–93. [CrossRef]
17. Thomas, K.W.; Dosemeci, M.; Coble, J.B.; Hoppin, J.A.; Sheldon, L.S.; Chapa, G.; Croghan, C.W.; Jones, A.; Knott, C.E.; Lynch, C.F.; et al. Assessment of a pesticide exposure intensity algorithm in the agricultural health study. *J. Expo. Sci. Environ. Epidemiol.* **2010**, *20*, 559–569. [CrossRef] [PubMed]
18. Coble, J.; Thomas, K.W.; Hines, C.J.; Hoppin, J.A.; Dosemeci, M.; Curwin, B.; Lubin, J.; Beane Freeman, L.E.; Blair, A.; Alavanja, M.C. An updated algorithm for estimation of pesticide exposure intensity in the Agricultural Health Study. *Int. J. Environ. Res. Public Health* **2011**, *8*, 4608–4622. [CrossRef]
19. Thouvenin, I.; Bouneb, F.; Mercier, T. Operator dermal exposure and protection provided by personal protective equipment and working coveralls during mixing/loading, application and sprayer cleaning in vineyards. *Int. J. Occup. Saf. Ergon.* **2017**, *23*, 229–239. [CrossRef]
20. Reffstrup, T.K.; Larsen, J.C.; Meyer, O. Risk assessment of mixtures of pesticides. Current approaches and future strategies. *Regul. Toxic. Pharmacol.* **2010**, *56*, 174–192. [CrossRef] [PubMed]
21. Wong, H.L.; Garthwaite, D.G.; Ramwell, C.T.; Brown, C.D. Assessment of exposure of professional agricultural operators to pesticides. *Sci. Total Environ.* **2018**, *619*, 874–882. [CrossRef]
22. Lu, J.L.D. Occupational safety of farmers in the vegetable industry. *Int. J. Occup. Saf. Ergon.* **2011**, *17*, 445–453. [CrossRef]
23. Databases for Vibration Machines, Umeå University, Department of Public Health and Clinical Medicine. Available online: http://www.vibration.db.umu.se/Default.aspx?lang=en (accessed on 5 January 2019).
24. Hand-Arm Vibration Database, PAF. Available online: https://www.portaleagentifisici.it/fo_hav_list_macchinari_avanzata.php?lg=EN&page=0 (accessed on 5 January 2019).
25. Fargnoli, M.; De Minicis, M.; Tronci, M. Design Management for Sustainability: An integrated approach for the development of sustainable products. *J. Eng. Technol. Manag.* **2014**, *34*, 29–45. [CrossRef]
26. Carpenter, D.O.; Arcaro, K.; Spink, D.C. Understanding the human health effects of chemical mixtures. *Environ. Health Perspect.* **2002**, *110*, 25–42. [CrossRef]
27. Kim, K.H.; Kabir, E.; Jahan, S.A. Exposure to pesticides and the associated human health effects. *Sci. Total Environ.* **2017**, *575*, 525–535. [CrossRef]
28. Nguyen, T.-H.-Y.; Bertin, M.; Bodin, J.; Fouquet, N.; Bonvallot, N.; Roquelaure, Y. Multiple Exposures and Co-exposures to Occupational Hazards among Agricultural Workers: A Systematic Review of Observational Studies. *Saf. Health Work* **2018**, *9*, 239–240. [CrossRef] [PubMed]
29. Damalas, C.A.; Eleftherohorinos, I.G. Pesticide exposure, safety issues, and risk assessment indicators. *Int. J. Environ. Res. Pub. Health* **2011**, *8*, 1402–1419. [CrossRef]
30. Lewis, K.A.; Tzilivakis, J.; Warner, D.J.; Green, A. An international database for pesticide risk assessments and management. *Hum. Ecol. Risk Assess. Int. J.* **2016**, *22*, 1050–1064. [CrossRef]
31. Maroni, M.; Fait, A.; Colosio, C. Risk assessment and management of occupational exposure to pesticides. *Toxicol. Lett.* **1999**, *107*, 145–153. [CrossRef]

32. Zhang, C.; Guanming, S.; Shen, J.; Hu, R.F. Productivity effect and overuse of pesticide in crop production in China. *J. Integr. Agric.* **2015**, *14*, 1903–1910. [CrossRef]
33. Sharifzadeh, M.S.; Abdollahzadeh, G.; Damalas, C.A.; Rezaei, R. Farmers' Criteria for Pesticide Selection and Use in the Pest Control Process. *Agriculture* **2018**, *8*, 24. [CrossRef]
34. Damalas, C.A.; Georgiou, E.B.; Theodorou, M.G. Pesticide use and safety practices among Greek tobacco farmers: A survey. *Int. J. Environ. Health Res.* **2006**, *16*, 339–348. [CrossRef] [PubMed]
35. Ye, M.; Beach, J.; Martin, J.; Senthilselvan, A. Occupational pesticide exposures and respiratory health. *Int. J. Environ. Res. Pub. Health* **2013**, *10*, 6442–6471. [CrossRef]
36. Fargnoli, M.; Lombardi, M.; Haber, N.; Puri, D. The Impact of Human Error in the Use of Agricultural Tractors: A Case Study Research in Vineyard Cultivation in Italy. *Agriculture* **2018**, *8*, 82. [CrossRef]
37. Damalas, C.A.; Abdollahzadeh, G. Farmers' use of personal protective equipment during handling of plant protection products: Determinants of implementation. *Sci. Total Environ.* **2016**, *571*, 730–736. [CrossRef] [PubMed]
38. Hashemi, S.M.; Hosseini, S.M.; Hashemi, M.K. Farmers' perceptions of safe use of pesticides: Determinants and training needs. *Int. Arch. Occup. Environ. Health* **2012**, *85*, 57–66. [CrossRef] [PubMed]
39. Abbassy, M.M.S. Farmer's Knowledge, Attitudes and Practices, and their Exposure to Pesticide Residues after Application on the Vegetable and Fruit Crops. Case Study: North of Delta, Egypt. *J. Environ. Anal. Toxicol.* **2017**, *7*, 2161-0525. [CrossRef]
40. Caffaro, F.; Cavallo, E. Comprehension of safety pictograms affixed to agricultural machinery: A survey of users. *J. Saf. Res.* **2015**, *55*, 151–158. [CrossRef] [PubMed]
41. Lichtenberg, B.; Mischke, U.; Scherf, S.; Röver, M.; Martin, S. Hazard and risk based allocation of safety instructions to operators handling pesticides. *J. für Verbraucherschutz und Lebensmittelsicherheit* **2015**, *10*, 373–384. [CrossRef]
42. Vitali, M.; Protano, C.; Del Monte, A.; Ensabella, F.; Guidotti, M. Operative modalities and exposure to pesticides during open field treatments among a group of agricultural subcontractors. *Arch. Environ. Contam. Toxic.* **2009**, *57*, 193–202. [CrossRef]
43. Cividino, S.R.S.; Pergher, G.; Gubiani, R.; Moreschi, C.; Da Broi, U.; Vello, M.; Rinaldi, F. Definition of a Methodology for Gradual and Sustainable Safety Improvements on Farms and Its Preliminary Applications. *Agriculture* **2018**, *8*, 7. [CrossRef]
44. Lombardi, M.; Fargnoli, M. Prioritization of hazards by means of a QFD-based procedure. *Int. J. Saf. Secur. Eng.* **2018**, *8*, 342–353. [CrossRef]
45. Cecchini, M.; Colantoni, A.; Monarca, D.; Cossio, F.; Riccioni, S. Survey on the status of enforcement of European directives on health and safety at work in some farms of central Italy. *Chem. Eng. Trans.* **2017**, *58*, 103–108. [CrossRef]
46. Vassie, L.; Tomàs, J.M.; Oliver, A. Health and safety management in UK and Spanish SMEs: A comparative study. *J. Saf. Res.* **2000**, *31*, 35–43. [CrossRef]
47. Micheli, G.J.; Cagno, E. Dealing with SMEs as a whole in OHS issues: Warnings from empirical evidence. *Saf. Sci.* **2010**, *48*, 729–733. [CrossRef]
48. Fargnoli, M.; Lombardi, M.; Haber, N.; Guadagno, F. Hazard Function Deployment: A QFD based tool for the assessment of working tasks–A practical study in the construction industry. *Int. J. Occup. Saf. Ergon.* **2018**, 1–53. [CrossRef] [PubMed]
49. Maroni, M.; Colosio, C.; Ferioli, A.; Fait, A. Biological monitoring of pesticide exposure: A review. Introduction. *Toxicology* **2000**, *143*, 1–118. [CrossRef] [PubMed]
50. Aktar, W.; Sengupta, D.; Chowdhury, A. Impact of pesticides use in agriculture: Their benefits and hazards. *Interdiscip. Toxicol.* **2009**, *2*, 1–12. [CrossRef] [PubMed]
51. Garcia, F.P.; Ascencio, S.Y.C.; Oyarzun, J.C.G.; Hernandez, A.C.; Alavarado, P.V. Pesticides: Classification, uses and toxicity. Measures of exposure and genotoxic risks. *J. Res. Environ. Sci. Toxicol.* **2012**, *1*, 279–293.
52. Barr, D.B. Biomonitoring of exposure to pesticides. *J. Chem. Health Saf.* **2008**, *15*, 20–29. [CrossRef]
53. Anwar, W.A. Biomarkers of human exposure to pesticides. *Environ. Health Perspect.* **1997**, *105*, 801–806. [CrossRef] [PubMed]

54. Colosio, C.; Rubino, F.M.; Alegakis, A.; Ariano, E.; Brambilla, G.; Mandic-Rajcevic, S.; Metruccio, F.; Minoia, C.; Moretto, A.; Somaruga, C.; et al. Integration of biological monitoring, environmental monitoring and computational modelling into the interpretation of pesticide exposure data: Introduction to a proposed approach. *Toxicol. Lett.* **2012**, *213*, 49–56. [CrossRef]
55. Harris, S.A.; Sass-Kortsak, A.M.; Corey, P.N.; Purdham, J.T. Pesticide exposures in professional turf applicators, job titles, and tasks performed: Implications of exposure measurement error for epidemiologic study design and interpretation of results. *Am. J. Ind. Med.* **2005**, *48*, 205–216. [CrossRef]
56. Marquart, J.; Brouwer, D.H.; Gijsbers, J.H.J.; Links, I.H.M.; Warren, N.; Van Hemmen, J.J. Determinants of dermal exposure relevant for exposure modelling in regulatory risk assessment. *Ann. Occup. Hyg.* **2003**, *47*, 599–607. [CrossRef]
57. Van Hemmen, J.J. EUROPOEM, a predictive occupational exposure database for registration purposes of pesticides. *Appl. Occup. Environ. Hyg.* **2001**, *16*, 246–250. [CrossRef]
58. Machera, K.; Tsakirakis, A.; Charistou, A.; Anastasiadou, P.; Glass, C.R. Dermal exposure of pesticide applicators as a measure of coverall performance under field conditions. *Ann. Occup. Hyg.* **2009**, *53*, 573–584. [CrossRef] [PubMed]
59. Dick, F.D.; Semple, S.E.; Van Tongeren, M.; Miller, B.G.; Ritchie, P.; Sherriff, D.; Cherrie, J.W. Development of a task-exposure matrix (TEM) for pesticide use (TEMPEST). *Ann. Occup. Hyg.* **2010**, *54*, 443–452. [CrossRef]
60. EFSA (European Food Safety Authority). Guidance on the assessment of exposure of operators, workers, residents and bystanders in risk assessment for plant protection products. *EFSA J.* **2014**, *12*, 3874. [CrossRef]
61. Ellis, M.C.B.; van den Berg, F.; van de Zande, J.C.; Kennedy, M.C.; Charistou, A.N.; Arapaki, N.S.; Butler, A.H.; Machera, K.A.; Jacobs, C.M. The BROWSE model for predicting exposures of residents and bystanders to agricultural use of pesticides: Comparison with experimental data and other exposure models. *Biosyst. Eng.* **2017**, *154*, 122–136. [CrossRef]
62. Sumon, K.A.; Rico, A.; Ter Horst, M.M.; Van den Brink, P.J.; Haque, M.M.; Rashid, H. Risk assessment of pesticides used in rice-prawn concurrent systems in Bangladesh. *Sci. Total Environ.* **2016**, *568*, 498–506. [CrossRef] [PubMed]
63. Protano, C.; Guidotti, M.; Vitali, M. Performance of different work clothing types for reducing skin exposure to pesticides during open field treatment. *Bull. Environ. Contam. Toxicol.* **2009**, *83*, 115–119. [CrossRef]
64. Rubino, F.M.; Mandic-Rajcevic, S.; Ariano, E.; Alegakis, A.; Bogni, M.; Brambilla, G.; De Paschale, G.; Firmi, A.; Minoia, C.; Micoli, G.; et al. Farmers' exposure to herbicides in North Italy: Assessment under real-life conditions in small-size rice and corn farms. *Toxicol. Lett.* **2012**, *210*, 189–197. [CrossRef]
65. Sieber, W.K., Jr.; Sundin, D.S.; Frazier, T.M.; Robinson, C.F. Development, use, and availability of a job exposure matrix based on national occupational hazard survey data. *Am. J. Ind. Med.* **1991**, *20*, 163–174. [CrossRef]
66. Perry, M.J.; Marbella, A.; Layde, P.M. Nonpersistent pesticide exposure self-report versus biomonitoring in farm pesticide applicators. *Ann. Epidemiol.* **2006**, *16*, 701–707. [CrossRef]
67. Baldi, I.; Carles, C.; Blanc-Lapierre, A.; Fabbro-Peray, P.; Druet-Cabanac, M.; Boutet-Robinet, E.; Soulat, J.M.; Bouvier, G.; Lebailly, P.; Barrau, M.; et al. A French crop-exposure matrix for use in epidemiological studies on pesticides: PESTIMAT. *J. Expos. Sci. Environ. Epidemiol.* **2017**, *27*, 56–63. [CrossRef] [PubMed]
68. Alavanja, M.C.; Sandler, D.P.; McMaster, S.B.; Zahm, S.H.; McDonnell, C.J.; Lynch, C.F.; Pennybacker, M.; Rothman, N.; Dosemeci, M.; Bond, A.E.; et al. The Agricultural Health Study. *Environ. Health Perspect.* **1996**, *104*, 362. [CrossRef]
69. Dosemeci, M.; Alavanja, M.C.; Rowland, A.S.; Mage, D.; Zahm, S.H.; Rothman, N.; Lubin, J.H.; Hoppin, J.A.; Sandler, D.P.; Blair, A. A quantitative approach for estimating exposure to pesticides in the Agricultural Health Study. *Ann. Occup. Hyg.* **2002**, *46*, 245–260. [CrossRef] [PubMed]
70. Blair, A.; Thomas, K.; Coble, J.; Sandler, D.P.; Hines, C.J.; Lynch, C.F.; Knott, C.; Purdue, M.P.; Zahm, S.H.; Alavanja, M.C.; et al. Impact of pesticide exposure misclassification on estimates of relative risks in the Agricultural Health Study. *Occup. Environ. Med.* **2011**, *68*, 537–541. [CrossRef]
71. Christensen, K.; Christensen, C.H.; Wright, J.M.; Galizia, A.; Glenn, B.S.; Scott, C.S.; Mall, J.K.; Bateson, T.F.; Murphy, P.A.; Cooper, G.S. The use of epidemiology in risk assessment: Challenges and opportunities. *Hum. Ecol. Risk Assess. Int. J.* **2015**, *21*, 1644–1663. [CrossRef]
72. Garzia, N.A.; Spinelli, J.J.; Gotay, C.C.; Teschke, K. Literature review: Dermal monitoring data for pesticide exposure assessment of farm workers. *J. Agromed.* **2018**, *23*, 187–214. [CrossRef] [PubMed]

73. Mandic-Rajcevic, S.; Rubino, F.M.; Ariano, E.; Cottica, D.; Neri, S.; Colosio, C. Environmental and biological monitoring for the identification of main exposure determinants in vineyard mancozeb applicators. *J. Expo. Sci. Environ. Epidemiol.* **2018**, *28*, 289–296. [CrossRef] [PubMed]
74. Van der Mark, M.; Vermeulen, R.; Nijssen, P.C.; Mulleners, W.M.; Sas, A.M.; van Laar, T.; Brouwer, M.; Huss, A.; Kromhout, H.; Kromhout, H. Occupational exposure to pesticides and endotoxin and Parkinson disease in the Netherlands. *Occup. Environ. Med.* **2014**, *71*, 757–764. [CrossRef]
75. Negatu, B.; Vermeulen, R.; Mekonnen, Y.; Kromhout, H. A method for semi-quantitative assessment of exposure to pesticides of applicators and re-entry workers: An application in three farming systems in Ethiopia. *Ann. Occup. Hyg.* **2016**, *60*, 669–683. [CrossRef] [PubMed]
76. ISSA (International Social Security Association). Assess your accident risk yourself! Risk evaluation at workplace. In *Brochure of the International Section Machine and System Safety, Mannheim*; ISSA: Geneva, Switzerland, 2000; ISBN 92-843-2130-1.
77. Regione Lombardia, Regional Decree n. 4580 of 29 April 2010 Concerning Good Practices of Pesticides' Use in Agriculture (In Italian: Decreto della Direzione Generale della Sanità n. 4580 del 29 Aprile 2010—Buona Pratica dell'Utilizzo dei Fitofarmaci in Agricoltura). Available online: http://www.consultazioniburl.servizirl.it/storicoBurl/burl/ElencoBollettini.aspx (accessed on 7 November 2018).
78. Cavallo, E.; Ferrari, E.; Bollani, L.; Coccia, M. Attitudes and behaviour of adopters of technological innovations in agricultural tractors: A case study in Italian agricultural system. *Agric. Sys.* **2014**, *130*, 44–54. [CrossRef]
79. Balsari, P.; Oggero, G.; Marucco, P. Pesticide application horticultural and floricultural farms of Liguria Region: Current situation and results of one year of sprayer inspections. *Julius-Kühn-Archiv* **2010**, *426*, 82–88.
80. Cividino, S.R.S.; Pergher, G.; Zucchiatti, N.; Gubiani, R. Agricultural Health and Safety Survey in Friuli Venezia Giulia. *Agriculture* **2018**, *8*, 9. [CrossRef]
81. Bevan, R.; Brown, T.; Matthies, F.; Sams, C.; Jones, K.; Hanlon, J.; La Vedrine, M. Human biomonitoring data collection from occupational exposure to pesticides—Final Report. *EFSA Support. Publ.* **2017**, *14*, 1–207. [CrossRef]
82. World Health Organization (WHO). The WHO Recommended Classification of Pesticides by Hazard and Guidelines to Classification. Available online: https://www.who.int/ipcs/publications/pesticides_hazard_2009.pdf (accessed on 5 January 2019).
83. Likert, R. *A Technique for the Measurement of Attitudes. Archives of Psychology*; The Science Press: New York, NY, USA, 1932.
84. *ISO/IEC 31010: 2009, Risk Management—Risk Assessment Techniques*; Edition 1.0; International Electrotechnical Commission: Geneve, Switzerland, 2009; ISBN 2-8318-1068-2.
85. Allahyari, M.S.; Damalas, C.A.; Ebadattalab, M. Farmers' technical knowledge about integrated pest management (IPM) in olive production. *Agriculture* **2017**, *7*, 101. [CrossRef]
86. Fargnoli, M.; De Minicis, M.; Di Gravio, G. Knowledge Management integration in Occupational Health and Safety systems in the construction industry. *Int. J. Prod. Dev.* **2011**, *14*, 165–185. [CrossRef]
87. Rijal, J.P.; Regm, R.; Ghimire, R.; Puri, K.D.; Gyawaly, S.; Poudel, S. Farmers' Knowledge on Pesticide Safety and Pest Management Practices: A Case Study of Vegetable Growers in Chitwan, Nepal. *Agriculture* **2018**, *8*, 16. [CrossRef]
88. Guarascio, M.; Lombardi, M. Massi, F.; Risk Analysis in handling and storage of petroleum products. *Am. J. Appl. Sci.* **2013**, *10*, 965–978. [CrossRef]
89. Colosio, C.; Mandic-Rajcevic, S.; Godderis, L.; van der Laan, G.; Hulshof, C.; van Dijk, F. Workers' health surveillance: Implementation of the Directive 89/391/EEC in Europe. *Occup. Med.* **2017**, *67*, 574–578. [CrossRef] [PubMed]
90. Damalas, C.A.; Koutroubas, S.D. Farmers' behaviour in pesticide use: A key concept for improving environmental safety. *Curr. Opin. Environ Sci. Health* **2018**, *4*, 27–30. [CrossRef]
91. Damalas, C.A.; Koutroubas, S.D. Farmers' training on pesticide use is associated with elevated safety behavior. *Toxics* **2017**, *5*, 19. [CrossRef]
92. Voss, C.; Tsikriktsis, N.; Frohlich, M. Case research in operations management. *Int. J. Oper. Prod. Manag.* **2002**, *22*, 195–219. [CrossRef]
93. Yin, R.K. *Case Study Research: Design and Methods*, 4th ed.; Sage: Thousand Oaks, CA, USA, 2008; ISBN 1412960991.

94. Kayyar, M.; Ameri, F.; Summers, J.D. A case study of the development of a design enabler tool to support frame analysis for Wright Metal Products, a US SME. *Int. J. Comput. Aided Eng. Technol.* **2012**, *4*, 321–339. [CrossRef]
95. Acquavella, J.F.; Alexander, B.H.; Mandel, J.S.; Burns, C.J.; Gustin, C. Exposure misclassification in studies of agricultural pesticides: Insights from biomonitoring. *Epidemiology* **2006**, *17*, 69–74. [CrossRef] [PubMed]

International Journal of
Environmental Research and Public Health

MDPI

Article

Correction Workers' Burnout and Outcomes: A Bayesian Network Approach

Jin Lee [1,*], Robert Henning [2] and Martin Cherniack [3]

1 Department of Psychological Sciences, Kansas State University, Manhattan, KS 66506, USA
2 Department of Psychological Sciences, University of Connecticut, Storrs, CT 06269, USA; robert.henning@uconn.edu
3 Department of Medicine, UConn Health, University of Connecticut, Farmington, CT 06030, USA; cherniack@uchc.edu
* Correspondence: jinlee@ksu.edu

Received: 3 December 2018; Accepted: 17 January 2019; Published: 20 January 2019

Abstract: The present study seeks to demonstrate how Bayesian Network analysis can be used to support Total Worker Health® research on correction workers by (1) revealing the most probable scenario of how psychosocial and behavioral outcome variables in corrections work are interrelated and (2) identifying the key contributing factors of this interdependency relationship within the unique occupational context of corrections work. The data from 353 correction workers from a state department of corrections in the United States were utilized. A Bayesian Network analysis approach was used to probabilistically sort out potential interrelations among various psychosocial and behavioral variables. The identified model revealed that work-related exhaustion may serve as a primary driver of occupational stress and impaired workability, and also that exhaustion limits the ability of correction workers to get regular physical exercise, while their interrelations with depressed mood, a lack of work engagement, and poor work-family balance were also noted. The results suggest the importance of joint consideration of psychosocial and behavioral factors when investigating variables that may impact health and wellbeing of correction workers. Also, they supported the value of adopting the Total Worker Health® framework, a holistic strategy to integrate prevention of work-related injury and illness and the facilitation of worker well-being, when considering integrated health protection and promotion interventions for workers in high-risk occupations.

Keywords: correction workers; stress; exhaustion; psychosocial and behavioral factors; Bayesian Network; Total Worker Health®

1. Introduction

Correction workers work under psychologically and physically demanding conditions [1–3]. They are frequently exposed to unexpected hold-over shift work that may result in circadian disruption, sleep loss, and increased fatigue. Also, correction workers experience constant threat of inmate assaults and riots, which can be emotionally draining due to hyper-alertness and anxiety [4]. Moreover, working conditions in the correctional setting are known to be associated with numerous types of health and performance outcomes, including immediate outcomes, like exhaustion and psychological distress, as well as more distant outcomes, like job dissatisfaction and impaired work ability [5]. According to the U.S. Department of Justice, correction workers, including correctional officers and administrative and support staff, are at higher risk of suicide, substance abuse, and divorce, while their mortality rate is the second highest of any occupation [6]. High turnover rates have also been reported [7].

The negative impact of demanding correctional work on correction workers' wellbeing can be explained by the classic stress-burnout model [8,9]. Adverse working conditions of correctional work act as stressors causing stress. These stressors lead to psychophysical strain symptoms, such as various forms of psychophysical burnout. Echoing this, empirical studies on correction workers have shown significant relationships between overwork and stress [8,10]. Also, studies have revealed that correction workers' stress is associated with burnout [8,11] and somatic symptoms [7].

These phenomena can also be understood within theoretical frameworks of the Job Demands-Resources model [12]. Exposure to the physically and psychologically demanding correctional working conditions with a lack of adequate resources is likely to deplete correction workers' psychological resources for socially adaptive and physically healthy self-regulatory behaviors [13]. Thus, correction workers' demanding work conditions can lead to exhaustion, which may then negatively influence healthy behaviors as well as socially adaptive behaviors. Additionally, Wright and Cropanzano showed that emotional aspects of exhaustion, which can be manifested in different forms, such as depression and stress, can undermine job performance [14].

In general, the negative impacts of demanding work conditions and subsequent psychophysical strain can be both extensive and derivative. Recent studies have shown various complications of stress. For example, stress can contribute to increased risk of cardiovascular diseases [15], while burnout, as an outcome of extended exposure to stress, can be associated with impairment of psychological resources, such as emotional intelligence and self-efficacy, as well as loss of social support [16]. Moreover, it was shown that burnout can negatively affect well-being at work, resources for coping, ability to work, and engagement [17]. Considering these findings, it can be inferred that specific adverse effects on workers' health in general (e.g., illnesses, psychological problems, obesity, etc.) are further compounded by compromised family health (e.g., marriage dysfunction, problematic children's behavior) and employer dissatisfaction (e.g., due to declined performance, increased health care costs). In corrections, work-related stress can lead to increased absentee rates, internal conflict, and suboptimal employee performance [18], all which may have reciprocal adverse influences on the work environment.

Our study attempts to elaborate the Job Demand-Resource model, which primarily focuses on stressors' impact on stress outcomes (strains), by examining the interrelations among the potential stress outcomes that are typical for correction workers. Our view is that the various stress outcomes do not simply occur in parallel, but instead are able to have synergistic effects when they occur in combination, in line with the view that stressor-strain relationships can be reciprocal [19,20]. Chronic exposure to the occupational context of correctional facilities, with its high demand that also lacks control or support, is likely to lead to various psychosocial and behavioral stress outcomes. In fact, Tennant found that enduring structural occupational stress can contribute to psychological disorders, like depression [21]. When confronted with different types of strain symptoms, one's resources, which are always limited in the case of correction workers, need to be used to cope with the extant symptoms first, whilst one's resources may not be adequately restored in a timely manner in order to respond to the emergence of additional strain symptoms. Subsequently, one's strain symptoms are likely to be exacerbated as more problems arise and as resources become more and more depleted.

The process of resource depletion is particularly concerning in situations in which strain symptoms are not simply end products but operate as derivative or secondary demands (or stressors). As various strain symptoms negatively affect a person in different ways when they are either within or outside the workplace, this suggests a person needs resources, including increased control and support, both within and outside the workplace to handle multiple strain symptoms. This inference aligns with the perspectives of Spillover Theory [22], as well as Conservation of Resources Theory [23]. Furthermore, when there is a lack of adequate resources, the stress-burnout process would accelerate because of the synergistic impact of multiple strain symptoms on resource depletion.

Our study explores the possible derivative or secondary role of strain symptoms as additional stressors. By doing so, the domains of stress intervention are also broadened from focusing exclusively on traditional stressors to also include strain symptoms themselves. This approach is not unlike secondary (i.e., reducing the impact of an injury and disease that has already occurred) or even tertiary (i.e., mitigating the impact of an ongoing injury and illness which has lasting effect) intervention approaches found in medical science and public health [24]. The dire implications of doing nothing to prevent any worsening or exacerbation of the health situation for correction workers was also a motivating factor.

1.1. Socio-Technical Systems Framework and Total Worker Health® Paradigm

The present study is based on a socio-technical systems framework which recognizes the interactions between behavior and the design of work system components and their potential to promote workers' health and safety [25,26]. Specifically, key principles of joint causation within the socio-technical systems framework [26] provide the rationale for examining the interplay among the organizational (i.e., workability, disengagement), social (i.e., work-family balance), psychological (i.e., stress, exhaustion, depression), and behavioral strain symptoms (i.e., limited physical exercises) in relation to the unique occupational context of correctional work. Understanding the interrelatedness of these various attributes can help in efforts to achieve compatibility of the work system's elements and goals in order to promote better organizational performance as well as employee safety, health, and wellbeing [27,28].

Socio-technical systems approaches emphasize contextual factors whenever relationships are examined among a specific set of variables used to represent the inherent complexity of the workplace. In this regard, the socio-technical systems approach represents a holistic approach that is consistent with the Total Worker Health® framework being advanced by the U.S. National Institute for Occupational Safety and Health (NIOSH) [29]. NIOSH defines Total Worker Health as "policies, programs, and practices that integrate protection from work-related safety and health hazards with promotion of injury and illness prevention efforts to advance worker well-being" [30]. Researchers and practitioners seeking to advance the Total Worker Health agenda are moving beyond conventional health protection and health promotion approaches by undertaking more comprehensive assessments of the health, safety, and wellbeing of workers, and also to design and test more integrated workplace interventions [31].

According to the socio-technical systems framework, how correction workers deal with the unusually demanding occupational conditions in corrections will be a key determinant of how this adversely impacts them. For example, working conditions in corrections may make it harder for correction workers to balance work and personal life. Subsequently, unique patterns of negative spillover effects [32] can be anticipated to impact both the psychosocial and behavioral states of correction workers, such that a disrupted work-family balance may exacerbate one's depression, stress, healthy eating, regular exercises, engagement to work, and workability. Meanwhile, the Total Worker Health paradigm speaks to the importance of integrated efforts both within (e.g., management commitment, working environment improvement) and outside the workplace (e.g., support from home and community) in order to effectively manage the adverse impact of the stressful work environment of corrections.

1.2. Analytic Approach: Bayesian Network Analysis

Bayesian Network analysis examines the relationships among variables based on their joint probability [33]. It utilizes machine learning algorithms that can efficiently cope with the uncertainty and complexity of component interactions within a system as a whole [34]. Bayesian Network analysis offers a network diagram (directed acyclic graph), which consists of nodes and arrows. The nodes are random variables that may consist of observed continuous or categorical quantities, or even latent variables. The arrows (i.e., edges or arcs) indicate probabilistic relationships. If two nodes are connected with an arrow, this suggests that the two nodes are conditionally dependent.

Bayesian Network analysis is efficient in examining the interactions of all system components included in the model, when individual, organizational, and physical factors co-exist and can jointly contribute, and this has the potential to provide valuable insights on the determinants of employee safety and health outcomes. This approach is remarkably suitable to socio-technical systems approaches, which emphasize the importance of examining the interplay among various system components in order to optimize their functioning for a healthy and sustainable workplace. The structural learning algorithm of Bayesian Network analysis is a type of greedy search algorithm [35], and this approach enables investigation of every possible structural association among selected variables to estimate the most probable model that satisfies the model selection criteria of a particular learning algorithm.

Moreover, Bayesian Network analysis is less susceptible to multicollinearity problems [36]. By leveraging the inter-correlations among variables, Bayesian Network analysis provides conditional probability distributions for the dependent relationships of study variables. A complex system can thus be viewed in a modular way by "breaking down the discovery process into the search for the specific components of a complex system, and thus avoiding ... multicollinearity" (p. 59) [37].

Bayesian Network analysis has been successfully applied in various settings that require quantitative modeling of complicated relationships among many variables, such as in genetic modeling and disease diagnosis [37]. Also, the Bayesian Network approach has already been used to unveil the mutual relationships among various organizational and psychosocial factors regarding stressors, stress, and strain in workplace. Specifically, more task demands were associated with more stress at work [38], while social support from both supervisors and co-workers was critical in workplace stress prevention [39]. All things considered, Bayesian Network analysis is therefore well suited to investigate complicated interrelationships among multiple psychosocial and behavioral outcomes of stress.

In summary, it is worth noting that there has been no scientific study which integrates the conceptual framework of Total Worker Health and the machine learning analytic framework as a means to promote workplace health and well-being. No publication was found under the keywords search of "Total Worker Health" and "machine learning" in PubMed and PsycINFO. To address this gap, the present study adopted the Total Worker Health framework and Bayesian Network analysis approach (1) to reveal the most probable ways that psychosocial and behavioral outcome variables in corrections work are interrelated, and (2) to identify the key contributing factors of this interdependency relationship within the unique occupational context of correctional work.

2. Method

2.1. Participants

Paper-and-pencil surveys were distributed at the correctional facilities with high (level 4) to highest (level 5) security. The data from 353 employees at the Connecticut Department of Correction was obtained from a study conducted by the Center for the Promotion of Health in New England Workplace (CPH-NEW), a NIOSH center of excellence for Total Worker Health. In return for completing the survey, monetary incentives were offered. Mean age of the sample was 42.84 (SD = 9.72) and 74.6% were males. Average job tenure was 11.96 yrs (SD = 6.46). In terms of ethnicity, 71.5% were white, 15.8% were black, and the remaining 12.7% included Hispanic, Asian, and others. The vast majority of the study participants were correctional officers (70.5%), followed by support staff, which included administrative staff, maintenance staff, food service staff, teachers, chaplains (11.7%), counselors (5.7%), medical staff (4.6%), lieutenants (4.3%), and others (3.2%). In general, the present study's participants were not considerably different from the correction workers from previous studies [40,41] in terms of their demographic characteristics, such as mean age, proportion of male workers, and average job tenure.

The total number of correction workers at the two correctional facilities in the present study was 862, and the number of total respondents in the final data set was 353 after removing the cases of incomplete responses (i.e., more than 50% missing responses to survey; no response to the key study variables), suggesting that the minimum response rate was 41.0%. This response rate might be partly explained by the fact that correction workers often engage in shift work, are already dedicating a high degree of their attention to the volatile and dangerous environments they work in, and experience high level of fatigue from this demanding work, all of which contribute to their lack of availability and interest in participating in scientific studies. It can be noted that extant research on correction worker samples reports similar response rates of 37% [40] and 43% [42].

2.2. Measures

Psychosocial and behavioral variables judged to be potential responses to stressful and demanding working conditions were selected for Bayesian Network modeling. Physical assessment variables such as systolic/diastolic blood pressure, waist circumference, hand grip strength, and body mass index were excluded because the primary focus of the present study was on psychosocial and behavioral factors of correction workers. Also, bio-physiological factors were excluded as they were more relevant to chronic disease, having indirect long-term negative effects across the lifespan.

2.2.1. Exhaustion

Work-related fatigue and exhaustion were assessed with three items adopted from the Burnout scale [43] and a 1–7 response scale (1: strongly disagree, 7: strongly agree). A sample item was; "After work, I have enough energy for leisure activities (reverse scored)". Internal consistency was satisfactory with $\alpha = 0.70$ [44].

2.2.2. Disengagement

Correction workers' perception of disengagement from their work was assessed with the two items adopted from the Burnout scale [43] and a 1–7 response scale (1: strongly disagree, 7: strongly agree). The items were; "More and more often I talk about my work in a negative way" and "Sometimes I feel really disgusted with my work." Internal consistency was satisfactory ($\alpha = 0.82$).

2.2.3. Depression

Depressed mood was measured with the 10 items of the Center for Epidemiologic Studies Depression Scale [45]. All items had a 1–4 response scale (1: rarely or none of the time, less than 1 day per week, 4: all of the time, 5–7 days per week). An example item was; "I was bothered by things that usually don't bother me." Internal consistency was satisfactory ($\alpha = 0.76$).

2.2.4. Stress

A slightly adapted single-item version of the Stress in General Scale, which was shown to be valid by Stanton et al. [46], was utilized to assess stress. The item "On average, how stressful is your work?" had a 1–5 response scale (1: not at all, 5: extremely).

2.2.5. Limitations to Regular Physical Leisure Exercise

Based on a series of focus group meetings with correction workers, and brainstorming with subject matter experts in psychophysical health, such as medical doctors, epidemiologists, ergonomists, as well as psychologists, a list of specific psychosocial and behavioral factors that are associated with workers' motivation and engagement to physical exercises was created by the CPH-NEW research team [47]. Using a yes-no answer format, 12 factors that limit correction workers' ability to get regular physical exercise were evaluated. Example items included "Fatigue or need to schedule sleep," "Pain in joints or muscles," and "Overtime or shift work."

2.2.6. Work–Family Balance (Work to Family and Family to Work Conflict)

Perceived level of conflict between demands from work and family was assessed with four items based on a 1–4 response scale (1: never, 4: always). The items were adopted from the questions used by Frone et al. [48]. An example item was "How often do things going on at work make you feel tense and irritable at home?" Internal consistency was satisfactory ($\alpha = 0.75$).

2.2.7. Workability

The Work Ability Index [49] was utilized to assess the correction workers' perceived ability to perform their work. The index consists of four items that are calibrated on a 0–10 response scale (0: cannot work, 10: work at best). An example item was "How many points would you give your current ability to work?". Internal consistency was satisfactory ($\alpha = 0.91$).

2.3. Analysis

Bayesian Network modeling was performed with GeNie [50], which is freely accessible to researchers and practitioners. The study variables were all discretized into five equal intervals by percent distribution (i.e., 0–20%, 21–40%, 41–60%, 61–80%, and 81–100%) in order to allow consistency in making interpretations and to simplify the probabilistic dependency relationship between all possible study variable pairs. By doing so, the strength of the probabilistic link between two variables X and Y is defined as the chance of the specific state of Y (e.g., top 20 percentile) given the specific state of X (e.g., bottom 20 percentile) in the identified Bayesian Network model. Furthermore, the presumption is that a randomly-selected response category will be correct 20% of the time by chance (i.e., one correct response out of five response options). Thus, if the classification accuracy of each study variable's state based on the Bayesian Network model is substantially greater than 20% (and closer to 100%), it can be concluded that the model is valid.

In the Bayesian Network analysis framework, "learning" represents successful estimation of probabilistic parameters and structure. After first randomly selecting half of the data ($n = 182$, 51.6%), a Bayesian Network model was learned without any prior assumptions about the interrelations among the interested psychosocial and behavioral factors. This enabled the modeling process to be completely data driven. Specifically, the "learn parameter" function of GeNie [50] was utilized; it is based on an expectation maximization (EM) algorithm with random restarts. EM is an iterative "hill-climbing" algorithm, which attempts to maximize the expected log likelihood of the probabilistic model [51,52]. It is one of the most widely used Bayesian Network learning techniques, and is particularly useful when data is incomplete (i.e., missing values) or when hidden variables are assumed.

The identified Bayesian Network model (learned with the first half of the data) was validated by testing the variables' state classification accuracy using the second half of the data ($n = 171$, 48.4%). Specifically, leave-one-out (LOO) cross-validation was utilized because it does not waste any data points in contrast to other cross-validation approaches (e.g., k-fold cross-validation). The LOO cross-validation attempts to answer how accurately the learned Bayesian Network model predicts the state of a left-out data point given the second data set minus one data point. Accuracy is computed as the percent of correct predictions, which can be compared with the minimum accuracy level, referred to as the random classification accuracy [53].

2.4. Ethical Approval

All subjects gave their informed consent for inclusion before they participated in the study. The study was conducted in accordance with the Declaration of Helsinki, and the protocol was approved by the Internal Review Board (IRB) of UConn Health (IE-13-033S-2).

3. Results

3.1. Bayesian Network Model Specification

Descriptive statistics of the study variables as well as their inter-correlations are presented in Table 1. Bayesian Network model was "learned" to reveal the mutual dependence of the seven psychosocial and behavioral factors. The final Bayesian Network model is presented in Figure 1. This model represents the most probable scenario of how these factors are jointly associated with the health and well-being of correction workers.

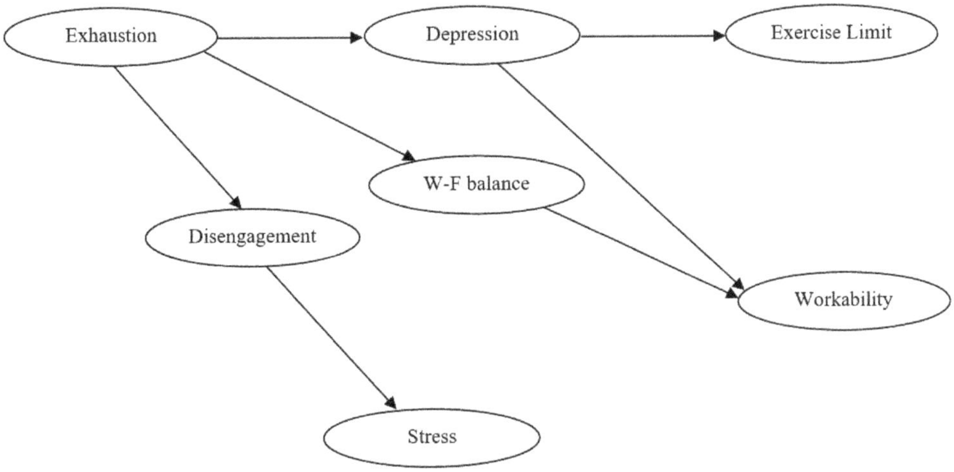

Figure 1. Final Bayesian Network model: the most probable scenario of the potential negative outcomes of correctional work. notes: W-F balance = Work-Family balance (work to family and family to work conflict); Exercise Limit = Limitations to regular physical leisure exercise.

3.2. Validation of the Bayesian Network Model

In the final Bayesian Network model, the accuracy of the study variables' state classification was well above the random classification level (in the present study, 20%), suggesting acceptable, but somewhat less than optimal, model validity. The specific classification accuracies were: 31.0% (3.7–65.9% across the states) for exhaustion, 35.7% (12.5–63.2% across the states) for disengagement, 27.5% (0–46.7% across the states) for stress, 41.5% (4.5–74.5% across the states) for depression, 56.1% (0–72.4% across the states) for work-family balance, 38.6% (0–66.7% across the states) for limitations to regular physical leisure exercise, and 40.9% (0–66.1% across the states) for workability. These accuracy levels were all greater than the random state, even though variations were detected across different states of each study variable. Relatively low accuracy levels for particular states of the study variables were primarily due to small observations for these particular states of the study variables, either in the learning or validation data sets.

3.3. Conditional Probabilities

The final Bayesian Network model suggested that work-related exhaustion may lead to derivative occupational stress as well as a loss of workability, and that work-related exhaustion also limits a correction worker's ability to get regular physical exercise. These three outcomes (i.e., stress, workability, and limitations to regular physical leisure exercise) were also consistently interrelated with the psychosocial factors of depressed mood, disengagement, and lack of work-family balance. Particularly, depressed mood served as an important "hub factor", being directly related to most of the study variables. The likelihood of having a high (top 20 percentile) depressed mood increased from 6 to 38% as the level of work-related exhaustion changed from low (bottom 20 percentile) to high (top 20 percentile). The likelihood of having poor (bottom 20 percentile) workability increased from 4% to 48%, as the level of depressed mood increased from low (bottom 20 percentile) to high (top 20 percentile). The likelihood of having poor (bottom 20 percentile) ability to get regular physical exercise increased from 4 to 17%. Graphical representation of the study variables' conditional probability distribution based on the final Bayesian Network model is presented in Figure 2.

Table 1. Means, Standard deviations (SD), and correlations of the study variables.

Study Variables	Mean (SD)	1	2	3	4	5	6	7	8	9	10
1. Exhaustion	30.88 (10.21)	-									
2. Disengagement	30.82 (10.53)	0.49 **	-								
3. Depression	10.63 (0.44)	0.51 **	0.40 **	-							
4. Stress	10.56 (10.02)	0.47 **	0.46 **	0.34 **	-						
5. Exercise Limit	20.36 (10.73)	0.40 **	0.29 **	0.40 **	0.22 **	-					
6. Work-Family balance	30.37 (0.79)	−0.40 **	−0.24 **	−0.45 **	−0.27 **	−0.23 **	-				
7. Workability	80.76 (10.40)	−0.38 **	−0.30 **	−0.54 **	−0.32 **	−0.35 **	0.43 **	-			
8. Healthy diet	20.95 (0.54)	−0.18 **	−0.10 ^{ns}	−0.19 **	−0.05 ^{ns}	−0.31 **	0.15 **	0.09 ^{ns}	-		
9. Nutrition	20.58 (0.84)	−0.18 **	−0.14 *	−0.29 **	−0.02 ^{ns}	−0.28 **	0.21 **	0.16 **	0.51 **	-	
10. Readiness to Improve Health	30.80 (10.00)	−0.17 **	−0.14 **	−0.27 **	−0.04 ^{ns}	−0.24 **	0.28 **	0.26 **	0.44 **	0.49 **	-

Notes: Exercise limit = Limitations to regular physical leisure exercise; ** $p < 0.01$; * $p < 0.05$; ^{ns} $p < 0.01$.

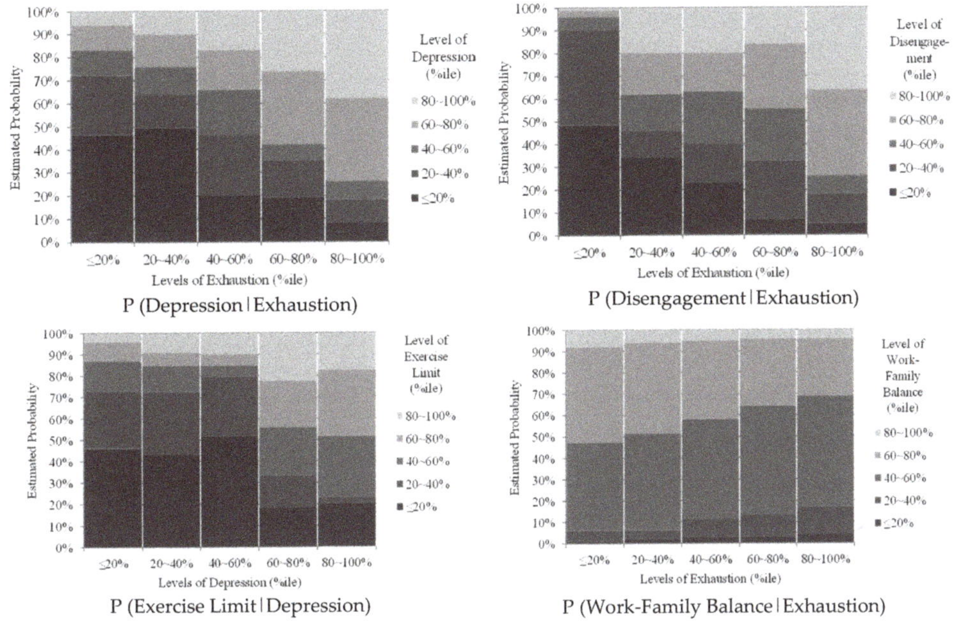

Figure 2. Conditional probability distribution based on the data-driven final Bayesian Network model. Notes: P(Y | X) = conditional probability of Y given X (i.e., probability of a particular state of Y given the particular state of X); Exercise Limit = Limitations to regular physical leisure exercise.

The establishment of a final model permits the simulation of many different "what if" scenarios, allowing the researcher to explore any revealed relationship in greater detail. In the present study, the probabilities of correction workers' stress, workability, and limitations to regular physical leisure exercise were calculated for two specific situations: (1) when other variables, such as exhaustion, disengagement, depression, and work–family balance are at their poorest (worst case scenario), and (2) when these same variables are optimal (best case scenario). As expected, the more desirable states of these variables—low stress, high workability, and reduced limitations to regular physical leisure exercise—were much more probable in the best case scenario than in the worst case scenario (Table 2).

Table 2. Probabilities at the Simulated Worst and Best Scenarios.

Outcome Variables	At Worst Scenario	At Best Scenario
Exercise Limit	Low (Bottom 20 percentile) = 20%	Low (Bottom 20 percentile) = 49%
Workability	High (Top 40 percentile) = 1%	High (Top 40 percentile) = 89%
Stress	Low (Bottom 20 percentile) = 3%	Low (Bottom 20 percentile) = 52%

Notes: Low = Bottom 20 percentile; High = Top 20 percentile; Exercise Limit = Limitations to regular physical leisure exercise.

4. Discussion

Psychological and physical health problems and concerns are diverse and prevalent among correction workers. In order to reveal the interplay among potential outcomes within their unique occupational context in a manner consistent with socio-technical systems approaches, the present study adopted the Bayesian Network analytic framework because of its flexibility and efficiency in exploring all possible interrelations among the study variables. Guided by well-established frameworks for workplace stress mechanisms, including the Job Demands-Resource Model [12], Spillover Theory [22,32], and Conservation of Resources Theory [23], study variables were selected based on assumptions about their potential interrelations. Subsequently, use of the data-driven Bayesian Network approach identified a model showing a probable scenario in which correction workers' exhaustion had dominant influence over a chain reaction that significantly raised the risk of several other negative psychosocial and behavioral outcomes. Correction workers' exhaustion was found to be associated with a lack of work engagement, depressed mood, and also interfered with work-family balance. Additionally, increased disengagement was found to be associated with work-related stress, while depressed mood was closely associated with less regular physical activity. At the same time, depressed mood and work-family imbalance were jointly associated with reduced work ability.

The results extend the previous finding of a close relationship between psychological distress and work-family imbalance among correction workers [54]. The identified joint processes of how the impact of exhaustion can be enhanced or mitigated by other factors also extends to previous findings regarding the impact of exhaustion on depression, absenteeism, depersonalization, and reduced personal accomplishment that were based on a French correctional officer sample [55].

4.1. Theoretical and Analytic Implications

First, the study findings complement relationships predicted by the Job Demands-Resource Model. In this model, job demands that result in exhaustion can negatively impact worker engagement, and this in turn is associated with work-related stress. Also, this model suggests that job demands that are closely associated with exhaustion will be negatively associated with psychosocial (i.e., mood and work-family imbalance) and organizational behavior outcomes (i.e., work ability). These same relationships were supported by the data-driven Bayesian Network model identified in the present study.

However contrary to relationships posited in the conventional stress models, relationships between stress to outcomes (i.e., engagement, workability) were not detected in the present study. This may be partly explained by the fact that other factors, such as depressed mood and work-family imbalance, were considered simultaneously along with the engagement and stress variables, speaking to the importance of examining psychosocial variables in combination with occupational context variables. Our findings indicate that the Job Demand-Resource Model may be a reasonable framework to first approach occupational health and safety issues, but it is also important to account for workers' adjustment to their particular work context, as is the case in the present study of correction workers.

Second, although a stress-to-burnout directional relationship has been widely accepted in previous studies [8,9], the present study showed that burnout (i.e., exhaustion) may be associated with derivative stress, which is subsequent to employee disengagement. In fact, there have been previous reports that disengagement, which may be followed by burnout, leads to more stress in workplace [56] and also a distressed mental state [57]. It should be noted that the finding here of a burnout-to-stress relationship doesn't necessarily reject the well-established causal link from stress to burnout, and also that our findings were based on the unique context of correctional work for which well-established causal linkages may not apply. Nonetheless, the results do suggest the need for adopting an unbiased perspective on how stress may be exacerbated by burnout in a particular population of workers. Within an autoregressive model framework [58], an outcome at one point in time can serve as a cause at another future point in time, and this may also be the case for the reciprocal stress and burnout relationship. Future studies could take a longitudinal approach to further examine the nature of the causal mechanisms behind the stress-burnout relationship.

4.2. Practical Implications

The results support use of the Total Worker Health framework for considering a wide range of factors impacting worker health and wellbeing. Integrated interventions that promote safety, health, and well-being among correction workers appear to be warranted, given the complex interplay of the psychosocial and behavioral factors reported on here. The results also suggest that taking steps to reduce the level of exhaustion in this working population may provide the most efficient way to reduce depressed mood, interruption of work-family balance, and a lack of work engagement. These factors were also shown to increase the risks of work-related stress, a reduction of regular physical exercise, and lowered work ability. Continued failure to manage workers' exhaustion would be ignoring an apparent primary risk factor.

However, management of this primary risk factor may prove particularly challenging if there is short staffing and also overtime requirements in an organization that functions 24/7 and that cannot afford to be understaffed at any time. If work-related exhaustion cannot be avoided, then intervention efforts can next focus on the proper management of workers' depressed mood because this was also shown to be strongly associated with the loss of work-family balance, increased negative attitudes toward their job, and reduced workability. Establishing a hierarchy of risk factors and then selecting the most attainable intervention is compatible with a participatory approach to intervention planning [28] which aims at identifying and addressing workers' needs and concerns that are most salient given their present circumstances.

4.3. Limitations and Suggestions for Future Study

Some limitations of the present study need to be addressed in future research. Generalizability of the findings is limited given the uniqueness and relatively small size of the sample. In particular, it can be noted that only half of the data was utilized for Bayesian Network model learning, while the remaining half of the data was utilized for the validation of the learned Bayesian Network model. Also, the present study was cross-sectional, which did not allow examination of the dynamic relationships among study variables across time. Moreover, the final Bayesian Network model's accuracy level was not at an ideal level, although it was found to be meaningfully above chance. To resolve this issue, a larger sample can be used for Bayesian Network model learning to enable more robust and reliable modeling. More data points generally ensure more reliable estimation of probability, particularly when the probability is smaller. Also, future studies are needed to more clearly demonstrate the distinct roles of job demands, job control, and support in the extended mechanisms affecting stressors, stress, strain, and the exacerbation of the strain symptoms. The role of individual differences, such as gender, age, and tenure in the interrelations among stress and stress outcomes can also be examined in future studies.

5. Conclusions

The present study demonstrated the value of using a machine learning algorithm, like Bayesian Network analysis, to explore the complicated interrelations among multiple psychosocial and behavioral factors in a specific socio-technical work context, and the ways these interrelations may be contributing to correctional officer health and wellness. Regardless of some limitations, like the relatively small sample size for a machine learning approach and the use of cross-sectional data, the findings of the present study suggest the importance of joint consideration of psychosocial and behavioral factors when investigating variables that may impact the health and wellbeing of correction workers. Moreover, the present study supported the value of adopting a Total Worker Health framework with integrated intervention approaches as a means to benefit workers in high-risk occupations.

Author Contributions: Conceptualization, J.L., R.H., and M.C.; methodology, J.L.; software, J.L.; validation, J.L., R.H., and M.C.; formal analysis, J.L.; investigation, M.C., R.H., and J.L.; resources, M.C., and R.H.; data curation, M.C., R.H., and J.L.; writing—original draft preparation, J.L.; writing—review and editing, M.C. and R.H.; visualization, J.L.; supervision, M.C. and R.H.; project administration, M.C. and R.H.; funding acquisition, M.C. and R.H.

Funding: This work was supported by grant no. U19-OH008857 from the National Institute for Occupational Safety and Health (NIOSH) at the Centers for Disease Control and Prevention. The contents of this article are solely the responsibility of the authors and do not necessarily represent the official views of NIOSH.

Acknowledgments: Publication of this article was funded in part by the Kansas State University Open Access Publishing Fund.

Conflicts of Interest: The authors the present study have no involvement in or affiliations with any organization or entity with any financial interest, such as employment, consultancies, stock ownership, or other equity interest, or non-financial interest, such as personal or professional relationships in the subject matter or materials discussed in this study.

References

1. Cherniack, M.; Dussetschleger, J.; Dugan, A.; Farr, D.; Namazi, S.; El Ghaziri, M.; Henning, R. Participatory action research in corrections: The HITEC 2 program. *Appl. Ergon.* **2016**, *53*, 169–180. [CrossRef] [PubMed]
2. Morse, T.; Dussetschleger, J.; Warren, N.; Cherniack, M. Talking about Health: Correction Employees' Assessments of Obstacles to Healthy Living. *J. Occup. Environ. Med.* **2011**, *53*, 1037–1045. [CrossRef] [PubMed]
3. Punnett, L.; Warren, N.; Henning, R.; Nobrega, S.; Cherniack, M. CPH-NEW Research Team. Participatory Ergonomics as a Model for Integrated Programs to Prevent Chronic Disease. *J. Occup. Environ. Med.* **2013**, *55*, S19–S24. [CrossRef] [PubMed]
4. Faghri, P.; Mignano, C. Overweight and Obesity in High Stress Workplaces. *J. Nutr. Disord. Ther.* **2013**, *3*, 3. [CrossRef]
5. Lazarus, R.S.; DeLongis, A.; Folkman, S.; Gruen, R. Stress and adaptational outcomes: The problem of confounded measures. *Am. Psychol.* **1985**, *40*, 770–779. [CrossRef]
6. U.S. Department of Justice. *Addressing Correctional Officer Stress Programs and Strategies: Issues and Practices*; NCJ No. 183474; U.S. Government Printing Office: Washington, DC, USA, 2000.
7. Armstrong, G.S.; Griffin, M.L. Does the job matter? Comparing correlates of stress among treatment and correctional staff in prisons. *J. Crim. Justice* **2004**, *32*, 577–592. [CrossRef]
8. Dignam, J.T.; Barrera, M.; West, S.G. Occupational stress, social support, and burnout among correctional officers. *Am. J. Community Psychol.* **1986**, *14*, 177–193. [CrossRef] [PubMed]
9. Pines, A.; Aronson, E. *Career Burnout: Causes and Cures*; Free Press: New York, NY, USA, 1988.
10. Triplett, R.; Mullings, J.L.; Scarborough, K.E. Work-related stress and coping among correctional officers: Implications from organizational literature. *J. Crim. Justice* **1996**, *24*, 291–308. [CrossRef]
11. Hurst, T.E.; Hurst, M.M. Gender differences in mediation of severe occupational stress among correctional officers. *Am. J. Crim. Justice* **1997**, *22*, 121–137. [CrossRef]
12. Bakker, A.B.; Demerouti, E. The job demands-resources model: State of the art. *J. Manag. Psychol.* **2007**, *22*, 309–328. [CrossRef]
13. Muraven, M.; Baumeister, R.F. Self-regulation and depletion of limited resources: Does self-control resemble a muscle? *Psychol. Bull.* **2000**, *126*, 247–259. [CrossRef] [PubMed]
14. Wright, T.A.; Cropanzano, R. Emotional exhaustion as a predictor of job performance and voluntary turnover. *J. Appl. Psychol.* **1998**, *83*, 486–493. [CrossRef]
15. Lecca, L.; Campagna, M.; Portoghese, I.; Galletta, M.; Mucci, N.; Meloni, M.; Cocco, P. Work Related Stress, Well-Being and Cardiovascular Risk among Flight Logistic Workers: An Observational Study. *Int. J. Environ. Res. Public Health* **2018**, *15*, 1952. [CrossRef] [PubMed]
16. Molero Jurado, M.; Pérez-Fuentes, M.; Gázquez Linares, J.; Simón Márquez, M.; Martos Martínez, Á. Burnout risk and protection factors in certified nursing aides. *Int. J. Environ. Res. Public Health* **2018**, *15*, 1116. [CrossRef] [PubMed]
17. Voltmer, J.B.; Voltmer, E.; Deller, J. Differences of Four Work-Related Behavior and Experience Patterns in Work Ability and Other Work-Related Perceptions in a Finance Company. *Int. J. Environ. Res. Public Health* **2018**, *15*, 1521. [CrossRef] [PubMed]
18. Auerbach, S.M.; Quick, B.G.; Pegg, P.O. General job stress and job-specific stress in juvenile correctional officers. *J. Crim. Justice* **2003**, *31*, 25–36. [CrossRef]
19. Leventhal, H.; Tomarken, A. *Stress Illness: Perspectives from Health Psychology In Stress and Health: Issues in Research Methodology*; Kasl, S.V., Cooper, C.L., Eds.; Wiley: Chichester, NY, USA, 1987; pp. 27–55.
20. Zapf, D.; Dormann, C.; Frese, M. Longitudinal studies in organizational stress research: A review of the literature with reference to methodological issues. *J. Occup. Health Psychol.* **1996**, *1*, 145–169. [CrossRef] [PubMed]

21. Tennant, C. Work-related stress and depressive disorders. *J. Psychosom. Res.* **2001**, *51*, 697–704. [CrossRef]
22. Zedeck, S.; Mosier, K.L. Work in the family and employing organization. *Am. Psychol.* **1990**, *45*, 240–251. [CrossRef]
23. Hobfoll, S.E. Conservation of resources: A new attempt at conceptualizing stress. *Am. Psychol.* **1989**, *44*, 513–524. [CrossRef]
24. Gordon, R.S., Jr. An operational classification of disease prevention. *Public Health Rep.* **1983**, *98*, 107–109. [PubMed]
25. Emery, F.E.; Trist, E. The causal texture of organizational environments. *Hum. Relat.* **1965**, *18*, 12–32. [CrossRef]
26. Kleiner, B.M. Macroergonomics: Analysis and design of work systems. *Appl. Ergon.* **2006**, *37*, 81–89. [CrossRef] [PubMed]
27. Haro, E.; Kleiner, B.M. Macroergonomics as an organizing process for systems safety. *Appl. Ergon.* **2008**, *39*, 450–458. [CrossRef] [PubMed]
28. Henning, R.; Warren, N.; Robertson, M.; Faghri, P.; Cherniack, M.; CPH-NEW Research Team. Workplace health protection and promotion through participatory ergonomics: An integrated approach. *Public Health Rep.* **2009**, *124* (Suppl. 1), 26–35. [CrossRef] [PubMed]
29. NIOSH. Total Worker Health® Program. 2015. Available online: http://www.cdc.gov/niosh/twh/ (accessed on 1 September 2015).
30. Tamers, S.L.; Goetzel, R.; Kelly, K.M.; Luckhaupt, S.; Nigam, J.; Pronk, N.P.; Rohlman, D.S.; Baron, S.; Brosseau, L.M.; Bushnell, T.; et al. Research Methodologies for Total Worker Health®: Proceedings from a Workshop. *J. Occup. Environ. Med.* **2018**, *60*, 968–978. [CrossRef] [PubMed]
31. Schill, A.L.; Chosewood, L.C. The NIOSH Total Worker Health® program: An overview. *J. Occup. Environ. Med.* **2013**, *55*, S8–S11. [CrossRef]
32. Westman, M. Crossover of stress and strain in the family and in the workplace. *Res. Occup. Stress Well-Being* **2002**, *2*, 143–181.
33. Korb, K.B.; Nicholson, A.E. *Bayesian Artificial Intelligence*; Chapman & Hall: Boca Raton, FL, USA, 2004.
34. Murphy, K. A Brief Introduction to Graphical Models and Bayesian Networks. 1998. Available online: http://www.cs.ubc.ca/~{}murphyk/Bayes/bayes.html (accessed on 19 November 2018).
35. Cooper, G.F.; Herskovits, E. A Bayesian method for the induction of probabilistic networks from data. *Mach. Learn.* **1992**, *9*, 309–347. [CrossRef]
36. Curtis, S.M.; Ghosh, S.K. A Bayesian Approach to Multicollinearity and the Simultaneous Selection and Clustering of Predictors in Linear Regression. *J. Stat. Theory Pract.* **2011**, *5*, 715–735. [CrossRef]
37. Sebastiani, P.; Perls, T.T. Complex Genetic Models. In *To Appear in Bayesian Belief Networks: A Practical Guide to Applications*; Pourret, O., Nam, P., Marcot, B.G., Eds.; Wiley: New York, NY, USA, 2007; pp. 53–72.
38. García-Herrero, S.; Mariscal, M.A.; Gutiérrez, J.M.; Ritzel, D.O. Using Bayesian networks to analyze occupational stress caused by work demands: Preventing stress through social support. *Acc. Anal. Prev.* **2013**, *57*, 114–123. [CrossRef]
39. García-Herrero, S.; Saldaña, M.Á.M.; Rodriguez, J.G.; Ritzel, D.O. Influence of task demands on occupational stress: Gender differences. *J. Saf. Res.* **2012**, *43*, 365–374. [CrossRef] [PubMed]
40. Brough, P.; Williams, J. Managing occupational stress in a high-risk industry: Measuring the job demands of correctional officers. *Crim. Justice Behav.* **2007**, *34*, 555–567. [CrossRef]
41. Finney, C.; Stergiopoulos, E.; Hensel, J.; Bonato, S.; Dewa, C.S. Organizational stressors associated with job stress and burnout in correctional officers: A systematic review. *BMC Public Health* **2013**, *13*, 82. [CrossRef] [PubMed]
42. Ghaddar, A.; Mateo, I.; Sanchez, P. Occupational stress and mental health among correctional officers: A cross-sectional study. *J. Occup. Health* **2008**, *50*, 92–98. [CrossRef] [PubMed]
43. Demerouti, E.; Bakker, A.B.; Nachreiner, F.; Schaufeli, W.B. The job demands-resources model of burnout. *J. Appl. Psychol.* **2000**, *86*, 499–512. [CrossRef]
44. Nunnally, J.C.; Bernstein, I.H. *Psychometric Theory*; McGraw-Hill Series in Psychology; McGraw-Hill: New York, NY, USA, 1994; Volume 3.
45. Radloff, L.S. The CES-D Scale: A Self-Report Depression Scale for Research in the General Population. *Appl. Psychol. Meas.* **1977**, *1*, 385–401. [CrossRef]

46. Stanton, J.M.; Blazer, W.K.; Smith, P.C.; Parra, L.F.; Ironson, G. A general measure of work stress: The stress in general scale. *Educ. Psychol. Meas.* **2001**, *61*, 866–888. [CrossRef]
47. University of Massachusetts Lowell, University of Connecticut. (n.d.). Center for the Promotion of Health in the New England Workplace (CPH-NEW). Available online: http://www.uml.edu/Research/centers/CPH-NEW/ (accessed on 19 November 2018).
48. Frone, M.R.; Russell, M.; Cooper, M.L. Antecedents and outcomes of work-family conflict: Testing a model of the work-family interface. *J. Appl. Psychol.* **1992**, *77*, 65–78. [CrossRef]
49. Ilmarinen, J.; Tuomi, K.; Eskelinen, L.; Nygård, C.H.; Huuhtanen, P.; Klockars, M. Background and objectives of the Finnish research project on aging workers in municipal occupations. *Scand. J. Work Environ. Health* **1991**, *17* (Suppl. 1), 7–11.
50. Druzdzel, M.J. SMILE: Structural Modeling, Inference, and Learning Engine and GeNIe: A development environment for graphical decision-theoretic models. In Proceedings of the AAAI/IAAI, Orlando, FL, USA, 18–22 July 1999; pp. 902–903.
51. Friedman, N. The Bayesian structural EM algorithm. In Proceedings of the Fourteenth Conference on Uncertainty in Artificial Intelligence, Madison, WI, USA, 24–26 July 1998; Morgan Kaufmann Publishers Inc.: Burlington, MA, USA, 1998; pp. 129–138.
52. Murphy, K. An Introduction to Graphical Models. 2001. Available online: http://www2.denizyuret.com/ref/murphy/intro_gm.pdf (accessed on 19 November 2018).
53. Cakmak, A.; Kirac, M.; Reynolds, M.R.; Ozsoyoglu, Z.M.; Ozsoyoglu, G. Gene ontology-based annotation analysis and categorization of metabolic pathways. In Proceedings of the 19th International Conference on Scientific and Statistical Database Management (SSBDM'07), Banff, AB, Canada, 9–11 July 2007; pp. 33–42.
54. Obidoa, C.; Reeves, D.; Warren, N.; Reisine, S.; Cherniack, M. Depression and work family conflict among corrections officers. *J. Occup. Environ. Med.* **2011**, *53*, 1294–1301. [CrossRef] [PubMed]
55. Neveu, J.P. Jailed resources: Conservation of resources theory as applied to burnout among prison guards. *J. Organ. Behav.* **2007**, *28*, 21–42. [CrossRef]
56. Wagner, R.; Harter, J. *The Elements of Great Managing*; Gallup Press: New York, NY, USA, 2006.
57. Robison, J. Disengagement Can Really Be Depressing. Gallup Business Journal Online. 2010. Available online: http://www.gallup.com/businessjournal/127100/disengagement-really-depressing.aspx (accessed on 19 November 2018).
58. MacCallum, R.C.; Austin, J.T. Applications of structural equation modeling in psychological research. *Annu. Rev. Psychol.* **2000**, *51*, 201–226. [CrossRef] [PubMed]

International Journal of
Environmental Research and Public Health

MDPI

Article

Differences in Metabolic Syndrome Prevalence by Employment Type and Sex

Duk Youn Cho [1] and Jung-Wan Koo [2,*]

1 Department of Rehabilitation and Assistive Technology, Korea National Rehabilitation Center, Seoul 01022, Korea; guylian77@gmail.com
2 Department of Occupational and Environmental Medicine, Seoul St. Mary's Hospital, College of Medicine, The Catholic University of Korea, Seoul 06591, Korea
* Correspondence: jwkoo@catholic.ac.kr; Tel.: +82-222-586-268

Received: 19 July 2018; Accepted: 20 August 2018; Published: 21 August 2018

Abstract: Workers may sometimes do the same work, but differ in their risk of health-related problems depending on whether the employment type is standard or non-standard. Furthermore, even with similar job and employment types, there may be differences in risk factors for health-related problems depending on sex. This study aimed to determine the prevalence of metabolic syndrome (MetS) by employment type and sex using data from the Fifth Korean National Health and Nutrition Examination Survey (KNHANES V) (2010–2012) and KNHANES VI (2013–2015) conducted by the Korea Centers for Disease Control and Prevention. Overall, 9523 adult wage workers (5523 standard workers and 4000 non-standard workers) aged $\geq$ 19 years were analyzed. To determine MetS prevalence odds ratios according to employment type, logistic regression analysis was performed disaggregated by sex. The prevalence of MetS significantly increased with age ($p < 0.001$), being married ($p < 0.05$), current smoking status ($p < 0.05$), and high-risk drinking ($p < 0.001$) among male subjects. The prevalence of MetS significantly increased among female manual workers ($p < 0.001$), those with lower educational level and household income ($p < 0.001$). Non-standard workers of either sex showed higher MetS prevalence than standard workers; only females showed significant difference ($p < 0.001$). Female non-standard workers showed 1.44, 1.33, and 1.34 (all $p < 0.001$) times higher odds of MetS prevalence in Models 1, 2, and 3, respectively, compared to standard workers, suggesting a difference in risk factors of MetS according to sex. Also, that employment type affects MetS prevalence suggests that employment pattern is an important risk factor especially in females. Therefore, to manage MetS in female non-standard workers, individual health care as well as social effort may be necessary.

Keywords: non-standard work; metabolic syndrome; Korean workers; socioeconomic status; sex

1. Introduction

Since the 2008 financial crisis, economic uncertainty has persisted throughout the world and this has resulted in continual job instability [1]. In Korea, unstable jobs such as non-standard employment began to emerge during the International Monetary Fund (IMF) economic crisis in 1997, and this trend has continued to this day [2]. Non-standard workers are mostly employed under working conditions with low wage levels and are treated differently regarding wages, including incentives and welfare benefits [3]. In addition, many non-standard workers have more than one job due to the low wages, and work during the weekend or late [4]. Long work hours, irregular lifestyle, and high risk of job stress exposure among non-standard workers seriously threatens their health and safety [4,5]. Long working hours or high occupational stress cause short-term problems such as stress, fatigue, lack of sleep, smoking, excessive drinking, and lack of exercise, leading to long-term problems such as digestive diseases, urogenital diseases, musculoskeletal diseases, and mental diseases [6]. The abovementioned short and long-term problems may individually threaten the health of workers, and various problems may be combined, resulting in chronic diseases.

Recently, the prevalence of metabolic syndrome (MetS) is rapidly increasing worldwide. The risk factors for MetS include aging, physical inactivity, Western diet, sedentary work, long working hours, and high occupational stress [7]. In other words, lifestyle and socioeconomic status are important risk factors for MetS [8]. The factors associated with MetS are closely related to cardiovascular risk factors or diabetes, including abdominal obesity, triglyceride levels, high-density lipoprotein (HDL) cholesterol levels, hypertension, and fasting plasma glucose levels [9]. Risk factors for MetS can be controlled and prevented through appropriate management. However, many non-standard workers are exposed to multiple risk factors regarding improper health management due to lack of money and time. In recent years, many studies have examined the differences among various occupational groups such as manual workers, non-manual workers, office workers, and firefighters concerning the effect of socioeconomic status on MetS [8,10–12]. In previous studies, there was no consensus on the association between job type and MetS prevalence. However, there was a consensus regarding a difference in risk factors affecting MetS prevalence according to sex [11,13,14]. However, even if they have the same occupation, health-related characteristics of workers may differ depending on whether the employment is standard or non-standard. Nevertheless, little research has been done on the difference in MetS prevalence according to employment type. Therefore, in this study, we aimed to determine the prevalence of MetS by employment type and by sex.

2. Materials and Methods

2.1. Subjects

This study used raw data from the Fifth Korean National Health and Nutrition Examination Survey (KNHANES V) (2010–2012) and the KNHANES VI (2013–2015) conducted by the Korea Centers for Disease Control and Prevention. A stratified multistage cluster probability sampling design was used to select representative samples of denormalized Korean civilians. A trained investigator visited subjects' homes directly for the standardized health evaluation and with a questionnaire. In order to assess the association between MetS and full-time employment, we used data regarding wage worker subjects aged 19 years or older with employment status. From 2010 to 2015, the final 9523 (5523 standard and 4000 non-standard) workers met the inclusion criteria, out of 48,482.

2.2. Definition of Variables

2.2.1. Metabolic Syndrome

The definition of MetS was based on the National Cholesterol Education Program Adult Treatment Panel (NCEP ATP III) criteria, in which three or more of the following five risk factors were considered: (1) abdominal obesity(defined for Koreans as a waist circumference of ≥90 cm in males and ≥85 cm in females); (2) triglyceride level ≥ 150 mg/dL; (3) HDL cholesterol level < 40 mg/dL in males and <50 mg/dL in females; (4) systolic blood pressure ≥ 130 mmHg or diastolic blood pressure ≥ 85 mmHg; and (5) fasting plasma glucose level ≥ 110 mg/dL [15].

For the measurement of waist circumference, the subject was allowed to comfortably rest his/her arms on his/her waist while looking forward with his/her bare skin exposed. The lower end of the last palpable rib and the upper points of the iliac crest on both sides were measured in the subject's midaxillary line. The subjects were asked to exhale; the tape was then pulled to such a point that the skin was not pressed, and measured to one decimal place. Fasting blood glucose, HDL cholesterol, and triglyceride levels were measured from blood samples. Blood pressure was measured using a mercury sphygmomanometer. Prior to blood pressure measurement, subjects rested for 5 min; then the blood pressure was measured once. They then rested for 30 s and the blood pressure was measured again. The average value was calculated from the two measurements. All measurements were made in accordance with the National Health and Nutrition Examination Guidelines.

2.2.2. Job-Related Variables

In the sixth survey (2013–2015), we distinguished between standard and non-standard workers using the variable "whether standard worker (EC_Wht_0)". However, no similar variable existed in the fifth survey (2010–2012) to confirm the standard worker status. Thus, standard and non-standard workers were distinguished using the variables "working hours (EC_WH)" and "employee status wage workers (EC_STT_2)". Standard workers were defined as "full-time and regular" workers. Non-standard workers were defined as "full-time and temporary", "full-time and daily", "hourly and regular", "hourly and temporary" or "hourly and daily workers" [16–18]. Non-manual and manual workers complied with the job classification of the Korean Standard Classification of Occupations [18,19]. Those classified as non-manual workers were managers, professionals, technicians, sales, and service workers. Those classified as manual workers were those engaged in agriculture, forestry, fishery, manufacturing, construction, mining and soldiers.

2.2.3. Lifestyle-Related Variables

Smoking status was classified as current smoker, ex-smoker, and non-smoker. Ex-smoker referred to a person who had smoked in the past but did not currently smoke, and a non-smoker referred to a person who had never smoked. Drinking was classified into high risk, moderate, or non-drinking. In Korea, high-risk drinking is defined as drinking more than 13 standard servings for men and over six standard servings for women on a weekly basis [20]. High-risk drinking was used in reference to males and females who drank more than 2–3 times in a week with more than 7–9 servings at a time and more than 5–6 servings, respectively, at a time. In 2014 and 2015, physical activity was confirmed using the practice rate of "aerobic physical activity". In the data before 2013, there was no variable for the practice rate of "aerobic physical activity", "high-intensity physical activity time" and "moderate physical activity time" were calculated according to the guideline on "aerobic physical activity practice rate". The "aerobic physical activity rate" guideline set the moderate physical activity for a week at more than 150 min, or the high-intensity physical activity at 75 min or more, or the previous two physical activities for a considerable amount of time. The denominator was set as the total number of subjects aged 19 years or older. High-intensity physical activity at 1 min was calculated as 2 min of moderate physical activity. Body mass index value was derived from the "anthropometric measurements". Stress was confirmed in four stages: "I feel stressed very much", "I feel stressed a lot", "I feel stressed a little" and "I rarely feel stressed". Depression was identified as a current disease.

2.2.4. Sociodemographic Characteristics

The sociodemographic characteristics of the subjects included age, educational level, marital status, and household income level. Educational level is divided into "elementary school", "middle school", "high school" and "$\geq$university". Marital status was classified into "married" if "married" or "living together" but as "others" regardless of the reason, if not living together. Household income level was divided into four stages from the first to the fourth quartiles. Data regarding the area of residence were identified in the results from Seoul to Jeju.

2.3. Statistical Analysis

In this study, a composite sample analysis was performed using raw data from the National Health and Nutrition Examination Survey, which was extracted using a two-stage stratified sampling design, rather than a simple random sample design. Stratification and cluster variables were applied and the composite sample design was conducted by applying the questionnaire survey weight. Frequency analysis was performed to report on the general characteristics and major variables of the study subjects. Chi-square analysis was used to determine the prevalence of MetS according to the general characteristics and MetS prevalence according to full-time employment. Odds ratios (ORs) were calculated by logistic regression analysis to determine the effects of age, lifestyle, and job-related factors on the prevalence of MetS. All statistical analyses were conducted using SPSS version 22.0 (IBM corp., Armonk, NY, USA). A p value < 0.05 was considered statistically significant. The study protocol was approved by the institutional review board of the Catholic University of Korea, College of Medicine (approval ID: KC18ZESI0410).

3. Results

3.1. General Characteristics of Subjects Included in the Study to Determine Metabolic Syndrome Prevalence

The study subjects were wage workers aged 19 years and older including 5006 men (52.6%), and 4517 women (47.4%), totaling 9523 workers. The prevalence of MetS differed significantly according to age and sex and seemed to increase significantly, for both sexes, with increasing age ($p < 0.001$). However, aside from age, other variables with significant differences in MetS prevalence differed between male and female workers (Table 1).

Table 1. General characteristics of subjects included in the study to determine metabolic syndrome prevalence (N = 9523).

Characteristics	Metabolic Syndrome, N (%)					
	Men (n = 5006)			Women (n = 4517)		
	Yes	No	p	Yes	No	p
Age (years)			<0.001			<0.001
19–29	35 (14.9)	211 (85.1)		14 (5.3)	315 (94.7)	
30–39	288 (21.9)	1038 (78.1)		79 (17.2)	896 (90.9)	
40–49	406 (28.8)	1035 (71.2)		202 (17.2)	1079 (82.8)	
50–59	364 (33.7)	752 (66.3)		322 (28.1)	816 (71.9)	
60–69	196 (29.9)	478 (70.1)		245 (45.0)	300 (55.0)	
≥70	53 (23.9)	160 (76.1)		118 (48.0)	131 (52.0)	
Education level			0.073			<0.001
≤Elementary school	115 (28.0)	331 (72.0)		398 (41.0)	544 (59.0)	
Middle school	147 (32.6)	306 (67.4)		160 (29.2)	368 (70.8)	
High school	461 (26.6)	1212 (73.4)		303 (18.4)	1322 (81.6)	
≥University	619 (25.5)	1815 (74.5)		119 (8.7)	1303 (91.3)	
Job type			0.244			<0.001
Non-manual worker	766 (27.4)	2010 (72.6)		454(15.3)	2388(84.7)	
Manual worker	576 (25.7)	1654 (74.3)		526(29.6)	1149(70.4)	
Marital status			0.019			0.271
Married	1247 (27.3)	3340 (72.7)		736 (19.9)	2810 (80.1)	
Others	95 (21.0)	324 (79.0)		244 (21.8)	727 (78.2)	
Household income level			0.386			<0.001
1st quartile	474 (27.7)	1221 (72.3)		208 (14.9)	1170 (85.1)	
2nd quartile	435 (26.4)	1270 (73.6)		265 (18.8)	1117 (81.2)	
3rd quartile	331 (25.0)	931 (75.0)		285 (22.1)	862 (77.9)	
4th quartile	102 (29.5)	242 (70.5)		222 (34.5)	388 (65.5)	
Smoking			0.003			0.273
Current smoker	596 (29.0)	1524 (71.0)		61 (22.4)	201 (77.6)	
Ex-smoker	516 (25.9)	1394 (74.1)		36 (15.7)	166 (84.3)	
Non-smoker	230 (22.6)	746 (77.4)		883 (20.4)	3170 (79.6)	
Drinking			<0.001			0.882
High risk drinking	365 (34.2)	711 (65.8)		43 (20.2)	170 (79.8)	
Moderate drinking or non-drinking	977 (24.4)	2953 (75.6)		937 (21.7)	3367 (78.3)	
Physical activity			0.261			0.111
Yes	613 (25.8)	1680 (74.2)		336 (21.9)	1151 (78.1)	
No	729 (27.4)	1984 (72.6)		644 (19.5)	2386 (80.5)	

Data were analyzed using Pearson's χ^2 test, $p < 0.05$.

Males showed significant differences in MetS prevalence in lifestyle-related variables such as smoking, drinking, and marital status. Among male subjects, MetS prevalence was significantly higher among current smokers ($p < 0.05$), the high-risk drinking group ($p < 0.001$), and among the married ($p < 0.05$). On the other hand, among female subjects, there were differences in socioeconomic variables. Lower educational level ($p < 0.001$), household income ($p < 0.001$), and manual work ($p < 0.001$) were related to a higher prevalence of MetS.

3.2. Metabolic Syndrome Prevalence According to Sex and by the Standard of Work

Among the male subjects, 3561 (71.1%) were standard workers and 1445 (28.9%) were non-standard workers. The prevalences of MetS among standard and non-standard workers were 26.1% and 28.2%, respectively, and the proportion of non-standard workers was high. However, there was no significant difference between the two groups. Among female subjects, 1962 (43.4%) were standard workers and 2555 (56.4%) were non-standard workers. The prevalences of MetS among the female subjects were 13.5% and 25.8% for standard and non-standard workers, respectively. Non-standard workers showed a statistically significant difference in MetS prevalence compared to standard workers ($p < 0.001$) (Table 2).

Table 2. Metabolic syndrome prevalence according to sex and by the standard of work.

Sex	Employment Type	Metabolic Syndrome, N (%)		Total	p
		Yes	No		
Male	Standard workers	942 (26.4)	2619 (73.6)	3561 (100.0)	0.174
	Non-standard workers	400 (28.2)	1045 (71.8)	1445 (100.0)	
	Total	1342 (26.6)	3664 (73.4)	5006 (100.0)	
Female	Standard workers	271 (13.5)	1691 (86.5)	1962 (100.0)	<0.001
	Non-standard workers	709 (25.8)	1846 (74.2)	2555 (100.0)	
	Total	980 (20.3)	3537 (79.7)	4517 (100.0)	

Data were analyzed using Pearson's χ^2 test, $p < 0.05$.

3.3. Factors Affecting Metabolic Syndrome

To determine the factors affecting MetS, logistic regression analysis was performed. The model consisted of three stages. Models 1, 2, and 3were adjusted for age, lifestyle factors, and factors related to economic activity, respectively. Regression analysis among male subjects showed that non-standard employment status in all models did not increase MetS prevalence. Among female non-standard workers, however, there was a 1.44 times increase in the risk of MetS in model 1 (OR = 1.44, $p < 0.001$), 1.33 times increase in risk in model 2 (OR = 1.33, $p < 0.001$), and 1.34 times increase in the risk in model 3 (OR = 1.34, $p < 0.001$) (Table 3).

Table 3. Prevalence odds ratios of factors affecting metabolic syndrome.

Sex	Model1 *		Model 2 **		Model 3 ***	
	Standard Workers	Non-Standard Workers	Standard Workers	Non-Standard Workers	Standard Workers	Non-Standard Workers
Males	Reference	0.97 (0.82–1.15)	Reference	0.94 (0.78–1.15)	Reference	0.97 (0.78–1.20)
Females	Reference	1.44 (1.18–1.77)	Reference	1.33 (1.07–1.65)	Reference	1.34 (1.07–1.67)

* adjusted for age. ** adjusted for age, smoking, drinking, physical activity, BMI, stress, and depression. *** adjusted for age, smoking, drinking, physical activity, BMI, stress, depression, household income, education level, job type, marital status, and region. BMI, body mass index.

4. Discussion

In recent studies, lifestyle-related factors such as age, unhealthy diet, and sedentary lifestyle, as well as socioeconomic status and environmental factors such as job type, occupational stress, and working hours have been reported as important causes of the increasing MetS prevalence [7,8,21,22]. In this study, we analyzed the differences in MetS prevalence with emphasis on employment type among the socioeconomic factors. As a result, MetS prevalence was shown among non-standard workers to be higher than that among standard workers. In particular, female subjects had a 1.34-fold higher risk of MetS prevalence among non-standard workers than among standard workers. This is consistent with the results of a study in which the risk of hypertension in non-standard female workers was 1.42 times higher than that of standard workers due to employment type and sex differences in cardiovascular health [18]. Hypertension is one of the risk factors for MetS, and might have affected the increased risk of MetS in female non-standard workers. The results of this study showed that female workers were more affected by socioeconomic factors than male workers. Among female workers, the lower the educational and household income levels, the higher the prevalence of MetS. Low educational and household income levels could cause differences in opportunities for workers to access health services and affect health-related behaviors [23,24]. In particular, the lower the socioeconomic status of female workers, the less they care about health care and hence, the higher the risk of MetS [12]. As a result of MetS prevalence according to job type, the prevalence among manual workers was higher than that among non-manual workers [25]. The highest MetS prevalence occurred among female skilled workers in the agricultural and fishing industries. MetS prevalence was higher among low-income and local residents [26,27]. These non-standard workers have low socioeconomic status and are treated poorly in wages, working conditions, and social safety [28]. Non-standard workers have limited working periods, resulting in unstable occupation that reduces perceived health condition, increases psychological stress, and affects physical health [29]. Psychological stress and physical health problems in non-standard workers increase the risk of chronic and acute diseases; furthermore, the social, physiological, and self-rated health of workers become lowered [30]. Finally, the difference in socioeconomic status due to unstable employment is a factor for health deterioration and social determinants of health [1]. Problems associated with low socioeconomic status among these non-standard workers have a greater impact on female workers than male workers, which ultimately increases the prevalence of MetS among female non-standard workers.

On the other hand, male workers showed no differences in economic level, educational level, and job type, and significant differences occurred in MetS prevalence among factors related to lifestyles such as smoking and drinking. Smoking increases the risks of low HDL cholesterol level, higher triglyceride level, and abdominal obesity, thus increasing the prevalence of MetS among male subjects [7]. Excessive drinking increases the risk of low HDL cholesterol level and cohort studies among Korean office workers over the past decade have also identified male sex as a risk factor for MetS [7,11]. Thus, unhealthy lifestyles such as smoking and drinking are closely related to the risk factors for MetS [31]. However, with smoking and drinking adjusted for, the two variables failed to show an increase in the prevalence of MetS among male non-standard workers. In other words, unhealthy lifestyle has a greater impact on MetS prevalence than differences in socioeconomic status. Thus, the inverse correlation between socioeconomic status and MetS in males was confirmed in previous studies [14,25,32]. Among males, non-manual workers with high levels of education and income had the highest risk of MetS, and the higher the socioeconomic status, the higher the risk of MetS [25,32]. In addition, male subjects were less likely to have MetS among workers with higher levels of physical activity [14]. The high prevalence of MetS among office workers is attributed to their long working hours, longer sitting periods, and more exposure to risk factors that can lead to MetS. Moreover, male office workers are known to have more opportunities for drinking [12,27,33–35]. A study of firefighters showed that men tend to enjoy healthier lifestyles with shift work and stressful job conditions, and that this lifestyle resulted in a lower prevalence of

MetS among them than office workers [36]. These results suggest that male workers have higher socioeconomic status than female workers, and that the type of work and their lifestyle are important factors for MetS prevalence. Similar to this study, previous studies have reported sex differences in the risk factors for MetS [11,13,25,37,38]. Hypertension, hyperglycemia, and high triglyceride level were major risk factors for MetS in males, and obesity and low HDL cholesterol level were the most common risk factors for females [13].

There are three possible reasons for the differences in MetS prevalence between male and female non-standard workers, based on previous studies on the difference in risk factors for MetS according to sex. The first is that female non-standard workers are more affected by work-related psychosocial factors due to lower socioeconomic classes. The proportion of non-standard workers among female workers is higher than that of non-standard male workers among male workers. In this study, 28.8% of males and 56.6% of females were classified as standard and non-standard workers from 2010 to 2015. Females often work as administrative support workers rather than managers, and often quit because of marriage, pregnancy, and childcare [11]. In addition, even after re-employment, it is difficult to resume in stable jobs because of the long leave period. For this reason, many females work as non-standard workers, and as temporary or part-time workers. With this low socioeconomic status, female workers are easily exposed to job-related psychological stress and eventually to MetS risk factors [25]. Female non-standard workers show poor mental health status such as high depression and suicidal ideation levels [39]. In addition, the ability to overcome psychological stress was lower than that among men [25,33]. Meta-analysis of the effects of work-related psychosocial factors on MetS revealed significant risk factors for some components associated with MetS such as weight gain, obesity, and hypertension [40].

The second reason is the high risk of obesity in female non-standard workers. Several studies have reported that the risk of obesity in female non-standard workers is higher than that in male non-standard workers [13,37]. Obesity and insulin resistance play a key role in the development of MetS [18,41]. Obesity increases the amount of free fatty acids in the body, which in turn increases insulin resistance, leading to cardiovascular diseases such as diabetes, lipid abnormalities, and hypertension [37]. Ultimately, the high risk of obesity affects the risk of cardiovascular disease and increases the risk of MetS [14].

The third reason is due to the physiological characteristics of female workers. In Korea, about 30% of female workers are mostly pink-collar workers such as nurses, stewardesses, nannies, babysitters, hairdressers, and administrative assistants [13]. These pink-collar workers engage more in shift work, and this results in a 5% higher prevalence of menstrual irregularity than among daily workers [6]. Females with menstrual irregularities are often diagnosed with polycystic ovary syndrome, and such females have a high risk of MetS [6]. However, the increased prevalence of MetS due to these hormonal problems may be due to shift work, which may be difficult to identify among differences in standard and non-standard workers. Nonetheless, the risk of MetS in non-standard workers is higher because they are unable to take immediate action concerning their problems, even if it occurs while doing the same thing [5]. These results suggest that the prevalence of MetS among female non-standard workers was higher than that among standard workers. Psychological problems caused by differences in socioeconomic status increase the risk of MetS in female non-standard workers, and the combination of physiological characteristics of females and that of being a non-standard worker lead to anxiety and consequent poor treatment.

The limitations of this study are as follows: First, the cross-sectional data used in the study may not clearly show a causal relationship between factors. Second, there might be information bias due to the self-reported questionnaire. For example, responses to smoking among female subjects may not be representative. Finally, the definitions of standard and non-standard work varied according to the survey period. In the sixth survey conducted between 2013 and 2015, there was a question to directly confirm standard and non-standard (EC_Wht_0) work, but there was no such question in the fifth survey conducted between 2010 and 2012. Therefore, the two items "job status wage worker (EC_STT_2)" and "working hours (EC_WH)" were defined according to non-standard worker standards. However, international standards for non-standard workers are not clear and there is a limit to how these apply in all countries [18]. Despite these limitations, this sample is representative of the results of the six-year data systematically surveyed in the entire Republic of Korea.

In this study, the prevalence of MetS in female non-standard worker was increased, and it was confirmed that the difference in socioeconomic status according to gender affects MetS prevalence. Thus, a fundamental change in employment patterns will be needed to address health-related problems that arise from non-standard work. The recent policy of converting non-standard work to standard work by the government will be a way to overcome the difference in health risk due to working style. However, there are difficulties in policy promotion due to various interests including current salary level, welfare problem, and reverse discrimination against standard workers. Employment stability and work environment improvement for non-standard workers are not only a matter of interest in payroll improvement but also an important solution to lower the social cost of health care and improve the quality of life and health care of all citizens. It is expected that the results of this study, showing the high risk of MetS in non-standard workers could be utilized as a basis for government policy promotion on health.

5. Conclusions

The results of this study confirm that the prevalence of MetS among non-standard female workers increased according to employment type. In addition, the risk factors leading to increases in the prevalence of MetS differed according to sex. In the future, direct research and long-term observation of psychosocial, lifestyle, and biological factors among non-standard workers will be needed using a cohort study of non-standard workers. It is necessary to clarify the cause of high MetS prevalence among female non-standard workers. In addition, among the factors affecting MetS, it is considered that lifestyle-related problems need to be investigated since these did not result in increased MetS prevalence among male non-standard workers.

Author Contributions: Conceptualization, D.Y.C.; Methodology, D.Y.C.; Formal analysis, D.Y.C., Data Curation, D.Y.C.; Writing—Original Draft preparation, D.Y.C. and J.-W.K.; Writing—Review & Editing, J.-W.K.; Supervision, D.Y.C. All authors have read and approved the submission.

Funding: This research received no external funding.

Acknowledgments: We thank the Korea Centers for Disease Control and Prevention for providing access to the raw data.

Conflicts of Interest: The authors declare no conflict of interest.

References

1. Inoue, M.; Minami, M.; Yano, E. Body mass index, blood pressure, and glucose and lipid metabolism among permanent and fixed-term workers in the manufacturing industry: A cross-sectional study. *BMC Public Health* **2014**, *14*, 207. [CrossRef] [PubMed]
2. Sohn, M.; Choi, M.; Jung, M. Working conditions, psychosocial environmental factors, and depressive symptoms among wage workers in South Korea. *Int. J. Occup. Environ. Health* **2016**, *22*, 209–217. [CrossRef] [PubMed]
3. Park, J.; Park, J.S.; Han, B.; Kim, Y. Vulnerability of employees in businesses with fewer than five workers (micro-enterprises) to occupational safety and health problems. *Am. J. Ind. Med.* **2017**, *60*, 1056–1065. [CrossRef] [PubMed]
4. Alali, H.; Braeckman, L.; Van Hecke, T.; De Clercq, B.; Janssens, H.; Wahab, M.A. Relationship between non-standard work arrangements and work-related accident absence in Belgium. *J. Occup. Health* **2017**, *59*, 177–186. [CrossRef] [PubMed]
5. Ray, T.K.; Kenigsberg, T.A.; Pana-Cryan, R. Employment arrangement, job stress, and health-related quality of life. *Saf. Sci.* **2017**, *100*, 46–56. [CrossRef] [PubMed]

6. Yu, J. Relationship between long working hours and metabolic syndrome among Korean workers. *Asian Nurs. Res. (Korean Soc. Nurs. Sci.)* **2017**, *11*, 36–41. [CrossRef] [PubMed]
7. Huang, J.H.; Li, R.H.; Huang, S.L.; Sia, H.K.; Chen, Y.L.; Tang, F.C. Lifestyle factors and metabolic syndrome among workers: The role of interactions between smoking and alcohol to nutrition and exercise. *Int. J. Environ. Res. Public Health* **2015**, *12*, 15967–15978. [CrossRef] [PubMed]
8. Mehrdad, R.; Pouryaghoub, G.; Moradi, M. Associationbetween metabolic syndrome and job rank. *Int. J. Occup. Environ. Med.* **2018**, *9*, 45–51. [CrossRef] [PubMed]
9. Oh, J.I.; Yim, H.W. Association between rotating night shift work and metabolic syndrome in Korean workers: Differences between 8-hour and 12-hour rotating shift work. *Ind. Health* **2018**, *56*, 40–48. [CrossRef] [PubMed]
10. Browne, R.A.V.; Farias-Junior, L.F.; Freire, Y.A.; Schwade, D.; Macêdo, G.A.D.; Montenegro, V.B.; Lopes, T.J.A.; Dantas, F.F.O.; Costa, E.C. Sedentary occupation workers who meet the physical activity recommendations have a reduced risk for metabolic syndrome: A cross-sectional study. *J. Occup. Environ. Med.* **2017**, *59*, 1029–1033. [CrossRef] [PubMed]
11. Ryu, H.; Kim, Y.; Lee, J.; Yoon, S.J.; Cho, J.H.; Wong, E.; Jung, J. Office workers' risk of metabolic syndrome-related indicators: A 10-year cohort study. *West. J. Nurs. Res.* **2016**, *38*, 1433–1447. [CrossRef] [PubMed]
12. Myong, J.P.; Kim, H.R.; Jung-Choi, K.; Baker, D.; Choi, B. Disparities of metabolic syndrome prevalence by age, gender and occupation among Korean adult workers. *Ind. Health* **2012**, *50*, 115–122. [CrossRef] [PubMed]
13. Lee, W.; Yeom, H.; Yoon, J.H.; Won, J.U.; Jung, P.K.; Lee, J.H.; Seok, H.; Roh, J. Metabolic outcomes of workers according to the international standard classification of occupations in Korea. *Am. J. Ind. Med.* **2016**, *59*, 685–694. [CrossRef] [PubMed]
14. Do, K.-A.; Jung, H.-S.; Chio, E.-H. Association between job-related factors and metabolic syndrome among male and female workers: Using the Korean national health and nutrition examination survey. *Korean J. Occup. Health Nurs.* **2015**, *24*, 39–47. [CrossRef]
15. Grundy, S.M.; Cleeman, J.I.; Merz, C.N.; Brewer, H.B.; Clark, L.T.; Hunninghake, D.B.; Pasternak, R.C.; Smith, S.C.; Stone, N.J. National Heart, Lung, and Blood Institute; American College of Cardiology Foundation; American Heart Association. Implications of recent clinical trials for the National Cholesterol Education Program Adult Treatment Panel III guidelines. *Circulation* **2004**, *110*, 227–239. [CrossRef] [PubMed]
16. Korea National Statistical Office. Glossary of Statistical Terminology 2006. Available online: http://lib1.kostat.go.kr/search/media/img/CAT000000054081?metsno=000000004259&fileid=M000000004259_FILE000002 (accessed on 1 May 2014).
17. Korea National Statistical Office. *Annual Report on the Economically Active Population in Korea*; Statistics Korea: Daejeon, Korea, 2004.
18. Seon, J.J.; Lim, Y.J.; Lee, H.W.; Yoon, J.M.; Kim, S.J.; Choi, S.; Kawachi, I.; Park, S.M. Cardiovascular health status between standard and nonstandard workers in Korea. *PLoS ONE* **2017**, *12*, e0178395. [CrossRef] [PubMed]
19. Korea National Statistical Office. *Korea Standard Classification of Occupations*; Statistics Korea: Daejeon, Korea, 2007.
20. Korea Centers for Disease Control & Prevention National Health Information Portal 2016. Available online: http://health.cdc.go.kr/health/HealthInfoArea/HealthInfo/View.do?idx=3700&subIdx=4&searchCate=&searchType=&searchKey=&pageNo=&category=&category_code=&dept=&sortType=&page=&searchField=&searchWord (accessed on 13 April 2018).
21. Sarebanhassanabadi, M.; Mirhosseini, S.J.; Mirzaei, M.; Namayandeh, S.M.; Soltani, M.H.; Pakseresht, M.; Pedarzadeh, A.; Baramesipour, Z.; Faraji, R.; Salehi-Abargouei, A. Effect of dietary habits on the risk of metabolic syndrome: Yazd healthy heart project. *Public Health Nutr.* **2018**, *21*, 1139–1146. [CrossRef] [PubMed]
22. Huang, J.H.; Li, R.H.; Huang, S.L.; Sia, H.K.; Lee, S.S.; Wang, W.H.; Tang, F.C. Relationships between different types of physical activity and metabolic syndrome among Taiwanese workers. *Sci. Rep.* **2017**, *7*, 13735. [CrossRef] [PubMed]
23. Zuo, H.; Shi, Z.; Hu, X.; Wu, M.; Guo, Z.; Hussain, A. Prevalence of metabolic syndrome and factors associated with its components in Chinese adults. *Metabolism* **2009**, *58*, 1102–1108. [CrossRef] [PubMed]

24. Park, M.J.; Yun, K.E.; Lee, G.E.; Cho, H.J.; Park, H.S. A cross-sectional study of socioeconomic status and the metabolic syndrome in Korean adults. *Ann. Epidemiol.* **2007**, *17*, 320–326. [CrossRef] [PubMed]
25. Ryu, J.Y.; Hong, S.; Kim, C.H.; Lee, S.; Kim, J.H.; Lee, J.T.; Kim, D.H. Prevalence of the Metabolic Syndrome among Korean Workers by Occupational Group: Fifth Korean National Health and Nutrition Examination Survey (KNHANES) 2010. *Ann. Occup. Environ. Med.* **2013**, *25*, 13. [CrossRef] [PubMed]
26. Shariff, Z.M.; Sulaiman, N.; Jalil, R.A.; Yen, W.C.; Yaw, Y.H.; Taib, M.N.; Kandiah, M.; Lin, K.G. Food insecurity and the metabolic syndrome among women from low income communities in Malaysia. *Asia Pac. J. Clin. Nutr.* **2014**, *23*, 138–147. [CrossRef] [PubMed]
27. Sánchez-Chaparro, M.A.; Calvo-Bonacho, E.; González-Quintela, A.; Fernández-Labandera, C.; Cabrera, M.; Sáinz, J.C.; Fernández-Meseguer, A.; Banegas, J.R.; Ruilope, L.M.; Valdivielso, P.; et al. Occupation-related differences in the prevalence of metabolic syndrome. *Diabetes Care* **2008**, *31*, 1884–1885. [CrossRef] [PubMed]
28. Cho, J.; Lee, J. Persistence of the gender gap and low employment of female workers in a stratified labor market: Evidence from South Korea. *Sustainability* **2015**, *7*, 12425–12451. [CrossRef]
29. Minelli, L.; Pigini, C.; Chiavarini, M.; Bartolucci, F. Employment status and perceived health condition: Longitudinal data from Italy. *BMC Public Health* **2014**, *14*, 946. [CrossRef] [PubMed]
30. Kang, S.H.; Song, J.H.; Koh, T.H.; Paek, D.M.; Park, J.T.; Chun, H. What causes the experience of discrimination in non-regular workers? *Ann. Occup. Environ. Med.* **2017**, *29*, 35. [CrossRef] [PubMed]
31. Tauler, P.; Bennasar-Veny, M.; Morales-Asencio, J.M.; Lopez-Gonzalez, A.A.; Vicente-Herrero, T.; De Pedro-Gomez, J.; Royo, V.; Pericas-Beltran, J.; Aguilo, A. Prevalence of premorbid metabolic syndrome in Spanish adult workers using IDF and ATPIII diagnostic criteria: Relationship with cardiovascular risk factors. *PLoS ONE* **2014**, *9*, e89281. [CrossRef] [PubMed]
32. Park, S.J.; Kang, H.T.; Nam, C.M.; Park, B.J.; Linton, J.A.; Lee, Y.J. Sex differences in the relationship between socioeconomic status and metabolic syndrome: The Korean National Health and Nutrition Examination Survey. *Diabetes Res. Clin. Pract.* **2012**, *96*, 400–406. [CrossRef] [PubMed]
33. Yamaoka, K.; Tango, T. Effects of lifestyle modification on metabolic syndrome: A systematic review and meta-analysis. *BMC Med.* **2012**, *10*, 138. [CrossRef] [PubMed]
34. Chandola, T.; Brunner, E.; Marmot, M. Chronic stress at work and the metabolic syndrome: Prospective study. *BMJ* **2006**, *332*, 521–525. [CrossRef] [PubMed]
35. Burton, N.W.; Turrell, G. Occupation, hours worked, and leisure-time physical activity. *Prev. Med.* **2000**, *31*, 673–681. [CrossRef] [PubMed]
36. Strauß, M.; Foshag, P.; Przybylek, B.; Horlitz, M.; Lucia, A.; Sanchis-Gomar, F.; Leischik, R. Occupation and metabolic syndrome: Is there correlation? A cross sectional study in different work activity occupations of German firefighters and office workers. *Diabetol. Metab. Syndr.* **2016**, *8*, 57. [CrossRef] [PubMed]
37. Lim, K.G.; Cheah, W.K. A review of metabolic syndrome research in Malaysia. *Med. J. Malay.* **2016**, *71*, 20–28.
38. Adeoye, A.M.; Adewoye, I.A.; Dairo, D.M.; Adebiyi, A.; Lackland, D.T.; Ogedegbe, G.; Tayo, B.O. Excess metabolic syndrome risks among women health workers compared with men. *J. Clin. Hypertens. (Greenwich)* **2015**, *17*, 880–884. [CrossRef] [PubMed]
39. Kim, I.H.; Muntaner, C.; Khang, Y.H.; Paek, D.; Cho, S.I. The relationship between nonstandard working and mental health in a representative sample of the South Korean population. *Soc. Sci. Med.* **2006**, *63*, 556–574. [CrossRef] [PubMed]
40. Sakuraya, A.; Watanabe, K.; Kawakami, N.; Imamura, K.; Ando, E.; Asai, Y.; Eguchi, H.; Kobayashi, Y.; Nishida, N.; Arima, H.; et al. Work-related psychosocial factors and onset of metabolic syndrome among workers: A systematic review and meta-analysis protocol. *BMJ Open* **2017**, *7*, e016716. [CrossRef] [PubMed]
41. Ford, E.S. Risks for all-cause mortality, cardiovascular disease, and diabetes associated with the metabolic syndrome: A summary of the evidence. *Diabetes Care* **2005**, *28*, 1769–1778. [CrossRef] [PubMed]

International Journal of
Environmental Research and Public Health

MDPI

Article

Relationships of Lower Lung Fibrosis, Pleural Disease, and Lung Mass with Occupational, Household, Neighborhood, and Slate Roof-Dense Area Residential Asbestos Exposure

Dongmug Kang [1,2], Yu-Young Kim [3], Minseung Shin [3], Min-Su Lee [3], Hee-Joo Bae [3], Se-Yeong Kim [2] and Young-Ki Kim [1,2,4,*]

1 Preventive, Occupational and Environmental Medicine, School of Medicine, Pusan National University, Yangsan 50612, Korea; kangdm@pusan.ac.kr
2 Occupational and Environmental Medicine, Pusan National University Yangsan Hospital, Yangsan 50612, Korea; 30white@hanmail.net
3 Premedical College, Pusan National University, Yangsan 50612, Korea; yyofficial96@naver.com (Y.-Y.K.); tls0264@naver.com (M.S.); leeguduk45@naver.com (M.-S.L.); heejoo700@hanmail.net (H.-J.B.)
4 Environmental Health Center for Asbestos, Pusan National University Yangsan Hospital, Yangsan 50612, Korea
* Correspondence: mungis@pusan.ac.kr; Tel.: +82-55-360-1281

Received: 26 June 2018; Accepted: 30 July 2018; Published: 2 August 2018

Abstract: This study aimed to evaluate the relationship between various asbestos exposure routes and asbestos-related disorders (ARDs). The study population comprised 11,186 residents of a metropolitan city who lived near asbestos factories, shipyards, or in slate roof-dense areas. ARDs were determined from chest X-rays indicating lower lung fibrosis (LFF), pleural disease (PD), and lung masses (LMs). Of the subjects, 11.2%, 10.4%, 67.2% and 8.3% were exposed to asbestos via occupational, household, neighborhood, and slate roof routes, respectively. The odds ratio (OR) of PD from household exposure (i.e., living with asbestos-producing workers) was 1.9 (95% confidence interval: 0.9–4.2), and those of LLF and PD from neighborhood exposure, or residing near asbestos factories) for <19 or >20 years, or near a mine, were 4.1 (2.8–5.8) and 4.8 (3.4–6.7), 8.3 (5.5–12.3) and 8.0 (5.5–11.6), and 4.8 (2.7–8.5) and 9.0 (5.6–14.4), respectively. The ORs of LLF, PD, and LM among those residing in slate-dense areas were 5.5 (3.3–9.0), 8.8 (5.6–13.8), and 20.5 (10.4–40.4), respectively. Substantial proportions of citizens residing in industrialized cities have potentially been exposed to asbestos, and various exposure routes are associated with the development of ARDs. Given the limitations of this study, including potential confounders such as socioeconomic status, further research is needed.

Keywords: asbestos; domestic; environmental; health impact survey; household; Korea; neighbor; roof; slate

1. Introduction

Asbestos, which is composed of long, thin fibers, has been used widely for decades because of its properties such as resistance to fire, heat, and electricity; tensile strength; and sound absorption. However, asbestos exposure can cause asbestos-related diseases (ARDs) such as malignant cancers, including lung cancer (LC), malignant mesothelioma (MM), laryngeal cancer, and ovarian cancer, as well as benign diseases such as asbestosis, pleural plaques, and pleural thickening [1]. Asbestos exposure via occupational, household, and neighborhood routes was reported as early as 1960 [2–4]. Occupational asbestos exposure occurs through the production of asbestos-containing products in settings such as mines and asbestos textile factories, or in workplaces that handle asbestos products, including shipyards and construction sites. Household exposure occurs when families exposed to asbestos at work come to their homes with work clothes. Neighborhood exposure occurs when living near to asbestos mines, asbestos factories, and shipyards. Although many studies have explored the extent of occupational exposure, including the associated disease burden [5,6], studies of household and neighborhood exposure to asbestos among ordinary citizens are rare. The majority of these studies indicate that ARDs consequent to household and neighborhood asbestos exposure are confined to MM [1,7]. However, most such studies did not control for other exposure routes, despite the possibility of overlap [1,2,7].

One exposure route that may be encountered during ordinary life is the asbestos slate roof, which is composed of 10–15% asbestos [8]. Asbestos slate has been widely used in western societies [9], and its use is increasing in developing countries [10]. In Korea, slate was widely used to replace roofing materials in rural areas during the period of rapid economic growth during the 1970s and 1980s, and was commonly used in poor urban areas [8]. However, few studies have addressed the health effects of living under or near slate roofs [8], even though the surrounding asbestos concentration in ambient air might be substantial [11].

In 2009, the Korean government banned asbestos. In 2011, the government began to compensate citizens for environmental asbestos diseases, and environmental health centers for asbestos (EHCA) began to conduct health impact surveys (HISs) of areas containing asbestos mines, factories, ship-building facilities, and large numbers of slate roofs [12,13]. Although HISs are based on the voluntary participation of citizens living near former sources of asbestos exposure, the responses elucidate the frequency of exposure and risks of occupational, household, and slate exposure among ordinary citizens.

The present study investigated the frequency of asbestos exposure via the occupational, household, neighborhood, and slate roof routes, and studied the relationships between these exposure routes and ARDs using HIS data of EHCA adjusted for other routes.

2. Materials and Methods

2.1. Study Subjects

The study subjects comprised participants in a HIS conducted by Pusan National University Yangsan Hospital (PNUYH) EHCA between 2009 and 2016. The majority of the participants currently reside in the Busan metropolitan area, which serves as the center of one of the most industrialized areas of Korea and traditionally housed many environmental asbestos exposure sources, such as asbestos textile factories and shipbuilding and ship repair industries [13]. For this study, the subjects were restricted to current citizens of Busan. Participants younger than 20 years were excluded to account for the long latency period of ARDs (median: 20 years) [14]. Accordingly, 2053 of the 13,433 PNUYH-EHCA HIS participants were excluded based on these criteria. After excluding an additional 194 cases because of incomplete questionnaire responses or chest radiography results, the final study comprised 11,186 subjects. The institutional review board of PNUYH approved this study (02-2009-037, 02-2012-018).

2.2. HIS Items: Questionnaire and Chest Radiograph

A structured questionnaire survey was administered by trained personnel through individual interviews during which informed consent was obtained from the subjects. Asbestos exposure was assessed qualitatively by the questionnaire. To determine occupational and household exposure, the subjects were asked whether they or someone in their household was exposed to structured asbestos-related work items during employment. To determine neighborhood exposure, the subject's life residential history was taken and verified using official residential records. Additionally, the subject's history of living under a slate roof was taken and compared to slate-dense areas predetermined by a previous study [13]. No exposure was defined as no exposure to occupational, household, or neighborhood sources, living under a slate roof, or living in slate-dense areas.

Posteroanterior chest radiography was performed using an FCR 5501 digital radiograph device (Fuji, Tokyo, Japan). Radiographs were read by two separate radiologists who had participated in a special reading session for ARDs provided by a Korean environmental corporation. The reading results were divided into three groups of ARDs: of asbestosis, pleural disease (PD), and LC. The reading results were categorized as follows: lower lung fibrosis (LLF) (asbestosis surrogate): asbestosis, diffuse lung disease, interstitial lung disease, nodular ground glass appearance; PD: pleural plaque, pleural thickening, loss of costo-phrenic angle; and LC: suspected malignancy, mass >1 cm, mediastinal enlargement. Any case of PD with a tuberculous history or reading opinion suggesting tuberculosis was excluded. Only screening results were analyzed in this study because the participation rates in secondary examinations to address abnormal screening results were low (4.6%) and not representative [14].

2.3. Data Analysis

The X^2-test and Fisher's exact test were used to conduct frequency analyses, and trends were assessed using the Cochran–Armitage trend test. Classes containing small numbers were merged into adjacent classes. Logistic regressions were conducted using the three radiography outcomes (LLF, PD, and LM) as the dependent variable. Simple, multiple (adjusted for sex, age, and smoking as confounders) [3,15], and full model logistic regressions (adjusted for other exposure routes and confounders) were conducted. The statistical analysis was performed using SAS, version 9.4 (SAS Institute, Cary, NC, USA).

3. Results

3.1. Prevalence Rates of LLF, PD, and LM by Subject Characteristics and Exposre

In our study, 120 (1.9%) and 211 (3.4%) cases of LLF and PD, respectively, were observed among women, with 264 (5.3%) and 295 (5.9%) cases, respectively, among men (p-values for sex-based comparisons < 0.0001). Furthermore, 61 (1.0%) and 45 (0.9%) cases of LM were observed among women and men, respectively (p-value for comparison = 0.6063). Most patients were between 50 and 79 years of age, and the proportions of LLF, PD, and LM differed by age (p-values for comparisons <0.0001). Compared to present and never smokers, ex-smokers were more likely to present with LLF and PD (p-value < 0.0001). Of the single exposure routes, neighborhood exposure was most frequent (53.3%), followed by slate roof (5.4%), occupational (3.4%), and household (2.4%) exposure. The total proportions of neighborhood, slate roof, occupational, and household exposure were 67.2%, 8.3%, 11.2%, and 10.4% respectively. Among subjects exposed to slate roofs, 2.7% lived in slate-roof-dense areas (data not shown).

The prevalence of LLF was highest among subjects exposed to all four sources (16.7%) followed by those exposed to occupational + neighbor + slate (13.0%) and occupational + neighbor (12.5%). Similarly, the prevalence of PD was highest among subjects exposed to all four sources (27.8%), followed by occupational + household + slate (25.0%). The prevalence of LM was highest among those exposed to slate roofs (4.2%), followed by occupational + slate (3.9%) (Table 1).

Table 1. Prevalence and rates of radiological abnormalities by characteristics and exposure routes.

Variable	LLF			PD			LM			Subjects Total	
	Case	Rate	p-Value	Case	Rate	p-Value	Case	Rate	p-Value	No.	%
Sex			<0.0001			<0.0001			0.6063		
Female	120	1.9		211	3.4		61	1		6160	55.1
Male	264	5.3		295	5.9		45	0.9		5026	44.9
Age (years)			<0.0001			<0.0001			<0.0001		
≤29	0	0		9	1		1	0.1		943	8.4
30–39	6	0.2		25	0.9		7	0.3		2777	24.8
40–49	2	0.2		15	1.8		3	0.4		848	7.6
50–59	44	2.1		88	4.3		12	0.6		2064	18.5
60–69	132	5		165	6.2		34	1.3		2643	23.6
≥70	200	10.5		204	10.7		49	2.6		1911	17.1
Smoking status			<0.0001			<0.0001			0.7679		
Never	156	2.1		268	3.7		66	0.9		7302	65.3
Ex-smoker	140	6.6		154	7.2		21	1		2131	19.1
Present smoker	88	5		84	4.8		19	1.1		1753	15.7
Exposure routes			<0.0001			<0.0001			<0.0001		
No exposure	11	0.5		10	0.5		7	0.4		2022	18.1
Occupational	9	2.4		8	2.1		1	0.3		378	3.4
Household	1	0.4		1	0.4		0	0.0		274	2.4
Neighbor	204	3.4		286	4.8		50	0.8		5960	53.3
Slate	30	5.0		42	7.0		25	4.2		599	5.4
Occupational + Household	2	3.1		0	0.0		0	0.0		65	0.6
Occupational + Neighbor	69	12.5		58	10.5		6	1.1		553	4.9
Occupational + Slate	4	7.8		6	11.8		2	3.9		51	0.5
Household + Neighbor	12	2.1		18	3.1		1	0.2		580	5.2
Household + Slate	2	4.0		4	8.0		0	0.0		50	0.4
Neighbor + Slate	19	4.6		47	11.5		10	2.4		410	3.7
Occupational + Household + Neighbor	10	7.9		8	6.4		3	2.4		126	1.1
Occupational + Household + Slate	0	0.0		3	25.0		0	0.0		12	0.1
Occupational + Neighbor + Slate	7	13.0		7	13.0		1	1.9		54	0.5
Household + Neighbor + Slate	1	2.9		3	8.8		0	0.0		34	0.3
Occupational + Household + Neighbor + Slate	3	16.7		5	27.8		0	0.0		18	0.2
Total	384	3.4		506	4.5		106	0.9		11,186	100.0 *

LLF: lower lung fibrosis, PD: pleural disease, LM: lung mass, * total percent.

3.2. Occupational and Household Exposures and Radiologic Abnormalities

A total of 1257 (11.2%) subjects were occupationally exposed to asbestos (data not shown). Among them, 104 (8.3%), 95 (7.6%), and 13 (1.0%) developed LLF, PD, and LM, respectively. The highest prevalence of LLF was observed among asbestos miners (21.4%), asbestos cement manufacturers (14.3%), and asbestos textile workers (11.9%) ($p < 0.0001$). The highest prevalence of PD was also observed among asbestos miners (17.9%), followed by asbestos friction material and joint sheet manufacturers (17.2%), and asbestos textile workers (11.9%) ($p < 0.0001$). By contrast, few subjects with occupational exposure developed LM, and no differences among occupations were observed ($p = 0.3889$). Differences in the prevalence of LLF and PD were also observed according to the duration of work ($p < 0.0001$ and $p < 0.0001$, respectively).

A total of 1159 (10.4%) subjects were exposed to asbestos by other household members with asbestos-related occupations (data not shown), and 31 (2.7%), 42 (3.6%), and 4 (0.3%) developed LLF, PD, and LM, respectively. Among the occupations of household members, the highest prevalence of LLF was associated with asbestos textile work (14.2%), followed by asbestos cement production (4.5%), and the highest prevalence of PD was associated with asbestos textile work (23.8%), and asbestos friction material and joint sheet manufacturing (8.3%) (Table 2).

Table 2. Prevalence and rates of radiological abnormalities among cases of occupational and household exposure by job type and exposure duration.

Variable		Occupational Exposure n (%)			Household Exposure n (%)		
		LLF	PD	LM	LLF	PD	LM
Occupation type	No exposure	280 (2.8)	411 (4.1)	93 (0.9)	353 (3.5)	464 (4.6)	102 (1.0)
Production	Mine	6 (21.4)	5 (17.9)	0 (0.0)	0 (0.0)	1 (4.4)	0 (0.0)
	Cement	4 (14.3)	1 (3.6)	1 (3.6)	1 (4.6)	1 (4.6)	0 (0.0)
	Friction, joint sheet	2 (6.9)	5 (17.2)	0 (0.0)	0 (0)	2 (8.3)	0 (0.0)
	Textile	5 (11.9)	5 (11.9)	2 (4.8)	3 (14.3)	5 (23.8)	1 (4.8)
Use	Construction	23 (9.9)	17 (7.3)	2 (0.9)	2 (1.3)	2 (1.3)	0 (0.0)
	Chemical, power plant	4 (5.6)	5 (6.9)	0 (0.0)	5 (4.0)	9 (7.2)	1 (0.8)
	Plumbing, insulation	7 (5.6)	11 (8.7)	1 (0.8)	0 (0.0)	8 (6.0)	0 (0.0)
	Automobile, train repair	2 (5.7)	3 (8.6)	0 (0.0)	1 (2.9)	2 (5.7)	1 (2.9)
	Shipbuilding, ship repair	37 (9.1)	27 (6.6)	5 (1.2)	8 (2.1)	7 (2.0)	1 (0.3)
	Others	14 (5.5)	16 (6.3)	2 (0.8)	11 (4.5)	5 (2.1)	0 (0.0)
	p-value (Fisher's exact)	<0.0001	<0.0001	0.3889	<0.0001	<0.0001	0.236
Duration	No exposure	280 (2.8)	411 (4.1)	93 (0.9)	353 (3.5)	464 (4.6)	102 (1.0)
	≤4 years	25 (5.7)	24 (5.4)	3 (0.7)	16 (2.4)	22 (3.3)	2 (0.3)
	5–9 years	15 (8.2)	18 (9.9)	3 (1.7)	1 (1.0)	4 (4.1)	1 (1.0)
	10–19 years	13 (5.7)	14 (6.1)	2 (0.9)	7 (5.3)	6 (4.5)	0 (0.0)
	≥20 years	51 (12.6)	39 (9.7)	5 (1.2)	7 (2.8)	10 (4.0)	1 (0.4)
	p-value (X^2 test)	<0.0001	<0.0001	0.7942	0.2052	0.5580	0.2244

LLF: lower lung fibrosis, PD: pleural disease, LM: lung mass

3.3. Neighborhood and Slate Roof Exposure and Slate Root-Dense Areas

A total of 7515 (67.2%) and 220 (2.0%) cases of neighborhood exposure from local asbestos factories and mines, respectively, were reported (data not shown). The prevalence of LLF, PD, and LM consequent to exposure to mines and factories were 302 (4.0%), 390 (5.2%), and 68 cases (0.9%) and 23 (10.5%), 42 (19.1%), and 3 cases (1.4%), respectively (p-value < 0.0001, p-value < 0.0001, and p-value = 0.6994, respectively).

Overall, 929 (8.3%) and 299 (2.7%) cases of slate roof exposure and residence in slate roof-dense areas were reported, respectively (data not shown). The prevalence of LLF, PD, and LM associated with slate roof exposure and residence in a slate roof-dense area were 35 (3.8%), 75 (8.1%), and 8 (0.9%); 390 (5.2%), and 68 (0.9%); and 31 (10.4%), 42 (14.0%), and 30 (10.0%), respectively (p-value < 0.0001). Differences in radiological abnormalities were observed with regard to the durations of neighborhood and slate roof exposure (p-value < 0.0001) (Table 3).

Table 3. Prevalence and rates of radiological abnormalities among cases of neighborhood, slate roof, and slate roof-dense area exposure and exposure durations.

Variable		Neighborhood Exposure			Slate Roof and Slate Roof-Dense Area		
		LLF	PD	LM	LLF	PD	LM
Exposure type	No exposure	59 (1.7)	74 (2.1)	35 (1.0)	318 (3.2)	389 (3.9)	68 (0.7)
	Category1 *	302 (4.0)	390 (5.2)	68 (0.9)	35 (3.8)	75 (8.1)	8 (0.9)
	Category2 **	23 (10.5)	42 (19.1)	3 (1.4)	31 (10.4)	42 (14.0)	30 (10.0)
	p-value	<0.0001	<0.0001	0.6994	<0.0001	<0.0001	<0.0001
Duration	No exposure	59 (1.7)	74 (2.1)	35 (1.0)	318 (3.2)	389 (3.9)	68 (0.7)
	<4 years	30 (1.3)	55 (2.5)	14 (0.6)	3 (2.2)	11 (8.0)	1 (0.7)
	5–9 years	41 (1.9)	80 (3.7)	5 (0.2)	8 (5.4)	12 (8.1)	3 (2.0)
	10–19 years	157 (6.5)	194 (8.0)	30 (1.2)	10 (5.0)	17 (8.5)	3 (1.5)
	≥20 years	97 (10.6)	103 (11.2)	22 (2.4)	45 (6.0)	77 (10.4)	31 (4.2)
	p-value	<0.0001	<0.0001	<0.0001	0.0003	<0.0001	<0.0001

LLF: lower lung fibrosis, PD: pleural disease, LM: lung mass. * Factory (Neighborhood exposure), Slate roof (Slate roof and slate roof-dense area). ** Mine (Neighborhood exposure), Slate roof in slate roof dense area (Slate roof and slate roof-dense area).

3.4. Trends in Combined Variables of Exposure Routes and Durations

Occupational, household, neighborhood, and slate roof exposures were classified as use vs. production, use vs. production, factory vs. mine, and slate roof only vs. slate roof in slate roof-dense area, respectively. Subsequently, the two categories for occupational, neighbor, and slate roof exposure were combined with durations of <20 vs. >20 years; the cut-off for household exposure duration was 5 years because many subjects did not reside with household members for as long as 20 years. The increasing trends in LLF differed among the categories for all exposure routes except household exposure (p-value < 0.0001). The trends in PD differed among the categories in all exposure routes and increased for all routes except household exposure. The trends in LM differed by categories for all exposure routes except household exposure, and increased with slate roof exposure (Table 4).

Table 4. Trend tests of combined exposure source and duration variables and chest radiographic abnormalities.

Type	Type and Duration (Year)	LLF *n* (%)		PD *n* (%)		LM *n* (%)	
		No	Yes	No	Yes	No	Yes
Occupational	No exposure	9649 (97.2)	280 (2.8)	9518 (95.9)	411 (4.1)	9836 (99.1)	93 (0.9)
	Use & ≤19 years	698 (94.7)	39 (5.3)	694 (94.2)	43 (5.8)	732 (99.3)	5 (0.7)
	Use & ≥20 years	345 (87.8)	48 (12.2)	357 (90.8)	36 (9.2)	388 (98.7)	5 (1.3)
	Production & ≤19 years	102 (87.9)	14 (12.1)	103 (88.8)	13 (11.2)	113 (97.4)	3 (2.6)
	Production & ≥20 years	8 (72.7)	3 (27.3)	8 (72.7)	3 (27.3)	11 (100.0)	0 (0.0)
p-value	χ^2	<0.0001		<0.0001		0.0013	
	Trend test	<0.0001		<0.0001		0.1428	
Household	No exposure	9674 (96.5)	353 (3.5)	9563 (95.4)	464 (4.6)	9925 (99.0)	102 (1.0)
	Use & ≤4 years	598 (97.7)	14 (2.3)	596 (97.4)	16 (2.6)	611 (99.8)	1 (0.2)
	Use & ≥5 years	444 (97.2)	13 (2.8)	440 (96.3)	17 (3.7)	455 (99.6)	2 (0.4)
	Production & ≤4 years	62 (96.9)	2 (3.1)	58 (90.6)	6 (9.4)	63 (98.4)	1 (1.6)
	Production & ≥5 years	249 (92.3)	2 (7.7)	23 (88.5)	3 (11.5)	26 (100.0)	0 (0.0)
p-value	χ^2	0.3341		0.0137		0.1778	
	Trend test	0.2009		0.4177		0.0876	
Neighbor	No exposure	3392 (98.3)	59 (1.7)	3377 (97.9)	74 (2.1)	3416 (99.0)	35 (1.0)
	Factory & ≤19 years	6399 (96.9)	205 (3.1)	6314 (95.6)	290 (4.4)	6558 (99.3)	46 (0.7)
	Factory & ≥20 years	814 (89.4)	97 (10.7)	811 (89)	100 (11.0)	889 (97.6)	22 (2.4)
	Mine & ≤19 years	192 (89.3)	23 (10.7)	176 (81.9)	39 (18.1)	212 (98.6)	3 (1.4)
	Mine & ≥20 years	5 (100.0)	0 (0.0)	2 (40.0)	3 (60.0)	5 (100.0)	0 (0.0)
p-value	χ^2	<0.0001		<0.0001		<0.0001	
	Trend test	<0.0001		<0.0001		0.7600	
Slate roof	No exposure	9640 (96.8)	318 (3.2)	9569 (96.1)	389 (3.9)	9890 (99.3)	68 (0.7)
	Roof & ≤19 years	427 (96.6)	15 (3.4)	408 (92.3)	34 (7.7)	438 (99.1)	4 (0.9)
	Roof & ≥20 years	467 (95.9)	20 (4.1)	446 (91.6)	41 (8.4)	483 (99.2)	4 (0.8)
	Roof in dense area & ≤19 years	39 (86.7)	6 (13.3)	39 (86.7)	6 (13.3)	42 (93.3)	3 (6.7)
	Roof in dense area & ≥20 years	229 (90.2)	25 (9.8)	218 (85.8)	36 (14.2)	227 (89.4)	27 (10.6)
p-value	χ^2	<0.0001		<0.0001		<0.0001	
	Trend test	<0.0001		<0.0001		<0.0001	

LLF: lower lung fibrosis, PD: pleural disease, LM: lung mass.

3.5. Logistic Regression Analysis

Given the small numbers of subjects in some categories, such as occupational exposure via production >20 years, household exposure via production <4 years, neighborhood mine exposure >20 years, and slate roof exposure in a dense area <19 years, these categories were merged with adjacent categories in the logistic regression analysis. The odds ratios (OR) of LLF following occupational exposure were increased in the categories of asbestos use >20 years and asbestos production. The ORs of LLF following neighborhood exposure were increased in all categories and in all models. However, for slate roof exposure, the OR of LLF was increased only in slate roof-dense areas.

The ORs of PD related to occupational exposure were similar to the ORs of LLF. The ORs were increased in the categories of asbestos use >20 years and asbestos production. However, the OR of PD following household exposure was increased only in the category of production. The ORs for

PD following neighborhood exposure and slate roof exposure were increased in all categories and in all models. Regarding LM, the OR following neighborhood exposure was increased in the category of factory exposure >20 years in all models, and factory exposure <19 years only in the full model. The ORs of LLF, PD, and LM in two categories, neighborhood factory exposure >20 years and slate roof exposure in a slate roof-dense area, were increased in all models (Table 5).

Table 5. Logistic regression of radiologic abnormalities by exposure route.

Variable	LLF									PD									LM								
	Simple			Multiple *			Full **			Simple			Multiple			Full			Simple			Multiple			Full		
	OR	95%CI		OR	95%CI		OR	95%CI		OR	95%CI		OR	95%CI		OR	95%CI		OR	95%CI		OR	95%CI		OR	95%CI	
Occupational																											
No exposure	1.0			1.0			1.0			1.0			1.0			1.0			1.0			1.0			1.0		
Use & ≤19 years	1.9	1.4	2.7	1.1	0.8	1.6	1.2	0.9	1.8	1.4	1.0	2.0	1.0	0.7	1.4	1.2	0.8	1.6	0.7	0.3	1.8	0.6	0.2	1.4	0.7	0.3	1.7
Use & ≥20 years	4.8	3.5	6.6	1.9	1.3	2.7	2.3	1.6	3.3	2.3	1.6	3.3	1.2	0.8	1.7	1.6	1.1	2.3	1.4	0.6	3.4	0.9	0.4	2.3	1.3	0.5	3.4
Production	5.3	3.2	9.0	2.8	1.6	4.9	3.1	1.7	5.6	3.3	2.0	5.7	2.1	1.2	3.6	1.8	1.0	3.2	2.6	0.8	8.2	1.8	0.6	5.9	2.1	0.6	7.6
Household																											
No exposure	1.0			1.0			1.0			1.0			1.0			1.0			1.0			1.0			1.0		
Use & ≤4 years	0.6	0.4	1.1	1.2	0.7	2.0	1.1	0.6	1.9	0.6	0.3	0.9	0.8	0.5	1.3	0.7	0.4	1.3	0.2	0.0	1.1	0.2	0.0	1.5	0.2	0.0	1.7
Use & ≥5 years	0.8	0.5	1.4	1.1	0.6	2.0	1.3	0.7	2.4	0.8	0.5	1.3	1.0	0.6	1.6	1.2	0.7	1.9	0.4	0.1	1.7	0.4	0.1	1.7	0.6	0.1	2.4
Production	1.3	0.5	3.5	1.3	0.4	3.6	1.0	0.3	3.0	2.3	1.1	4.6	2.3	1.1	4.7	1.9	0.9	4.2	1.1	0.2	7.9	1.0	0.1	7.1	0.7	0.1	5.6
Neighbor																											
No exposure	1.0			1.0			1.0			1.0			1.0			1.0			1.0			1.0			1.0		
Factory & ≤19 years	1.8	1.4	2.5	2.7	2.0	3.6	4.1	2.8	5.8	2.1	1.6	2.7	2.7	2.1	3.5	4.8	3.4	6.7	0.7	0.4	1.1	1.0	0.6	1.5	2.7	1.4	5.2
Factory & ≥20 years	6.9	4.9	9.6	5.1	3.6	7.2	8.3	5.5	12.3	5.6	4.1	7.7	4.4	3.2	6.0	8.0	5.5	11.6	2.4	1.4	4.1	1.9	1.1	3.2	5.6	2.8	11.4
Mine	6.7	4.1	11.1	2.9	1.7	4.8	4.8	2.7	8.5	10.8	7.2	16.2	5.6	3.7	8.6	9.0	5.6	14.4	1.3	0.4	4.4	0.7	0.2	2.3	2.2	0.6	8.1
Slate roof																											
No exposure	1.0			1.0			1.0			1.0			1.0			1.0			1.0			1.0			1.0		
Roof & ≤19 years	1.1	0.6	1.8	0.8	0.4	1.3	0.7	0.4	1.3	2.1	1.4	3.0	1.7	1.2	2.5	1.6	1.1	2.3	1.3	0.5	3.7	1.1	0.4	3.0	1.1	0.4	3.0
Roof & ≥20 years	1.3	0.8	2.1	0.5	0.3	0.9	0.8	0.5	1.3	2.3	1.6	3.2	1.2	0.9	1.8	1.8	1.2	2.6	1.2	0.4	3.3	0.6	0.2	1.8	0.9	0.3	2.7
Roof in dense area	3.5	2.4	5.2	1.6	1.1	2.4	5.5	3.3	9.0	4.0	2.9	5.7	2.4	1.7	3.4	8.8	5.6	13.8	16.2	10.4	25.3	8.7	5.4	14.2	20.5	10.4	40.4

LLF: lower lung fibrosis, PD: pleural disease, LM: lung mass. * Adjusted for sex, age, smoking. ** Adjusted for sex, age, smoking + other exposure route.

4. Discussion

In the present study, 11.2%, 10.4%, and 8.3% of subjects were exposed to asbestos through slate roof, occupational, and household routes, respectively. We note that these exposures were identified incidentally, as the subjects participated in a HIS focused on neighborhood exposure and slate roof-dense areas. As noted, despite many previous studies of ARDs and various asbestos exposure routes [1,3,4], studies on the extent of exposure among ordinary residents are rare. The proportions in this study might have been over-estimated because individuals who were well aware of asbestos, such as occupationally exposed workers and their families, may have participated at high rates. As the proportions of various non-occupational exposure routes have not been routinely studied [6,16], the authors could not compare the frequencies of exposure via various routes with those of other studies.

Occupational exposure in the asbestos mining and asbestos textile industries was associated with higher prevalence of LLF and PD. In general, occupational exposure during the production of asbestos-containing materials was associated with higher prevalence of LLF and PD, compared to the occupational use of asbestos products [17]. A previous finding that low levels of occupational, household, and neighborhood exposure may induce pleural plaques [18] is consistent with our results. In this study, household exposure correlated only with PD. Previous studies of household exposure have reported similar results, indicating a significant relationship between household exposure and pleural abnormalities not related to lung cancer [19]. Although many studies identified pleural abnormalities related to household exposure without controlling for confounders [19], the present study adjusted for both confounders and other exposure routes.

The prevalence levels of PD were similar among those who resided near mines for <19 years and near factories for >20 years. Although the ambient concentrations of asbestos fibers may differ according to the source [13], previous studies have not addressed the effects of various exposure sources, including mines, factories, and ship-building facilities, on environmental exposure. Furthermore, the prevalence of PD increased among people who resided in slate roof-dense areas. Although asbestosis normally occurs at relatively high exposure levels, with the exception of mild fibrosis occasionally occurring at lower levels [18], the high prevalence of PD resulting from neighborhood exposure and slate roof exposure in a slate-dense area was unusual. The U.S. Occupational Safety and Health Administration has set a permissible exposure limit for workers of 0.1 asbestos fibers/cc in a time weighted average of 8 h [20]. However, a reference dose for non-malignant ARDs is not available, and it is difficult to determine the concentration or exposure level required to induce asbestosis.

Slate roofs can be damaged by age, rain, and wind [21]. Although a previous ecological study predicted future mortality due to asbestos slate roofs, particularly due to malignant mesothelioma [8], the study focused on asbestos consumption in general, and not on slate roof exposure. Another study found that some of the indoor air concentrations of asbestos in slate roof houses in Busan city exceeded 1×10^{-4} f/mL [22]; although this might not support a high incidence of PD in in slate roof-dense areas, it might support the development of LC. According to the US Environmental Protection Agency, specific risk levels of combined LC and MM that cause extra cancer in relation to air concentrations are 1 in 10,000 for 4×10^{-4} f/mL, 1 in 100,000 for 4×10^{-5} f/mL, and 1 in 1,000,000 for 4×10^{-6} f/mL [23].

In short, this study indicated an increased cancer risk of >1 in 10,000 among residents with slate roofs. Therefore, living under a slate roof might lead to ARDs. However, given the low sensitivity and specificity of chest X-rays, the radiologic results in the present study might not have detected genuine ARDs. People who live under slate roofs and/or in slate-dense areas tend to have a lower socioeconomic status (SES), which is associated with other lung diseases such as idiopathic pulmonary fibrosis [24,25]. Accordingly, the relationship between LM and a slate-dense area in the present study may be attributable to a lower SES [26]. We note that ours may have been the only study to investigate ARDs consequent to living under a slate roof and/or in a slate-roof-dense area.

This study had some limitations of note. First, both exposures and outcomes may have been misclassified. Occupational, household, and slate roof exposure data relied on the memories of the research subjects. However, as information about residential histories and slate roof-dense areas was verified using official records, this bias might not apply to neighborhood exposure and slate-roof-dense areas. Additionally, this study was based on the results of screening tests such as chest radiography, rather than on specific confirmatory tests such as computed tomography and clinical diagnosis. This may have led to the over- or under-estimation of disease prevalence. To avoid the misclassification of tuberculosis sequelae such as pleural plaques or costo-phrenic angle blunting, we excluded cases with histories of tuberculosis from the PD category. Despite these efforts to prevent misclassification, the inherent limitations of the HIS dataset may have introduced substantial bias. Second, a subject with respiratory symptoms might have been more likely to recall exposure sources, leading to information bias. Third, although age, sex, and smoking status were controlled as confounders, SES was not investigated, despite its role as a potential confounder. This variable should be controlled in future studies, as subjects exposed to asbestos may have had a lower SES. Fourth, the study subjects were voluntary participants, which reduces the generalizability of the results. Finally, exposure should require the evaluation of the fiber number in the living area and/or the patient sputum, our study is speculative and presently only indicative. It should be subsequently confirmed by the objective evaluation of the exposure. Also, Korea used almost chrysotile asbestos, so the results cannot be generalized to other situations in which amphiboles were mainly used.

These limitations warrant further studies that include objective exposure and specific outcome measures, as well as a representative population in which to evaluate various asbestos exposure routes. In addition, a well-designed study of exposure status should adjust for SES and the health outcomes associated with slate roofs, including residence in a slate-dense area.

Despite these limitations, the observed asbestos exposure of ordinary citizens through various routes has provided new insights. Previously, industrialized areas containing many factories and poor urban areas may have housed working populations with greater exposure to asbestos, and residents in those areas might have had a lower SES, which has been associated with respiratory disease.

5. Conclusions

Substantial proportions of study subjects who had lived near asbestos factories, shipbuilding facilities, and slate roof-dense areas were exposed to asbestos through occupational, household, and slate roof routes. After controlling for sex, age, smoking status, and other asbestos exposure routes, we found that the occupational, household, neighborhood, and slate roof exposure routes were associated with LLF and PD; PD; LLF, PD, and LM; and LLF, PD, and LM, respectively. To our knowledge, this may be the first report of the health effects of slate roof exposure. However, this study is vulnerable to misclassifications of exposure and outcome measurements, information bias, and other potential confounders, including SES. A well-designed study is needed to overcome those limitations.

Author Contributions: Conceptualization, D.K.; Methodology, Y.-K.K.; Software, S.-Y.K.; Validation, Y.-K.K. and S.-Y.K.; Formal Analysis, Y.-Y.K., M.S., M.-S.L., and H.-J.B.; Writing-Original Draft Preparation, D.K.; Writing-Review and Editing, Y.-K.K. and S.-Y.K.; Visualization, D.K.; Supervision, D.K.; Project Administration, D.K.; Funding Acquisition, D.K.

Funding: This research was funded by a two-year research Grant of Pusan National University, Ministry of Environment, Busan Municipal Government.

Conflicts of Interest: The authors declare no conflict of interest. The founding sponsors had no role in the design of the study; in the collection, analyses, or interpretation of data; in the writing of the manuscript; or in the decision to publish the results.

References

1. Valenzuela, M.; Giraldo, M.; Gallo-Murcia, S.; Pineda, J.; Santos, L.; Ramos-Bonilla, J.P. Recent scientific evidence regarding asbestos use and health consequences of asbestos exposure. *Curr. Environ. Health Rep.* **2016**, *3*, 335–347. [CrossRef] [PubMed]
2. Wagner, J.C.; Sleggs, C.A.; Marchand, P. Diffuse pleural mesothelioma and asbestos exposure in the North Western Cape Province. *Occup. Environ. Med.* **1960**, *17*, 260–271. [CrossRef]
3. Bourdès, V.; Boffetta, P.; Pisani, P. Environmental exposure to asbestos and risk of pleural mesothelioma: Review and meta-analysis. *Eur. J. Epidemiol.* **2000**, *16*, 411–417. [CrossRef] [PubMed]
4. Mensi, C.; Riboldi, L.; De Matteis, S.; Bertazzi, P.A.; Consonni, D. Impact of an asbestos cement factory on mesothelioma incidence: Global assessment of effects of occupational, familial, and environmental exposure. *Environ. Int.* **2015**, *74*, 191–199. [CrossRef] [PubMed]
5. World Health Organization. Asbestos: Use, Bans and Disease Burden in Europe. 2014. Available online: http://www.who.int/bulletin/volumes/92/11/13-132118/en/ (accessed on 25 November 2017).
6. Kauppinen, T.; Uuksulainen, S.; Saalo, A.; Mäkinen, I.; Pukkala, E. Use of the Finnish Information System on Occupational Exposure (FINJEM) in epidemiologic, surveillance, and other applications. *Ann. Occup. Hyg.* **2014**, *58*, 380–396. [PubMed]
7. D'Agostin, F.; Michieli, P.; Negro, C. Pleural mesothelioma in household members of asbestos-exposed workers in Friuli Venezia Giulia, Italy. *Int. J. Occup. Med. Environ. Health* **2017**, *30*, 419–431. [PubMed]
8. Kim, S.Y.; Kim, Y.C.; Kim, Y.; Hong, W.H. Predicting the mortality from asbestos-related diseases based on the amount of asbestos used and the effects of slate buildings in Korea. *Sci. Total Environ.* **2016**, *542 Pt A*, 1–11. [CrossRef]
9. Frassy, F.; Candiani, G.; Rusmini, M.; Maianti, P.; Marchesi, A.; Rota Nodari, F.; Via, G.D.; Albonico, C.; Gianinetto, M. Mapping asbestos-cement roofing with hyperspectral remote sensing over a large mountain region of the Italian Western Alps. *Sensors* **2014**, *14*, 15900–15913. [CrossRef] [PubMed]
10. Li, J.; Dong, Q.; Yu, K.; Liu, L. Asbestos and asbestos waste management in the Asian-Pacific region: Trends, challenges and solutions. *J. Clean. Prod.* **2014**, *81* (Suppl. C), 218–226. [CrossRef]
11. Kim, Y.C.; Hong, W.H.; Zhang, Y.L. Development of a model to calculate asbestos fiber from damaged asbestos slates depending on the degree of damage. *J. Clean. Prod.* **2015**, *86*, 88–97. [CrossRef]
12. Kang, D.M.; Kim, J.E.; Lee, Y.J.; Lee, H.H.; Lee, C.Y.; Moon, S.J.; Kang, M.S. Environmental health centers for asbestos and their health impact surveys and activities. *Ann. Occup. Environ. Med.* **2016**, *28*, 68. [CrossRef] [PubMed]

13. Kang, D.M.; Kim, J.E.; Kim, J.Y.; Lee, H.H.; Hwang, Y.S.; Kim, Y.K.; Lee, Y.J. Environmental asbestos exposure sources in Korea. *Int. J. Occup. Environ. Health* **2016**, *22*, 307–314. [CrossRef] [PubMed]
14. Frost, G. The latency period of mesothelioma among a cohort of British asbestos workers (1978–2005). *Br. J. Cancer* **2013**, *109*, 1965–1973. [CrossRef] [PubMed]
15. Courtice, M.N.; Wang, X.; Lin, S.; Yu, I.T.S.; Berman, D.W.; Yano, E. Exposure-response estimate for lung cancer and asbestosis in a predominantly chrysotile-exposed Chinese factory cohort. *Am. J. Ind. Med.* **2016**, *59*, 369–378. [CrossRef] [PubMed]
16. Choi, S.; Kang, D.; Park, D.; Lee, H.; Choi, B. Developing asbestos job exposure matrix using occupation and industry specific exposure data (1984–2008) in Republic of Korea. *Saf. Health Work* **2017**, *8*, 105–115. [CrossRef] [PubMed]
17. Feletto, E.; Schonfeld, S.J.; Kovalevskiy, E.V.; Bukhtiyarov, I.V.; Kashanskiy, S.V.; Moissonnier, M.; Straif, K.; Schüz, J.; Kromhout, H. A comparison of parallel dust and fibre measurements of airborne chrysotile asbestos in a large mine and processing factories in the Russian Federation. *Int. J. Hyg. Environ. Health* **2017**, *220*, 857–868. [CrossRef] [PubMed]
18. Tossavainen, A. Asbestos, asbestosis, and cancer: The Helsinki criteria for diagnosis and attribution. *Scand. J. Work Environ. Health* **1997**, *23*, 311–316. [CrossRef]
19. Goswami, E.; Craven, V.; Dahlstrom, D.L.; Alexander, D.; Mowat, F. Domestic asbestos exposure: A review of epidemiologic and exposure data. *Int. J. Environ. Res. Public Health* **2013**, *10*, 5629–5670. [CrossRef] [PubMed]
20. Agency for Toxic Substances and Disease Registry. Asbestos Toxicity: What are U.S. Standards and Regulations for Asbestos Levels? ATSDR Environmental Medicine & Environmental Health Education—Case Studies in Environmental Medicine. 2016. Available online: https://www.atsdr.cdc.gov/csem/csem.asp?csem=29&po=8 (accessed on 3 December 2017).
21. Tadas, P.; Dainius, M.; Edvinas, K.; Linas, K.; Maksim, K.; Axel, Z. Comparative characterization of particle emissions from asbestos and non-asbestos cement roof slates. *Build. Environ.* **2011**, *46*, 2295–2302. [CrossRef]
22. Jeong, J.W.; Cho, S.; Park, G.T.; Lee, S.J. Health risk assessment and evaluation of asbestos release from asbestos-cement slate roofing buildings in Busan. *J. Environ. Sci. Int.* **2013**, *22*, 1579–1587. [CrossRef]
23. United States Environmental Protection Agency, Office of Research and Development. Asbestos CASRN 1332-21-4 1988. Available online: https://cfpub.epa.gov/ncea/iris2/chemicalLanding.cfm?substance_nmbr=371 (accessed on 3 December 2017).
24. Hegewald, M.J.; Crapo, R.O. Socioeconomic status and lung function. *Chest* **2007**, *132*, 1608–1614. [CrossRef] [PubMed]
25. Sahni, S.; Talwar, A.; Khanijo, S.; Talwar, A. Socioeconomic status and its relationship to chronic respiratory disease. *Adv. Respir. Med.* **2017**, *85*, 97–108. [CrossRef] [PubMed]
26. Aldrich, M.C.; Selvin, S.; Wrensch, M.R.; Sison, J.D.; Hansen, H.M.; Quesenberry, C.P., Jr.; Seldin, M.F.; Barcellos, L.F.; Buffler, P.A.; Wiencke, J.K. Socioeconomic status and lung cancer: Unraveling the contribution of genetic admixture. *Am. J. Public Health* **2013**, *103*, e73–e80. [CrossRef] [PubMed]

International Journal of
Environmental Research and Public Health

MDPI

Article

Aberrant Driving Behaviour, Risk Involvement, and Their Related Factors Among Taxi Drivers

Javadreza Vahedi [1], Afshin Shariat Mohaymany [1,*], Zahra Tabibi [2] and Milad Mehdizadeh [1]

[1] Transportation Planning, School of Civil Engineering, Iran University of Science & Technology, Tehran 16846-13114, Iran; vahedi@ub.ac.ir (J.V.); milad_mehdizadeh@ymail.com (M.M.)

[2] Psychology, Department of Clinical Psychology, Ferdowsi University of Mashhad, Mashhad 91779-48974, Iran; tabibi@um.ac.ir

* Correspondence: shariat@iust.ac.ir; Tel.: +98-21-7724-0098; Fax: +98-21-7322-3143

Received: 7 June 2018; Accepted: 28 July 2018; Published: 1 August 2018

Abstract: The current study aims to investigate the aberrant driving behaviour and risk involvement of Iranian taxi drivers. The sample comprised 405 Iranian taxi drivers, who were recruited with a cross-sectional design, using a self-completion questionnaire survey during October and November 2016. We contribute to the literature by understanding how and to what extent the socioeconomic, demographic, driving, and aberrant driving behaviours influence risk involvement (accident involvement and traffic tickets). The validated 27-item Driver Behaviour Questionnaire (DBQ) was applied to measure aberrant driving behaviour. The results from valid observations ($n = 381$) explored a four-factor solution (including errors, ordinary violations, lapses, and aggressive violations) of the DBQ. The results also showed that being a single driver, having a high annual driving mileage, and a high number of daily taxi trips were positively associated with accident involvement. Furthermore, there was a positive correlation between the more ordinary violations and aggressive violations and accident involvement. Establishing better training and qualification mechanisms for taxi drivers could be considered by traffic safety experts in order to reduce ordinary and aggressive violations.

Keywords: aberrant driving behaviour; accident involvement; taxi drivers; driver behaviour questionnaire

---

1. Introduction

A growing interest has emerged in exploring the principal human factors of the driving behaviour in road transport studies. Road traffic accidents are recognised as a major source of fatality in the world. Several studies have shown that human factors play a critical role in road traffic accidents [1–3].

However, little is known about the aberrant driving behaviour of the taxi drivers, despite its importance [4–7], particularly among taxi drivers in the Middle Eastern context. Firstly, taxi drivers drive in a work-related context [8]. A small body of studies have investigated an occupational context [6,9], and most of them have examined the driving behaviour among the general driving population. Taxi drivers are mostly males and spend most of their time in urban traffic. In addition, the taxi is recognised as a private mode of transportation in western countries, while taxi services are seen as a mode of public transport (PT) in some eastern countries like Iran. This type of taxi has become the main dimension of the integrated transport system in Iranian cities and is playing an important role in passengers' daily urban travel. Taxi drivers do not have to undergo specific training and qualification in Iran. Any person with an ordinary driver's license and no major criminal record can be employed as a taxi driver. As taxi fares as a public transport mode are relatively low in Iran, taxi drivers often comprise the low-income strata of society. Because of the higher workload and spending greater time in traffic congestions, these drivers usually commit more risky driving compared with the general driving population. Furthermore, the taxi industry in Iran, as an organisation related to municipalities, is responsible for the management of taxis by taking measures such as determining the number of required taxis in each traffic analysis zone (TAZ) based on demand.

Most previous studies have been conducted in countries with good traffic safety performance. There might be an increase in the negative consequences of road traffic accidents in regions with low transport safety performance in the Middle East context, such as Iran [10,11]. For example, the global status report on road safety shows that the share of pedestrians in traffic-related mortalities in Iran is 23% [12]. Surprisingly, the national statistics of Iran show a high rate of fatality and injuries in road traffic accidents between taxis and young pedestrians [13]. Dalziel and Job [14] also found that taxi–pedestrian collisions were ranked as the fifth cause of all traffic accidents in Australia. A study by Shi et al. [4] revealed that passengers and police appear to have a very negative impression of the taxi drivers' driving behaviours in Beijing, China. Hence, understanding how demographic variables (e.g., age), socioeconomic characteristics (e.g., educational background and car ownership status), and the driving experiences of taxi drivers are related to their aberrant driving behaviour and risk involvement, could be interesting in countries with a similar traffic safety performance and work-related context, such as Iran.

Given the importance of public health in occupational contexts, the current study aims to overcome this deficiency by investigating the aberrant driving behaviour and risk involvement of Iranian taxi drivers. For this purpose, we used the information of 405 Iranian taxi drivers, recruited with a cross-sectional design, using a self-completion questionnaire survey during October and November 2016. We contribute to the literature by (1) identifying the principal dimensions of aberrant driving behaviour (Driver Behaviour Questionnaire [DBQ] factors) and confirming the factor structure of the DBQ among taxi drivers; (2) exploring socioeconomic, demographic, and driving factors, explaining the identified DBQ factors; and (3) understanding how and to what extent the socioeconomic, demographic, driving, and identified DBQ factors influence risk involvement (accident involvement and receiving traffic tickets).

The remaining sections are organised as follows: Firstly, a review of the literature is presented in the following section. Secondly, we describe the participants, data, and statistical procedure used in this study. Thirdly, the results of the statistical analysis used in this study are discussed. Fourthly, an in-depth discussion of the results is provided. The paper is concluded by summarising the key findings and offering planning suggestions.

2. Literature Review

A critical review of previous studies showed that (1) most of the efforts were focussed on identifying the principal dimensions of the DBQ, (2) a few studies have examined the determinants of the identified DBQ factors through demographic variables (e.g., age and gender) and driving characteristics (e.g., annual mileage), and (3) several papers have investigated the role of the DBQ factors, as well as the demographic variables (e.g., age, gender) and driving characteristics in risks, including in accident involvement and receiving traffic tickets. We classify the review based on the aforesaid three findings. Then, the study's contribution and research gaps are highlighted at the end of this section.

2.1. The Driver Behaviour Questionnaire

The Driver Behaviour Questionnaire is one of the instruments widely used to measure the human factors related to driving (i.e., aberrant driving behaviour) in different parts of the world [15]. The DBQ has played a prominent role in the realm of traffic psychology. The notion traces back to 1990, when Reason and colleagues [16] represented the DBQ's first version, by including 50 items in an instrument. The authors explored three principal factors (violations, dangerous errors, and relatively harmless lapses) for this instrument. Later, the DBQ was abridged or extended to cover new driving factors (e.g., aggressive violation) [17–22]. Several studies have applied the 28- or 27-item version of the DBQ in recent years. The DBQ's extended version has been mostly reported by a four-factor solution, including ordinary or rule violations, aggressive violations, errors, and lapses [23–26]. Violations refer to a driver's intention to infringe on the regulations of safe driving (e.g., overtaking a slow driver on the inside). Aggressive violations are hostile motivations for aggressive driving (e.g., getting angry at a driver and expressing your anger in some ways). Errors refer to misjudgements and observational failures in driving (e.g., failing to notice that pedestrians are crossing when turning into a side street); while lapses refer to limitations in memory and attention (e.g., hitting something overlooked when reversing).

2.2. Correlates of the Driver Behaviour Questionnaire Factors

Gender and age are the demographic factors that are reported to be correlated with the DBQ factors. Mesken et al. [27] found that men report fewer lapses and more violations than women do. Shi et al. [28] also showed that aggressive violation behaviours in male drivers are more common compared with female drivers. On the other hand, the authors found that male drivers make fewer errors and violations. Furthermore, Rimmö and Hakamies-Blomqvist [29] reported that males and females had similar results in the DBQ structure. Batool and Carsten [30] also found no significant gender differences in the violation score. Sullman et al. [23] indicated that younger drivers tend to have higher ordinary and aggressive violation. Batool and Carsten [30] found that younger drivers display more dangerous driving behaviours. Among other variables, some studies found that a high annual mileage, greater violations, and fewer lapses were correlated [16,23]. Batool and Carsten [30] found that middle-income group drivers were more likely to display aggressive driving behaviour. Furthermore, de Winter and Dodou [15], through a meta-analysis, showed that age and annual mileage could be important correlates of errors and violations. The authors concluded that younger drivers tend to have more violations and error scores, while more driving exposure was positively associated with violations and errors.

2.3. Predictors of the Risks (Accident Involvement)

Several studies have shown that older drivers have a lower rate of accident involvement [23,31], while an increased annual mileage (or driving exposure) escalate accident risks [31,32]. However, studies have not found any definitive and significant association between the driver's gender, age, annual mileage, level of education, and accident risks, including accident involvement and receiving traffic tickets [24,33]. In addition to accident involvement, traffic tickets can be used as a risk indicator. A traffic ticket is the primary means of traffic law enforcement. Both types of tickets (either by a police officer or by traffic cameras) have been included in this study.

Regarding the relationship between the DBQ factors and accident risks, studies have found that ordinary violations [23,24,34–37], aggression [35], and pushing-speeding [38], as well as lapses and errors [39] are related to accident risks. For instance, Gras et al. [24] found that higher violation scores were positively related to accident involvement. Rowe et al. [36] reported that higher violations were related to the bus drivers' accident involvement. Bener et al. [39] showed that higher scores of errors, aggression-speeding, and lapses were positively related to accident involvement.

2.4. Contribution of the Current Study

The literature suggests that (1) most of the previous studies have been conducted on samples obtained from the general driving population, including car, bus, and truck drivers; (2) a large body of studies has examined the DBQ in Western and European countries and areas with good safety performances, such as Denmark [40], the United Kingdom [36], France [41], New Zealand [23], Australia [26,32], and North America [25]; and (3) most of the previous studies have limited themselves to an examination of the correlation between a few demographic variables (e.g., age and gender) and driving characteristics (e.g., annual mileage), and DBQ factors and accident risks. Despite extensive review, we did not find any study that focused on the DBQ factors of taxi drivers in a Middle Eastern context. Machin and De Souza [42] showed that 29.7% of the accidents were caused by unsafe driving behaviours of taxi drivers in Australia. Also, they found that the major variables contributing to the unsafe driving behaviours were aberrant driving behaviours and personal factors. Hence, this study contributes to the literature by examining a wide range of socioeconomic variables in predicting high scores of the DBQ factors and accident risks among Iranian taxi drivers.

2.5. Aims and Hypotheses

The aim of this study was to examine the association between different background variables and the DBQ factors of Iranian taxi drivers, and their accident involvement and receiving traffic tickets. It was hypothesized that the drivers with different taxi driving experiences, demographics, and socioeconomic features might display different aberrant driving behaviour (e.g., lapses and ordinary violations). For example, well-educated and older drivers often commit fewer violations. We were also interested in investigating the role of a several variables such as years of taxi driving experience, household size, and economic status of drivers (e.g., income status and car ownership), as well as the DBQ factors in the accident involvement and traffic tickets.

3. Materials and Methods

3.1. Procedure and Respondents

A sample of Iranian taxi drivers was recruited during October and November 2016. A cross-sectional design using a self-completion questionnaire survey was employed for data collection in this study. Based on local data resources such as the number of taxi drivers and taxi stations in the urban network, 20 taxi stations were selected for data collection in two Iranian cities. The study areas were in Bojnurd and Neyshabur in the northeast of Iran. Bojnurd and Neyshabur have a population of 324,083 and 451,780, respectively [43]. Public transport (PT) in the cities includes urban buses and taxis (shared taxi). The taxis have specific stations (origins and destinations) across the cities. However, they do not have dedicated paths and hence drive on all main streets and roads similar to other private vehicles in the cities. The taxi stations are usually fixed-point waiting locations for picking up and dropping off passengers. Taxis usually have a capacity of four passengers and as soon as a taxi picks up its four passengers, the driver heads for the destination. The selected cities have some interesting features, which motivated us to select them for in this study. For example, their public transport system and the general urban traffic patterns are representative of most Iranian cities and other less developed regions in the Middle East.

A convenience sampling method was employed to collect data in the taxi stations. Of the 405 distributed questionnaires among taxi drivers in the selected stations, 24 had not answered the questions relevant to risk involvement and DBQ. Hence, these cases were removed from the analysis, leaving 381 valid observations for further analysis. It is important to note that almost all of the Iranian taxi drivers are males. Therefore, the present sample only included male taxi drivers.

Participation in the study was on an anonymous and voluntary basis. The taxi drivers were ensured that the survey and responses would have no influence on their driving assessment by the traffic police or taxi industry management. They were also assured that no information would be delivered to their employing firms.

3.2. Measures

3.2.1. Demographic, Socioeconomic, and Driving Characteristics

Information regarding the drivers' demographic and socioeconomic variables and driving characteristics were gathered in the first part of the questionnaire. The age, educational background (above high school = 1, high school or lower = 0), marital status (single = 1, other = 0), household size, car ownership status, and income level of the participants were recorded. The driving characteristics including the annual mileage (km), years of driving' experience, and hours of driving in a week, and the number of respondent's daily taxi trips were also recorded.

3.2.2. Driver Behaviour Questionnaire Measurement

The validated 27-item DBQ [17,19] was used to measure aberrant driving behaviour. The original version of DBQ in Persian, which has been used in this study, was already tested and validated on a group of professional lorry drivers in Iran [20]. The content validity of the original questionnaire was checked by a panel of experts. In addition, before data collection, a pilot survey was conducted among 30 taxi drivers in the study area, to examine whether the survey instruments and procedures yielded the desirable outcomes. The pilot study led to minor corrections in the questionnaire. For instance, the wording of some background variables was revised and one DBQ-item was changed. The original English items were translated into Persian by two native Persian co-researchers; these were then translated back into English by another English expert. A six-point Likert scale (0 = never, 1 = hardly ever, 2 = occasionally, 3 = quite often, 4 = frequently, and 5 = nearly all the time) was used for measuring all of the items. The taxi drivers were questioned to report how often they had engaged in each of the 27 behaviours in the past year. The instrument included eight items relevant to lapses (L) like, "Realise that you have no clear memory of the road you have been travelling on". Aggressive violations (AV) contained six items, such as, "Become angry at another driver and chase them with the intention of showing them how angry you are". Ordinary violations (V) included five items, such as, "Disregard the speed limit on a residential road". Errors (E) also contained eight items, such as, "When turning left, nearly hit a bicycle rider who has come up on your left".

3.2.3. Risk Involvement

The information regarding the taxi drivers' accident involvement and the number of traffic tickets was queried. The survey assessed how many accidents the taxi drivers had been involved in during the last year. The definition of accidents also covered injury to the participant (and any other person, such as pedestrians) and damage to property or vehicles [23]. The number of received traffic tickets of the taxi drivers was also recorded for the past year.

3.3. Statistical Analysis

To reveal the profiles of the background variables (demographic, socioeconomic, and driving characteristics) and the overall scores of the DBQ items, descriptive statistics were applied. To test the DBQ's dimensional structure, the instrument principal component analyses (PCA) with a varimax rotation and iteration were applied. To determine the number of extracted components, the Scree-plot and Kaiser criterion (an eigenvalue above 1.00 was considered to be a significant value) were used. A factor loading above 0.40 was used as a criterion for items to be retained in the DBQ components. To test the internal consistency and reliability of the scales, Cronbach's α (alpha) was calculated. Furthermore, the average corrected inter-item total correlations (Aiic) were calculated as indicators of reliability, because Cronbach's α tends to be biased when the scales contain few or many items [44]. The cut-off value of 0.30 was considered for the Aiic. In addition to the PCA, a confirmatory factor analysis (CFA) was utilized to confirm the factors identified in the current study and in the literature. The factor structure of the 27-item DBQ was confirmed using CFA with Amos 23. The root mean square error of approximation (RMSEA), the comparative fit index (CFI), and the Tucker–Lewis index (TLI) were applied as fit indices to determine the fitness of the data with the specified model [45]. RMSEA values below 0.06 and CFI and TLI values between 0.90 and 0.95 reflected an adequate fit [46]. The chi-square (χ^2) with corresponding significance level was also reported.

To predict the scores of the identified DBQ-factors across the background variables (demographic, socioeconomic variables, and driving characteristics), four linear regression models were employed.

The multiple linear regression model with the k predictor variables ($x_1, x_2, x_3, \ldots, x_K$) and a continuous (or interval scale) dependent variable, y, can be written as Equation (1), as follows:

$$y = \beta_0 + \beta_1 x_1 + \beta_2 x_2 + \ldots \beta_k x_k + \varepsilon \quad (1)$$

where ε is the residual terms of the model and β_i is the regression coefficient. The ordinary least squares method was used for estimation. Furthermore, two binary logistic regression models were applied to predict the accident involvement and received traffic tickets. The binary logistic regression model is a type of predictive modelling that can be applied when the dependent variable is binary; that is, when there are only two possible outcomes (e.g., accident involvement = 1, otherwise = 0). The general form of the logistic regression model is Equation (2), as follows:

$$\log(\frac{p_1}{1-p_1}) = \beta_0 + \beta_1 x_1 + \beta_2 x_2 + \ldots \beta_k x_k \quad (2)$$

where, p_1 is the probability that $x_1, x_2, x_3, \ldots, x_K$ are predictors, and β_i is the regression coefficient. To estimate this model, the maximum likelihood method was employed.

Furthermore, the dichotomous variable (yes/no) about accident involvement and ticket involvement was defined as the dependent variable in the binary logistic models. The dependent variable of the self-report accident involvement was set to 1 if the drivers had been involved in at least one accident over the past year, and zero otherwise (no accident). Furthermore, the dependent variable for the self-report traffic tickets was set to 1 if they had received at least one traffic ticket during the past year, and zero otherwise (no ticket).

In addition to the variables found statistically significant in a 95% confidence interval, all of the non-significant tested variables have been adjusted for and been reported in the models. To calculate the marginal effect of each explanatory variable on the outcome variable, the odds ratio (OR) was reported. The OR for an explanatory variable indicates the relative amount by which the odds of a dependent variable increase (OR >1) or decrease (OR <1) when the value of the explanatory variable is increased by 1.0 unit. These statistical analyses were carried out in SPSS 22.0.

4. Results

4.1. Characteristics of the Driver Behaviour Questionnaire Items

Table 1 shows the descriptive statistics of the background variables. On average, the taxi drivers were 36.26 years old (standard deviation (SD) = 11.57). The mean annual driving mileage was 79,143.31 km (SD = 72875.12) (see Table 1). The drivers had an average of 81.32 (SD = 62.67) hours of driving in a week, and 13.42 (SD = 14.21) years of experience driving a taxi. On average, 38.03% of the respondents reported that they had been involved in at least one accident during the last year.

Table 2 shows the means and standard deviations of all of the DBQ items reported by the taxi drivers. Among the 27 DBQ items, on the aggressive violation item, "Get angry at a certain type of driver and express your anger any way you can" (mean (M) = 2.24, SD = 1.97) and an ordinary violation item, "Drive so close to the car in front that it would be difficult to stop in an emergency" (M = 2.11, SD = 1.78), were the highest reported aberrant driving behaviours (Table 2). The item, "Misread signs and exit roundabout on the wrong road" (M = 1.43, SD = 1.32) was the highest reported lapse among taxi drivers. Furthermore, the item, "Queuing to turn left onto a main road, you pay such close attention to the traffic on the main road that you nearly hit the car in front" (M = 2.01, SD = 1.69) was the most prevalent reported error.

4.2. Dimensionality and Reliability Indices of the Driver Behaviour Questionnaire Items

The PCA with iteration and varimax rotation showed that the DBQ segmented into four dimensions in the sample of the Iranian taxi drivers. Table 3 shows the results of the PCA solution.

This solution explained 55.12% of the variance. The first dimension, the errors, included eight items (Cronbach $\alpha = 0.76$, average corrected inter-item correlation = 0.61, explained variance = 22.33%). Ordinary violations, the second dimension, contained six items (Cronbach $\alpha = 0.83$, average corrected inter-item correlation = 0.69, explained variance = 13.47%). The third dimension, lapses, included four items (Cronbach $\alpha = 0.71$, average corrected inter-item correlation = 0.50, explained variance = 10.77 %). The fourth dimension, the aggressive violations, included three items (Cronbach $\alpha = 0.74$, average corrected inter-item correlation = 0.51, explained variance = 8.55%). The results of a CFA for the DBQ displayed good fitness ($\chi^2 = 750.14$, degree of freedom = 203, $p < 0.001$, RMSEA = 0.052, CFI = 0.92, TLI = 0.92) with a four-factor structure, which was similar to the PCA results. As for the distribution, all of the variables used in the CFA were shown to have normal distribution. Furthermore, the Shapiro–Wilk (S–W) test for all of the variables did not indicate any significant deviation from normality.

4.3. Predictors of the Driver Behaviour Questionnaire Factor Scores

Table 4 shows that four multiple linear regression models significantly predicted four factors of the DBQ as four dependent variables (DV) (e.g., the model summary for the model with DV 'error' *F-value* = 2.20, $p < 0.01$, $R^2 = 0.11$, *Adjusted* $R^2 = 0.08$). Older taxi drivers reported more errors (Beta (B) = 0.24, $p < 0.001$), and lower ordinary ($B = -0.83$, $p < 0.05$) and aggressive violations ($B = -0.48$, $p < 0.001$). A higher educational background had a negative effect on aggressive violations ($B = -0.82$, $p < 0.001$). Drivers who were single were more likely to commit ordinary ($B = 0.15$, $p < 0.01$) and aggressive violations ($B = 1.21$, $p < 0.001$). A higher level of car ownership ($B = -0.25$, $p < 0.05$) and income ($B = -0.41$, $p < 0.05$) were positively associated with more aggressive violations. A higher annual driving mileage was related to more ordinary ($B = 0.51$, $p < 0.001$) and more aggressive violations ($B = 0.28$, $p < 0.05$). Furthermore, more hours of driving were positively associated with greater violations, while more years of driving experience were correlated with fewer violations. The taxi drivers who had more daily trips tended to report more violations.

4.4. Predictors of the Risk Involvement

Table 5 shows that two binary logistic models significantly predicted accident involvement (Model $\chi^2 = 203.91$, $p < 0.001$) and traffic tickets (Model $\chi^2 = 198.12$, $p < 0.001$). The old age of taxi drivers (OR = 0.78, $p < 0.001$) and high-income level of households (OR =0.86, $p < 0.05$) were negatively related to a traffic accident. The results showed that driver's marital status (OR = 1.61, $p < 0.001$), higher annual driving mileage (OR = 2.12, $p < 0.001$), higher hours of driving (OR = 1.75, $p < 0.001$), and higher number of daily taxi trips (OR = 1.83, $p < 0.001$) were positively associated with the accident involvement. Regarding the relationship between the DBQ-factor and accident involvement, more ordinary violations (OR = 1.63, $p < 0.001$) and aggressive violations (OR = 1.92, $p < 0.001$) were positively related to accident involvement.

The results also showed that being a single driver (OR = 1.85, $p < 0.05$), having a higher annual mileage (OR = 2.75, $p < 0.001$), higher hours of driving in a week (OR = 2.10, $p < 0.001$), a higher number of daily trips (OR = 1.48, $p < 0.001$), more errors (OR = 1.34, $p < 0.001$), and more ordinary violations (OR = 1.28, $p < 0.05$) were positively associated with receiving traffic tickets. Also, a higher level of car ownership (OR = 0.83, $p < 0.05$) and higher income level (OR = 0.92, $p < 0.05$) were negatively related to traffic tickets involvement.

Table 1. Descriptive statistics of the background variables and risk involvement (n = 381). SD—standard deviation.

Variable	Description	Mean	SD
Age of driver	Continuous variable	36.26	11.57
Educational background of driver	High (higher than high school) = 1, low = 0	0.37	0.47
Driver's marital status	Single = 1, otherwise = 0	0.14	0.34
Driver's household size	Number	2.90	1.82
Number of owned private car in household	Number	0.94	0.35
Driver's income status	Higher than two million Tomans * = 1, otherwise = 0	0.14	0.35
Annual driving mileage	Continuous variable (kilometres in the last year)	79,143	72,875
Hours of driving in a week	Continuous variable (hours in a week)	81.32	62.67
Years of driving experience of a taxi	Continuous variable (unit: year)	13.42	14.21
Number of respondent's taxi trips in each day	Number	47.34	45.57
Accident involvement in the last year (self-reported)	At least one accident = 1, no accident = 0	0.38	0.48
Traffic tickets involvement in the last year (self-reported)	At least one ticket = 1, no ticket = 0	0.43	0.49

* 1 Euro = 3496 Tomans (August 2017).

Table 2. Means and standard deviations of all Driver Behaviour Questionnaire (DBQ) items reported by the taxi drivers ($n = 381$).

Item	Mean	SD
Errors (E)		
Queuing to turn left onto a main road, you pay such close attention to the traffic on the main road that you nearly hit the car in front	2.01	1.69
Fail to notice that pedestrians are crossing when turning into a side street from a main road	1.97	1.43
Brake too quickly on a slippery road	1.85	1.27
Fail to check your rear-view mirror before pulling out, changing lanes, etc.	1.52	1.33
When turning left, nearly hit a bicycle rider who has come up on your left	1.21	1.06
Attempt to overtake someone that you had not noticed was signaling a right turn	0.97	1.10
Miss seeing a "give way" sign and just avoid colliding with traffic having the right of way	0.83	0.97
Underestimate the speed of an oncoming vehicle when overtaking	0.67	0.88
Lapses (L)		
Misread signs and exit roundabout on the wrong road	1.43	1.32
Switch on one thing, such as the headlights, when you meant to switch on something else, such as the wipers	1.24	1.32
Attempt to drive away from traffic lights in the wrong gear	0.91	1.19
Forget where left taxi/car in a taxi/car park	0.78	0.96
Having set out to drive to one place, you suddenly realize you are on the road to somewhere else	0.75	1.03
Get in the wrong lane approaching a roundabout or junction	0.69	0.90
Realize that you have no clear memory of the road you have been travelling on	0.64	0.87
Hit something when reversing that you had not previously seen	0.58	0.94
Ordinary violations (OV)		
Drive so close to the car in front that it would be difficult to stop in an emergency	2.11	1.78
Enter an intersection knowing that the traffic lights have already changed against you	1.91	1.66
Overtake a slow driver on the inside	1.45	1.55
Disregard the speed limit on a residential road	1.31	1.22
Disregard the speed limit on a freeway or rural highway	0.96	1.05
Aggressive violations (AV)		
Get angry at a certain type of driver and express your anger any way you can	2.24	1.97
Use your horn to indicate your annoyance to another road user	2.03	1.84
Become angry at another driver and chase them with the intention of showing them how angry you are	1.93	1.75
Stay in a lane that you know will be closed ahead until the last minute before forcing your way into the other lane	1.79	1.52
Race away from traffic lights with the intention of beating the driver next to you	1.73	1.44
Pull out of an intersection so far you force your way into the traffic	0.93	1.01

Table 3. Principal component analysis (PCA) for the DBQ items.

Dimensions	Loadings			
	Errors	Ordinary Violations	Lapses	Aggressive Violations
1—Errors (Cronbach α = 0.765, Aiic = 0.61, Ev = 22.33%, Dimension's mean (SD) = 1.38 (0.50))				
Fail to notice that pedestrians are crossing when turning into a side street from a main road (E)	0.82			
Attempt to overtake someone that you had not noticed was signalling a right turn (E)	0.76			
Queuing to turn left onto a main road, you pay such close attention to the traffic on the main road that you nearly hit the car in front (E)	0.73			
Miss seeing a "give way" sign and just avoid colliding with traffic having the right of way (E)	0.71			
Fail to check your rear-view mirror before pulling out, changing lanes, etc. (E)	0.70			
When turning left, nearly hit a bicycle rider who has come up on your left (E)	0.64			
Brake too quickly on a slippery road (E)	0.59			
Get in the wrong lane approaching a roundabout or junction (L)	0.41			
2—Ordinary violations (Cronbach α = 0.832, Aiic = 0.69, Ev = 13.47%, Dimension's mean (SD) = 1.40 (0.50))				
Drive so close to the car in front that it would be difficult to stop in an emergency (OV)		0.74		
Enter an intersection knowing that the traffic lights have already changed against you (OV)		0.70		
Disregard the speed limit on a freeway or rural highway (OV)		0.65		
Disregard the speed limit on a residential road (OV)		0.61		
Overtake a slow driver on the inside (OV)		0.55		
Underestimate the speed of an oncoming vehicle when overtaking (E)		0.46		
3—Lapses (Cronbach α = 0.710, Aiic = 0.50, Ev = 10.77%, Dimension's mean (SD) = 0.92 (0.34))				
Misread signs and exit roundabout on the wrong road (L)			0.68	
Hit something when reversing that you had not previously seen (L)			0.62	
Realise that you have no clear memory of the road you have been travelling on (L)			0.57	
Having set out to drive to one place, you suddenly realise you are on the road to somewhere else (L)			0.51	
4—Aggressive violations (Cronbach α = 0.742, Aiic = 0.51, Ev = 8.55%, Dimension's mean (SD) = 2.06 (0.13))				
Use your horn to indicate your annoyance to another road user (AV)				0.74
Get angry at a certain type of driver and express your anger any way you can (AV)				0.71
Become angry at another driver and chase them with the intention of showing them how angry you are (AV)				0.63

Notes: Factor loadings <0.40 not reported. E—error; L—lapse; OV—ordinary violation; AV—aggressive violation; Aiic—average corrected inter-item correlation; Ev—explained variance.

Table 4. Predictors of the four DBQ factors.

Variable	Error		Ordinary Violation		Lapses		Aggressive Violation	
	B	*t*-Test	B	*t*-Test	B	*t*-Test	B	*t*-Test
Constant	2.05	117	3.05 ***	3.89	−2.21	−1.04	2.76	1.43
Age of driver	0.24 ***	3.81	−0.83 **	−2.45	−0.09	−1.27	−0.48 ***	−3.46
Educational background of driver	0.13	0.92	−0.22	−1.50	0.17	1.34	−0.82 ***	−3.02
Driver's marital status	−0.33	−1.40	0.15 *	2.22	−0.04	−0.42	1.21 ***	4.21
Driver's household size	0.16	1.02	−0.08	−1.25	0.12	1.31	−0.11	−1.84
Number of owned private car in household	0.07	1.32	−0.12	−1.76	−0.05	−0.42	−0.25 *	−2.21
Driver's income status	0.18	1.09	−0.30	−1.60	0.02	0.19	−0.41 *	−2.23
Annual driving mileage	−0.37	−1.51	0.51 ***	3.12	0.14	1.25	0.28 *	2.19
Hours of driving in a week	−0.08	−0.97	0.71 ***	3.80	−0.57***	−3.52	0.89 ***	4.12
Years of driving experience of a taxi	−0.10	−1.30	−0.45 *	−2.21	−0.23	−1.34	−0.13 *	−2.15
Number of respondent's taxi trips in each day	0.12	1.41	0.94 ***	3.91	−0.12	−1.11	1.51 ***	4.83
Model summary	$F = 2.20$ **, $R^2 = 0.11$, *Adjusted* $R^2 = 0.08$		$F = 3.91$ ***, $R^2 = 0.27$, *Adjusted* $R^2 = 0.18$		$F = 2.18$ **, $R^2 = 0.10$, *Adjusted* $R^2 = 0.07$		$F = 2.20$ **, $R^2 = 0.11$, *Adjusted* $R^2 = 0.08$	

*: $p < 0.05$, **: $p < 0.01$, ***: $p < 0.001$. B—regression coefficient of variables in the model.

Table 5. Predictors of the accident involvement and receiving traffic tickets.

Variable	Accident Involvement			Tickets Involvement		
	B	OR	Wald	B	OR	Wald
Constant	1.18	-	1.23	3.19 ***	-	10.45
Age of driver	−0.25 ***	0.78	6.12	−0.11	0.89	1.48
Educational background of driver	−0.12	0.92	1.57	−0.08	0.93	1.39
Driver's marital status	1.27***	1.61	9.42	1.34 *	1.85	4.38
Driver's household size	0.11	1.08	1.35	0.09	1.02	1.12
Number of owned private car in household	0.24	0.91	1.55	−0.34 *	0.83	4.84
Driver's income status	−0.12*	0.86	4.31	−0.08 *	0.92	4.27
Annual driving mileage	0.80 ***	2.12	12.44	0.93 ***	2.75	10.91
Hours of driving in a week	0.54 ***	1.75	11.21	0.63 ***	2.10	13.41
Years of driving experience of a taxi	0.13	1.24	1.61	0.24	1.12	1.39
Number of respondent's taxi trips in each day	0.64 ***	1.83	10.34	0.53 ***	1.48	13.11
Error (factor1)	0.34	1.21	1.67	0.25 ***	1.34	14.21
Ordinary violation (factor2)	0.71 ***	1.63	12.01	0.18 *	1.28	4.41
Lapse (factor3)	0.07	1.19	1.20	0.11	1.04	1.13
Aggressive violation (factor4)	0.81 ***	1.92	11.67	0.29	1.12	1.71
Model summary	Chi-square = 203.91 (degree of freedom (df) = 15), enter method, sig = 0.000. R^2 = 0.28 (Cox and Snell), 0.43 (Nagelkerke). 82.3% correctly predicted, HL: Chi-square (df = 8) = 4.80, sig = 0.779.			Chi-square= 198.12 (df = 15), enter method, sig = 0.000. R^2 = 0.21 (Cox and Snell), 0.39 (Nagelkerke). 71.2% correctly predicted, HL: Chi-square (df = 8) = 3.57, sig = 0.628.		

*: $p < 0.05$, **: $p < 0.01$, ***: $p < 0.001$. B—regression coefficient of variables in the model. OR—odds ratio; the OR for an explanatory variable tells us the relative amount by which the odds of a dependent variable increase (OR >1) or decrease (OR <1) when the value of the explanatory variable is increased by 1.0 unit. Wald—the Wald test is the test of significance for individual regression coefficients in logistic regression. HL: Hosmer–Lemeshow test.

5. Discussion

The purpose of the current study was to examine the predictors of risk involvement and aberrant driving behaviour among Iranian taxi drivers. The study attempted to identify the barriers of public health in the professional or occupational context of taxi drivers.

Firstly, in accordance with several previous studies that have been conducted among the general driving population of car, bus, and truck drivers in other countries, the current study identified and confirmed a four-factor solution of the DBQ for taxi drivers [19,24,26]. Secondly, the study explored several predictors of drivers' aberrant driving behaviours. Thirdly, the study examined whether the demographic, socioeconomic, driving characteristics, and the DBQ factors (error, lapse, ordinary violation, and aggressive violation) could predict two outcomes of risk involvement (accident and traffic tickets).

The majority of studies conducted on the general driving population in countries with a Western cultural orientation showed that some of the DBQ factors, such as ordinary violation and demographic characteristics (e.g., age), were predictors of accident involvement [15]. In contrast to several previous studies, and in accordance with the hypotheses of the study, the findings of the current study showed that several socioeconomic variables and aberrant driving factors were significant predictors of risk involvement among Iranian taxi drivers. The findings indicated that, in addition to ordinary violations, the reported errors and aggressive violations of taxi drivers could be seen as significant and positive predictors of risk involvement in Iran. These findings support our hypotheses that drivers with different taxi driving experiences, demographics, and socioeconomic features as well as different DBQ factors might influence risk involvement among taxi drivers.

Somewhat expectedly, the mean scores of the DBQ-items, including items relevant to ordinary violation such as, "drive so close to the car in front that it would be difficult to stop in an emergency", and aggressive violations such as, "get angry at a driver and express your anger any way you can", were higher among Iranian taxi drivers compared with the general driving population [24,26], bus drivers [37], and truck drivers [23] in Western countries. A plausible explanation may be the nature of the study population (urban taxi drivers versus general public). In particular, a higher exposure of Iranian taxi drivers and also more hours of driving in urban road traffic influenced aberrant driving behaviours. A potential explanation for this relationship may be the negative influence of factors related to driver's work-related physical and mental characteristics, such as fatigue, sleepiness, anger, and stress [9,47]. Additionally, heavy traffic, narrow streets, the overall chaotic driving environment in the study area, delays and traffic congestion might increase such mental and physical features. Nordfjærn et al. [48] also speculated that professional drivers might perceive significantly more control and be involved in more accidents compared with non-professional drivers. This suggests that professional drivers like taxi drivers may constitute a risk group in the road traffic.

Regarding the relationship between the aberrant driving behaviour and different background variables, the four DBQ factors were significantly predicted by several explanatory variables, such as the age and income status of drivers. In contrast to several previous studies [15], and in line with the results of Tabibi et al. [49] and the hypotheses of this study, the findings showed that older taxi drivers were more likely to commit driving errors. Interestingly, high-income drivers were less likely to commit aggressive violations. To decrease violations, the finding highlights that policymakers should consider the income status of taxi drivers, such as the development of taxi trade unions and developing salary regulations in Iran. Additionally, single taxi drivers were more likely to report ordinary and aggressive violations. These drivers might generally be more likely to engage in risk-taking behaviours and excitement-seeking behaviours [50].

In line with previous studies [23,24], the probability of involvement in a traffic accident tended to increase with the more reported ordinary violations. In addition to ordinary violations, the study found that more aggressive violations of taxi drivers were strong and positive predictors of accident involvement. This study also investigated the predictors of other measures of risk involvement (i.e., receiving traffic ticket). More errors and ordinary violations were positively related to greater traffic ticket involvement.

Among the background variables, the young age of taxi drivers was associated with involvement in accidents, which is congruent with the literature [23]. The authors found the positive influence of young age on the higher accident involvement of truck drivers in New Zealand. Single drivers are more likely to be involved in an accident and receive traffic tickets. Previous findings have also shown that single drivers are more prone to risk-taking behaviours (e.g., [51]). The findings also showed that a higher annual mileage, higher hours of driving, and a higher number of daily trips were related to higher accidents and tickets. Lourens et al. [31] also showed that accidents were positively correlated with annual mileage (exposure) in the general driving population in the Netherlands. Policymakers could aim to reduce accident involvement of their taxi drivers by controlling the road traffic exposure among the drivers.

To summarise, among the different demographic, socioeconomic, and driving factors, being a young and single driver alone, with factors such as a high income, high annual driving mileage and hours of driving, higher number of daily taxi trips, and reported ordinary and aggressive traffic violations were positively related to a higher accident involvement among taxi drivers. However, educational background, household size, car ownership status, driving experiences, errors, and lapses were not associated with accident involvement. Furthermore, the non-ownership of the cars, low income, high annual driving mileage and hours of driving, high number of daily taxi trips, more errors, and ordinary traffic violations were positively associated with receiving more traffic tickets. Meanwhile, the age of drivers, educational background, household size, driving experiences, lapses, and aggressive violations did not significantly affect the relationship between the explanatory variables and receiving traffic tickets.

Limitations

The present study has limitations such as the self-reported nature of measurements, the cross-sectional design, and convenience sampling. The questionnaire was based on self-reports including demographic variables, socioeconomic characteristics, risk involvement, and psychological instruments such as aberrant driving behaviour (the 27-item DBQ). This may impose limitations regarding potential socially desirable responses, causal explanations between the variables, and issues regarding representativity. However, in the present study, we examined a rather large sample (10% of the study population) of taxi drivers scattered in all regions of Bojnurd and Neyshabur (two cities in Iran). This may increase the likelihood of a representative sample. A great deal of underreporting and forgetting about driving accidents has been pointed out in a study [24]. This issue also reduces the strength of any potential relationship and the variability in accident involvement.

6. Conclusions

Much of the previous research on aberrant driving behaviour has focussed on examining the factor-solution of the DBQ among the general driving population in Western settings. Little evidence exists to investigate a wide-range of demographic variables, socioeconomic characteristics, and driving factors on the DBQ factors, as well as on the accident involvement among taxi drivers as public transport drivers in the Middle East context. This research augmented the literature by exploring the predictors of the DBQ factors and the risk involvement among Iranian taxi drivers. The study explored a four-factor solution of a 27-item DBQ including errors, ordinary violations, lapses, and aggressive violations. The study further indicated that several variables such as the drivers' age, marital status, annual mileage, number of daily trips, and ordinary and aggressive violations could influence accident involvement.

The findings of the current study could be utilized for implementing and planning safe driving behaviour interventions among taxi drivers. For example, interventions aimed to enhance the traffic safety of taxis, as public transport, could tackle these risk by careful management of the work schedules, including the number of daily trips, hours of driving (see [52]), and improving the economic conditions of taxi drivers [5]. This encourages more country-specific studies in the future. This may also require an attitude change in the taxi industry management, where safety is equally important or prioritized over economic profits and efficiency. Furthermore, establishing improved training and qualification mechanisms for taxi drivers could be implemented by traffic safety experts to reduce the ordinary and aggressive violations among the specific groups of taxi drivers, such as young and single drivers.

Author Contributions: The authors' contributions in the article are as follows: J.V.: Conceived the study, literature review, research design, data collection, manuscript writing; A.S.M.: Content planning, procedure management, research methodology and analysis; Z.T.: Content planning and research methodology; M.M.: Content planning, manuscript writing and editing and analysis.

Funding: This research received no external funding.

Acknowledgments: The authors would like to acknowledge the contributions of taxi drivers, who in different ways, helped us to conduct the research.

Conflicts of Interest: The authors declare no conflict of interest.

References

1. PIARC—World Road Association (WRA). *Road Safety Manual [CD-ROM]*; Piarc Technical Committee on Road Safety: Harrogate, UK, 2003.
2. Walshe, E.A.; Ward McIntosh, C.; Romer, D.; Winston, F.K. Executive function capacities, negative driving behavior and crashes in young drivers. *Int. J. Environ. Res. Public Heaith* **2017**, *14*, 1314. [CrossRef] [PubMed]
3. Zhu, M.; Rudisill, T.M.; Rauscher, K.J.; Davidov, D.M.; Feng, J. Risk Perceptions of Cellphone Use While Driving: Results from a Delphi Survey. *Int. J. Environ. Res. Public Heaith* **2018**, *15*, 1074. [CrossRef] [PubMed]
4. Shi, J.; Tao, L.; Li, X.; Xiao, Y.; Atchley, P. A survey of taxi drivers' aberrant driving behavior in Beijing. *J. Transp. Saf. Secur.* **2014**, *6*, 34–43. [CrossRef]
5. Wang, Y.; Li, L.; Prato, C.G. The relation between working conditions, aberrant driving behaviour and crash propensity among taxi drivers in China. *Accid. Anal. Prev.* **2018**. [CrossRef] [PubMed]
6. Razmara, A.; Aghamolaei, T.; Madani, A.; Hosseini, Z.; Zare, S. Prediction of safe driving behaviours based on health belief model: The case of taxi drivers in Bandar Abbas, Iran. *BMC Public Health* **2018**, *18*, 380. [CrossRef] [PubMed]
7. Razmara, A.; Aghamolaei, T.; Madani, A.; Hosseini, Z.; Zare, S. Risky behaviors of taxi drivers in Bandar Abbas, Iran. *Electron. Phys.* **2018**, *10*, 6588. [CrossRef] [PubMed]
8. Poó, F.M.; Ledesma, R.D.; López, S.S. The taxi industry: Working conditions and health of drivers, a literature review. *Transp. Rev.* **2018**, *38*, 394–411. [CrossRef]
9. Bener, A.; Lajunen, T.; Özkan, T.; Yildirim, E.; Jadaan, K.S. The impact of aggressive behaviour, sleeping, and fatigue on road traffic crashes as comparison between minibus/van/pick-up and commercial taxi drivers. *J. Traffic Transp. Eng.* **2017**, *5*, 21–31. [CrossRef]
10. Mehdizadeh, M.; Nordfjaern, T.; Mamdoohi, A.R.; Mohaymany, A.S. The role of parental risk judgements, transport safety attitudes, transport priorities and accident experiences on pupils' walking to school. *Accid. Anal. Prev.* **2017**, *102*, 60–71. [CrossRef] [PubMed]
11. Şimşekoğlu, Ö.; Nordfjærn, T.; Rundmo, T. Traffic risk perception, road safety attitudes, and behaviors among road users: A comparison of Turkey and Norway. *J. Risk Res.* **2012**, *15*, 787–800. [CrossRef]
12. World Health Organization. Global Status Report on Road Safety 2015. Available online: http://www.who.int/violence_injury_prevention/road_safety_status/2015/en/ (accessed on 17 May 2018).
13. Adl, J.; Dehghan, N.; Abbaszadeh, M. The survey of unsafe acts as the risk factors of accidents in using taxis for intercity travelling in Tehran. *Saf. Promo. Inj. Prev. (Tehran)* **2014**, *2*, 39–46.
14. Dalziel, J.; Job, S. Taxi drivers and road safety. In *A Report to the Federal Office of Road Safety*; Department of Transport and Regional Development: Canberra, Australia, 1997.
15. De Winter, J.; Dodou, D. The driver behaviour questionnaire as a predictor of accidents: A meta-analysis. *J. Saf. Res.* **2010**, *41*, 463–470. [CrossRef] [PubMed]
16. Reason, J.; Manstead, A.; Stradling, S.; Baxter, J.; Campbell, K. Errors and violations on the roads: A real distinction? *Ergonomics* **1990**, *33*, 1315–1332. [CrossRef] [PubMed]

17. Lawton, R.; Parker, D.; Stradling, S.G.; Manstead, A.S. Predicting road traffic accidents: The role of social deviance and violations. *Brit. J. Psychol.* **1997**, *88*, 249–262. [CrossRef]
18. Parker, D.; Lajunen, T.; Stradling, S. Attitudinal predictors of interpersonally aggressive violations on the road. *Transp. Res. Part F Traffic Psychol. Behav.* **1998**, *1*, 11–24. [CrossRef]
19. Lajunen, T.; Parker, D.; Summala, H. The Manchester driver behaviour questionnaire: A cross-cultural study. *Accid. Anal. Prev.* **2004**, *36*, 231–238. [CrossRef]
20. Mehdizadeh, M.; Shariat-Mohaymany, A.; Nordfjaern, T. Accident involvement among Iranian lorry drivers: Direct and indirect effects of background variables and aberrant driving behaviour. *Transp. Res. Part F Traffic Psychol. Behav.* **2018**, *58*, 39–55. [CrossRef]
21. Maslać, M.; Antić, B.; Lipovac, K.; Pešić, D.; Milutinović, N. Behaviours of drivers in Serbia: Non-professional versus professional drivers. *Transp. Res. Part F Traffic Psychol. Behav.* **2018**, *52*, 101–111. [CrossRef]
22. Maslać, M.; Antić, B.; Pešić, D.; Milutinović, N. Behaviours of professional drivers: Validation of the DBQ for drivers who transport dangerous goods in Serbia. *Transp. Res. Part F Traffic Psychol. Behav.* **2017**, *50*, 80–88. [CrossRef]
23. Sullman, M.J.; Meadows, M.L.; Pajo, K.B. Aberrant driving behaviours amongst New Zealand truck drivers. *Transp. Res. Part F Traffic Psychol. Behav.* **2002**, *5*, 217–232. [CrossRef]
24. Gras, M.E.; Sullman, M.J.; Cunill, M.; Planes, M.; Aymerich, M.; Font-Mayolas, S. Spanish drivers and their aberrant driving behaviours. *Transp. Res. Part F Traffic Psychol. Behav.* **2006**, *9*, 129–137. [CrossRef]
25. Beanland, V.; Sellbom, M.; Johnson, A.K. Personality domains and traits that predict self-reported aberrant driving behaviours in a southeastern US university sample. *Accid. Anal. Prev.* **2014**, *72*, 184–192. [CrossRef] [PubMed]
26. Stephens, A.; Fitzharris, M. Validation of the driver behaviour questionnaire in a representative sample of drivers in Australia. *Accid. Anal. Prev.* **2016**, *86*, 186–198. [CrossRef] [PubMed]
27. Mesken, J.; Lajunen, T.; Summala, H. Interpersonal violations, speeding violations and their relation to accident involvement in finland. *Ergonomics* **2002**, *45*, 469–483. [CrossRef] [PubMed]
28. Shi, J.; Bai, Y.; Ying, X.; Atchley, P. Aberrant driving behaviors: A study of drivers in Beijing. *Accid. Anal. Prev.* **2010**, *42*, 1031–1040. [CrossRef] [PubMed]
29. Rimmö, P.-A.; Hakamies-Blomqvist, L. Older drivers' aberrant driving behaviour, impaired activity, and health as reasons for self-imposed driving limitations. *Transp. Res. Part F Traffic Psychol. Behav.* **2002**, *5*, 47–62. [CrossRef]
30. Batool, Z.; Carsten, O. Self-reported dimensions of aberrant behaviours among drivers in Pakistan. *Transp. Res. Part F Traffic Psychol. Behav.* **2017**, *47*, 176–186. [CrossRef]
31. Lourens, P.F.; Vissers, J.A.; Jessurun, M. Annual mileage, driving violations, and accident involvement in relation to drivers' sex, age, and level of education. *Accid. Anal. Prev.* **1999**, *31*, 593–597. [CrossRef]
32. Davey, J.; Wishart, D.; Freeman, J.; Watson, B. An application of the driver behaviour questionnaire in an Australian organisational fleet setting. *Transp. Res. Part F Traffic Psychol. Behav.* **2007**, *10*, 11–21. [CrossRef]
33. Nordfjærn, T.; Hezaveh, A.M.; Mamdoohi, A.R. An analysis of reported driver behaviour in samples of domestic and expatriate Iranians. *J. Risk Res.* **2015**, *18*, 566–580. [CrossRef]
34. Şimşekoğlu, Ö.; Nordfjærn, T. The role of safety culture/climate and social cognitive factors for driving behaviors of Turkish professional drivers transporting petroleum products. *J. Risk Res.* **2017**, *20*, 650–663. [CrossRef]
35. Hassan, H.M. Investigation of the self-reported aberrant driving behavior of young male Saudi drivers: A survey-based study. *J. Transp. Saf. Secur.* **2016**, *8*, 113–128. [CrossRef]
36. Rowe, R.; Roman, G.D.; McKenna, F.P.; Barker, E.; Poulter, D. Measuring errors and violations on the road: A bifactor modeling approach to the driver behavior questionnaire. *Accid. Anal. Prev.* **2015**, *74*, 118–125. [CrossRef] [PubMed]
37. Mallia, L.; Lazuras, L.; Violani, C.; Lucidi, F. Crash risk and aberrant driving behaviors among bus drivers: The role of personality and attitudes towards traffic safety. *Accid. Anal. Prev.* **2015**, *79*, 145–151. [CrossRef] [PubMed]
38. Mohamadi Hezaveh, A.; Nordfjærn, T.; Mamdoohi, A.R.; Şimşekoğlu, Ö. Predictors of self-reported crashes among Iranian drivers: Exploratory analysis of an extended driver behavior questionnaire. *Promet Traffic Transp.* **2018**, *30*, 35–43. [CrossRef]

39. Bener, A.; Ozkan, T.; Lajunen, T. The driver behaviour questionnaire in arab gulf countries: Qatar and United Arab Emirates. *Accid. Anal. Prev.* **2008**, *40*, 1411–1417. [CrossRef] [PubMed]
40. Martinussen, L.M.; Hakamies-Blomqvist, L.; Møller, M.; Özkan, T.; Lajunen, T. Age, gender, mileage and the dbq: The validity of the driver behavior questionnaire in different driver groups. *Accid. Anal. Prev.* **2013**, *52*, 228–236. [CrossRef] [PubMed]
41. Gueho, L.; Granie, M.-A.; Abric, J.-C. French validation of a new version of the driver behavior questionnaire (DBQ) for drivers of all ages and level of experiences. *Accid. Anal. Prev.* **2014**, *63*, 41–48. [CrossRef] [PubMed]
42. Machin, M.A.; De Souza, J.M. Predicting health outcomes and safety behaviour in taxi drivers. *Transp. Res. Part F Traffic Psychol. Behav.* **2004**, *7*, 257–270. [CrossRef]
43. Iran National Census. The Statistical Center of Iran. 2016. Available online: http://irandataportal.syr.edu/wp-content/uploads/Population-and-Households.xlsx (accessed on 17 March 2018).
44. Hair, J.F.; Black, W.C.; Babin, B.J.; Anderson, R.E. *Multivariate Data Analysis*, 7th ed.; Pearson Prentice Hall: Upper Saddle River, NJ, USA, 2009; ISBN 978-013-894-858-045.
45. Kline, R.B. *Principles and Practice of Structural Equation Modeling*, 4th ed.; The Guilford Press: New York, NY, USA, 2015; pp. 265–280. ISBN 978-14-6252-334-4.
46. Kim, K.H.; Bentler, P.M. Data modeling: Structural equation modeling. In *Handbook of Complementary Methods in Education Research*; Green, J.L., Camilli, G., Elmore, P.B., Eds.; Lawrence Erlbaum Associates Publishers: Mahwah, NJ, USA, 2006; pp. 161–175. ISBN 978-080-585-932-4.
47. Montoro, L.; Useche, S.; Alonso, F.; Cendales, B. Work environment, stress, and driving anger: A structural equation model for predicting traffic sanctions of public transport drivers. *Int. J. Environ. Res. Public Health* **2018**, *15*, 497. [CrossRef] [PubMed]
48. Nordfjærn, T.; Jørgensen, S.H.; Rundmo, T. Safety attitudes, behaviour, anxiety and perceived control among professional and non-professional drivers. *J. Risk Res.* **2012**, *15*, 875–896. [CrossRef]
49. Tabibi, Z.; Borzabadi, H.H.; Stavrinos, D.; Mashhadi, A. Predicting aberrant driving behaviour: The role of executive function. *Transp. Res. Part F Traffic Psychol. Behav.* **2015**, *34*, 18–28. [CrossRef]
50. Nordfjærn, T.; Şimşekoğlu, Ö.; Can, S.; Somer, O. Social cognition and personality traits related to risky driving in a Turkish sample. *J. Risk Res.* **2015**, *18*, 452–466. [CrossRef]
51. Shinar, D.; Schechtman, E.; Compton, R. Self-reports of safe driving behaviors in relationship to sex, age, education and income in the us adult driving population. *Accid. Anal. Prev.* **2001**, *33*, 111–116. [CrossRef]
52. Shi, J.; Xiao, Y.; Tao, L.; Atchley, P. Factors causing aberrant driving behaviors: A model of problem drivers in China. *J. Transp. Saf. Secur.* **2017**, 1–15. [CrossRef]

MDPI
St. Alban-Anlage 66
4052 Basel
Switzerland
Tel. +41 61 683 77 34
Fax +41 61 302 89 18
www.mdpi.com

International Journal of Environmental Research and Public Health Editorial Office
E-mail: ijerph@mdpi.com
www.mdpi.com/journal/ijerph